M000251400

Pickwell's Binocular Vision Anomalies

BRUCE J.W. EVANS, BSC, PHD, FCOPTOM, FAAO, FEAOO, FBCLA, DIPCLP, DIPORTH

Director of Research, Institute of Optometry
Visiting Professor, City, University of London
Visiting Professor of Optometry, London South Bank University
London, UK

ELSEVIER

Elsevier
1600 John F. Kennedy Blvd.
Ste 1800
Philadelphia, PA 19103-2899

PICKWELL'S BINOCULAR VISION ANOMALIES,
SIXTH EDITION

ISBN: 978-0-323-73317-5

Notice

Practitioners and researchers must always rely on their own experience and knowledge in evaluating and using any information, methods, compounds or experiments described herein. Because of rapid advances in the medical sciences, in particular, independent verification of diagnoses and drug dosages should be made. To the fullest extent of the law, no responsibility is assumed by Elsevier, authors, editors or contributors for any injury and/or damage to persons or property as a matter of products liability, negligence or otherwise, or from any use or operation of any methods, products, instructions, or ideas contained in the material herein.

Library of Congress Control Number: 2020948303

Senior Content Strategist: Kayla Wolfe
Content Development Specialist: Kevin Travers
Content Development Manager: Meghan B. Andress
Publishing Services Manager: Deepthi Unni
Senior Project Manager: Manchu Mohan
Design: Bridget Hoette
Illustrator: Narayanan Ramakrishnan
Marketing Manager: Kate Bresnahan

Printed in China

Last digit is the print number: 9 8 7 6 5 4 3 2 1

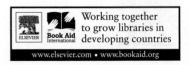

This sixth edition, like previous editions, concentrates on the practical and clinical aspects of binocular vision for students and practitioners. The 'how-to-do-it' approach has been retained and extended by new tables, summaries of test procedures, and case studies. The theory of binocular vision has been kept to the minimum necessary to understand the investigative and therapeutic procedures.

The first and second editions drew largely on Professor Pickwell's enormous clinical and research experience. This new edition, which is the fourth completed by the present author, continues to contain a great deal of Professor Pickwell's sound advice. Most of the alterations have been revisions and updates in view of recent research, and over 500 new references to recent research have been added to this edition.

Sadly, Professor Pickwell died in 2005. Professor Pickwell's systematic and rigorously scientific approach played an important part in the evolution of optometry and orthoptics into subjects with an ever-strengthening evidence base. It is hoped that this book will be a lasting tribute to his enormous contribution to this field.

The fact that contemporary research has not necessitated any major changes in emphasis is a tribute to Professor Pickwell's original work. There has been an evolution of binocular vision tests and treatments from using artificial instruments that create unnatural viewing conditions towards more natural methods that are less disruptive to normal binocular vision. This evolution is desirable, and some of the older techniques that do not add useful additional clinical information and are not in common use have been omitted from this edition.

A great many theories and therapies have been suggested for binocular vision anomalies and it can be difficult to 'sort the wheat from the chaff'. This requires an 'evidence-based approach', although for many optometric activities the evidence is not as strong as is desirable (Rowe and Evans, 2018). In this approach, rigorous scientific research is used to investigate old and new techniques alike. Investigative approaches and treatments that have been validated in this way are taken most seriously, and others are acknowledged as unproven. In this book, greatest weight is given to approaches that have been validated with double-masked randomised placebo-controlled trials (RCTs).

The RCT is a powerful tool, but one tool cannot solve all problems (Hill, 1966). In some scenarios, 'pragmatic trials' can have greater relevance than RCTs (Patsopoulos, 2011), and although RCTs are prioritised in this book, other relevant research is also included. In common with other workers in this field (Joyce et al., 2015), where 'top tier' evidence is not available from RCTs, a pragmatic approach has been adopted of moving down the hierarchy of evidence to the next level. Case studies represent a weak form of scientific evidence and are included in this book only to illustrate management approaches that are supported by stronger evidence.

In well-researched topics (e.g., amblyopia treatment), systematic reviews and meta-analyses provide a very high level of evidence. Where appropriate, topics that were extensively reviewed in previous editions of this book are now abbreviated to a summary of relevant reviews.

A few brief suggestions are given now for those undertaking research on binocular vision anomalies. Where data can be gathered as a continuous variable they should, wherever possible, be analysed as a continuous variable and not dichotomised into normal or abnormal binary variables (Cumberland et al., 2014), or into grades of normality. An obsession with p-values is a commonplace example of dichotomising inappropriately, and confidence intervals should be quoted (Amrhein, Greenland, & McShane, 2019). Variables should be recorded on a linear scale wherever possible. For example, accommodation and convergence should be recorded in dioptres and prism dioptres rather than centimetres. In research on optometric correlates of academic underachievement, it is important to control for confounding variables such as IQ and attention deficit disorder and researchers should be masked.

The book is divided into four parts: the general investigation of binocular anomalies, heterophoria, strabismus, and incomitant deviations and nystagmus. In the parts on heterophoria and strabismus, the main features of these conditions are summarised in a general introductory chapter, then discussed in more detail in subsequent chapters.

A comprehensive glossary of orthoptic terminology is included at the end of the book. It includes abbreviations in an attempt to bring some standardisation to clinical practice. The appendices include clinical worksheets and diagnostic algorithms to help the practitioner adopt a logical approach to investigation, diagnosis, and treatment. The appendices also include test norms, highlight confusing aspects, and list suppliers of clinical equipment. The final appendix is a guide to the **Digital Resource** that accompanies this book. The **Digital Resource** includes video clips of commonly encountered incomitant deviations and key clinical tests.

In this book, the term **squint** is avoided and replaced by **strabismus** or, synonymously, heterotropia. The term squint is ambiguous because it is commonly used to refer to half-shut eyes. The term **deviation** is used as a generic term to describe both heterophoria and strabismus.

I wish to acknowledge the contributions of my colleagues at the Institute of Optometry, in clinical practice, and research collaborators. Special thanks to Dr Robert Yammouni for many thought-provoking discussions about binocular vision. I am also grateful to Dr Dorothy Thompson, Josephine Evans, Tasnim Rashid, and Fardip Rashid for their assistance. Finally, my thanks to the staff of Elsevier for their support and encouragement.

Bruce J.W. Evans

Declaration of interest

The author developed the IFS exercises (described in Chapter 10) at the Institute of Optometry, which is a charity. The exercises are marketed by I.O.O. Sales Ltd., which exists to raise funds for the Institute of Optometry. I.O.O. Sales Ltd pays the author a small 'award to inventor' based on sales of the IFS exercises.

This book is intended to provide a clinical text on the investigation and management of binocular vision anomalies by methods other than medicine and surgery. It is hoped that it will be useful to the student facing the subject for the first time, and also to the established practitioner seeking a reference to the binocular anomalies likely to be seen in everyday practice. The aim has been to produce a 'how-to-do-it' book. It is not a textbook on the theory of binocular vision. There are several excellent books which cover the anatomy, physiology, and mechanisms of binocular vision. The theory has therefore been kept to the minimum necessary for an adequate appreciation of the anomalies, their investigation, and treatment. I have assumed that the reader has a basic knowledge of normal binocular vision or is acquiring this simultaneously with clinical studies. I also assume a knowledge of the general procedures of eye examination and refractive methods.

The history and past literature of orthoptics seems to be full of descriptions of unsubstantiated methods which have come and gone as it was found that they did not work. At times it has appeared to have been a maze of suggested procedures which have varied from 'cure-alls' to useful clinical ideas. I cannot claim to have explored all of them. What I have tried to do is describe the methods which I have found effective, and where possible provided the references for practical evaluations. I have tried to write from my own particular experience which has extended over thirty years. In doing so, I am very aware of others whose experience has been parallel, but not necessarily the same. As far as possible, I have also tried to reflect some of their views, and acknowledge their contributions to the ongoing development of clinical practice.

To help the student, I have tried to provide a recognisable pattern in dealing with the conditions described, and I hope thereby to have produced a mnemonic approach to the subject which will aid learning and application in a clinical setting. Each condition is dealt with in the general order of definition, investigation, evaluation, and management. Under the heading of management, I have considered five nonmedical possibilities: removing any general cause, correcting refractive error, orthoptics, relieving prisms, and referral. These patterns will be obvious in the early chapters, and are assumed in the later ones.

I wish particularly to acknowledge the work and encouragement given to me by my colleagues in the binocular vision clinics at the University of Bradford, who have stimulated my thoughts and actions over many years. I would mention Mr M. Sheridan and Dr W. A. Douthwaite. I am particularly indebted in this respect to Dr T. C. A. Jenkins who also read the manuscript and made many helpful suggestions. I wish to thank Mrs J. Paley for interpreting the initial draft and for typing the manuscript, and also the staff of the Graphics Unit of the University of Bradford for their help with the illustrations.

David Pickwell

CONTENTS

PART 1

Investigation

CHAPTER 1

Nature of Binocular Vision Anomalies

Introduction

Binocular vision is the coordination and integration of what is received from the two eyes separately into a single binocular percept. Proper functioning of binocular vision without symptoms depends on several factors which can be considered under three broad headings:

1. The anatomy of the visual apparatus.
2. The motor system that coordinates movement of the eyes.
3. The sensory system through which the brain receives and integrates the two monocular signals.

Anomalies in any of these can cause difficulties in binocular vision, or even make it impossible. This is illustrated schematically in Fig. 1.1. In considering the binocular difficulties of a patient, therefore, all three parts of the total system need to be investigated:

1. *Anatomy.* Abnormalities in the anatomy of the visual system can be either developmental, occurring in the embryological development of the bony orbit, ocular muscles, or nervous system, or acquired through accident or disease.
2. *Motor system.* Even if the motor system is anatomically normal, anomalies can occur in the functioning which can disturb binocular vision or cause it to break down. These may be due to disease, or they may be malfunctions of the physiology of the motor system. For example, excessive accommodation due to uncorrected hypermetropia can result in excessive convergence due to the accommodation–convergence relationship. This is a frequent cause of binocular vision problems. Examples of disease affecting the motor system are haemorrhages involving the nerve supply to the extraocular muscles, changes in intracranial pressure near the nerve nuclei, or pressure on the nerves or nerve centres from abnormal growths of intracranial tissue. Such conditions require urgent medical attention to the primary condition and early recognition is therefore essential. The investigation for this type of pathology is discussed in Chapter 17.
3. *Sensory system.* Anomalies in the sensory system can be caused by such factors as a loss of clarity of the optical image in one or both eyes, an image larger in one eye than the other (aniseikonia), anomalies of the visual pathway or cortex, or central factors in the integrating mechanism. The ultimate goal of binocularity is stereopsis (DeAngelis, 2000), which improves motor skills at near distances (O'Connor, Birch, Anderson, & Draper, 2010), but has a minimal effect beyond about 40 m (Bauer, Dietz, Kolling, Hart, & Schiefer, 2001).

   Stereopsis is not the only benefit from binocularity: there is a binocular advantage in terms of visual acuity and contrast sensitivity. The benefit in terms of contrast sensitivity is underestimated in the ideal conditions of visual acuity testing. For example, when driving in snow or with a dirty windshield, binocularity markedly outperforms monocular vision (Otto, Bach, & Kommerell, 2010). Binocular performance is better than monocular at a wide range of tasks (Sheedy, Bailey, Buri, & Bass, 1986). Difficulties in the coordinating mechanism of the motor system can also be accompanied by adaptations and anomalies in the sensory system, such as suppression, abnormal retinal correspondence, or amblyopia. These may occur to lessen the symptoms caused by the motor anomaly, as adaptations of the sensory system.

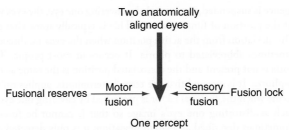

Fig. 1.1 Simplified schematic model illustrating the interaction of an ocular motor function (fusional reserves) with a sensory system (sensory fusion) to achieve binocular single vision.

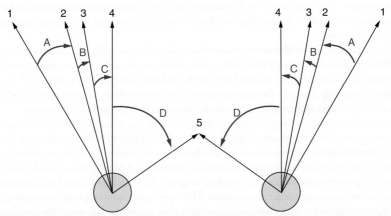

Fig. 1.2 Schematic diagram illustrating binocular positions of the eyes and types of vergence. *1*, Anatomical position of rest; *2*, physiological position of rest (passive position); *3*, position of functional rest; *4*, active position for distance vision or primary position; *5*, active position for near vision; *A*, tonus; *B*, initial convergence; *C*, fusional vergence; *D*, the sum of accommodative convergence, proximal vergence and fusional vergence for near vision. (Modified from Solomons, 1978, *Binocular Vision: a Programmed Text*, Heinemann, London.).

The anatomical, motor, and sensory systems must be normal for good binocular vision. The position of the eyes relative to each other is determined first by their anatomical position. Humans have forward-looking eyes placed in the front of the skull, and this brings the visual axes of the two eyes almost parallel to each other. In most cases, they are slightly divergent when the position is determined only by anatomical factors, and this is known as the **position of anatomical rest** (Fig. 1.2, position 1). In normal circumstances, this state seldom exists, as physiological factors nearly always operate. When a person is conscious, muscle tone and postural reflexes usually make the visual axes less divergent: the **position of physiological rest** (Fig. 1.2, position 2). The **fixation reflex** triggers **initial convergence** which takes the eyes to the **position of functional rest** (Fig. 1.2, position 3). For distance vision, **fusional vergence** then acts to bring the eyes to the **active** or **primary position**.

For emmetropes, there is negligible accommodation during distance vision but significant accommodation for near vision. Therefore, for near vision another physiological factor affecting the position of the eyes is the accommodation—convergence relationship: the eyes will converge as accommodation is exerted, and this is **accommodative convergence**. An awareness of the proximity of an object induces **proximal vergence** and, finally, for near vision there is, as with distance vision, **fusional (disparity) vergence**, which positions the retinal images on corresponding points (or within corresponding Panum's areas). In Fig. 1.2, the angle D is the sum of accommodative convergence, proximal vergence, and fusional vergence for near vision.

If fusional vergence is suspended, for example by covering one eye, the eyes will adopt a **dissociated position** at the position of functional rest. This is typically somewhat deviated from the active position. This deviation from the active position when the eyes are dissociated is known as **heterophoria**, sometimes abbreviated to phoria. It occurs in most people. The rare situation where a heterophoria is not present and the dissociated position is the same as the active position is known as **orthophoria**. It is stressed that the term 'heterophoria' applies only to the deviation of the eyes that occurs when the fusional factor is prevented by covering one eye or dissociated by other methods such as distorting one eye's image so that it cannot be fused with the other. Heterophoria is sometimes described as a latent deviation; it is only detected on dissociation of the two eyes. Sometimes the eyes can be deviated even when no dissociation is introduced. This more permanent deviation is called **heterotropia** or **strabismus**. Other, less favoured terms include **squint** (a confusing term because it is often used by patients to refer to half closed eyes) or **cast**. Ocular deviations can, therefore, be classified as either heterophoria or strabismus, but there are other important practical classifications that need to be considered in investigating the binocular vision of a patient.

The symptoms and clinical features of most binocular vision anomalies fit into recognisable patterns. The recognition of these patterns is the process of diagnosis and this is an obvious preliminary to treatment. The classifications adopted here are intended to assist diagnosis (Fig. 1.2). The term **deviation** is used generically to describe strabismus and heterophoria. Cyclotorsional and vertical deviations often occur together when they may be described as **cyclovertical deviations**.

Accommodation and convergence are closely linked, and this interaction needs to be considered when investigating binocular vision anomalies. For example, a patient with a problematic exophoria may use accommodative convergence to reduce the deviation, causing the accommodative lag to be lower under binocular than monocular conditions (Momeni-Moghaddam, Goss, & Sobhani, 2014b). Conversely, a patient with a problematic esophoria requires divergence to achieve binocular vision and exhibits decreased convergence accommodation. This may explain why esophoric cases typically have greater accommodative lag under binocular conditions than monocular (Momeni-Moghaddam et al., 2014b). A study found accommodative errors greater than 1 D in 11% of patients with decompensated exophoria and 22% of patients with decompensated esophoria (Hasebe, Nonaka, & Ohtsuki, 2005). This is one reason why blurred vision can be a symptom of binocular vision anomalies: patients may manipulate accommodation to avoid diplopia, but at the expense of blur.

Prevalence of Binocular Vision Anomalies

Strabismus affects between 2% (Hashemi et al., 2019) and 3% (Robaei et al., 2006) and amblyopia 3% (Adler, 2001) of the population. The prevalence of strabismus varies in different countries and ethnicities (Hashemi et al., 2019).

Between 18% (Pickwell, Kaye, & Jenkins, 1991) and 20% (Karania & Evans, 2006a, 2006b) of patients consulting a primary care optometrist have a near heterophoria which has the signs and symptoms suggestive of decompensated heterophoria. Some authors give higher prevalence figures (Montes-Mico, 2001), although prevalence estimates are strongly influenced by diagnostic criteria and referral bias. There is a need to guard against 'pathologising' large proportions of the nonclinical population. For example, one study with the laudable aim of evaluating screening tools for nonstrabismic binocular/accommodative anomalies suggested nearly one-third of all children may have such anomalies, and yet included no assessment of symptoms (Hussaindeen et al., 2018). A thorough review concluded 7% of the population are stereoblind (Chopin, Bavelier, & Levi, 2019).

A large North American clinical study found that, other than refractive error, the most prevalent ophthalmic conditions in the clinical paediatric population are binocular and accommodative disorders (Scheiman et al., 1996). Binocular and accommodative conditions were 10 times more prevalent than eye diseases.

Before undertaking a surgical procedure that will significantly change the refractive error, it is important to check the binocular status and consider the likely effect of surgery on any binocular vision anomaly (Finlay, 2007). Binocular vision anomalies are an uncommon cause of nontolerance to spectacles (Freeman & Evans, 2010).

Classifications of Binocular Vision Anomalies

There are several different approaches to the classification of binocular vision anomalies (Darko-Takyi, Khan, & Nirghin, 2016). A simplified classification is illustrated in Fig. 1.3.

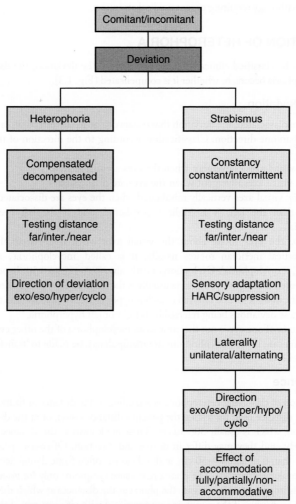

Fig. 1.3 Simplified classification of ocular deviations. *Cyclo*, Cyclophoria or Cyclotropia; *eso*, esophoria or esotropia; *exo*, exophoria or exotropia; *HARC*, harmonious anomalous retinal correspondence; *hyper*, hyperphoria or hypertropia; *hypo*, hypotropia; *inter.*, intermediate.

COMITANCY

Ocular deviations can be classified as comitant (concomitant) or incomitant. Comitant deviations are the same in all directions of gaze for a given fixation distance. Incomitant deviations vary with the direction of gaze, that is, as the patient moves the eyes to fixate objects in different parts of the field of fixation, the angle of the deviation will vary (Chapter 17). There may be no deviation in one part of the motor field, but a marked deviation in other parts. In incomitant deviations, the angle of deviation will also vary depending on which eye is fixating. Incomitant deviations are also referred to as paralytic, paretic, or palsied: a paresis is a partial paralysis. Usually they are caused by abnormalities of anatomy or functioning of the motor system due to accident or disease, or abnormal development. It is important to distinguish incomitant deviations from comitant as the management is different and has different priorities. An incomitant deviation of sudden onset is usually caused by trauma or active pathology requiring urgent medical attention.

CLASSIFICATION OF HETEROPHORIA

Heterophoria can be classified clinically by the direction of the deviation, the fixation distance at which the heterophoria occurs, or whether it is compensated (Fig. 1.3).

Direction of Deviation

When the eyes are dissociated, the deviation that occurs can be in any direction, or may be a combination of more than one direction. Classification according to the direction of the deviation is as follows:

1. *Esophoria:* visual axes convergent when the eyes are dissociated.
2. *Exophoria:* visual axes divergent when the eyes are dissociated.
3. *Hyperphoria:* visual axes vertically misaligned when the eyes are dissociated: if the right eye is higher than the left, it is 'right hyperphoria', and if the left eye is higher, 'left hyperphoria'.
4. *Cyclophoria:* the eyes rotate about the visual axes when dissociated: if the top of the primary vertical meridian rotates nasally, it is called 'incyclophoria', and if it rotates temporally, 'excyclophoria'. Cyclophoria nearly always co-occurs with hyperphoria.

It should be noted that right hyperphoria usually is the same as a dissociated deviation of the left eye downwards. It can therefore be referred to as 'left hypophoria'. In practice, the term 'hypophoria' is seldom used, these deviations being referred to as right or left hyperphoria.

An excyclophoria of one eye is not the same as an incyclophoria of the other eye. For example, a right excyclophoria can, if the test conditions are manipulated, be made to 'transfer' to an excyclophoria of the other eye.

Fixation Distance

The second method of classifying heterophoria is according to the distance of fixation. This is usually either at 6 m, the distance used for testing the patient's distance vision, or at the distance the patient uses for near vision, which is usually 30—50 cm. These are known as the 'distance phoria' and 'near phoria', respectively, and they may differ in degree and direction. Of course, people fixate objects at distances other than 6 m and 30—50 cm, and individuals often fixate digital devices at intermediate distances for prolonged periods. The phoria may cause symptoms only for visual tasks at a particular distance. It is important to investigate the phoria at the distances at which the patient normally uses the eyes, and to discover if the symptoms are associated with vision at any of these distances.

Most children are orthophoric at distance and orthophoric, or have a low degree of exophoria, at near (Walline, Mutti, Zadnik, & Jones, 1998). On average, between the ages of 5—10 years there is a very slight shift in the near heterophoria of decreasing exophoria and increasing esophoria

(Walline et al., 1998). During adult life, the average phoria for distance vision remains the same, but at 65 years the mean near exophoria has increased by 6Δ (Δ is the symbol for prism dioptres). This exophoria for near vision is called **physiological exophoria** (Freier & Pickwell, 1983).

One way of conceptualising motor fusion is to link these mean heterophorias to the resting position of the vergence system, **tonic vergence** (Rosenfield, 1997). If a person is in a totally darkened room with no visual stimuli then, typically, the eyes take up a position where they are aligned on a plane about 1 m away from the observer (although there is considerable intersubject variation). If this is taken to be the resting position of the vergence system, then distance vision can be thought of an active divergence and near vision as an active convergence away from the resting position. This model explains why the average heterophoria at distance is a very slight esophoria and the average heterophoria at near is an exophoria (Freier & Pickwell, 1983), and the effect of some drugs is to produce an eso-shift at distance and an exo-shift at near (Rosenfield, 1997).

Duane (1896) suggested a method of classification for strabismus based on whether the deviation is greater for distance or near vision. This became known as the Duane-White classification and is applied below in a modified form for heterophoria.

1. Esophoria
   (a) Divergence weakness esophoria: usually considered an anomaly of distance vision: the degree of esophoria is greater for distance than for near vision.
   (b) Convergence excess esophoria: a higher degree of esophoria for near vision than for distance.
   (c) Basic (or mixed) esophoria: the degree of esophoria does not differ significantly with the fixation distance.
2. Exophoria
   (a) Convergence insufficiency exophoria: a higher degree of exophoria for near vision than for distance. This is typically diagnosed as a syndrome, and in this book (Chapter 8) is given the term CIES to differentiate it from an isolated finding of a remote near point of convergence (near point of convergence insufficiency, NPCI).
   (b) Divergence excess exophoria: a larger deviation for distance vision than for near. This type often breaks down intermittently into a strabismus for distance vision and can also be classified as an intermittent exotropia.
   (c) Basic (or mixed) exophoria: the degree of exophoria does not differ significantly with the fixation distance.

Von Noorden (1996) pointed out that it is best to consider the Duane-White classification as descriptive rather than aetiological.

Compensation

The third and clinically very important classification of heterophoria is as either compensated or decompensated (Marton, 1954). As already stated, heterophoria is a physiological (normal) condition, as in most cases it is not harmful and causes no symptoms. In these circumstances it is described as compensated. Sometimes, there are abnormal stresses on the binocular vision which result in symptoms and the heterophoria is decompensated. This is more likely to happen if there are developmental abnormalities in the anatomical, motor, or sensory systems. These may not in themselves make the phoria decompensated and in very many cases do not. The trigger, or catalyst, that causes a heterophoria to decompensate is often a change in the patient's general or visual conditions. The factors that may bring about such a change are listed in Chapter 4. The first consideration in treatment is to remove as many as possible of these decompensating factors.

CLASSIFICATION OF STRABISMUS

As well as deciding whether strabismus or heterotropia is comitant or incomitant, it can be classified according to constancy, eye preference, and the direction of deviation (Fig. 1.3). In some patients the angle varies markedly with the accommodative state. Strabismus may be present for both distance vision and for near vision, or at only one fixation distance. The angle of deviation may vary with the fixation distance, giving classifications of divergence weakness, convergence excess, or basic (mixed) types of convergent strabismus; and convergence weakness, divergent excess, or basic types of divergent strabismus. These correspond with the classifications of heterophoria on p. 7. An attempt was made to standardise terminology and classification in 2001 (Committee for the Classification of Eye Movement Abnormalities and Strabismus, 2001). Some of the new terminology that this committee suggested seems not to have impacted on common usage (e.g., replacing Duane's retraction syndrome with cocontractive retraction syndrome).

Constancy

Strabismus can be classified as either constant, if present all the time and under all circumstances, or intermittent, if present only sometimes. Some cases of strabismus are intermittent in the sense that patients have coordinated binocular vision most of the time, but when the visual system or general well-being is under stress, the strabismus occurs. In these cases, binocular vision may not show the signs of decompensated heterophoria but breaks down into a strabismus. In some cases, an intermittent strabismus will develop into a constant strabismus if left untreated, but in others it remains intermittent. A rare form of intermittent strabismus in which the patient has a large convergent strabismus on alternate days only is referred to as 'cyclic strabismus' or 'alternate day squint'. Costenbader and Mousel (1964) found it to be less than 0.1% of all strabismus. The cyclic strabismus usually becomes constant after a few months.

In the case of intermittent strabismus, it is useful to enquire about the proportion of time the strabismus is present. This is likely to depend on tiredness and can be highly variable (Hatt, Leske, Kirgis, Bradley, & Holmes, 2007). A patient who has binocular vision for most of the time may have a better prognosis.

Direction of Deviation

The classification by the direction of the deviation is illustrated in Fig. 1.4.

Eye Preference

In strabismus, some patients always use the same eye for fixation, and others can fixate with either eye. Strabismus then can be classified as (1) unilateral or (2) alternating.

In alternating strabismus, the eye chosen for fixation at any given time can depend on:

1. *Fixation distance.* Some patients will use one eye for distance vision and the other for near.
2. *Direction of gaze.* In some patients, the eye used for fixation will depend on the direction of gaze. In convergent strabismus, this may indicate a congenital impairment in the abducting function of one or both eyes. The right eye fixates objects in the left of the field, and the left eye in the right; this is known as 'crossed fixation'.
3. *Vision and refraction.* If the vision and the refractive error are equal or nearly equal, the choice of eye for fixation may appear indiscriminate. Some cases of this type are considered to lack the ability to fuse, and these have been called 'essentially alternating' (Worth, 1903). These are often divergent strabismus, and very rarely respond to treatment to establish binocular vision. Some other alternating strabismus will become unilateral if left untreated. In young children this is undesirable because it can result in amblyopia.

Accommodative State

The angle of the strabismus may vary with the amount of accommodation exerted. In hypermetropes this is an important factor in the treatment, so that strabismus may be classified as: fully accommodative, partially accommodative, or nonaccommodative. The strong association between

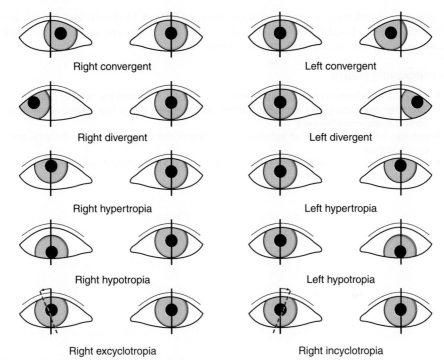

Right convergent   Left convergent

Right divergent   Left divergent

Right hypertropia   Left hypertropia

Right hypotropia   Left hypotropia

Right excyclotropia   Right incyclotropia

Fig. 1.4 Classification of strabismus by direction of deviation.

esotropia and hypermetropia raises the question of whether the hypermetropia leads to esotropia or the strabismus impairs the emmetropisation process. A thorough review concluded that in children, the emmetropisation process fails (causing hypermetropia) prior to the onset of esotropia (Smith et al., 2017).

It is estimated that about two-thirds of cases of comitant convergent strabismus have an accommodative element. The angle will be reduced by refractive correction of hypermetropia, fully in some cases, and partially in others. In such cases, the refractive correction forms a major part of the treatment of the deviation.

In about one-third of cases of comitant convergent strabismus, the refractive correction does not appear to change the angle of deviation. These are nonaccommodative strabismus. Some patients who overconverge for near vision have nonaccommodative strabismus. In these cases, the convergence excess is not stimulated by the accommodative effort.

IMPORTANCE OF CLASSIFICATION

In the clinical assessment of both heterophoria and strabismus, the classification assists in deciding what can be done to help the patient: the clinical management.

In cases of heterophoria, for example, the most important consideration is whether the deviation is compensated or decompensated (Chapter 4). Compensated heterophoria usually requires no action. The management of esophoria is different from that of exophoria. It will also differ if the heterophoria is present for near vision as accommodation is normally active compared to distance vision. In the same way, the management of strabismus will depend first on the classification. This is further elaborated in Chapter 15.

Although classification is important, some cases are difficult to classify, and may be best described by their clinical features. Classifications often merge into one another, for example decompensated exophoria and intermittent exotropia.

CLINICAL KEY POINTS

- Binocular coordination depends on anatomy, the motor system, and the sensory system
- Binocular vision anomalies are likely to affect approximately one in five patients consulting primary eyecare practitioners
- Heterophoria can be classified according to the direction of deviation, fixation distance, and compensation
- Strabismus can be classified according to constancy, direction of deviation, eye preference, and accommodative state

Detecting Binocular Vision Anomalies in Primary Eyecare Practice

Introduction

The routine for examining the eyes and vision of every patient in primary eyecare should have three objectives: to detect the presence of anomalies, indicate when further investigative tests are required, and to determine the management. In some cases, the presenting symptoms or history indicate that a binocular anomaly is likely to be the cause of the trouble. With other patients, binocular vision anomalies will be discovered during the examination, although these were not obvious to the patient.

When all the results of the eye examination are considered together, they may fit into a recognisable pattern, which is called the diagnosis. It is unhelpful that various diagnostic criteria apply to some binocular vision and accommodative anomalies (Cacho-Martinez, Garcia-Munoz, & Ruiz-Cantero, 2010); the issue of diagnostic uncertainty is returned to on p. 13. Based on the diagnosis, a decision can be reached on what to do for the patient: the management of the case. This process can be summarised as follows:

$$\text{Investigation} + \text{Evaluation} \rightarrow \text{Diagnosis} \rightarrow \text{Management}$$

Management options for primary eyecare practitioners include further investigation, refractive or prismatic correction, treatment (e.g., eye exercises or patching), or referral for medical attention.

An outline of the routine procedures is illustrated in Fig. 2.1. The type of investigation of the binocular functions will depend on whether a strabismus or heterophoria has been found. Whereas a routine examination will have broader objectives, the description in this chapter emphasises the binocular vision aspects. This chapter does not describe all the clinical procedures that routinely are used to investigate heterophoria and strabismus; most of these are described in later chapters. However, certain tests, such as the cover test, are fundamental to the investigation of binocular function and are best described at this stage.

Tests should be explained to patients as they are carried out, so that patients understand the general aspects of a routine eye examination. It is best to leave a detailed explanation of the results until the end of the eye examination, when a full picture emerges.

SHOULD BINOCULAR VISION TESTS CREATE NATURAL OR ARTIFICIAL VIEWING CONDITIONS?

There are often several different tests that can be used, for example to measure the magnitude of heterophoria at a given distance. The various tests will create differing conditions and will therefore produce different results. Tests which create less natural viewing conditions and dissociate the eyes to a greater degree tend to produce higher estimates of the deviation. This raises the question of whether it is better to know the deviation that occurs under natural viewing conditions or the 'full' deviation that occurs under artificial viewing conditions.

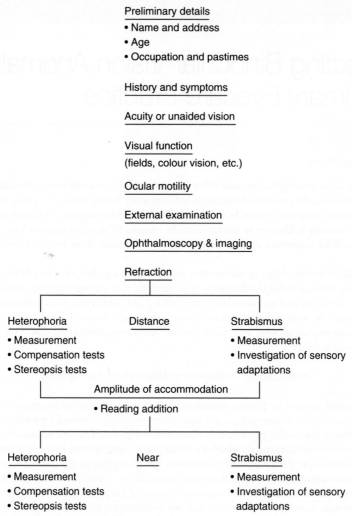

Preliminary details
• Name and address
• Age
• Occupation and pastimes

History and symptoms

Acuity or unaided vision

Visual function
(fields, colour vision, etc.)

Ocular motility

External examination

Ophthalmoscopy & imaging

Refraction

Heterophoria	**Distance**	Strabismus
• Measurement		• Measurement
• Compensation tests		• Investigation of sensory
• Stereopsis tests		adaptations

Amplitude of accommodation
• Reading addition

Heterophoria	**Near**	Strabismus
• Measurement		• Measurement
• Compensation tests		• Investigation of sensory
• Stereopsis tests		adaptations

Fig. 2.1   Summary of routine eye and vision examination.

If the purpose of a binocular vision test is to detect what is happening with that person's visual system under everyday conditions, the binocular vision test should mimic everyday visual conditions. For example, the practitioner may wish to know whether symptoms that a patient has reported when gaming on their smartphone are attributable to a binocular vision anomaly. The most relevant tests are those that mimic the viewing conditions when they view the smartphone and include a cover test and Mallett fixation disparity test at the appropriate distance (pp. 74—79). It is best to carry out the most naturalistic tests (e.g., fixation disparity) before more dissociative tests (Brautaset & Jennings, 1999).

If, on the other hand, the purpose of a binocular vision test is to reveal information about the aetiology of a binocular vision anomaly, it may be helpful to fully dissociate the patient. For example, in a patient who is complaining of vertical diplopia when reading it may be necessary to perform a double Maddox Rod Test to fully investigate the characteristics of the vertical diplopia (p. 133).

REFRACTIVE CORRECTION DURING BINOCULAR VISION TESTS

A common question from students and practitioners is 'what refractive correction (if any) should be worn when carrying out binocular vision tests?' The answer to this question depends on what the clinician wishes to know. To discover whether symptoms in everyday life are related to a binocular vision anomaly, the binocular vision tests should be carried out with the patient wearing the optical correction, if any, that they would use most often for that task in everyday life. Conversely, if the clinician wishes to determine what effect a proposed refractive correction will have on a patient's binocular vision status, they should carry out the tests with the patient wearing the proposed refractive correction. It will sometimes be appropriate to test patients under both conditions.

DIAGNOSTIC UNCERTAINTY: EFFECTS OF TEST REPEATABILITY, DIAGNOSTIC STABILITY, REGRESSION TO THE MEAN

The diagnostic process was described at the beginning of this chapter, and it was noted that disagreement over diagnostic criteria leads to uncertainty over diagnosis. Several other confounding factors influence diagnosis, and these will now be briefly considered. Fundamental properties of any clinical test are its repeatability (variation in measurements by the same person under the same conditions) and reproducibility (variation in measurements by different clinicians). There has been relatively little research on the reproducibility of many tests for diagnosing binocular vision anomalies.

Even if a clinical test perfectly measures the clinical status, it is possible that this status changes in an individual on different occasions. For example, fatigue may cause the angle of deviation to increase and/or a heterophoria to break down to a strabismus. Physical and mental activities can also influence test results (Vera, Jiménez, García, & Cárdenas, 2017), as can the instructions given to the patient (Karania & Evans, 2006a, 2006b).

The two factors just described will contribute to random errors on repeated measurements, which in turn lead to an effect described as **regression to the mean**. This statistical effect means that when a clinical measurement is repeated, individuals with extreme values (e.g., poor performance) at the first measurement are likely to change towards the population mean at the second reading. Regression to the mean occurs even when the person tested receives no treatment (Yu & Chen, 2014). This has consequences for researchers (Barnett, van der Pols, & Dobson, 2005) and clinicians (Morton & Torgerson, 2003). If a binocular vision anomaly is diagnosed from one measurement and then treatment is instigated, some patients may appear to have improved on treatment solely because of this statistical effect. One approach that will minimise this error is sequential testing (Morton & Torgerson, 2003). For example, in a prevalence survey, Stidwill (1997) made a diagnosis of decompensated heterophoria only when the Mallett fixation disparity test detected an aligning prism on at least two separate occasions. As a rule, repeat testing is recommended before a binocular vision anomaly is diagnosed. In exceptional cases, this may not be required; for example, if a patient reports intermittent diplopia and is found to have a very large exophoria that breaks down rapidly on the cover-uncover test.

The importance of repeat testing was highlighted in research (Adler, Scally, & Barrett, 2013) measuring the amplitude of accommodation (pp. 30–32), a test which is prone to many measurement errors (Burns, Allen, Edgar, & Evans, 2020). Adler and colleagues found, of 26 children who 'failed' the test at the first visit, with no treatment 58% passed at a second visit and 81% passed at a third visit. This highlights not only the importance of repeat testing to confirm a diagnosis, but also the problems inherent in converting a continuous variable (amplitude of accommodation) into a binary, pass/fail, variable (see Preface).

Randomised controlled trials (RCTs) will control for regression to the mean, but will nonetheless lead to an overestimation of treatment effects (Yudkin & Stratton, 1996). It is therefore preferable to use the mean of several measurements as the basis for selection in RCTs, and this approach has been used in a trial of vision therapy (Evans, Evans, Jordahl-Moroz, & Nabee, 1998).

Preliminary Details

Preliminary details will include such information as the name and address. More important clinically, however, is the age of the patient. This must be noted in relation to the age of onset of any strabismus, as it is likely to influence the extent of the sensory adaptations and the prognosis.

The patient's occupation and pastimes should also be noted, so the visual demands are understood. Some patients have a greater need for stereopsis, and others use their eyes in conditions that put a greater stress on binocular vision. Changes in the workplace can also help understand the cause of the patient's problem.

Symptoms and History

SYMPTOMS

General Comments About Symptoms

Many patients will attend for examination at regular intervals, although they are not complaining of symptoms. This can result in the early detection of anomalies as symptoms often occur at an advanced stage in the progression of a condition. In children, binocular anomalies can occur without any serious symptoms, due to sensory adaptations. The onset of a strabismus at an early age is seldom accompanied by symptoms. Older patients may attend because of symptoms which they associate with the eyes and vision, or come for a check because they have a history of binocular vision problems. Patients often underestimate the role of symptoms: the most powerful single factor in determining whether optometrists prescribe interventions are the symptoms that the patient reports (O'Leary & Evans, 2003).

The eyes are just one organ in a complex organism and visual symptoms should not be considered in isolation. As discussed on p. 18, psychogenic factors can be the source of many visual symptoms and can indeed cause some ocular motor anomalies (see Case Study 2.1 on p. 35). Practitioners should be sensitive to anything that is causing anxiety, such as family problems, bullying at school or in the workplace, and health worries. Anxious people do not always appear anxious and sometimes, a gentle enquiry about whether there is anything causing the patient anxiety or stress can be revealing.

Headache

Headache is a common symptom. It may be caused by a very large variety of problems, many of which are unrelated to the eyes or vision. It is important to determine if any headache is associated with the use of eyes. Decompensated heterophoria can cause headache which occurs after prolonged use of the eyes, often under adverse visual conditions. Some authors have observed that the headache is most likely to be frontal (Pickwell, 1984a), but others say headache from asthenopia can be of any type (Duke-Elder & Abrams, 1970). Usually, headache due to binocular vision problems is less intense or absent in the morning after a night's sleep and gets worse as the day wears on. Refractive error is a risk factor for headache in children (Hendricks, De Brabander, van Der Horst, Hendrikse, & Knottnerus, 2007) and adults (Akinci et al., 2008). Appendix 11 is a headache diary that can be given to patients to help them identify whether there are any visual triggers.

An unusual source of headache that may present to the eyecare practitioner is trochlear headache, from inflammation to one of the structures in the trochlear region, related to trochleodynia and trochleitis (Tran, McClelland, & Lee, 2019). The condition can be misdiagnosed as migraine or tension-type headache, with which it can coexist. Referral is required for medical investigation and management.

It has long been claimed that migraine can be a symptom of heterophoria (Worth, 1905) and this is discussed further on p. 64. On average, patients with migraine have a slightly higher than usual prevalence of heterophoria, fixation disparity, and reduced stereopsis (Harle & Evans, 2006). There is no good evidence that these anomalies are a common cause of migraine.

Palinopsia, the persistence or recurrence of visual images after the stimulus has been removed, is an uncommon symptom which may need careful questioning to differentiate from diplopia. There are two types (Gersztenkorn & Lee, 2015). **Illusory palinopsia** describes after-images that are unformed, indistinct, or of low resolution and are affected by ambient light. This represents a dysfunction in visual perception resulting from migraine, drugs, or head trauma. In contrast, **hallucinatory palinopsia** describes after-images that are not usually affected by environmental conditions of light or motion and are long-lasting, isochromatic, and of high resolution. This category represents a dysfunction in visual memory and is caused by posterior cortical lesions or seizures (Gersztenkorn & Lee, 2015).

Diplopia

Diplopia is uncommon in long-standing strabismus, as sensory adaptations occur. Its presence therefore suggests a deviation of recent onset, although about two-thirds of cases of acquired strabismus from brain damage (usually stroke or trauma) do not report diplopia (Fowler, Wade, Richardson, & Stein, 1996). Deviations of recent onset may have a pathological cause. The patient should also be asked if the doubling is constant or intermittent, whether it is horizontal, vertical, or both (diagonal), and if it is associated with any particular visual tasks or directions of gaze. Incomitant deviations are more likely to have a vertical component.

Double vision in heterophoria indicates that it is intermittently breaking down into a strabismus. This may be because the factors causing the decompensation have reached a serious state and sometimes it is an early indication of an active pathological cause. In the latter case, the onset of intermittent diplopia is likely to be more sudden and dramatic. A simple questionnaire has been developed for quantifying diplopia (Holmes, Liebermann, Hatt, Smith, & Leske, 2013).

Blurred Vision

Blurred vision is a common symptom in heterophoria. It can be associated with accommodative difficulties such as undercorrected presbyopia or hypermetropia. In these cases, blurred vision is more likely to be noticed by the patient during close work. The significance of blurred vision should not be underestimated: having blurred vision more than once or twice a month has a detectable and significant impact on functional status and well-being (Lee, Spritzer, & Hays, 1997).

Poor Stereopsis

Poor stereopsis occurs with some binocular vision problems in which the patients report difficulty in judging distances. Patients often do not notice this symptom because of the many monocular clues to depth perception (Rabbetts, 2007).

Asthenopia

Asthenopia describes any symptoms associated with the use of the eyes, typically eyestrain and headache, including general tiredness or soreness of the eyes or lids. Asthenopic symptoms may be unrelated to the eyes and vision (Ip, Robaei, Rochtchina, & Mitchell, 2006), or can result from either internal (binocular and accommodative factors) or external (e.g., dry eye) factors (Sheedy, Hayes, & Engle, 2003). In this research, one of the conditions triggering internal asthenopia is induced astigmatism and Sheedy and colleagues assumed the mechanism was stressed accommodation and convergence from 'accommodative uncertainty and fluctuation'. An alternative hypothesis might be the direct effect of blur.

Literally, the term asthenopia means weakness, or debility, of the eyes or vision, so the term may be best confined to describing symptoms arising from a visual or ocular anomaly, rather than from purely extrinsic (e.g., environmental) factors. Asthenopic symptoms associated with the use of digital displays (desktop and laptop PCs, tablets, smartphones) have been collectively referred to as digital eye strain (DES) or computer vision syndrome (Rosenfield, 2016; Sheppard & Wolffsohn, 2018). The aetiology of DES can be divided into the same external and internal factors as conventional asthenopia (Gowrisankaran & Sheedy, 2015). Viewing distances are closer and asthenopic symptoms worse after reading from a smartphone for 60 minutes (Long, Cheung, Duong, Paynter, & Asper, 2017). Low power adds (+ 0.75) often improve symptoms and sometimes performance in DES (Yammouni & Evans, 2020).

A Swedish study suggested that asthenopia in school children is largely attributable to refractive error (Abdi, Lennerstrand, Pansell, & Rydberg, 2008). However, these authors did not use a standardised questionnaire for detecting asthenopia and graded their orthoptic test results rather than treating them as continuous variables (Cumberland et al., 2014). Another study argued that asthenopia is present in one-quarter of unselected children aged 6—16 years. Asthenopia is more likely to occur when there is a combination of visual compromise and cognitively demanding tasks (Nahar, Gowrisankaran, Hayes, & Sheedy, 2011).

There is considerable overlap between symptoms related to dry eye and binocular/accommodative anomalies and this emphasises the need for careful differential diagnosis (Rueff, King-Smith, & Bailey, 2015). Indeed, these researchers found that the correlation between the results of two dry eye questionnaires is lower than the correlation between a dry eye questionnaire and a questionnaire designed to detect binocular vision anomalies.

Dizziness and Vertigo

Dizziness and vertigo may occur in incomitant heterophoria (Chapter 17). Vertigo can also be caused by variations to the blood supply to the brain, middle ear defects, or alterations in magnification from spectacle changes, particularly astigmatic changes (Rabbetts, 2007).

Monocular Eye Closure or Occlusion

Monocular eye closure (eyelid squinting) is used by patients with refractive error to improve acuity and in other cases to reduce illumination, particularly glare from the superior visual field (Sheedy, Truong, & Hayes, 2003). It is a common symptom in sunlight and in strabismus, particularly intermittent exotropia, and occurs to reduce photophobia rather than to avoid diplopia (Wiggins & von Noorden, 1990). Photophobia commonly occurs in intermittent exotropia, and successful surgery only alleviates the photophobia in about half of cases (Lew, Kim, Yun, & Han, 2007).

Monocular eye closure under normal lighting conditions can occur to avoid diplopia or other visual symptoms associated with binocular vision anomalies. This is a relatively common sign of a binocular anomaly and some patients adopt an unusual head posture, so the nose occludes the view of one eye (e.g., reading or writing with the head on the page).

HISTORY

When strabismus is reported or detected, it is important to discover how long it has been present and if it is constant or intermittent. The history or symptoms may suggest trauma or pathological conditions which contribute to the cause of the strabismus (Chapter 17). Questions should be asked about the possibility of birth trauma (e.g., the use of forceps) and whether the birth was full term. Prematurity is associated with an increased risk of hypermetropia and anisometropia (Lindqvist, Vik, Indredavik, & Brubakk, 2007) and a fivefold increased risk of esotropia (Robaei, Huynh, Kifley, & Mitchell, 2006). If postnatal trauma is suspected, the practitioner should always be mindful of the possibility of nonaccidental injury (child abuse). An estimated 40% of cases of physically abused children exhibit ocular complications, and any serious or suspicious injuries should be reported to the general medical practitioner (Barnard, 1995).

Another important part of the history is to gain an understanding of any previous treatment. This may have included spectacles, occlusion, eye exercises, or surgery. In each case, it is necessary to discover the type and effect of treatment given. Generally, if a treatment has been tried and proved unsuccessful, it is not worth trying again. An exception is a child whose motivation to undertake eye exercises or wear spectacles might change over time.

The patient's general health may also be significant in binocular vision anomalies. Poor general health may contribute to heterophoria becoming decompensated and will make treatment more difficult.

Many developmental conditions are associated with a higher than usual prevalence of binocular and accommodative anomalies and these are summarised in Table 2.1. Dyslexia (specific reading difficulty) affects about 7% of children (Hulme & Snowling, 2016). The main predictors of reading performance are nonvisual (e.g., phonemic awareness) and the relative contribution of visual-motor skills is small (Santi, Francis, Currie, & Wang, 2014). Dyslexia is sometimes associated with binocular instability (Chapter 5) although, in most cases, this is not a major cause of the dyslexia (Evans, Drasdo, & Richards, 1994). If patients with reading difficulties report asthenopia, this can be the result of binocular or accommodative anomalies or might be a sign of sensory visual stress (p. 64). As highlighted in the Preface, much research on this subject is of limited value for one or more of the following reasons (Evans, 2001a): excluding a high proportion of the relevant population (Shin, Park, & Park, 2009), lack of a control group (Christian, Nandakumar, Hrynchak, & Irving, 2018), not randomly allocating participants to treatment and control groups (Dusek, Pierscionek, & McClelland, 2011), not controlling for confounding variables (Palomo-Alvarez & Puell, 2010), dichotomising continuous variables (Shin et al., 2009), or assuming a correlation indicates a causal relationship (Hopkins, Black, White, & Wood, 2019).

Research on normal students may help to understand the relationship between binocular vision anomalies and dyslexia. For normal participants, when researchers induced a vergence conflict with prism or spherical lenses, performance at a cognitive task was impaired (Daniel & Kapoula, 2019). It is as if students had to reallocate some of their cognitive resources to maintain single and clear vision, causing a decrease in performance at the cognitive task. Tolerance to vergence/accommodation mismatch was lower in more difficult cognitive tasks. These researchers did not investigate dyslexics, but it could be speculated from this research that binocular instability might be more problematic for a dyslexic than for a good reader.

TABLE 2.1 ■ **Some Developmental Conditions Associated With Binocular and Accommodative Anomalies.**

Condition	Binocular and Accommodative Anomalies That are Prevalent in the Condition
Albinism	Low amplitude of accommodation (Karlén, Milestad, & Pansell, 2019) Nystagmus Stereoblindness, strabismus
Autism	Strabismus and amblyopia (Gowen et al., 2017) Reduced convergence and high accommodative lag (Little, 2018) Abnormal smooth pursuit and saccades (Gowen et al., 2017) (also, refractive errors [Little, 2018; Neuenschwander, Rohrbach, & Schroth, 2018], sensory visual stress [Ludlow, Wilkins, & Heaton, 2008])
Down syndrome	Reduced accommodative response; bifocals successful in 65% (Al-Bagdady, Stewart, Watts, Murphy, & Woodhouse, 2009) 29% risk of strabismus (Cregg et al., 2003); bifocals reduce the proportion with strabismus and the angle of strabismus (de Weger, Boonstra, & Goossens, 2019) Incomitant deviations Infantile nystagmus syndrome (also, keratoconus, cataract, iris pigmented spots, blepharitis, refractive errors, colour vision defects)
Fragile X syndrome	30% exhibit strabismus (also, refractive errors and visual motion processing)

Attention deficit/hyperactivity disorder (ADHD) has a higher prevalence in children with visual problems not correctable with spectacles or contact lenses (DeCarlo et al., 2014). Children with reading or other learning problems need a thorough vision assessment and vision screening is inadequate for these cases (Solebo, 2019).

FAMILY HISTORY

The highest familiar association is for hypermetropic accommodative esotropia where 26% of first-degree relatives are affected, compared with 15% in infantile esotropia, 12% in anisometropic eso-tropia, and 4% in exotropia (Ziakas, Woodruff, Smith, & Thompson, 2002).

Acuity or Unaided Vision

The unaided vision of each eye or the corrected acuity with the patient's present refractive correction is usually measured with a standard letter chart. For young children, other methods may be more appropriate (Chapter 3). If the patient does not wear a refractive correction all the time, it is useful to record the vision with and without the correction. It is important to record the acuities early in the examination, as this often gives a clue to what may be expected in subsequent investigation. For example, an eye with reduced acuity is more likely to be the deviated eye in strabismus. When visual acuity is carefully measured, the 95% limits are approximately ±1 line (Smith, 2006). In children aged 6−11 years, 95% of cases are repeatable to within ±1.5 lines (Manny, Hussein, Gwiazda, Marsh-Tootle, & COMET study group, 2003).

In amblyopia, other details may be inferred from the way in which the patient reads the chart. Difficulty in reading the middle letters of a line in the correct order may suggest eccentric fixation with the small accompanying scotoma, a common feature of strabismic amblyopia (Chapter 13).

Patients with low vision, for example in age-related maculopathy, may be particularly prone to symptomatic binocular vision anomalies and need careful evaluation of their binocular status (Rundstrom & Eperjesi, 1995). In older people, binocular vision anomalies may increase the risk of falls (Evans & Rowlands, 2004).

VISUAL CONVERSION REACTION (PSYCHOGENIC VISUAL LOSS; FUNCTIONAL VISION LOSS)

Reduced vision can result from a **visual conversion reaction** (VCR; psychogenic visual loss, func-tional visual loss). Typically, a child complains of blurred vision (Middleton, Sinason, & Davids, 2007) and the practitioner detects reduced visual acuity for no apparent reason. In about one-third of cases (Lim, Siatkowski, & Farris, 2005), the problem only affects one eye and might be misdiag-nosed as amblyopia. It can occur at any age, affects mostly females, and may be associated with psy-chosocial events, primarily social in children and trauma in adults (Lim et al., 2005). One-fifth of cases have migraine, facial pain, or coexisting organic pathology (Lim et al., 2005).

Up to half of adults and a quarter of children with VCR have coexisting real pathology (Scott & Egan, 2003). Therefore, the term VCR is appropriate: it is as if the patient has subconsciously converted a real anomaly into a nongenuine anomaly with symptoms. For the practitioner, this means the presence of illogical or inconsistent symptoms should motivate them to redouble their efforts at searching for a genuine problem and monitor the patient closely. There is a complex interaction between psychogenic factors and visual function: sometimes there may be a measur-able visual problem that nonetheless is thought to have a psychogenic function (see Case Study 2.1 on p. 35).

A vertical prism dissociation test has been shown to rapidly differentiate VCR from poor vision due to pathology (Golnik, Lee, & Eggenberger, 2004). The procedure is summarised in

TABLE 2.2 ■ **Test Routine and Norms for the 4Δ Vertical Prism Test.**

1. Have the child view an isolated letter from two lines larger than the visual acuity of their better eye, wearing any refractive correction required.
2. Hold a 4Δ trial lens base down in front of the better eye.
3. Ask the patient what they see.
4. If they only see one letter, they have very poor vision in one eye.
5. If they see two letters, ask how they are orientated and to describe the letters.
6. If they see one clear letter and one blurred letter, they have poor vision in one eye.
7. In visual conversion reaction (VCR), they will see two letters and will not comment that one is clearer than the other.

TABLE 2.3 ■ **Test Routine for the Paired Cylinders Test.**

1. A plus cylinder and a minus cylinder of the same power (e.g., 4 DC) are placed at parallel axes in front of the 'normal' eye in a trial frame.
2. The patient's normal correction is placed in front of the eye with poor acuity.
3. The patient is asked to read, with both eyes open, text that previously could be read with the normal eye but not with the poor eye.
4. As the patient begins to read, the axis of one of the cylinders is rotated about 10–15 degrees. The axes of the two cylinders thus will no longer be parallel, blurring vision in the normal eye.
5. If the patient continues to read the line or can read it again when asked to do so, he or she must be using the affected eye.

Table 2.2. An ingenious approach is the **paired cylinders test** in Table 2.3 (Miller, 2011). Another useful test is to measure the visual acuity twice, once at half the full testing distance (Zinkernagel & Mojon, 2009).

A useful way to explain VCR is that some people cannot describe their emotional difficulties in words and can only express them physically (Middleton et al., 2007). Counselling or psychiatric referral can be helpful.

Ocular Motor Investigation

The term **motor** refers to that which imparts motion so that **ocular motor** is used to describe the neurological, muscular, and associated structures and functions involved in movements of part or all of one or both eyes. Strictly speaking, the term **oculomotor** refers only to the functioning of the third cranial nerve. Confusingly, some authors use **oculomotor** variously as a synonym of **ocular motor**, to describe saccadic eye movements, or to describe saccadic and pursuit eye movements (Simmons, 2017).

A basic investigation of ocular motor function normally includes:

1. *Cover test:* revealing whether any deviation is strabismus or heterophoria, the degree of deviation, and some indication of compensation in heterophoria.
2. *Motility test:* which investigates any restrictions of eye movements and comitancy.
3. *Near triad:* convergence, accommodation, and pupillary miosis occur during near vision and are called the near triad. Another associated motor reflex is the movement of the eyelids during eye movements.

COVER TEST

This is largely an objective test relying on the critical observation of the practitioner. It is the only way to distinguish between heterophoria and strabismus unless there is a very marked deviation.

The cover test requires considerable skill, but this can be acquired by practice. Essentially it consists of covering and uncovering each eye in turn, whilst the other eye fixates a letter on a distance chart or a suitable near fixation target. The basic cover/uncover test will be described first, and then various modifications discussed. A summary of the procedure with this most important of binocular vision tests can be found at the end of this section.

As one eye is covered, the practitioner watches the other: any movement indicates that it was deviated (strabismic) and had to move to take up fixation. As the cover is removed, the practitioner watches the eye which has been covered: any movement of this eye indicates that it was deviated under the cover and recovers when the cover is removed and it is free to take up fixation. In the absence of strabismus, this shows heterophoria.

The test should be carried out for distance vision using a letter on the Snellen chart from the line above the visual acuity threshold of the eye with lowest acuity, so that precise accommodation is required. It is repeated for near vision at the patient's usual working distance. If the visual acuity is worse than about 6/36 at the relevant distance, a spotlight should be used for fixation. For preschool children, an animated cartoon movie may be an appropriate target (Troyer, Sreenivasan, Peper, & Candy, 2017). If it is known from previous eye examinations that a patient has a permanent or intermittent strabismus in one eye, the nonstrabismic eye should be covered first. Translucent occluders are available which allow the practitioner to observe the approximate position of the eye behind the occluder, without allowing the patient any form vision. It is important that the covered eye is fully occluded, particularly from bright lights in the periphery which can stimulate abnormal movements in some patients. In performing the cover test, the eye is usually covered only for 1 or 2 seconds, so that the response to momentary dissociation is observed, although longer occlusion (up to 10 seconds) will be more likely to reveal the full deviation (Barnard & Thomson, 1995).

The cover test should not be repeated unnecessarily since the deviation increases with repeated covering and can break down into a strabismus. In cases where it is suspected that the heterophoria may be breaking down into strabismus, the cover test should be performed as the first step before the visual acuity is assessed. The practitioner will have to estimate the appropriate target and repeat the cover test if the target proves to be too small when the visual acuity is later assessed. The effect of repeated and longer dissociation can be observed by the alternating cover test method (below), and by holding the occluder in place for longer.

Cover Test in Strabismus

This is illustrated in Fig. 2.2, which shows the movements in right convergent strabismus (esotropia), and in Fig. 2.3, which shows right divergent strabismus (exotropia) with right hypertropia. The cover test will also help in investigating other aspects of strabismus:

1. *Constancy.* An intermittent strabismus may be present sometimes and binocular vision recovered at other times. Often this type of strabismus is not present until the cover test is performed, but the momentary dissociation is sufficient to make the strabismus manifest.
2. *Direction of deviation.* Indicated by the direction of the movement; for example, in convergent strabismus the deviated eye will be seen to move outwards to take up fixation when the other eye is covered.
3. *Eye preference.* In alternating strabismus, covering one eye will transfer the strabismus to the other eye which will continue to fixate when the cover is removed. In such cases, a preference for fixation with one eye may be found, although fixation can be maintained with either eye: if the patient blinks or changes fixation momentarily, the fixation typically reverts to the preferred eye. In other cases, the patient may be able to maintain fixation with either eye at will.
4. *Degree of deviation.* With practice, the angle of the strabismus can be estimated from the amount of the movement. This is the preferred method of assessing the deviation and can be made easier by comparing the movement during the cover test to a version movement

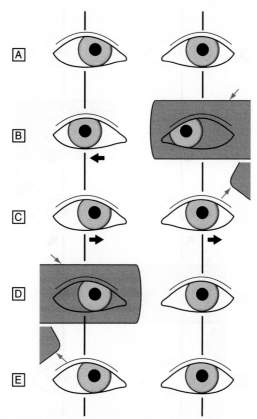

Fig. 2.2 Cover test in right convergent strabismus. (Movement of the eye is signified by the *bold black arrow*, movement of the cover by the *grey arrow*.) (A) Deviated right eye; (B) left eye covered, both eyes move to the right so that the right eye takes up fixation; (C) left eye uncovered, both eyes move to the left as the left eye again takes up fixation; (D) right eye covered, no movement of either eye; (E) cover removed, no movement. Note: both eyes move together in accordance with Hering's law (see Glossary).

of known magnitude. For example, an eye will make a version movement of 1Δ when the person looks between two objects 6 cm apart at 6 m. The width of a line of letters on most Snellen charts for acuities from 6/18 to 6/6 is 12 cm. Hence, if the patient looks from a letter at one end of the line to one on the other end, then the resulting saccadic eye movement is 2Δ. On a typical LogMAR (ETDRS) chart, an eye movement from letters at one end of the 6/9 line (LogMAR 0.2) to the other end is equivalent to approximately 2Δ.

Cover Test in Heterophoria

This is illustrated with respect to esophoria in Fig. 2.4. The eyes are straight until they are dissociated by covering one. Then the covered eye deviates into the heterophoric position behind the cover. It will be seen to make a recovery movement when the cover is removed. In the simplest cases (Fig. 2.4A—C), the eye which is not covered will continue to fixate without making any movements when the other is covered or when the cover is removed. It should be noted that this is not in accordance with Hering's law of equal eye movements (see Glossary).

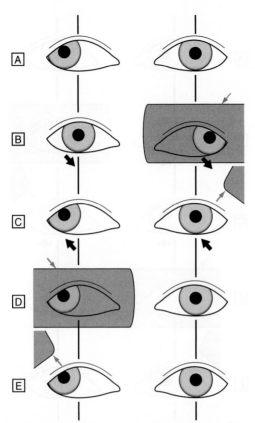

Fig. 2.3 Cover test in right divergent strabismus with right hypertropia. (Movement of the eye is signified by the *bold black arrow*, movement of the cover by the *grey arrow*.) (A) Right eye deviated out and up;
(B) left eye covered − both eyes move left and downwards for the right eye to take up fixation; (C) left eye
uncovered − both eyes move right and upwards as the left eye again takes up fixation; (D) and (E) no movement of either eye as the strabismic right eye is covered and uncovered.

Movements of both eyes may be seen on the removal of the cover in some cases (Fig. 2.4D−F).
This is particularly noticeable in large degrees of heterophoria and cases of strong ocular dominance
(Peli & McCormack, 1983). When the cover is removed, both eyes are seen to make a versional
movement of about half the total phoria deviation, that is, they both move in the same direction, to
the left or to the right. This versional movement is relatively quick and is followed by a slower
change of vergence of about the same magnitude. For the eye which has been covered, the second
part of the recovery will be in the same direction as the versional movement. For the noncovered
eye, the second movement will be a return to its fixation position. That is to say, the eye which is
not covered will be seen to make an apparently irrelevant movement outwards (for esophoria) and
back again to its fixation position. In the cases which show this pattern of movements, it will be
noted that Hering's law does apply.

In heterophoria, the cover test movements are usually the same whether the left or the right eye
is covered. In some cases, however, this is not so. In uncorrected anisometropes, the movement can
be larger in one eye if a change in accommodation is required to keep the fixation target in focus
when one eye is covered, but not when the other is covered. Another cause of asymmetry of eye
movements during cover testing is incomitancy (see Chapter 17).

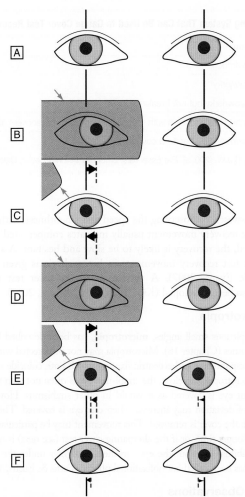

Fig. 2.4 The cover test in esophoria. (Movement of the eye is signified by the *bold black arrow*, movement of the cover by the *grey arrow*.) (A–C) From the 'straight' active position, the right eye moves inwards when dissociated by covering (B); it moves outwards to resume fixation with the other eye when the cover is removed (C). Note that the left (uncovered) eye does not move during the simple pattern of movements. (D–F) The 'versional pattern': the right eye moves inwards under the cover, as in the simple pattern (D); on removing the cover, both eyes move to the right by the same amount (about half the degree of the esophoria) (E); both eyes then diverge to the straight position (F).

In some patients, the versional pattern of movements may show when one eye is covered, but the simple pattern if the cover is applied to the other eye. These patients have marked ocular motor dominance. The versional pattern is seen on removing the cover from the dominant eye: fixation is quickly transferred to the dominant eye by the versional movement, and the recovery from the heterophoric position occurs in the nondominant eye. These patients often have slight amblyopia with a small central suppression area in the nondominant eye and are considered by some to be a variant of microtropia (below).

The cover test helps in the investigation of heterophoria by giving information about:

1. *Direction of deviation:* esophoria, exophoria, hyperphoria, or cyclophoria.
2. *Degree of deviation:* estimated from the amount of movement seen on removing the cover.

TABLE 2.4 ■ A Grading System That Can Be Used to Gauge Cover Test Recovery in Heterophoria.

Grade	Description
1	Rapid and smooth
2	Slightly slow/jerky
3	Definitely slow/jerky but not breaking down
4	Slow/jerky and breaks down with repeat covering, or only recovers after a blink
5	Breaks down readily after 1—3 covers

Reproduced from Evans, B.J.W. [2005a]. *Eye Essentials: Binocular Vision*. Elsevier, Oxford.

3. *Compensation:* assessed by observing the speed and smoothness of the recovery movement. A smooth quick recovery movement usually indicates compensated heterophoria, but if it is decompensated, the recovery is likely to be slow and hesitant. A schema for grading the quality of cover test recovery movements in heterophoria is given in Table 2.4 (Evans, 2005a; Tang & Evans, 2007). A system based on cover test result in intermittent exotropia has also been developed (Kim, Kim, Ahn, & Lim, 2017).

Cover Test in Microtropia

Strabismus with inconspicuous small angles, **microtropia**, has been described by several terms and as having various characteristics (Chapter 16). Microtropia may not be detected with the cover test because of abnormal retinal correspondence and eccentric fixation which both coincide in degree with the angle of the strabismus. In microtropia, therefore, the strabismic eye is often not seen to move to take up fixation when the dominant eye is covered as it would in other strabismus. However, in some cases of microtropia, the angle of deviation may increase when one eye is covered. There may be an apparent 'phoria movement' when the cover is removed. This movement may be particularly noticeable if the cover is held in place for a longer time, or if the alternating cover test (see next) is used. It may be assumed that in the active or habitual position, the eyes are held straighter under the influence of peripheral fusion. This condition has been called 'monofixational phoria' (Parks & Eustis, 1961; Chapter 16).

Other Cover Test Observations

Failure of an eye to take up fixation sometimes occurs in both strabismus and heterophoria. The experienced practitioner can see that an eye is deviated. The eye will move to take up fixation if the patient is asked to 'look very hard at' the target, or is asked to look at a point a little higher than but close to the original fixation point; say 2 or 3 mm for near vision. The eye can then be seen to make a horizontal movement as well as the necessary very small vertical one. Alternatively, the head can be moved by 1—2 cm, or during near fixation the fixation target can be moved by this amount. The patient will then make a pursuit movement with, if he has failed to take up fixation, a refixation movement superimposed upon it.

Latent nystagmus may also be revealed by the cover test. It shows a conjugate oscillation of both eyes when one is covered (Chapter 18).

The cover test described above is the basic method, sometimes called the **cover/uncover test**. There are several modifications to the cover test which will give further useful information in some cases.

Alternating Cover Test

When the cover/uncover test has been carried out as described above, it is useful then to transfer the cover from one eye to the other and back several times (typically, 6—10 covers or 3—5 cycles). The degree of the deviation usually increases, making it easier to see.

Where no obvious strabismus is seen, the eyes should be observed to see if any recovery movement takes place when the cover is finally removed after the alternating cover test. This gives an indication of the degree of compensation, as poorly compensated heterophoria does not recover so readily or as smoothly after the alternating cover test. If as the cover is removed, the eye that is being uncovered does not appear to take up fixation, the cover should be reintroduced in front of the other eye. This is to see if the repeated covering has induced a strabismus, in which case the recently uncovered eye will be seen to move to take up fixation when the other eye is covered.

The alternating cover test is sometimes called the alternate cover test. This is potentially confusing, because there are several variations to the cover test, rather than two alternatives.

Prism Measurement

Measurement of the deviation can be carried out by placing a relieving prism before an eye to neutralise the cover test movement. This can be done using single prisms from a trial case, or more conveniently with a prism bar. The lowest power of prism that neutralises the movement is taken as a measure of the deviation. This can be done in heterophoria or in strabismus but, for larger deviations, potential inaccuracies associated with the use of prisms should be borne in mind (Firth & Whittle, 1994, 1995).

In the case of strabismus, the habitual angle is measured by the **simultaneous prism cover test**, which should be carried out after the cover/uncover test and before the alternating cover test, to avoid increasing the angle by dissociation. The cover/uncover test will have revealed the strabismic eye and the likely size of deviation. The practitioner simultaneously approaches the fixating eye with the cover and the strabismic eye with the prism estimated to neutralise the deviation. If no movement is observed, the size of the habitual deviation has been correctly estimated. If a movement is seen, the test is repeated with the new estimate of the required prism.

Once the **habitual angle** has been measured in this way, the **total angle** can be measured by neutralising the movement during the alternating cover test without removing the prism bar between movements of the cover.

When the correct relieving prism is in place, the corneal reflections of a fixation light appear symmetrically placed in the two eyes. Before applying the cover therefore, an estimate of angle can be made by increasing the prism power until the corneal reflections appear to be symmetrically placed. This is called the Krimsky test (Krimsky, 1943), but is not as accurate as the cover test.

Subjective Cover Test ('Phi' Test)

If there is a deviation, either heterophoria or strabismus, the patient will observe an apparent jump of the fixation point when the cover is transferred from one eye to the other. This apparent jump is known as 'phi' movement. In convergent deviations, the jump will appear to be against the movement of the cover, that is, if the cover is moved from the right eye **to the left**, the fixation point will appear to the patient to move to the **right**. A 'with' movement occurs in divergent deviations (Appendix 1). Prisms can be introduced to eliminate this movement and provide a subjective measure of the deviation. As the phi test involves repeated covering (usually an alternating cover test), the angle of deviation is likely to increase beyond that usually measured with the cover/uncover test.

Value and Accuracy of the Cover Test

Although this section describing the cover test is quite lengthy, the cover test is probably the most important binocular vision test. Because it is so valuable as a diagnostic procedure and takes so little time, it should be incorporated in all routine eye examinations. The time taken to acquire the necessary skill in observation is well worth while. Minimal training is required for the efficient detection of small eye movements (Fogt, Baughman, & Good, 2000).

Rainey, Schroeder, Goss, and Grosvenor (1998) noted that 99% of observers could detect eye movements of less than 2Δ. These authors examined the interexaminer repeatability of variations of the alternating cover test. The 95% confidence limits were 3.3Δ when the eye movements were estimated, 3.6Δ when measured with prisms, and 2.5Δ for the subjective cover test. In intermittent exotropia, differences of less than 6Δ are likely to represent test-retest variability (Yang & Hwang, 2011). Other research indicates, the accuracy of prism measurement with the alternating cover test is such that changes of 10Δ or more are likely to represent a real change (Holmes, Leske, & Hohberger, 2008; de Jongh, Leach, Tjon-Fo-Sang, & Bjerre, 2014), or 13Δ for large-angle (> 20Δ) exodeviations at near (Hatt, Leske, Liebermann, Mohney, & Holmes, 2012).

An automated cover test with eye tracking apparatus (Barnard & Thomson, 1995) produces more repeatable results (Mestre, Otero, Díaz-Doutón, Gautier, & Pujol, 2018).

Rabbetts (2007) advised that the practitioner should watch the limbus and noted that because the lateral borders of the limbus are most easily seen between the patient's eyelids, it is easier to detect horizontal than vertical movements of the eyes. He suggested that other methods should be used to double check for vertical imbalances. The examiner should also watch for any eyelid movements as a slight vertical movement of the eyelashes may help detect vertical deviations. For young or uncooperative patients, there are alternative methods of assessing ocular alignment and these are discussed in Chapter 3.

Summary of Cover Test Procedure and Recording of Results

The basic cover test procedure is summarised in Table 2.5 and Table 2.6. A simplified approach to recording cover test results in given in Table 2.7.

MOTILITY TEST (OCULAR MOVEMENTS)

An examination of binocular function needs to explore the ability of the patient to move the eyes into all parts of the motor field. The test method is described here, and the interpretation of results is discussed in Chapter 17.

The motility test is usually carried out by asking the patient to look at a pen torch light, which is moved in the motor field, while the patient is asked to follow it with the eyes and keep the head still.

TABLE 2.5 ■ Summary of Basic Cover Test Procedure in Strabismus.

1. As the cover moves over one eye then the practitioner should watch the uncovered eye. It is the behaviour of the uncovered eye that reveals whether the patient has a strabismus.
2. For example, as the left eye is covered the practitioner should watch the right eye. If the right eye moves, this indicates a strabismus in this eye (Fig. 2.2).
3. The direction and amplitude of the movement should be estimated. The cover is then slowly removed from the eye that has been covered and this eye is observed to see if a movement occurs, signifying heterophoria (see Table 2.6).

TABLE 2.6 ■ Summary of Basic Cover Test Procedure in Heterophoria.

1. As the cover is slowly removed from the eye that has been covered, this eye is observed for any movement. If a movement occurs as an eye regains fixation after being covered, this indicates a heterophoria (Fig. 2.4).
2. The direction and amplitude of the movement should be estimated.
3. The quality of the recovery movement should also be noted. This gives an objective indication of how well the patient can compensate for the heterophoria (Table 2.4).

TABLE 2.7 ■ **Example of a Recording of Cover Test Results.**

D 2Δ XOP G1 → 2Δ XOP G2
N 8Δ XOP G1 → 12Δ XOP G3
Key: at distance, the cover/uncover test reveals 2Δ exophoria with good (grade 1) recovery. After the alternating cover test the angle does not change but the recovery becomes a little slower (grade 2 recovery).
At near, the cover/uncover test reveals 8Δ exophoria with good recovery. After the alternating cover test the angle builds to 12Δ exophoria with quite poor recovery, but not quite breaking down into a strabismus (grade 3 recovery).

The pen light should be kept at approximately a constant distance from the patient's head (about 50 cm). It is easier to detect any incomitant deviations if the light is not moved too fast: typically the light is moved from the centre to the periphery in about 2–4 s. Spectacles are not usually worn, unless there is a very marked accommodative strabismus (e.g., high hypermetropia with a marked convergent strabismus).

The motility test is usually performed binocularly, and if there is any suspicion of abnormality, it is repeated monocularly. The binocular motor field is restricted by the patient's brow and nose to eye movements of about 25 degrees from the primary position. It can be useful, however, to move the light into the monocular fixation area, as this is similar to carrying out a cover test in peripheral directions of gaze. Latent deviations and incomitancies can sometimes be detected by doing this. If there is any doubt, an actual cover test can be carried out in the peripheral gaze position. The cover will eliminate peripheral fusion when this is done. A quick useful routine is as follows, and a recording sheet for the results is given in Appendix 8:

1. *Fixation* is checked first, in each eye, by asking the patient to fixate the pen torch with the eyes in the primary position, while the other eye is occluded. Each eye is observed to see that steady fixation is maintained, with no wandering. The position of the pen torch reflection in the cornea is also noted with respect to the pupil. It should be symmetrical between the two eyes; usually slightly nasal if the angle lambda is normal (Fig. 3.2). Any asymmetry may indicate eccentric fixation (Chapter 13).

2. *Pursuit eye movements* should be smooth with no jerks as the light is moved horizontally. Both eyes should follow the light evenly across the binocular motor field and out into the area of monocular fixation, first one way and then the other. The lid apertures should not vary appreciably as this is carried out. In crossed alternating fixation, a jump of both eyes can be seen as the patient changes fixation to the other eye on moving from one half of the motor field to the other (Chapter 3).

3. *Vertical movement of the eyes and lids* are checked by moving the pen torch slowly about 25 cm above the horizontal, and then 25 cm below. Both eyes should follow the movement with corresponding lid movements. This may detect an A- or V- syndrome (Chapter 17).

4. *Comitancy* is next examined. This is done by moving the light across the upper part of the motor field to the right and then to the left. This includes the area of binocular fixation and the monocular part of the field. The patient is asked to say if any doubling occurs in the binocular area, and the practitioner observes any underaction or overshooting of one eye compared with the other. Incomitancy may be detected either by subjective diplopia or by the practitioner's observation. The process is repeated across the lower part of the motor field and then the central part (Chapter 17). Alternatively, some authorities recommend that a 'star' technique is used where the pen torch is moved in the horizontal (at eye level), vertical (looking for gaze palsies), and four oblique positions (Mallett, 1988a).

	4Δ R hypert	4Δ R hypert	4Δ R hypert		
LEFT GAZE	6Δ R hypert	4Δ R hypert	4Δ R hypert	**RIGHT GAZE**	
	12Δ R hypert	8Δ R hypert	8Δ R hypert		

Fig. 2.5 Example of method of recording objective (cover test in peripheral gaze) or subjective deviation in the cardinal positions of gaze. The results are suggestive of a right superior oblique palsy. Note: the record is made as perceived by the patient and it is important to label right gaze and left gaze (see text). *hypert.*, hypertropia.

5. *Cover testing in peripheral gaze* will help identify areas of overaction or underaction. It is important to watch the pupil reflexes to ensure that both eyes can see the target in all positions, and to ensure that the cover fully occludes the eye. A proforma for recording results is given in Appendix 8 and an example of the recording of results is given in Fig. 2.5.

6. *Reports of diplopia.* Patients should be asked about any diplopia they perceive during the test (Appendix 8). The position of gaze where there is maximum diplopia will usually identify the primary problem, and the image that is furthest out originates from the underacting eye (Chapter 17). It is again essential to watch reflections of the light to be certain that the patient is fixating. Reports of diplopia are in some cases inconsistent with the other clinical findings. Some patients appear to suppress the diplopic image in certain directions of gaze, others seem to be inconsistent and easily confused in describing diplopia.

7. *Monocular motility* can be useful in some cases. In mechanical (restrictive) incomitancies, there will be a restriction of monocular motility, but not usually in neurogenic incomitancies.

8. *Saccadic movements* can be checked by asking the patient to change fixation from the pen torch held at the right of the field to the practitioner's finger held in the left of the field, pause and back to the pen torch. These movements should be smooth, quick and accurate.

The motility test provides a great deal of information, and the interpretation of the results can be difficult for inexperienced practitioners. Initially, it can be simpler to carry out the test three times (Evans, 2000a), first looking solely at the corneal reflections of the pen torch, second carrying out cover tests in peripheral positions of gaze, and third asking the patient about diplopia (Appendix 8).

The motility test is the only objective routine clinical test for incomitant eye movements, but there are several subjective methods. These are particularly useful in recently acquired deviations where suppression is unlikely, and they are described in Chapter 17.

TESTS OF SACCADIC EYE MOVEMENTS

Objective instruments for assessing saccadic eye movements (e.g., by measuring the reflection of light from the limbus) are discussed further in Chapter 18. Some clinical tests exist which, it is claimed, can assess saccadic eye movements in digit reading tasks. An early example of this type of test is the New York State Optometric Association King-Devick Test. This used randomly spaced numbers in horizontal rows, and it is argued that good saccadic eye movement control is required to perform well. However, many other skills are also required to perform the test, so it is unlikely that the test has a high sensitivity or specificity for diagnosing saccadic dysfunction.

To control for some confounding variables, the Developmental Eye Movement test (DEM) was developed which has vertical columns of numbers as a control condition (Taylor-Kulp & Schmidt, 1997). Although an improvement, this test is still likely to be influenced by confounding variables such as digit recognition, attention (Coulter & Shallo-Hoffmann, 2000), sequencing and intelligence. The test has been shown to have poor repeatability (Rouse, Nestor, Parot, & DeLand, 2004) and its results do not correlate with results from an objective eye movement tracker (Ayton, Abel, Fricke, & McBrien, 2009). Further research indicates performance at the DEM test does not indicate a deficit causing poor reading, but rather is the effect of reading practice (Medland, Walter, & Margaret Woodhouse, 2010). These authors concluded that the DEM test should not be used to diagnose eye movement difficulties in patients with poor reading. A third study confirmed that 'the DEM is not a measure of saccadic eye movements' (Webber, Wood, Gole, & Brown, 2011).

It has been suggested that poor performance at the DEM may correlate with academic performance because it taps into other factors that link with academic performance (Wood, Black, Hopkins, & White, 2018). These authors emphasised that their results do not support a causative relationship between DEM results and poor reading.

In any event, the need for the routine clinical assessment of saccadic eye movements is questionable. Saccadic eye movements are the fundamental method of using the visual system to analyse or search any visual scene. For example, saccadic eye movements are used when walking down a street, driving a car, playing a ball sport, or watching television. It seems intuitively unlikely that saccadic dysfunction is a common clinical finding, and the author is unaware of any well-controlled studies that have demonstrated this. Simmons criticised the concept of 'oculomotor dysfunction' and noted that studies investigating 'oculomotor training' are conspicuously absent from the literature, in contrast to the 'casualness with which primary oculomotor dysfunction is diagnosed and treated in clinical practice' (Simmons, 2017), referring to the situation in North America. Simmons challenged the belief that 'oculomotor therapy' is effective, suggesting that symptoms attributed to saccadic dysfunction are explained by vergence dysfunction.

It has been argued that saccadic dysfunction is a feature of specific reading difficulties (dyslexia), but the evidence for this is weak. Saccadic irregularities when reading are most likely to be secondary to impaired linguistic processing (Evans, 2001a). The evidence for a beneficial effect of saccadic training programs is equivocal at best (Evans, 2001a).

There are some rare pathological conditions which affect saccadic eye movements, and these are discussed in Chapter 18. It may be helpful to assess eye movements, including saccades, pursuit, and vergence, in young children suspected of diseases affecting the central nervous system and an algorithm for combining observations into an 'ocular motor score' has been suggested for this (Olsson, Fahnehjelm, Rydberg, & Ygge, 2015). Vision therapy has been advocated to improve eye movements following traumatic brain injury, but the evidence is 'very low-certainty' (Rowe et al., 2018).

NEAR

The third aspect of the motor investigation is concerned with the near triad (associated reflexes): convergence, accommodation, and pupil reflexes. These constitute three synkinetic actions which normally come into play during near vision. The oculomotor (third cranial) nerve serves all of these, and disturbances of one may be accompanied by the others (see Chapter 17 for pathological causes). Clinicians often encounter isolated anomalies of convergence or of accommodation and these will be considered in isolation.

Convergence

There are two aspects of convergence movements. The first is pursuit (ramp) convergence: following an object brought slowly closer to the eyes by converging to retain a foveal image in both eyes. The second involves changing fixation from one object to another at a different distance: a refixation task for which there is the added stimulus of physiological diplopia. This second convergence movement is jump (step) vergence. The investigation of convergence can include both pursuit and jump convergence.

Near Point of Convergence (Pursuit Convergence)

A suitable target is brought slowly towards the eyes from about 50 cm and on the median line until the patient reports that it doubles and/or the practitioner sees that one eye has ceased to converge. It may be instructive to note if the patient reports or demonstrates excessive discomfort during the test (Adler, 2001). The RAF rule is typically used, but this has several limitations and holding a target in free space seems less variable (Adler, Cregg, Viollier, & Woodhouse, 2007), as long as the endpoint is carefully measured with a tape measure.

The target should be detailed (accommodative), of a size that is resolvable by each eye, and the patient should wear reading glasses where appropriate. Eighty-five percent of children aged 5—11 years have a near point of convergence of 6 cm or less (Hayes, Cohen, Rouse, & DeLand, 1998). Other authors have recommended stricter norms for younger children: 5 cm or less for children aged 0—7 years (Chen, O'Leary, & Howell, 2000) and based on a population of (mostly) young adults (Scheiman et al., 2003). Olsson and colleagues described <10 cm as an adequate response (Olsson et al., 2015). There is considerable debate about what is an acceptable near point of convergence, but the answer to this question is likely to relate to the distance at which the patient habitually works and the closest distance at which they are likely to need to fixate. People using smartphones sometimes use these at close viewing distances, that shorten with prolonged use (Long et al., 2017). It has been suggested that a 'convergence reserve' of half the required working distance seems reasonable (Rae, 2015).

With many patients, the near point of convergence will be closer to the eyes than the near point of accommodation, and the target will be seen to blur before it doubles. The convergence should still be investigated even if the target is blurred.

Jump Convergence Test

The patient is asked to fixate a small object placed at about 50 cm from the eyes, and then to change fixation to a second object introduced at 15 cm (p. 145). The patient's eyes should be seen to converge promptly and smoothly from the more distant object to the nearer one. Abnormal findings are version movements of both eyes, hesitant or slow convergence, or no movement (Pickwell & Hampshire, 1981a, 1981b). A quantitative measurement can be obtained by repeating the test whilst gradually bringing the near target closer to the patient. The closest distance to which the patient can 'jump converge' is recorded.

The assessment of convergence by clinical tests needs to indicate if it will be adequate to cope with the needs of the patient in near vision. This can be decided by considering both convergence tests together: a near point of convergence less than 8—10 cm and good jump convergence are taken as adequate for most patients. A fuller discussion of convergence anomalies is given in Chapter 8 and other tests of vergence function are described in more detail elsewhere in this book, including fusional reserve testing (pp. 69—73) and vergence facility (p. 73).

Accommodation

Amplitude of Accommodation

The amplitude of accommodation is a measure of the closest point at which the eyes can focus: it is the range from the far point to the near point in dioptres. Because it is measured from the far point, the measurement needs to be taken with the distance correction in place.

The usual method is to ask the patient to look at small print which is moved slowly towards the eye until the patient reports that clear vision cannot be maintained. When a just noticeable blur occurs, the card is moved in further to confirm that it becomes worse and is then moved back until it clears. The midpoint between the first blur and first clear positions is the near point (Reading, 1988). Typically, the text is mounted on a near-point rule so that the dioptral distance can be read from the rule. In the case of a young patient with a near point close to the eyes, a negative sphere (−4.00 D) can be held before the eyes so that the accommodative range is moved to the middle of the rule. The value of this sphere is then added to the reading. This is a subjective method and its accuracy depends on the patient's ability to distinguish a blur point, on the depth of focus, and other variables (Burns et al., 2020), but it is a standard clinical procedure. Accuracy can be improved by using smaller text as the target approaches, which reveals conventional norms to be an overestimate (Aitchison, Capper, & McCabe, 1994).

A subject which rarely receives the attention it deserves is the speed at which the target is moved. Evans et al. (1994) moved the target at 0.50 diopters per second (D/s), but Evans, Wilkins et al. (1996) used 1 D/s which seems more practical in a clinical setting. Note, the target moves slower when it is nearer the patient. Patient instructions are also important (Stark & Atchison, 1994) and it is best to ask patients to carefully look at the target. Literate patients can read text and preliterate patients can describe a detailed picture: when they make errors, the endpoint has been passed.

The amplitude of accommodation can also be measured monocularly using negative lenses. This will give a different result to the push-up method because the cue of proximity will be lacking. A small proportion of people do not seem to accommodate normally to minus lenses (Anderson & Stuebing, 2014).

Routine clinical methods of measuring the amplitude of accommodation (Burns, Evans, & Allen, 2014) are prone to a number of errors (Burns et al., 2020), which no doubt contributes to the large test-retest variability of up to approximately 5 D. Indeed, the dissimilarity of push-up measurements to objective estimates of accommodation has led some to argue that subjective methods should not be described as tests of accommodation, but rather as assessing the 'near point of clear vision' (Anderson & Stuebing, 2014).

The expected amplitudes of accommodation (Table 2.8) for a given age can be calculated from the Hofstetter formulae (Reading, 1988):

$$\text{Minimum amplitude (D)} = 15.0 - (0.25 \times \text{age in years})$$
$$\text{Probable amplitude (D)} = 18.5 - (0.3 \times \text{age in years})$$

The values in Table 2.8 generally seem to be appropriate for European races living in temperate climates. There is evidence of a racial variation or differences caused by geographical area of upbringing (Duke-Elder, 1970), with lower amplitude of accommodation in people of Chinese race (Edwards, Law, Lee, Leung, & Lui, 1993). Otherwise, an amplitude lower than the value in Table 2.8 is suspicious, indicating accommodative insufficiency. A large study in Brazil found 2.8% of children showed amplitude of accommodation less than 2 D lower than Hofstetter's minimum reference value (Castagno et al., 2016).

Accommodative insufficiency can result from some medications, such as antihistamines (Wright, 1998) and alcohol abuse (Campbell, Doughty, Heron, & Ackerley, 2001), but accommodation is only minimally reduced in patients undergoing heroin detoxification (Firth, Pulling, Carr, & Beaini, 2004). Interestingly, a case has been reported where a minimal dose of alcohol significantly improved combined accommodative and convergence insufficiency (Sturm, Berger, & Zangemeister, 2007).

Abnormalities of accommodation related to binocular vision are considered in later chapters. Accommodative insufficiency (a lower than expected amplitude of accommodation) can be a

TABLE 2.8 ■ Expected Minimum Accommodative Amplitudes for Various Ages, Given in Dioptres and Centimetres, Rounded to the Nearest 0.25 Units. It is recommended that dioptres are used clinically.

Age (yrs)	Minimum (D)	Minimum (cm)
4	14.00	7.00
6	13.50	7.50
8	13.00	7.75
10	12.50	8.00
12	12.00	8.25
14	11.50	8.75
20	10.00	10.00
30	7.50	13.25
40	5.00	20.00
50	2.50	40.00

common cause of symptoms (Sterner, Gellerstedt, & Sjostrom, 2006) and accommodation is an important part of the assessment of any pre-presbyopic patient with a suspected binocular vision anomaly.

The interaction between accommodation and convergence should be considered in any patient with an apparent accommodative dysfunction. For example, 'pseudo-accommodative insufficiency' associated with asthenopia can result from low divergent fusional reserves with a high AC/A ratio (Houston, Jones, & Weir, 2000). There is a remote near point of accommodation and when this is reached, a sudden transient esotropia or esophoria is apparent. It is believed that these patients underaccommodate to prevent a manifest deviation. These authors recommend training divergent fusional reserves and negative relative vergence rather than prescribing convex lenses (Houston et al., 2000).

Accommodation is often deficient in Down syndrome and many of these patients benefit from bifocals, which can act as a treatment as well as a correction (Al-Bagdady et al., 2009). Albinism is often associated with poor accommodation (Karlén et al., 2019). A visual conversion reaction (pp. 18–19) can sometimes present as accommodative insufficiency (Middleton et al., 2007).

Facility of Accommodation
Jump accommodation can be assessed using flippers, and this assesses the accommodative facility, or rate of change of accommodation (Fig. 2.6 and p. 145). This form of accommodative facility testing has been criticised because it is prone to a number of confounding variables (Kedzia, Pieczyrak, Tondel, & Maples, 1999), but the test may be useful for children who report difficulties changing focus in class between the board and a book, or pre-presbyopic adults with similar symptoms. First, refractive errors should be excluded. Typically, flippers with ± 2.00 lenses are used at 40 cm, and Zellers, Alpert, and Rouse (1984) found that the normal response for this test was 7.7 cycles per minute (cpm) with a standard deviation of 5 cpm. One cycle is a change from plus to minus and back to plus (i.e., two 'flips'). As 68% of a normal population lie within one standard deviation of the mean, patients whose accommodative facility is 2.5 cpm or less are in the bottom 16% of performance at this test. An early study assessed the reliability of this test using three measurements over 3 weeks (McKenzie, Kerr, Rouse, & DeLand, 1987). Most people who pass an arbitrary cut-off pass successive testing, but only one-third of participants who failed the first testing continued to

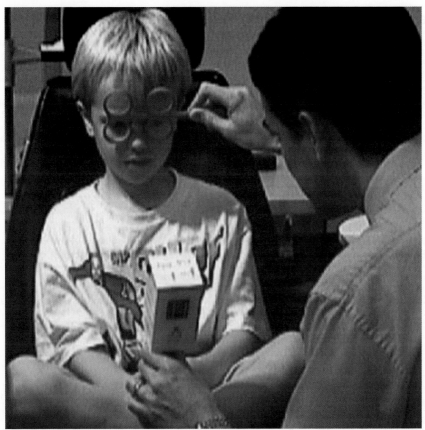

Fig. 2.6 'Flippers', as used to test or train accommodative or vergence facility. The patient is wearing polarised glasses and views the vertical fixation disparity target of the near Mallett unit to monitor for suppression.

fail on all three trials. This is likely to result from a regression to the mean effect (p. 13) and from the fact that accommodative facility testing exhibits a large practice effect (Horwood & Toor, 2014). Therefore, it is recommended that treatment is not started until a patient has demonstrated symptoms and an anomaly on at least two occasions.

Eperjesi (2000) recommended using the vertical OXO target on the near Mallett unit for this test, since it allows a check on suppression. Disappearance, but not movement, of a Nonius strip is significant: the flip lenses should only be 'flipped' when the patient reports that the OXO is clear and single and that both Nonius strips are present. Some patients struggle when they are asked to report on suppression, as well as the targets clearing.

Binocular vision problems are more likely to influence binocular than monocular accommodative facility, although there are many exceptions to this rule (Garcia, Cacho, Lara, & Megias, 2000). The test procedure for flippers is summarised in Table 2.9.

Accuracy of Accommodation

A useful test for assessing accommodative accuracy is MEM (monocular estimate method) retinoscopy (Cooper, 1987). The patient binocularly fixates a detailed target on the retinoscope and is asked to keep this clear. Retinoscopy is carried out along the horizontal meridian and lenses are very

TABLE 2.9 ■ Procedure for Testing Accommodative Facility With Flippers.

1. Usually, ±2.00 D lenses are used, although ±1.50 or ±1.00 can be used if the ±2.00 cannot be cleared.
2. Start with the plus lenses, explaining to the patient that the target may blur or double and they should report when the target becomes clear and single.
3. If possible, use a target that allows a control for suppression, such as the OXO target that is designed to test for vertical fixation disparity.
4. As soon as the target is described as clear and single with no suppression, flip the lenses to the pair of minus lenses. Ask the child to again report when the target is clear, single, and both strips are present.
5. Repeat 4, flipping to the plus lenses.
6. Continue, measuring how many cycles can be completed in 1 minute (cycles per minute; cpm). Note, one cycle is two flips.
7. The binocular test norms are that about 90% of the population perform better than 2 cpm and about 50% of the population perform better than 7 cpm. If there is an abnormal test result binocularly, the test can be repeated monocularly.
8. Only treat cases where there are symptoms and a repeatable finding of low facility.

TABLE 2.10 ■ Procedure for Measuring Accommodative Lag With MEM Retinoscopy.

1. The retinoscopy is carried out at the patient's usual reading distance.
2. The patient wears any refractive correction they usually use for reading.
3. The patient fixates a target on the retinoscope; no correction needs to be made for working distance.
4. The target is viewed binocularly.
5. Retinoscopy is usually only carried out in the horizontal meridian.
6. Typically, a 'with' movement is seen indicating that the accommodation lags behind the target (plus lenses need to be added). An 'against' movement suggests accommodative spasm.
7. Spherical lenses are introduced of a power that it is thought will neutralise the reflex. For a typical 'with' movement, the first lens might be +0.50.
8. The lens is introduced monocularly and is rapidly interposed: it should be present for no more than ½ second. This should be just long enough for a 'sweep' of the retinoscope to see if the reflex is now neutralised.
9. If the reflex is not neutralised, then steps 7–8 are repeated until the reflex is neutralised.
10. Steps 4–9 are then repeated for the other eye.
11. Norms for mean ±1 SD are plano to +0.75 D.

MEM, Monocular estimate method; SD, standard deviation.

briefly held in front of each eye to neutralise the retinoscope reflex. Each lens should only be present monocularly and for a split second so as not to disrupt the status of the patient's accommodation. The accommodative lag is usually about +0.50 D, values greater than +1.00 D may represent accommodative insufficiency (Appendix 9). If a negative lens is required to neutralise the reflex, this indicates accommodative spasm. This test is particularly useful when there is a low amplitude of accommodation, and with uncooperative patients.

A different approach (Nott retinoscopy) involves the fixation target being held in a constant position and the retinoscope being moved to and fro to obtain reversal. Typically, this reveals a slightly lower degree of accommodative lag (Cacho, Garcia-Munoz, Garcia-Bernbabeu, & Lopez, 1999), especially in those with high lags (Goss, Groppel, & Dominguez, 2005), although results of the two approaches are comparable (Locke & Somers, 1989; Goss et al., 2005). The interexaminer reliability 95% limits of agreement are ±0.17 D and ±0.31 for Nott and MEM, respectively.

Another test, the dynamic cross cylinder test, does not seem to provide an accurate measurement of the accommodative response to a near target in a young population (Benzoni, Collier, McHugh, Rosenfield, & Portello, 2009). MEM retinoscopy is most common, and the procedure is summarised in Table 2.10.

Accommodative Anomalies

Accommodative anomalies are variously classified into three, five, or six different categories (Darko-Takyi et al., 2016). The main types of anomaly are summarised here. For all these, a diagnosis can only be made if the condition is not explained by uncorrected refractive error.

1. *Accommodative paralysis*, characterised by the absence of accommodation (see also paralysis of the near triad, p. 124). This can occur spontaneously as an idiopathic condition in children or adults, typically returning to normal within 3—15 months (Almog, 2008). Cycloplegic refraction and reading glasses or bifocals are required. Referral to exclude pathology is a sensible precaution, although it is doubtful whether neuroimaging is indicated (Almog, 2008).

2. *Accommodative insufficiency*, in which there is a low amplitude of accommodation for the patient's age.

3. *Accommodative infacility (inert accommodation):* the accommodation responds only slowly to changes of fixation, and the patient reports that when looking from near to distance vision, or the other way, objects come into focus only after a short delay. This can also be an early sign of spasm of accommodation caused by excessive amounts of work at too close a working distance, often accompanied by uncorrected hypermetropia (convergence excess esophoria in Chapter 7). If patients only report that distance is slow to clear after near vision, this can be a sign of a myopic change in their refractive error.

4. *Accommodative fatigue (ill-sustained accommodation)* is indicated when a patient reports that accommodation cannot be sustained for long periods of near vision, but reports blurring after a short time. Some authors consider this to be a subclassification of accommodative insufficiency (Darko-Takyi et al., 2016).

5. *Accommodative spasm (accommodative excess)* can result in pseudomyopia. Case Study 2.1 is an unusually extreme example of this condition.

CASE STUDY 2.1

BACKGROUND

10-year-old girl referred to the author 2 years ago, who reported blurred vision. Family optometrist had carried out cycloplegic refraction and diagnosed pseudomyopia. Referred to ophthalmologist who diagnosed overactive ciliary muscle causing pseudomyopia, and prescribed course of cycloplegic agents. Problems persisted, mother noticed transient esotropia and consulted paediatric ophthalmologist who stopped cycloplegic agents and said psychogenic, after confirming that MRI and electrophysiological tests were normal, and discharged.

SYMPTOMS

Patient describes diplopia since the problem started 2 years ago, which she says is constant, horizontal, at all distances, but does not bother her as she has 'got used to it'. DV OK as sits at front in class. NV OK, if she holds text close. Infrequent (monthly) headaches which are mild. School progress OK. Parents mentioned patient has some bullying at school. General health good and no medication. Family history of corneal problem in father requiring grafts.

Clinical Findings

Normal: ocular health (biomicroscopy of corneas and topography normal), OCT, pupil reactions,NPC, ocular motility, Ishihara.

Spectacles:	R +1.75/−0.75 × 21	L +1.75/−0.50 × 158
Vision/VA:	Very variable, each eye varying from 6/12 to 6/48	
Retinoscopy:	R −4.75/−0.50 × 180 Both eyes result highly variable, sudden changes in reflex	L −2.25/−1.25 × 5

Subjective:	R −2.50/−0.25 × 150 6/15 −	L −2.75/−1.25 × 206/15−
	Both eyes result highly variable, sudden changes in Rx and VA	
Cover test (no Rx):	DV orthophoria	NV orthophoria
Cover test (with subjective findings):	DV 5Δ L SOT	NV 2Δ SOP Grade 1 recovery
Amp. Acc.:	Highly variable, 14 D monocularly at times	
Stereoacuity:	None recordable with Randot 2 shapes and circles	
Cyclo Retinoscopy:	R + 1.25/ − 0.25 × 20 6/7.5	L + 1.50/ − 0.25 × 175 6/7.5

Comment, Management, Follow-Up. During the examination there were clear signs of cyclospasm causing pseudomyopia. The patient was seen twice more and the findings similar. Vision therapy to improve accommodative function was described as beneficial by the patient but did not change the clinical findings. The cycloplegic Rx was prescribed and the patient reported this cured the diplopia and improved the vision, but clinical findings seemed little improved and the child still had to sit at the front in class to see the board and hold near text very close. With these adaptations, she and the teachers reported no difficulties, indicating that the cyclospasm was probably worse in the consulting room. The patient was clearly anxious about her father's visual problem, reports of bullying at school persisted, and behavioural difficulties at home were reported. The author referred the patient to a child psychologist at a children's hospital that also has ophthalmology services.

Amp. Acc, Accommodative amplitude; *D*, dioptre; *DV*, distance vision; *L*, left; *N*, near; *NPC*, near point of convergence; *NV*, near vision; *OCT*, optical coherence tomography; *R*, right; *SOP*, esophoria; *SOT*, esotropia; *VA*, visual acuity.

A comparison of vision therapy with convex lenses showed both interventions were associated with an improvement in reading (Brautaset et al., 2008). Eye exercises were associated with greater improvement in function, but also with high rates of discontinuation.

An RCT investigated reading additions as a treatment for accommodative insufficiency, comparing +1.00 with +2.00 additions (Wahlberg, Abdi, & Brautaset, 2010). Both additions improved symptoms, but only the +1.00 addition was associated with an improvement in accommodative amplitude.

An RCT showed that eye exercises can be effective at improving accommodative amplitude and facility in children with symptomatic convergence weakness exophoria and accommodative dysfunction (Scheiman et al., 2011).

Pupil Reflexes

Anomalies of pupil reflexes may help in the diagnosis of binocular difficulties due to neural disturbances. It is necessary therefore to check the pupil reflexes to light, and in near vision. The direct light reflex is checked by shining a light into one eye and observing the pupil constriction. At the same time, the consensual reflex is checked by observing the constriction of the pupil of the other eye. This is repeated by shining the light into the other eye. The near-vision pupil reflex is checked by asking the patient to look at a distant object and then at one about 25 cm from the eyes: the pupil constriction accompanying the accommodation and convergence is observed.

A 'swinging flashlight' test should be carried out to detect relative afferent pupillary defects (RAPD); this has been described as the single most important test in eye examination (Kosmorsky & Diskin, 1991). Each pupil is stimulated by a bright pen torch light which is swung to alternately illuminate each eye, pausing for just 1−2 s for an eye to equilibrate with the light stimulus (Bremner, 2000). If an eye has a RAPD then, when stimulated in this way, its pupil will dilate instead of constricting. This is because when the abnormal eye is stimulated the consensual reflex from the other eye will outweigh the direct response from the abnormal eye. The presence of a RAPD in the absence of gross ocular disease indicates a neurological lesion in the afferent visual system (Spalton, Hitchings, & Hunter, 1984). A cataract will not produce a RAPD, but a major retinal lesion or neurological lesion of the afferent visual pathway will. Dense amblyopia may also produce a RAPD.

When checking the pupil reflexes, abnormalities in size, irregularities in shape, or inequalities between the right and left pupils should be noted.

Sensory Investigation

STEREOACUITY

Stereoacuity tests (Fig. 3.3) can be classified in a number of ways (Chopin et al., 2019), typically as random dot and contoured, which are sometimes described as measuring **global** and **local** stereoacuity respectively (Saladin, 2005; Vancleef et al., 2017). It has been argued that constant strabismus is always associated with markedly reduced random dot stereoacuity, but not necessarily with greatly reduced contoured stereoacuity. However, one study suggests that patients who have fusion but lack stereoacuity, as may occur following patching in infancy, can do surprisingly well on random dot tests (Charman & Jennings, 1995).

Monocular cues have been shown to influence results in the following tests: Titmus circles (Cooper & Warshowsky, 1977), Titmus fly, animals, and circles (Leske & Holmes, 2004), Frisby (Cooper & Feldman, 1979), Random dot E (Cooper, 1979), and TNO (Cooper, 1979). The Lang II stereotest is not a reliable method of screening for strabismus or amblyopia (Ohlsson, Villarreal, Sjostrom, Abrahamsson, & Sjostrand, 2002). Indeed, a large study of 12−13-year-old children suggests that none of the commonly used stereotests (Titmus, Frisby, Lang 2, TNO, Randot) are suitable for screening for amblyopia or strabismus (Ohlsson et al., 2001). This view was supported by a study which found that performance on the Randot circles test improved by about one level at a second test and within subject variability is up to three levels on repeat testing (Adler, Scally, & Barrett, 2012). On tests free of monocular cues (defined as a pass on the Frisby test, better than 800″ on the preschool Randot test, or better than 140″ on the Titmus circles test), stereopsis is rare in strabismus where the horizontal deviation is more than 4Δ (Leske & Holmes, 2004).

Clinical stereotests do not fully describe patients' ability to use stereopsis in everyday life, where monocular cues may be integrated with binocular cues (Harwerth, Moeller, & Wensveen, 1998). Patients who perform poorly on clinical tests may still have stereoperception for dynamic (moving) scenes in real life (Rouse, Tittle, & Braunstein, 1989). Clinical stereotests suffer from a ceiling effect: the most difficult stimuli are easily attainable for most people (Heron, Dholakia, Collins, & McLaughlan, 1985). Nonetheless, stereotests can provide useful information when the results are considered together with those of other clinical tests.

The development of stereoacuity in young children is discussed in Chapter 3. Stereoacuity declines in advancing years owing to alterations in early stages of visual processing (Schneck, Haegerstrom-Portnoy, Lott, & Brabyn, 2000). Impaired stereoacuity is correlated with a history of falls in older people (Lord & Dayhew, 2001), indicating a need for binocular vision anomalies to be detected in this age group. Multifocal spectacles impair depth perception and edge-contrast sensitivity at critical distances for detecting obstacles in the environment and may contribute to the risk of falls when negotiating stairs and in unfamiliar settings outside the home (Lord, Dayhew, & Howland, 2002). Compared with other tests, the TNO test seems to underestimate stereoacuity (Vancleef et al., 2017), especially in older people (Garnham & Sloper, 2006). Tests that use random dots are more degraded by reduced monocular visual acuity than real depth tests, such as the Frisby test (Odell, Hatt, Leske, Adams, & Holmes, 2009).

As various stereoacuity tests produce different results (Vancleef et al., 2017), it is essential for the clinician to record the test used. Research with the TNO test shows a significant variation between different editions and so the edition should be recorded (van Doorn, Evans, Edgar, & Fortuin, 2014).

A little should be said about the scale of stereoacuity measurement, which is nonlinear. Typically, the measurement levels in a test involve a doubling at successive levels (e.g., in the TNO test, 15″, 30″, 60″, etc.). Each doubling is sometimes referred to as an octave step (Adams, Leske, Hatt, & Holmes, 2009). For researchers, stereoacuity results should be analysed after $\log_{10}$ transformation: each doubling of the stereoacuity threshold corresponds to an approximately 0.3 change of the log transformed value and a tenfold increase in the stereoacuity threshold (e.g., from 12″ to 120″ corresponds to a 1.0 change in the log stereoacuity value).

OTHER SENSORY INVESTIGATION

The Mallett foveal suppression (binocular status) test can sometimes detect a range of problems, including reduced visual acuity, foveal suppression in heterophoria, and strabismus. The test is described on pp. 83−84 and other suppression tests in the chapters on strabismus.

External and Ophthalmoscopic Examinations

During the early part of the examination, general observation of the patient can take place. With respect to binocular vision it is appropriate to notice:

1. Compensatory head postures that may be adopted in incomitant deviations or nystagmus (Chapters 17 and 18): a head-tilt, a rotation of the face to the left or right, or the face turned up or down.
2. Any obvious strabismus.
3. Exophthalmos: protrusion of one or both eyes.
4. Epicanthus: a fold of skin across the inner angle of the lids seen in some European children, and frequently in oriental races, which may give the appearance of a convergent strabismus; the cover test should confirm whether a strabismus is present.
5. Anatomical asymmetries, malformations, or signs of injury.
6. Ptosis or other anomalies of the lid openings. Patients may attempt to compensate for ptosis by using their frontalis muscle. This can be prevented by asking the patient to close their eyes when the practitioner presses against the frontal bone: pressure is maintained when the eyes are opened, and significant frontal muscle activity is thus weakened.
7. Scleral signs of previous strabismus operations, which may show as a scar or a local reddening.

It is essential that a fundus examination is carried out to discover any signs of active pathology, before proceeding to treat a functional deviation. An assessment of the visual fields is also advisable in patients who are old enough, as it will help to detect certain pathological abnormalities. Sensory fusion could be impaired by any pathology that degrades one eye's image (Fig. 1.1); for example, patients with cataract are more likely to develop exotropia, and heterophoric status is improved following cataract surgery (Spierer, Priel, & Sachs, 2005).

Retinoscopy and Subjective Refraction

In many binocular vision anomalies, correction of the refractive error is important in the treatment. In many heterophoria cases no other treatment is required, and in fully accommodative strabismus, refractive correction cures the strabismus. Exact and full determination of the refractive error is often essential. The function of the refractive correction in specific anomalies is described in later chapters, and it is not the function of this book to give details of different methods of refraction. However, it is emphasised that great care must be taken to ensure that each eye is given the correction that will provide a sharp retinal image. This correction should be balanced between the two eyes in the sense that it is equally clear without one eye accommodating more than the other. This can be done objectively by passing the retinoscope light quickly from one eye to the other to ensure that, at the conclusion of the retinoscopic examination, both eyes are neutralised simultaneously. In heterophoria where there is binocular fixation, this is best done by asking the patient to fixate the retinoscope once the monocular error has been neutralised with distance fixation (Barrett, 1945; Hodd, 1951). Balancing can be carried out subjectively by several methods (Rabbetts, 2007): Humphriss fogging, polarised duochrome, Turville infinity balance or septum, or by an equalizing technique using alternating occlusion.

In strabismus or amblyopia, retinoscopy is more important as an accurate subjective test may not be possible on the amblyopic eye. Extra care must be taken to ensure that refraction is on the visual axis. In divergent or larger angle convergent strabismus, the practitioner can move to align with the visual axis. The correct position can be judged by centring the reflection in the cornea of the retinoscope light. In the case of cycloplegic refraction, the patient can be asked to look at the retinoscope and the other eye occluded.

CYCLOPLEGIC REFRACTION

There is a broad range of opinion on when cycloplegic refraction is necessary (Doyle, McCullough, & Saunders, 2019). Noncycloplegic refraction is adequate for the diagnosis and determination of astigmatism in children aged 6–13 years (Doherty, Doyle, McCullough, & Saunders, 2019). Concerning hypermetropia, the same study found a cut-off with noncycloplegic refraction of +1.50 D or more detecting 87% of children (aged 6–13 years) with cycloplegic hypermetropia of +2.50 D or more (Doherty et al., 2019). These findings support the view that cycloplegic refraction is not necessary for all children consulting primary eyecare practitioners but as noncycloplegic refraction misses 13% of cases with significant hypermetropia, the indications for cycloplegia in Table 2.11 need to be applied.

It is important to ensure that all appropriate tests have been carried out before cycloplegic agent is instilled. For example, if a small/moderate degree of hypermetropia is found on 'dry' retinoscopy in a patient with an esodeviation, check how the cover test result changes with this prescription corrected before instilling cycloplegia. If this prescription does not correct the eso-deviation, try additional convex lenses. Such testing will not be useful once the ciliary muscle has been paralysed, and yet this information is crucial when it comes to prescribing.

Cyclopentolate is typically used for cycloplegic refraction, but tropicamide is adequate for most healthy, nonstrabismic infants (Twelker & Mutti, 2001). It has been suggested that children with neurological impairment could have seizures elicited by cyclopentolate (Coulter et al., 2014). Ideally, cycloplegic refractions should be carried out in the late afternoon so that the binocularly stressful period of increased AC/A ratio occurs while the child is asleep (Jennings, 1996). Additionally, photophobia caused by the cycloplegia will be less of a problem towards dusk. The child will need to be excused any homework.

Cycloplegia affords the opportunity of a dilated pupil and fundus examination should be timed to take advantage of this. If a parent has noticed any white in the pupillary reflex at any time, careful dilated fundoscopy is essential. If a good view of the fundus cannot be obtained, referral is a sensible precaution in view of the small but devastating risk of a retinoblastoma.

TABLE 2.11 ■ Indications for Cycloplegic Refraction.

Indication
Symptom of 'turning eye'
Other suspicious symptom (e.g., young child closing or covering one eye)
Family history suspicious for high hypermetropia
Esotropia
Significant esophoria
Apparent low accommodation
Reduced visual acuity
Abnormal stereoacuity
Unstable objective or subjective refraction (including from poor cooperation)
Large discrepancy between objective and subjective results
High hypermetropia for age
Significant anisometropia in young child
Spasm of the near triad or of accommodation alone

PRESCRIBING CRITERIA FOR REFRACTIVE ERROR (SEE ALSO PP. 47–48)

Hypermetropia in infants of 4 D or more is associated with increased risk of strabismus and worse acuity at age 4 years (Atkinson, Braddick, Nardini, & Anker, 2007). In this research, partial spectacle correction in infancy produced better outcomes and did not affect emmetropisation. The hypermetropic group showed poorer performance on visuoperceptual, cognitive, motor, and attention tests.

An association between mild or moderate hypermetropia and poor reading has been known for many years (Stewart-Brown, Haslum, & Butler, 1985). Other studies have linked hypermetropia to impaired literacy (Williams, Latif, Hannington, & Watkins, 2005) and hypermetropia and/or astigmatism to impaired visual-motor integration, which normalises following refractive correction (Roch-Levecq, Brody, Thomas, & Brown, 2008). In 4–5-year-old children, uncorrected hypermetropia of 4.00 D or more or hypermetropia between 3.00 D and 6.00 D associated with reduced binocular near visual acuity or reduced stereoacuity is associated with significantly worse performance on a test of early literacy (Kulp et al., 2016). In the same study, significant hypermetropia was associated with deficits of attention and, if the near acuity is reduced, with impaired visual-motor integration and visual perception (Kulp et al., 2017). However, correlations do not prove causality and as these studies did not control for potentially confounding variables (e.g., IQ), there could be a noncausal explanation.

Children aged 9–10 years demonstrated significantly improved speed of reading 4–6 months after full correction of hypermetropia compared with a group who had a partial correction and another group with no correction (van Rijn et al., 2014). There is a need for more randomised controlled trials, but when considering whether to prescribe for hypermetropia, it is appropriate to consider not just visual acuity but also accommodation, vergence, stereopsis, and education (Cotter, 2007).

Mutti notes that, on average, children experience an acuity benefit from the correction of hypermetropia from +2.00 to +3.00 D and higher and argues that as most emmetropisation occurs in the first year and hypermetropia is usually fairly stable after that, the visual benefit from correction should trump concern over interference with emmetropisation (Mutti, 2007). In contrast, one study found that full correction of hypermetropia may inhibit emmetropisation during early and late childhood (Yang, Choi, Kim, & Hwang, 2014). The degree of hypermetropia may be important when considering emmetropisation. Children around the age of 3–4 years whose hypermetropia is less than +3.00 are likely to experience a reduction in the hypermetropia over the next 6 years and outgrow the need for glasses, but those with hypermetropia over +5.00 will not experience a significant reduction in the refractive error (Mezer et al., 2015).

It is important to discover the full extent of anisometropia, usually with cycloplegic refraction. As the degree of anisometropia increases, then so the risk of amblyopia and impaired binocularity increases (Rutstein & Corliss, 1999).

In lower degrees of hypermetropia where the child is compensating well without correction, it is sometimes acceptable to monitor the child closely and not prescribe glasses, unless symptoms (e.g., intermittent esotropia, problems at school) or signs (e.g., decompensated esophoria, reduced acuity) develop. This strategy is only appropriate for straightforward compensated cases where the parents are observant, understand the risks, and are prepared to attend for very frequent examinations. As always, full clinical records need to be kept.

Leat (2011) reviewed prescribing criteria for refractive errors in infants and children, noting challenges owing to limitation in the evidence. Prescribing criteria, based on Leat (2011), are summarised in Table 2.12 and Appendix 2. Leat stressed that other factors need to be considered. For example, hypermetropia is fully corrected if necessary, to control an esotropia and symptoms and other test results (e.g., visual acuity, stereoacuity) will influence the decisions whether to prescribe and whether to fully correct. Of course, unusual refractive errors that do not meet the threshold for prescribing should be monitored. In producing these guidelines, Leat followed the principle in the preschool years of assisting emmetropisation (Hung, Crawford, & Smith, 1995) by partially correcting refractive errors unless other factors (e.g., strabismus, amblyopia) required full correction.

TABLE 2.12 ■ **Prescribing Criteria for Refractive Errors in Infants and Children.**

Refractive error	Age (years)	Criterion	Adjustment
Hypermetropia	1+	≥3.50 D in any meridian	Give partial Rx
	4+	≥2.50 D in any meridian	Reduce by 1 to 1.50 D
	School	≥1.50 D	Nearly fully correct
Astigmatism	1¼+	≥2.50 DC	Give partial Rx
	2+	≥2.00 DC	Give partial Rx
	4+	≥1.50 DC	Give full cylinder
Oblique astigmatism	School	≥0.75	Fully correct
	1+	≥1.00 DC	Correct ∼ ¾
Anisometropia	If amblyopia, correct the full level of anisometropia		
	1+	≥3.00	Reduce by 1.00 D aniso
	3½+	≥1.00 if hypermetropia	Fully correct the anisometropic element of Rx
		≥2.00 if myopia	
		≥1.50 if astigmatism	
Myopia	0–1	<−5.00	Undercorrect by 2.00 D
	1–walking	<−2.00	Undercorrect by 0.50 to 1.00
	4–school	<−1.00	Full correction
	School	any myopia	Full correction[a]

[a] Consider myopia control (p. 101).

DC, Dioptre cylinder; *Rx*, prescription.

Based on Leat, S.J. [2011]. To prescribe or not to prescribe? Guidelines for spectacle prescribing in infants and children. *Clinical and Experimental Optometry* **94**(6), 514–527.

Leat stressed that in hypermetropia this required close monitoring. The emmetropisation process appears to be deficient in strabismus (Ingram, Gill, & Lambert, 2000), so the full hypermetropic correction can be prescribed in these cases.

Measurement and Assessment of Deviation

In heterophoria, the first requirement is to assess if it is compensated when any appropriate correction is in place. If the heterophoria was not compensated before the refractive correction was found, but it is now better compensated, the correction is indicated as a part of the management of the heterophoria and in alleviating symptoms. Assessing the degree of compensation with and without the spectacles is discussed in Chapter 4. The assessment should be made for distance and/or for near vision, according to when decompensation occurs. The measurement of the degree of heterophoria and investigation of stereopsis may be required as part of the assessment (Chapters 3 and 4).

In strabismus, the angle of deviation is measured for distance and for near vision with the refractive correction in place, so that its effect on the angle can be determined. The measurement can be made with the cover test, as described above. In the case of long-standing strabismus, binocular sensory adaptations may have developed to alleviate diplopia and confusion. The extent and nature of these adaptations may need to be determined. Sensory adaptations and their investigation are covered in the chapters on strabismus, but a routine is summarised here.

1. Retinal correspondence can be investigated with Bagolini striate lenses or with a polarised test (e.g., the Mallett ARC and suppression in strabismus [MARCS] test). The depth of abnormal retinal correspondence can be assessed with a filter bar before the deviated eye until diplopia or suppression occurs.
2. Suppression can be investigated by the ease with which the patient gets diplopia, and the depth of suppression determined with a filter bar in front of the undeviated eye until diplopia occurs.
3. In esotropia, physiological diplopia may be elicited at a distance where the visual axes cross; this can indicate a good prognosis.

AC/A RATIO

The AC/A ratio is the amount of convergence which occurs reflexly in response to a change of accommodation of 1 D. It can be measured in several ways, but the usual method is the **gradient test**. The degree of heterophoria for near vision is measured using a dissociation test with an accommodative target (e.g., Maddox wing test), with any habitually worn refractive correction in place. It is then measured with binocular spherical lenses (e.g., +2.00) to change the accommodation. The change in convergence per dioptre of accommodation is assessed. For example, if the heterophoria measurement with the prescription is 6Δ esophoria, with an addition of +2.00 DS (dioptre sphere) changes to 4Δ exophoria, the vergence is changing by 5Δ per dioptre of accommodation, that is, an AC/A ratio of 5. The AC/A ratio may be different at distance and near (Rosenfield & Ciuffreda, 1991; Spiritus, 1994), but is little affected by the length of period of dissociation (Rosenfield, Rappon, & Carrel, 2000) or by previous adaptation to prisms (Rainey, 2000). The effect of age on the ratio (Tait, 1951) is slight, suggesting that the effort to produce a unit change in accommodation remains fairly constant with age (Ciuffreda, Rosenfield, & Chen, 1997). The 95% limits of repeatability are between ± 1 and ± 2, with the modified Thorington method giving the best repeatability (Escalante & Rosenfield, 2006).

Another method of measuring the AC/A ratio is the **heterophoria comparison method**, in which the distance heterophoria is compared with the near heterophoria. The total change in vergence angle from distance to near is divided by the dioptric change. The change in vergence needs to take into account the interpupillary distance and the heterophorias. The dioptric change, for example, is approximately 3 D from 6 m to 0.3 m. The formula is given in Appendix 10 (for derivation, see Jennings, 2001a).

The heterophoria comparison method usually gives a higher value of the AC/A ratio since the awareness of the proximity of the near target will increase the convergence at near (proximal convergence). In the gradient method there is no change in the proximal cue and this method is more relevant for predicting the effect of a refractive correction on the deviation at a given distance. The phoria method is confounded by changes in tonic vergence (Bobier & McRae, 1996) and does not correlate with the true (response; the gradient method when accommodation is measured objectively) AC/A ratio (Bhoola, Bruce, & Atchison, 1995). These authors found that the usual stimulus gradient AC/A ratio does correlate significantly with the response AC/A ratio, but the correlation is only modest. It was concluded that the clinical method is best considered as useful only in detecting very high and very low AC/A ratios.

The Dominant Eye

Eyecare practitioners often refer to 'the dominant eye', for example when prescribing spectacles or prisms. However, there are many different methods of assessing ocular dominance (Fig. 2.7) and, for most people, the eye that is dominant will vary depending on the task (Ehrenstein, Arnold-Schulz-Gahmen, & Jaschinski, 2005). For example, the eye with best acuity is not necessarily the same as the sighting dominant eye (Pointer, 2001). An exception to this is unilateral strabismus when the dominant eye will be the nonstrabismic eye, probably regardless of test.

With normal subjects, ocular dominance will even vary at different points in the visual field (Fahle, 1987). Not only does the dominant eye vary with task, but sensory dominance appears insignificant in most individuals with normal vision (Suttle et al., 2009).

The significance of Fig. 2.7 is that when practitioners consider the question 'which is the dominant eye', they should choose a test to assess ocular dominance that is relevant to the reason for asking the question. For example, if the practitioner wishes to prescribe a prism just in front of one eye (the 'nondominant' eye), the most appropriate test for determining which eye requires the prism is the test that is used to determine the prism (e.g., Mallett fixation disparity test). If a contact lens practitioner or surgeon is prescribing monovision, the best method to determine which eye is preferred for

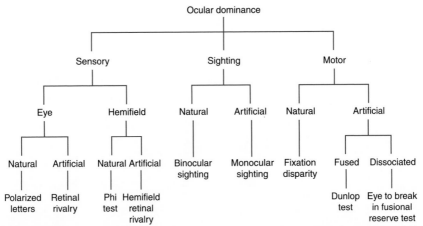

Fig. 2.7 Classification of tests of ocular dominance. (From Evans, B.J.W. [2001a]. *Dyslexia and Vision*. Wiley: London.)

distance is to simulate the monovision situation whilst the patient fixates in the distance and to see whether the patient is more comfortable and clear when the left or right eye is blurred with a near vision lens (Evans, 2007a).

CLINICAL KEY POINTS

■ For all patients with two eyes, a thorough eye examination must always include an assessment of binocular function

■ An assessment of binocular function is best carried out as a part of a complete eye examination. A careful assessment of ocular health and refractive status is an important part of the investigation of binocular vision anomalies

■ The act of measuring binocular coordination usually influences the binocular status

■ The orthoptic tests which best predict the binocular status during everyday visual function are those which most closely mimic everyday viewing conditions

■ The best time to explain a test is as you do it. The best time to explain a result is when you have finished all your tests and have the complete picture

CHAPTER 3

Examination of Young Children

Objectives

In examining the eyes and vision of preschool children, under the age of 4–5 years, the approach and method should be modified from the routine appropriate to older children and adults. It is likely that there will be much less cooperation on the part of the very young patient so clinicians need to use quick simple tests that can be applied for the short attention span. Precise measurements may not always be possible, and clinicians need to look for significant departures from normal.

A young child cannot give subjective symptoms and we rely on the observation and impressions of the parent. The family history will be very important. Children whose parents or siblings have strabismus or amblyopia are very much more likely to develop these conditions. Birth history is also important (e.g., prematurity, complications, birth weight).

This chapter is mainly concerned with the professional eyecare of young children, rather than with screening methods. No visual acuity test is likely to be adequate for screening by itself, even for refractive errors (O'Donoghue, Rudnicka, McClelland, Logan, & Saunders, 2012): binocular vision tests and ophthalmoscopy are essential for detecting a wide range of potential problems (Rydberg & Ericson, 1998). Regular eye examinations or vision screening throughout school life seems important as 70% of children who have significant ocular conditions go undetected by their parents or teachers (Rose, Younan, Morgan, & Mitchell, 2003). Screening methods for preschool children are discussed on p. 175.

Unfortunately, many areas of the UK do not have good preschool or school screening programmes and, in the absence of these, optometrists should seek to examine all children (from neonates onwards) at routine intervals. This may not be necessary if there is a local screening programme that is thorough, properly audited, and repeated at periodic intervals to detect developing problems. However, even the best screening programme may fail to detect some anomalies and children with risk factors (family history, birth factors, symptoms) should always receive professional eyecare.

Active Pathology

Anomalies of binocular vision in children, as in adults, may be a sign of active pathology. The first responsibility of the practitioner is to investigate this possibility. It is particularly important to check for incomitancy, note the palpebral openings, and carry out careful ophthalmoscopy. Where there is any doubt, the patient will need to be referred for medical investigation before proceeding. It must be remembered that there are methods of investigation which are available in some hospitals but are seldom possible in primary eyecare practices.

Development of Vision

To assess the eyes and the vision of infants, it is important to know how vision normally develops from birth through infancy and childhood. Normal vision requires a good optical system with a focused image and good resolution. Optical resolution has also to be matched with a neural receptor system capable of good resolution and a neural image processing ability leading to perception. The perceptive level itself is very dependent on previous visual and other sensory experience. Obviously, this sensory experience cannot be present at birth. As experience grows, reflexes are reinforced and associations between different sensory input and experiences are formed. For example, it is clear that very early in life an infant learns to recognise the mother's face and the meaning of different facial expressions. All visual functions are built as they are reinforced by experience acting on the anatomical and physiological systems which, although not complete at birth, mature early in life and allow the full potential of the visual system to develop.

The macular region of the retina is poorly developed at birth and both this and the visual cortex continue developing after birth. One would expect, therefore, that the spatial visual functions of neonates are significantly below the accepted norms for adults, and this is the case. It should be stressed that there is a wide variability in the development of visual functions and the figures given below are illustrative typical values from the literature. All aspects of visual development, normal and abnormal, have been reviewed (Fulton, Hansen, Moskowitz, & Mayer, 2013). In contrast to major spatial resolution deficits seen in young infants, temporal resolution (e.g., flicker detection) is remarkably good (Teller, 1990). Some theories account for this and other findings by considering the development of parallel pathways, including cortical and subcortical components (Teller, 1990).

Contrast sensitivity at birth is far below adult levels and it improves rapidly over the first 6 months, achieving adult levels at the age of 3 months for low spatial frequencies, but taking more than 8 years to reach adult levels at high spatial frequencies (Gwiazda, Bauer, Thorn, & Held, 1997). Faces are attractive to infants, and studies have shown that these are fixated at the age of 2 months but not at 1 month. Infants have some ability to discriminate between expressions at about 3 months and between faces at about 5 months.

VISUAL ACUITY

The rate at which visual acuity develops in human infants depends on how it is defined and how it is investigated. Using the objective assessment of the visually evoked potential (VEP), it appears that the infant's ability to resolve patterns improves from a level equivalent to about 6/38 at the age of 1 month to the equivalent of 6/15 at about the age of 6 months (Teller, 1990). Another method, physiological optokinetic nystagmus (OKN), is mediated via a different nervous pathway to normal visual acuity. OKN methods are not in common clinical use and will not be covered here.

The most common approach to assessing visual acuity in infants is based on 'preferential looking' when the practitioner observes whether the infant turns the head or eyes to look at a grating or picture rather than a grey patch of equal size and luminance. If no preference is shown for the grating, it is assumed that it cannot be resolved, although it should be noted that this approach assesses extrafoveal vision. This method indicates that visual acuity is approximately equivalent to 6/180 to 6/90 at age 1 month, 6/90 to 6/36 at 3 months, and 6/60 to 6/18 at 6 months (Appendix 2).

Obviously, a Snellen type acuity measurement cannot be made until the child is older even if specially designed tests are used which employ pictures (see pp. 50—52). These tests suggest that 6/6 acuity is not achieved until over the age of 3 years. All these Snellen type tests, however, involve an element of form perception. At the simplest, the child must be able to recognise the difference between shapes. Form perception is developed later than simple resolution, so Snellen type measurements assess a more advanced form of vision than preferential looking tests (p. 177). Kay pictures overestimate acuity (Anstice and Thompson, 2014) and other picture charts (e.g., Lea) are better for predicting letter charts (Anstice et al., 2017). Lea symbols are designed along the Bailey-Lovie LogMAR principles (Hyvarinen, Nasanen, & Laurinen, 1980), but still typically produce about one LogMAR line better than with Snellen (Laidlaw et al., 2003). Most children can complete a recognition acuity task by the age of 4 years (Anstice & Thompson, 2014). Monocular acuities are possible only in two-thirds of children aged 3—4 years and nearly all over 4 years (Salt, Sonksen, Wade, & Jayatunga, 1995).

TABLE 3.1 ■ **Various Estimates of the Development of Visual Acuity (VA) with Age. Approximate Snellen equivalents are given.**

Age (months)	Test	VA (Snellen equivalent)	Source
Newborn	Preferential looking	6/360 to 6/120	Stidwill (1998)
	Unspecified	6/240	Ansons & Davis (2001)
1	Preferential looking	6/180	Teller (1990)
	Preferential looking	6/360 to 6/90	Fulton et al. (2013)
3	Preferential looking	6/120 to 6/30	Fulton et al. (2013)
4	Preferential looking	6/50	Teller (1990)
	Preferential looking	6/120 to 6/30	Stidwill (1998)
6	Preferential looking	6/30	Teller (1990)
	Preferential looking	6/60 to 6/19	Fulton et al. (2013)
9	Preferential looking	6/46 to 6/12	Fulton et al. (2013)
12	Preferential looking	6/24	Teller (1990)
	Preferential looking	6/38 to 6/9	Fulton et al. (2013)
12–17	Cardiff cards preferential looking	6/48 to 6/12	Adoh & Woodhouse (1994)
18	Preferential looking	6/30 to 6/7.5	Fulton et al. (2013)
18–23	Cardiff cards preferential looking	6/24 to 6/7.5	Adoh & Woodhouse (1994)
24	Preferential looking	6/12 to 6/9	Teller (1990)
	Preferential looking	6/24 to 6/6	Fulton et al. (2013)
24–29	Cardiff cards preferential looking	6/15 to 6/7.5	Adoh & Woodhouse (1994)
30–36	Cardiff cards preferential looking	6/12 to 6/6	Adoh & Woodhouse (1994)
36	Preferential looking	6/6	Teller (1990)
	Preferential looking	6/12 to 6/5	Stidwill (1998)
	Single optotypes	6/6	Ansons & Davis (2001)
36–48	Single optotypes	6/6	Atkinson, Anker, and Evans (1988)
	Crowded optotypes (Cambridge cards)	6/12 to 6/9	Atkinson et al. (1988)
36–48	Crowded optotypes (Cambridge cards)	6/6	Atkinson et al. (1988)

The ranges given by Fulton et al. (2013) are the 95% limits.

With computerised letter charts, testing is much simpler with single optotypes surrounded by crowding bars, and this approach is necessary for some younger children. However, this method produces less pronounced crowding than linear tests (Anstice & Thompson, 2014), which should be used as soon as the child is able (p. 177). Some norms for various clinical visual acuity tests can be found in Table 3.1 and a guide for clinical use is given in Appendix 2.

REFRACTIVE ERROR

The refractive error during the first year of life is very variable in most infants. At birth it is approximately +2.00 DS (dioptre sphere) (standard deviation = 2.00 DS). Hypermetropic astigmatism is present in 29% and myopia in 23% (Cook & Glasscock, 1951). In many infants, high degrees of astigmatism are observed during the first year, but this is variable and usually disappears before the end of the first year. On average, hypermetropia decreases rapidly during the first year to a mean level of about +1.50 D at age 1 year, and then decreases slowly at the average rate of about 0.1 D per year, until the age of 10−12 years when the typical rate of change slows even more. Myopia over 5 D in children under the age of 10 years can be associated with systemic or ocular pathologies and it has been recommended that these cases are referred (Logan, Gilmartin, Marr, Stevenson, & Ainsworth, 2004), preferably to a paediatric ophthalmologist.

Nearly three-quarters of children with esotropia and/or amblyopia have a 'significant' refractive error (myopia, hypermetropia ≥ + 2.00 D, anisometropia ≥ 1.00 D, astigmatism ≥ 1.50 DC [dioptre cylinder]) and children with these refractive errors have a one in four chance of developing strabismus and/or amblyopia (Bishop, 1991). Hypermetropic children are at higher risk of developing accommodative esotropia if there is a positive family history of esotropia, subnormal random dot stereopsis, or hypermetropic anisometropia (Birch, Fawcett, Morale, Weakley, & Wheaton, 2005).

Leat (2011) reviewed prescribed criteria for infants and children and recommended the criteria reproduced in Table 2.12 and Appendix 2.

UNIOCULAR FIXATION

Normally, the peripheral retina is well-developed at birth, but the central five degrees of the retina is at best partially functional at birth. Hence, in the first few weeks of life precise foveal fixation is unlikely, but fixation of suitable targets may take place at nonfoveal retinal locations. The tendency to fixate new objects increases during the first 3 months of life. The fixation reflex requires reinforcement by active vision if it is to develop normally. If the system is faulty in some way, this may prevent normal development of central fixation and therefore normal acuity.

The fixation reflex does not become firmly established until later and if anything impedes it during the first 2−3 months of life, central fixation can easily be lost. This period of 2 or 3 months of rapid maturation is known as the critical period for fixation. In comparison, the critical period for acuity development is 2 or 3 years. The critical period is followed by a further interval during which the system can easily break down: the plastic period. Central fixation can still be lost up to the age of 3 years if anything disturbs the system.

Occasionally there are abnormalities in the foveal nervous system which are present from birth, but these account for only a very small number of eyes with fixation failure. Most loss of fixation arises from the lack of a central image in a strabismic eye or, occasionally, from a very blurred image. If either of these is present during the critical period there will be a failure of development of normal fixation and acuity and, unless treatment is given before the end of the plastic period, it is unlikely that central fixation can ever be achieved. The longer the strabismus or the blurred vision is left untreated, the less chance there is of ever achieving central fixation with full acuity. This emphasises the need for early detection and treatment. It has also been shown that if an eye is occluded for a significant period (e.g., ptosis or cataract) during the critical period, this impedes acuity development (deprivation amblyopia). If the occlusion occurs before the age of several months, central fixation will also be lost.

BLINKING REFLEX, VESTIBULO-OCULAR REFLEX, SACCADIC AND PURSUIT EYE MOVEMENTS

At birth, a blinking response to bright lights should be present (Mehta, 1999). The vestibulo-ocular reflex is present (in full term infants) by the seventh day (Mehta, 1999). Saccades are readily apparent in neonates but tend to be small and are relatively unresponsive to novel stimuli in the periphery. By the second week of life, small saccadic eye movements can reliably direct the line of sight towards a peripheral target and after the second month, large single saccades occur. Although this resembles the situation in adults, adult levels of saccadic accuracy are still being reached at 7 months of age (Harris, Jacobs, Shawkat, & Taylor, 1993). Compared with adults, saccadic latencies are prolonged in infants, preschool children, and possibly even older children.

Pursuit eye movements are present in neonates, but are brief, intermittent, and frequently interspersed with saccades. Parents and clinicians should be able to detect the behavioural sign of infants fixating and following targets of interest by the age of 2 months. The visual system becomes better at pursuing faster targets beyond the first 10—12 weeks. In infantile esotropia, there is usually crossed fixation so that fixation occurs with the right eye for objects in the left field and with the left eye for objects in the right of the field. Under these circumstances, the pursuit reflex may develop normally in each eye for half the field. In the other half, the eye may not follow correctly if the other eye is covered. This will give the appearance of a lateral rectus palsy. As the crossed fixation is a form of alternating strabismus, it usually allows the development of good acuity.

FUSION, VERGENCE, AND STEREOPSIS

Rudimentary binocular alignment without cosmetically noticeable strabismus is often present at birth, but true bifoveal fixation probably does not occur until the age of about 2—3 months. Occasional (<15% of the time) **neonatal misalignments** of the visual axes are common and usually innocuous in the first month of life but should become much less common in the second month (Horwood, 2003b). These are most often convergent, probably reflect the normal development of vergence control, and only require referral if they worsen after 2 months or if there is an intermittent deviation at 4 months (Horwood, 2003a).

Conjugate eye movements may or may not occur in neonates, although convergence may not occur for 2 months. One view (Schor, 1993) is that tonic, proximal, and accommodative vergence are present at birth, but fusional vergence develops later (at about 4 months), possibly in line with improved visual acuity. A clinical implication of this is that infants are unlikely to show a vergence response to horizontally orientated prisms until fusional vergence develops. One would expect the development of sensory fusion to be closely interlinked with motor fusion, and this appears to be the case. Several measures of cortical binocularity confirm that sensory fusion is, on average, first found at the age of 3—4 months (Birch, Shimojo, & Held, 1985). The ultimate goal of binocularity is stereoacuity and it is not surprising that research techniques have shown that stereoacuity is initially absent and then develops abruptly and rapidly from the age of about 3—4 months (Birch et al., 1985). Clinically, stereopsis is detected at different times using different tests and these are discussed later in this chapter.

Cortical cells require an input from both eyes if they are to become the 'binocularly driven' cells of the normal adult system. This must occur during the critical period. A strabismus or occlusion of one eye will prevent this bifoveal stimulation and, if not checked during the critical period for this function, binocular vision may never be possible as the binocularly driven cells will not develop but will become monocular cells. Nelson's (1988a) review on the 'risk of binocularity loss' concluded that 'relative plasticity' was at its maximum between the ages of 1 and 3 years. The plasticity then reduced rapidly at first (to 50% of its maximum at age 4 years) and then more gradually, to 20% of its maximum at age 6 and about 10% at age 8. Obviously, 'infantile esotropia syndrome' (Chapter 15) with its onset under the age of 6 months needs early referral. If such patients are not seen until they are over a year old, it is very unlikely that anything other than a cosmetic operation will help. Indeed, the prognosis for achieving binocular vision in infantile esotropia is never very good.

ACCOMMODATION

Accommodation is probably present from birth but is initially (until the age of about 3 months) inaccurate and principally operative over a short range (from about 20—75 cm). It is thought the main constraints on accommodative function in infants are attention and detection of the blur signal. Under ideal conditions of attention, accommodative function varies from one infant to another (Hainline, 2000), but is probably good enough to give them the acuity that their sensory system can resolve (Aslin, 1993).

Examination

During the examination, young children usually sit on the carer's knee, where they will feel more secure in otherwise strange surroundings. The parent or carer may be able to help in eliciting the child's attention when required, or in steadying the head. Give time for the patient to get used to the situation while you are taking the history and symptoms from the parent or carer. Try to relate to the child in a friendly way at appropriate moments before carrying out any 'tests'. Where possible, tests are presented as games to be played. A third adult in the room may be helpful for holding test cards and fixation targets for distance vision. Do not darken the room unless absolutely necessary, and then it is better to adjust the lighting slowly. It is sometimes advantageous to wear informal clothing, avoiding clinical white coats. Picture books may be useful and small attractive toys to hold attention for fixation are necessary, preferably ones that make a noise to give reinforcement. It is also useful to have toys in the reception area, and ideally a children's area with a small table and chairs as this helps children to feel at home from the beginning of their visit. For toddlers, it is useful to have a car booster seat to place on the consulting room chair.

METHODS AND EQUIPMENT

For preschool children, the practitioner must decide the minimum test results they need to obtain and the most direct way of gathering this information. It is important to be quick and to frequently change tests to maintain interest. If a strabismus is suspected, the priorities are to address the following questions:

1. Is binocular vision present?
2. Are there any signs of a strabismus?
3. Is the unaided vision the same in the two eyes?
4. Is the refractive error normal for the age?
5. Is the corrected acuity normal for the age?

It may not be possible to answer all these questions for every child. With others, much more can be done in addition. A lot will depend on the level of cooperation of the young patient. Patience and more than one visit may be required. The following procedures are typical of those that can be used in preschool children. The order of testing will depend on the child's cooperation and the practitioner's personal preference.

Vision and Visual Acuity

A variety of clinical tests allow the practitioner to measure uncorrected vision and visual acuity in children of any age, although monocular testing is particularly difficult at about 1–2 years (Shute, Candy, Westall, & Woodhouse, 1990). For infants, preferential looking cards are usually the best method of assessment (Fig. 3.1), and a single presentation is used when the looking behaviour is clear, with a maximum of three presentation when equivocal (McCulloch, 1998). Classic grating pattern preferential looking cards, such as the Keeler acuity cards or Lea gratings paddles, are required for infants below the age of about 6 months. After this age, children become bored with these tests (Teller, 1990) and, especially over the age of 1 year, children usually respond to the more interesting vanishing optotype cards (Cardiff Acuity Test; Adoh & Woodhouse, 1994). The Cardiff test is not good at detecting amblyopia (Geer & Westall, 1996), so crowded optotype tests should be used as soon as the child is capable. Like any visual acuity test, the Cardiff test will not detect all cases of refractive error (Howard & Firth, 2006).

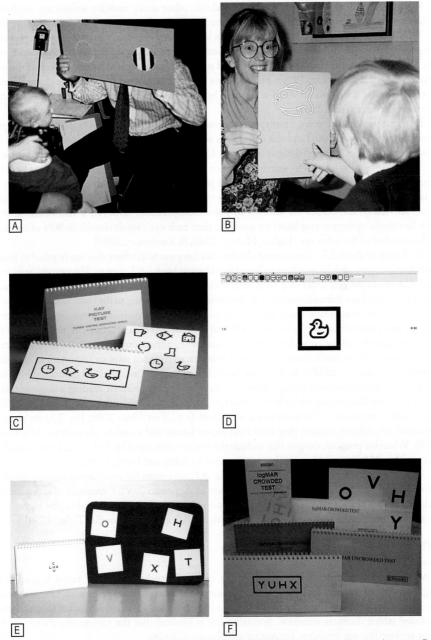

Fig. 3.1 Some visual acuity tests used with children. (A) Preferential looking grating test (courtesy Prof. Simon Barnard); (B) Cardiff acuity cards; (C) Kay Three Metre Crowded Book (courtesy Hazel Kay); (D) A Kay symbol presented in a crowding box on Test Chart 2000 (reproduced with permission from Thomson Software Solutions and Kay Pictures); (E) Cambridge crowding test; (F) Glasgow acuity card.

Where preferential looking tests are not available, other acuity tests for infants are to observe behaviour when one eye is covered, OKN, and the **fixation preference test**, also known as the 10Δ (or 12Δ) base down test. In this test, a 10Δ lens is introduced vertically in front of one eye whilst the patient fixates an accommodative target. Spontaneous alternation of fixation should occur, or if one eye is preferred, the nonpreferred eye should maintain fixation for at least 5 seconds if the preferred eye is covered (Mehta, 1999). This test does not accurately identify children with two lines or more interocular difference in visual acuity and better visual acuity tests should be used whenever possible (Friedman et al., 2008).

By about the age of 2 years, optotype tests should be possible with most children. Initially, pictorial optotypes may be used and the main types are Kay, Lea, and Patti Pics (similar to Lea). All these are available in crowded designs (see later). One approach is to give the child a near card with all the pictures and ask them to match a distance optotype with one on the near card. The other approach is to teach the child the names of the pictures, starting with large pictures. The key to obtaining cooperation is to give the child plenty of praise and make the process into an enjoyable game. Inevitably, test results are affected by patient cooperation; however, if monocular acuities with Lea single optotypes (see later) are possible, then each eye's result should, in 90% of cases, be within one line of the other eye (Becker, Hubsch, Graf, & Kaufmann, 2002).

By the age of about 2.5−3 years most children can carry out tests where they are required to match letter acuity targets with large reference letters in a chart or book held close to. Historically, tests were used that presented one letter at a time with no control of crowding. This is undesirable because uncrowded tests have reduced sensitivity at detecting amblyopia owing to the crowding phenomenon, or contour interaction. These terms describe the effect of adjacent contours at reducing target detection. Contour interaction occurs when an adjacent contour is placed at a distance equivalent to the width (or diameter) of the target letter and is maximal when adjacent contours are 0.4 letter diameters away. Contour interaction is most marked in strabismus, so crowded tests are important to maximise detection of strabismic amblyopia. Most paediatric letter charts are available in a crowded design and these should be used and isolated optotypes avoided. For younger children, reading a single optotype is a simpler task than coping with a line of optotypes, and a single letter with 'crowding bars' (Fig. 3.1) is a sensible compromise. Computerised acuity charts (e.g., Test Chart 2000; Fig. 3.1) are strongly advocated for children because they offer randomised letters and a variety of optotypes (Thomson, 2000). Wherever possible, designs that include the features advocated by Bailey and Lovie should be used and LogMAR scoring has much to recommend it (Bailey and Lovie, 1976).

Various visual acuity tests are illustrated in Fig. 3.1 and norms for visual acuity tests are given in Table 3.1 and summarised in the clinical worksheet in Appendix 2. VEP measures of acuity are not included as they are not generally used in primary eyecare practice, but they tend to give higher estimates than preferential looking, with acuities as high as 6/9 at 6 to 12 months (Teller, 1990).

Binocular Vision

Cover Test

A cover test is usually possible in most infants, if a sufficiently 'interesting' target is used (e.g., brightly coloured squeaky toy). As children become older more detailed targets, and more accurate results, can be obtained. The palm of the hand or thumb is used for occlusion rather than the usual 'occluder' which distracts attention. Sometimes, it is obvious that the patient objects to one eye being covered but not the other, suggesting a difference in acuity.

The most common deviation in young children, which usually presents in the first 6 months of life, is 'infantile esotropia syndrome' (Chapter 15). It usually has a large angle, over 40Δ, which is similar for distance and near fixation. There is often a higher degree of hypermetropia than normal for the age and the deviation may be partially accommodative. There is usually crossed alternating fixation, that is, the right eye tends to fixate objects in the left part of the visual field, and the left eye fixates in the right field. The change of fixation can be seen if the patient can be persuaded to follow a target moved across the horizontal. It seems that about half the patients have amblyopia with eccentric fixation (Dale, 1982). There may be latent nystagmus (Chapter 18), and sometimes dissociated vertical deviation (Chapter 9).

Congenital exotropia is rarer than congenital esotropia and is different in that congenital exotropia is typically present from birth. The angle is usually large and constant and may be associated with neurological abnormalities (Chapter 15).

Another infantile anomaly is 'nystagmus compensation (or blocking) syndrome' (von Noorden, 1976). In this condition, the convergent strabismus seems to be adopted in order to lessen nystagmoid movements which are reduced on convergence of the eyes. The patient's head is usually turned away from the side of the fixating eye to produce further convergence of this eye, and there may be the appearance of a lateral rectus palsy (Chapter 17). Neither of these conditions can be treated by refractive or orthoptic means alone, and a surgeon's opinion should be obtained as soon as possible.

Occasionally, with very young children a reliable cover test result cannot be obtained and other methods of assessing ocular alignment are required. Three such methods are described. It is stressed that these methods are much less accurate than a cover test and, whenever possible, the cover test should be used in preference.

Hirschberg's Method and Krimsky's Method

Hirschberg's method uses the position of the corneal reflection of a pen torch. Fig. 3.2A shows, for two deviations, how the reflection of a light in the cornea appears displaced from the centre of the pupil by 1 mm for each 20Δ (11 degrees) of deviation of the eye (various estimates range from 7 to 15 degrees; Spector, 1993; Pearson, 1994). Fig. 3.2B shows the appearance for a left divergent strabismus of about 20Δ. Fig. 3.2 assumes that the angle lambda (Glossary) is zero, and the reflex is central in the right undeviated eye. Angle lambda at birth is typically 13.75Δ, reducing to 9Δ by 5 years old (Pearson, 1994). The position of the reflex in the nonamblyopic eye (with the other eye covered) should be noted before the angle of strabismus is estimated binocularly by judging the difference in position of the reflex in the strabismic eye. In a right convergent strabismus with a large angle lambda, the reflexes would therefore appear in the same positions as those shown in Fig. 3.2B.

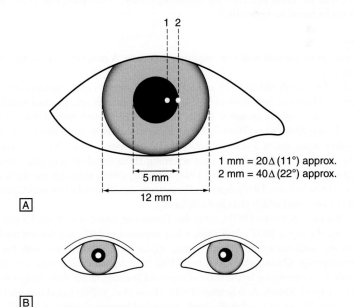

Fig. 3.2 **Hirschberg estimation method for the angle of strabismus.** See text for details.

Krimsky's method is a modification of Hirschberg's method where prisms are placed in front of the deviating eye until the prism power is found which makes the corneal reflexes appear to occupy the same relative positions (Krimsky, 1943). These methods are imprecise: deviations of up to 14Δ may be overlooked (Spector, 1993).

Bruckner's Test

The practitioner views both eyes through a direct ophthalmoscope at 75–100 cm. If the fundus reflexes are equally bright, this suggests that there is no strabismus. If they are not equally bright, there is either a strabismus (in the eye with the brighter reflex), pigmentary difference, unequal pupil size, or anisometropia (Griffin & Grisham, 1995). Von Noorden (1996) said that asymmetric fundus reflexes may be normal in infants up to the age of 10 months.

Motility

The presence of an incomitancy will increase the risk of pathology being present. It is usually possible to check for incomitancy by holding the child's head still and attracting the attention so that the eyes turn into the tertiary positions of gaze. With infants it is generally better not to hold the head but to move the motility target further than usual and allow the patient to move their head. Alternatively, the parent can rotate the child whose attention is held on a stationary fixation target.

Convergence and Motor Fusion

Convergence can be assessed by moving the target towards the nose after near cover testing.

Motor fusion can be assessed by testing for convergence when base out prisms are introduced monocularly. A convergent movement of the eye shows that binocular single vision, at least in the periphery (Kaban, Smith, Beldavs, Cadera, & Orton, 1995), is present; a versional movement suggests that the other eye is not fixating, and the prism should be tried before this eye. If no movement is seen, it suggests that binocular vision may be abnormal, or the child is inattentive. Most infants can overcome 20Δ base out by 6 months of age (Riddell, Horwood, Houston, & Turner, 1999). By the age of 4–5 years, it should be possible to measure full fusional reserves; the eyes should be observed to check the break and recovery points objectively. Some paediatric norms for fusional reserve tests can be found in Appendix 2.

Stereoacuity

Sensory fusion can be assessed with tests requiring stereopsis. A range of stereoacuity tests are illustrated in Fig. 3.3.

About half of 6-month-old children and 80% at 9–17 months give a positive response to the Lang Stereotest. However, only 65% of 9–11-month-old infants give positive responses to the Frisby Stereotest, although by the age of 2 years 100% of children with normal vision responded to the Frisby and Lang Stereotests (Westall, 1993). Successful stereoacuity testing is possible in virtually all children at the age of 3 years (Shute et al., 1990). Several studies have suggested that the Random Dot E test is particularly good for screening (Hammond & Schmidt, 1986; Ruttum, Bence, & Alcorn, 1986; Pacheco & Peris, 1994; Schmidt, 1994), although the method of use is important (Fricke & Siderov, 1997). Specifically, patients should be asked on which plate the 'E' is present, and not just asked which plate looks different.

Romano, Romano, & Puklin (1975), using the Titmus test, found that at age 3.5 years the lower limit of the normal range is 3000". At 5 years, it had improved to 140", and did not reach a normal adult value of 40" until the age of 9 years. Norms appear to be a little better with the Toegepast Natuurwetenschappelijk Onderzoek (TNO) test. With conventional clinical tests, the improvement from 18 months to 5.5 years may be the result of improved attention rather than changes in neurophysiology (Ciner, Schanel-Klitsch, & Scheiman, 1991). Heron et al. (1985) found that with the Frisby, Randot, TNO, and Titmus tests, adult-like levels are reached between the ages of 5 and 7 years.

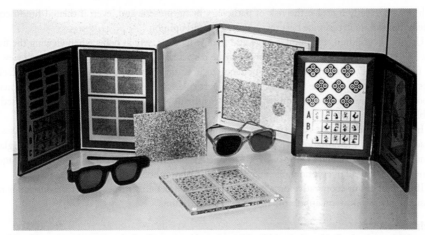

Fig. 3.3 Stereoscopic tests. In the foreground is a plate of the Frisby test and in the background, from left to right, the Randot, Lang, TNO, and Titmus tests (sometimes called the Wirt test, which was in fact a precursor of the Titmus circles test). *TNO,* Toegepast Natuurwetenschappelijk Onderzoek test.

In one study, the Lang stereotest detected every case of constant large angle strabismus, 90% of cases of microtropia, and 65% of cases of anisometropic amblyopia (Lang and Lang, 1988). The future of stereoacuity testing for young children (Ciner, Schanel-Klitsch, & Herzberg, 1996) or children with a learning disability (Ciner et al., 1991) may be preferential looking methods. Using a preferential looking technique, Schmidt (1994) found that the Random Dot E test was better for screening preschool children than a visual acuity stimulus. Preferential looking stereoacuity cards are not widely available at present, but show promise as a test for children in the first year of life (Calloway, Lloyd, & Henson, 2001).

The distinction between global (random dot) and contoured stereotests was discussed on p. 37. Some norms for stereotests for young children can be found in Appendix 2.

Ocular Health

As some strabismus in children under the age of 5 years may be due to pathology, it is very important to do everything possible to examine ocular health. For example, the palpebral openings should be noted: the two lid openings should be equal and symmetrical. Any inequality in a strabismic child may indicate a growth of extra tissue in the orbit, causing proptosis and abnormal eye movements. It could be caused, for example, by a dermoid cyst, sarcoma of the muscles, or glioma of the optic nerve. All these conditions require referral.

An attempt should be made to look at the media and fundus but, even if a full ophthalmoscopic examination is not possible, look at the colour of the fundus reflex. This may be done with an ophthalmoscope, or with a retinoscope moved around so that all areas of the fundus are checked: the retinoscope gives a narrow concentrated beam of light, and can be used from a greater distance, which may more readily be tolerated by the patient. White areas of the fundus can be a sign of retinoblastoma, and a strabismus may be the first sign of this condition (Abramson et al., 2003), which usually begins before the age of 4 years. A white reflex that the parent reports and the practitioner confirms, whatever the cause, requires urgent referral. Congenital cataract should be removed as early as possible, ideally within 6 weeks of birth (Birch & Stager, 1995). It is not uncommon for parents to obtain a white reflex in one eye in a photograph and for no pathology to be found. This may be because the child looks away from the camera and the flash image is focussed on the optic nerve head. However, even one such image indicates the need for careful dilated fundoscopy. Two such images greatly increase the risk of pathology being present and, even if dilated fundoscopy appears normal, such cases are best referred for a second opinion.

Usually, in children, the pupil is large and the media clear, which helps when viewing the fundus. Indirect ophthalmoscopic techniques may be particularly appropriate to get an overall view of the fundus quickly, and mydriasis may be required in some cases. Indirect ophthalmoscopy facilitates comparison of the size of the optic discs, particularly when a graticule is used. Optic nerve hypoplasia is a cause of poor vision which may be difficult to recognise and hence misdiagnosed as amblyopia (Chapter 13).

In infants where the eyes appear large, or there is the suspicion of asymmetry or of pale discs, it is useful to record the horizontal visible iris diameter. This is likely to be abnormal in infantile glaucoma and norms are given in Appendix 2. Other signs of infantile glaucoma include hazy, opaque, corneas and the triad of epiphora, blepharospasm, and photophobia.

If an infant is uncooperative on a particular day and a detailed inspection of the fundus is not possible, then a follow-on appointment can be arranged soon.

Refraction

With preschool children, a realistic goal may be to discover if there is any significant refractive error, rather than to measure the exact refraction. Refractive errors outside the normal ranges (Appendix 2) indicate a need for further investigation.

Lens racks are available for children who are too young to wear a trial frame. The most common method for refracting infants is to hold single trial lenses before the eye and this is reasonably effective. Refractor heads and phoropters are not appropriate for young children, but sometimes can be used from the age of about 4 years if introduced in a child-friendly way.

The refraction will need to be carried out objectively. Careful retinoscopy is important, and some practitioners prefer to work at a distance of half a metre for very young patients, with an appropriate working distance adjustment. An 'against' movement may indicate less hypermetropia or that the patient is accommodating. A cycloplegic refraction can follow at a second appointment. The corrected acuity can also be measured. During the cycloplegic examination, the patient can be encouraged to fixate the retinoscope light.

There is some debate over when to carry out a cycloplegic refraction. On one extreme, some authors recommend carrying out a cycloplegic refraction to determine the full refractive error as a matter of course in young patients; others argue that a cycloplegic refraction represents an abnormal state and is hardly ever appropriate in optometric practice. A sensible 'middle-ground' approach is not to perform a cycloplegic refraction on every child, but rather when a preliminary examination reveals one of the risk factors in Table 2.11. In infants a greater reliance will be placed on the objective signs in Table 2.11. Even when a cycloplegic refraction is performed, it is still important for the practitioner to know the noncycloplegic refraction, as this can influence the sensory status (Kirschen, 1999). Patients under the age of 3 months who need a cycloplegic refraction are best examined in the hospital environment because of the risk of systemic effects of the cycloplegic agent (Edgar & Barnard, 1996).

Some practitioners use Mohindra's technique of retinoscopy as an alternative to cycloplegic refraction (Mohindra & Molinari, 1979). This is carried out in darkness with one eye occluded and with the child fixating the retinoscope light. To take account of the patient's accommodation, for a working distance of 0.5 m an allowance of 0.75 D is subtracted from the result (Stafford & Morris, 1993).

A fairly reliable objective assessment of the refractive state can also be obtained by photorefraction. This term covers three different techniques which all involve the analysis of a photograph of the image of a flash source that has been refracted on entry and exit from the eye (Thompson, 1993). The sizes of the photographed light patches depend both on the defocus of the eye relative to the camera distance and on the pupil diameter so that a computerised system can calculate the refractive error from the reflex sizes. Photorefraction is claimed to be particularly useful for screening large numbers of infants, although it may lack sensitivity for detecting anisometropia (Fern, Manny, & Garza, 1998). Recently, an iPhone App using photorefraction has shown promising results at detecting the risk factors for amblyopia (Walker et al., 2020).

Management

First, the question of a referral for medical investigation should be considered, and this is essential if there is any doubt about the presence of pathology. It should also be recommended for significant binocular vision anomalies if the aetiology is unknown or the circumstances would not allow a reasonable prognosis to management by the optometrist. If the patient is going to require medical attention, the sooner the referral the better.

Preschool children are often too young to cooperate with any form of orthoptic exercises. Some can carry out simple exercises and a range of suitable exercises is described by Wick (1990). Refractive error should be corrected if possible, and amblyopia may need treatment by occlusion (Chapter 13). The importance of correcting significant hypermetropia to prevent amblyopia is discussed in Chapter 13.

Children with a parent (or other close relative) with amblyopia or strabismus are particularly at risk of amblyopia. It is therefore important that these children should be seen as early in life as possible, and that young adult patients with amblyopia should be advised that eye examinations are recommended for their children.

The general principles of strabismus management are described in Chapter 15.

CLINICAL KEY POINTS

- Precise results are usually not possible with young children and frequent appointments are often appropriate
- Visual acuity is readily assessed in young children by preferential looking and norms vary for different tests
- Refractive errors are very variable in the first year, but at the age of 1 year, more than 3 D of hypermetropia is a risk factor for strabismus
- Binocular functions, including stereoacuity, are usually present by the age of about 4 months
- Always attempt a cover test and motility test. Stereotests and the 20∆ base out prism tests are also useful

PART 2

Heterophoria

CHAPTER 4

Evaluation of Heterophoria

Introduction

A heterophoria only requires treatment if it is causing symptoms or impaired performance, if the binocular status is likely to deteriorate if it is not treated, or if the condition might in the future need treatment and would be more effectively treated now (Evans, 2010). A heterophoria that is causing symptoms or impaired performance or is breaking down to a strabismus is called a **decompensated heterophoria**. If it is decompensated, the evaluation should identify which factors have caused it to become so. In general, it is a heterophoria that has been fully compensated but becomes decompensated that gives rise to symptoms. After identifying the factors that cause the heterophoria to decompensate, the management consists of removing or relieving as many of them as possible.

Some heterophoria can be secondary to an active disease, pathological process, or recent injury. This type will be called 'pathological' heterophoria. It is usually incomitant. In some directions of gaze, it may even break down into a strabismus and double vision occurs. As already explained (Chapter 2), some parts of the routine eye examination are particularly important in the detection of pathological deviations, and these assume more significance in the total evaluation when pathology is suspected. These aspects are summarised in Table 15.1 and the detection of incomitant deviations is covered in Chapter 17. At this stage, the emphasis is on nonpathological heterophoria.

Factors Affecting Compensation

As most people have some degree of heterophoria, it is obviously important to decide which cases require treatment. That is to say, it is necessary to distinguish compensated from decompensated heterophoria. If the heterophoria is compensated, there is no need to evaluate it further. If it is decompensated, further evaluation is required to see which of the classifications describes the appearance presented, which may help to reveal the reason for the decompensation and the appropriate treatment.

The factors that influence whether a heterophoria is compensated can be broadly classified under three headings: the size of the heterophoria, sensory fusion, and motor fusion. These are illustrated schematically in Fig. 4.1, which is derived from Fig. 1.1. It is important to identify and remove as many as possible of the decompensating factors. The factors listed in the next section may contribute to heterophoria becoming decompensated, particularly if there is a marked change in them. In the list, factors 1 (a–d), 2, and 3 are motor factors and 1 (e) and 4 and 5 are sensory factors.

STRESS ON THE VISUAL SYSTEM

1. Excessive use of vision under adverse circumstances
   (a) Work held too close to the eyes for long periods. A comfortable working distance depends on the amplitude of accommodation, and therefore on the patient's age. As the amplitude decreases with age, stress on accommodation and convergence can occur if a proper working distance is not adopted. The near distance can also present stress in early presbyopia (Pickwell, Jenkins, & Yekta, 1987). Prolonged use of

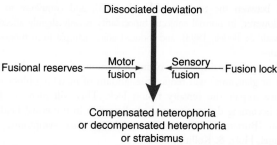

Fig. 4.1 Factors influencing whether a person can overcome a dissociated deviation to cause it to be a compensated heterophoria, or whether it becomes decompensated or breaks down to a strabismus.

computer display screen equipment, which is typically further out than the usual reading distance, can cause a deterioration in the near point of convergence and near point of accommodation (Gur, Ron, & Heicklenklein, 1994).

(b) A sudden increase in the amount of close work. This can occur with a change in the workplace, or students nearing examination time.

(c) Increased use of the pursuit reflexes: for example, playing or watching ball games, or reading when travelling.

(d) Tasks which dissociate accommodation and convergence. Several features of virtual reality displays can disrupt the normal relationship between convergence and accommodation (Wann, Rushton, & Mon-Williams, 1995) and cause stress on the visual system (Mon-Williams, Wann, & Rushton, 1993) associated with symptoms (Morse & Jiang, 1999). Similar effects can occur with 3-D displays, when symptoms occur in a minority of users (Fortuin et al., 2011) but are more likely in those with subtle binocular vision anomalies (Lambooij, Fortuin, Ijsselsteijn, Evans, & Heynderickx, 2010). One cause of this motor visual stress is inappropriate vertical gaze angle (Mon-Williams, Plooy, Burgess-Limerick, & Wann, 1998), but visually-induced motion sickness (VIMS) also contributes to symptoms with 3-D displays (Howarth, 2011).

(e) Inappropriate illumination or contrast (Pickwell, Yekta, & Jenkins, 1987). Visual conditions in the home or workplace are sometimes inappropriate, involving too little or too much illumination or contrast or glare. Night driving conditions may produce long periods of looking into a dark field with very reduced fusion stimulus at a time when the patient is fatigued. Reduced illumination does not influence the degree of heterophoria (Kromeier, Schmitt, Bach, & Kommerell, 2001), but presumably reduces sensory fusion and perhaps also fusional reserves.

2. *Accommodative anomalies.* Because of the relationship of accommodation and convergence, anomalies of accommodation can put stress on binocular vision. The additional accommodation required by an uncorrected hypermetrope to permit clear vision or the high accommodative effort in incipient presbyopia are examples of this. Both conditions may show decompensated phoria until the appropriate refractive correction is given.

3. *Imbalanced and/or low fusional reserves.* Where there is stress on binocular vision, the fusional reserves are often found to be imbalanced and/or low. It is not known if this is a cause of the stress or the result of it, but the fusional reserves of individuals are known to vary from time to time. This is related to Sheard's and Percival's criteria, described later.

4. *Refractive error.* Refractive errors, such as astigmatism and anisometropia (and sometimes myopia), can make fusion more difficult due to image blur (Irving & Robertson, 1996), particularly if it is unequal between the two eyes (Wood, 1983), and contribute to decompensation of the phoria. However, in normal subjects, binocularity is only slightly affected by blur, reduced contrast (Ukwade & Bedell, 1993), and induced anisometropia from monovision contact lenses (Evans, 2007a).

5. *Visual loss.* A visual impairment involving a portion of the visual field (e.g., in macular degeneration or glaucoma) will reduce the amount of matching binocular field from each eye and hence impair the sensory fusion lock. This will increase the likelihood of a heterophoria becoming decompensated. A distortion in the visual field can interfere with central fusion (Burian, 1939) and this might produce symptoms, including diplopia (Steffen, Krugel, Holz, & Kolling, 1996).

STRESS ON THE WELL-BEING OF THE PATIENT

1. *Poor general health.* A deterioration in the patient's health can result in decompensation of the phoria (Pickwell & Hampshire, 1984). This is particularly true if other decompensating factors are also present.

2. *Worry and anxiety.* It is helpful to know if there are major worries that may contribute to the binocular vision symptoms, even if the problems themselves are not visual. If the situation is temporary, as with a student's pre-examination stress, this may affect the type or the timing of treatment. For example, a student approaching examinations may be prescribed prismatic spectacles to temporarily correct an anomaly that might usually be treated in the first instance with exercises.

3. *Old age.* This can be important for decompensation of near phoria. Presbyopic patients can respond to eye exercises but frequently require 'top up' exercises (Wick, 1977). In some cases, prism relief may be required. Distance heterophoria varies little with age (Palomo, Puell, Sanchez-Ramos, & Villena, 2006).

4. *Emotional and temperamental problems.* Psychological difficulties and personality problems are difficult to assess during an eye examination, but they may be relevant factors. The treatment of psychological difficulties lies outside the scope of eyecare practitioners, although it may be necessary to take such difficulties into account. This is a useful reminder that we are not dealing just with eyes, but with people.

5. *Adverse effect of alcohol and pharmacological agents.* Alcohol decreases convergent and divergent fusional reserves (Watten & Lie, 1996). Alcohol and some prescribed and abused drugs can cause patients to become relatively esophoric at distance and exophoric at near (Rosenfield, 1997). Some drugs reduce the amplitude of accommodation and can therefore affect binocular vision indirectly.

6. *Traumatic brain injury (TBI).* TBI, even when mild, can be associated with diffuse axonal injury (DAI) resulting in abnormal vergence and accommodation, hyperphoria (Doble, Feinberg, Rosner, & Rosner, 2010), and other eye movement deficits (Thiagarajan, Ciuffreda, & Ludlam, 2011).

In deciding if heterophoria is compensated, the results of all parts of the eye examination need to be considered, but some sections or tests are particularly important. Sometimes the routine eye examination may also suggest that supplementary tests should be carried out to assist the evaluation. The following parts of the routine or supplementary tests are particularly useful in assessing heterophoria:

1. Symptoms
2. Cover test
3. Refraction
4. Measurement of the degree of heterophoria
5. Fusional reserves

6. Partial dissociation tests
7. Fixation disparity tests
8. Suppression tests
9. Stereoscopic tests
10. Binocular acuity

Diagnosis of Decompensated Heterophoria

Many optometric procedures, including the careful taking of symptoms, have been proposed as useful methods of diagnosing whether a heterophoria is decompensated. These will now be discussed and, at the end of this chapter, and of the next chapter, conclusions will be drawn about which tests are the most useful.

SYMPTOMS

Symptoms are usually present in decompensated heterophoria (McKeon, Wick, Aday, & Begley, 1997). Less commonly, suppression develops to such an extent that symptoms are avoided. There is no set of symptoms that is pathognomic of heterophoria, and the symptoms that are sometimes associated with decompensated heterophoria can also be caused by other problems. It can, however, be said that in the absence of symptoms and of suppression, any heterophoria is compensated, at least at that point in time. When symptoms are present, the practitioner must decide if these are due to the heterophoria or to some other cause. It is only by considering the symptoms together with the other findings that the total picture enables the diagnosis of decompensated heterophoria. In general, symptoms from decompensated heterophoria are associated with some particular use of the eyes for prolonged periods, and these symptoms are lessened or alleviated by resting the eyes. It follows that, in general, the symptoms will be less in the morning and increase during the day. In heterophoria, they are more frequently associated with near visual tasks.

Decompensated heterophoria can give rise to the symptoms detailed here, which are summarised in Table 4.1. The symptoms can be broadly classified into three categories: visual perceptual distortions (numbered in Table 4.1 and below as 1−3), binocular factors (4−6), and asthenopia (7−10).

1. *Blurred vision.* Uncorrected refractive error may put stress on the accommodation−convergence relationship, which results in decompensated heterophoria. Conversely, in other

TABLE 4.1 ■ Summary of Symptoms of Decompensated Heterophoria.

Symptom	Generic description
1. Blurred vision 2. Diplopia 3. Distorted vision	Visual perceptual symptoms
4. Difficulty with stereopsis 5. Monocular comfort 6. Difficulty changing focus	Binocular symptoms
7. Headache 8. Aching eyes 9. Sore eyes	Asthenopic symptoms
10. General irritation	Referred symptom

cases, where there is no refractive error, high degrees of phoria can influence accommodation resulting in blurred vision. Some patients interpret small amounts of diplopia as blur.

2. *Diplopia.* In heterophoria, any diplopia is intermittent and is worse after prolonged use of the eyes, particularly for concentrated tasks. The diplopia that accompanies a pathological deviation is usually more sudden in onset and is less often associated with any particular use of the eyes for lengthy periods.

3. *Distorted vision.* In some cases of decompensated heterophoria (and in binocular instability, discussed in the next chapter), the precise binocular alignment may be variable. This can be seen during the fixation disparity test: even if the patient does not experience diplopia, there may be a transient fixation disparity with the visual axes showing a variable misalignment of several minutes of arc. This may cause the patient to perceive visual perceptual distortions (Gibson, 1947), such as letters or words moving, flickering, or jumping. They may see shapes or patterns on the page and may skip or omit words or lines. This condition needs to be differentially diagnosed from sensory visual stress (Meares-Irlen Syndrome; see next section).

4. *Stereopsis problems.* Occasionally there are difficulties in depth perception reported by the patient; e.g., in ball games, pouring liquids into receptacles.

5. *Monocular comfort.* A patient may notice that vision is more comfortable if one eye is closed or covered. This can be due to photophobia, but also seems to be associated with heterophoria problems, especially divergence excess (Chapter 8). Patients, especially children, may adopt an abnormal head posture when they are reading (e.g., lay their head on the page) so that their nose is acting as an occluder to give monocular vision.

6. *Difficulty changing focus.* Patients may report that distance vision is blurred immediately following prolonged periods of close work. This can also be a sign of a myopic shift.

7. *Headache.* Rabbetts (2007) stated that horizontal heterophorias tend to give frontal headaches. These frontal headaches are said to occur, in exophoria, during concentrated vision but, in esophoria, at other times, possibly the day after concentrated work. A survey found that the commonest symptom in children consulting an optometric clinic was headache (8%) and for a quarter of these cases the headache was commonly associated with study or reading (Barnard & Edgar, 1996). One study suggests that 10% of an unselected university student population report headaches associated with studying (Porcar & Martinez-Palomera, 1997).

8. *Aching eyes.* The patient says that the eyes hurt after intensive use of the eyes for demanding visual tasks at the relevant distance. In heterophoria, this is usually a dull pain, and is therefore described by the patient as an ache, sometimes saying that the eyes 'feel tired'.

9. *Sore eyes.* The patient may describe a feeling of soreness.

10. *General irritation.* The difficulty in maintaining comfortable single vision may result in the patient reporting a feeling of irritability or of nervous exhaustion.

Sensory Visual Stress

Sensory visual stress was previously called 'scotopic sensitivity syndrome' or Meares-Irlen syndrome (Evans, 2001a) and is also known as **pattern-related visual stress** or **visual stress**. Visual stress is also used to describe visually stressful conditions relating to binocular vision anomalies (Yekta, Pickwell, & Jenkins, 1989; Wilmer & Buchanan, 2009), which is more motor in origin. Therefore, the word sensory may be more appropriate when describing the form of visual stress described here.

Sensory visual stress is controversial, but some evidence indicates it is a visual processing anomaly associated with a hyperexcitability of the visual cortex. The condition appears to be prevalent in people with autism (Ludlow, Wilkins, & Heaton, 2008), and affects approximately 20% of people with dyslexia (Evans & Allen, 2016) and some individuals with migraine (Wilkins, Patel, Adjamian, & Evans, 2002) and epilepsy (Wilkins et al., 1999). Sensory visual stress is alleviated with individually prescribed coloured filters and the hue and saturation of the required tint seems to vary from one sufferer to another and sometimes needs to be highly specific (Wilkins et al., 1994). It is believed tinted lenses redistribute the excitation in the cortex so as to avoid local regions that are hyperexcitable (Wilkins, 2018). Diagnostic criteria have been suggested following a Delphi study (Evans, Allen, & Wilkins, 2017). The condition is characterised by reports of asthenopia and visual perceptual distortions: sufferers typically perceive words appearing to move, shimmer, or blur and report similar effects from mid-spatial frequency striped patterns (Evans & Stevenson, 2008).

In a small minority (Monger, Wilkins, & Allen, 2015) of cases of sensory visual stress (Case Study 4.1), the situation is further complicated by a heterophoria that may be decompensating (Evans, 2005b), or by binocular instability (Chapter 5) (Evans, Wilkins et al., 1996). This can make the differential diagnosis difficult, as it may not be clear whether the unstable visual perception from sensory visual stress is causing the binocular vision anomaly, or whether the binocular vision anomaly is a primary cause of the symptoms. The diagnostic criteria outlined in the next chapter can be helpful in these cases and significant optometric anomalies are corrected before colour is used (Evans, 2018a, 2018b). This is important because accommodative (Drew, Borsting, Stark, & Chase, 2012) or binocular (Evans & Allen, 2016) anomalies could explain some reports of a benefit from coloured filters owing to effects on longitudinal chromatic aberration.

In some cases, symptoms may only be completely alleviated by correction of any ocular motor anomaly in addition to coloured filters (Evans, 2001a). Indeed, it is interesting to note that in some of the most thorough studies of vision therapy for decompensated convergence weakness exophoria, 58% of adults (Scheiman, Mitchell, Cotter, Kulp et al., 2005) and 56% of children (CITT, 2008) were still symptomatic after 12 weeks of intensive vision therapy. A factor analysis of the symptoms of visual discomfort concluded that symptoms may be attributable in some cases to sensory visual stress and in others to binocular vision anomalies or refractive errors (Borsting, Chase, & Ridder, 2007). It seems likely that the best approach to alleviating symptoms that may be attributable to ocular motor anomalies or sensory visual stress is an holistic approach, in which all potential causes of the symptoms are detected (Evans, 2018a). A flow chart for the investigation of visual factors for people with (suspected) dyslexia is given in Appendix 4.

CASE STUDY 4.1

BACKGROUND
Boy, aged 8, with specific learning difficulties.

SYMPTOMS
After reading for 20 mins: words 'jump around on the page', trouble following the line, and eyestrain. Skips or omits words or lines and light sensitive. No headaches.

Clinical Findings
Normal: ocular health, visual acuities, refractive error (low hypermetropia), accommodative function. Large decompensated exophoria at near.

Management
Given eye exercises for convergent fusional reserves.

Follow-up 2 Months Later. Exercises done but make eyes hurt and symptoms unchanged. Ocular motor status improved and exophoria now compensated. Tested with coloured overlays and showed consistent response, so issued coloured overlay and significant improvement in reading speed.

Follow-up 3 Months Later, Returned for Testing with Intuitive Colorimeter. Overlay definitely helps: less 'hurting eyes' and less movement of text. Consistent response to testing with Intuitive Colorimeter and Precision Tints. Precision Tints prescribed.

Follow-up 9 Months Later. Precision Tints used voluntarily for reading, writing, etc. No symptoms when wearing tinted glasses; symptoms without glasses unchanged. Refraction, ocular motor tests, ocular health, and visual fields all normal. Colorimeter checked and new tint prescription found which further improved perception. This was prescribed.

Follow-up 24 Months Later. No symptoms when wearing tints. Reading and spelling greatly improved. Refraction, ocular motor tests, ocular health, visual fields all normal. Colorimetry checked and no change to tint required. Advised yearly checks.

Comment. In this case, correction of the ocular motor problem had no effect on symptoms, which seem to originate from sensory visual stress. The tint initially changed, but then stabilised.

Migraine

Nearly 8% of the population suffer from migraine (Bates, Blau, & Campbell, 1993) and a literature review (Harle &Evans, 2004) found claims that migraine can be triggered by low convergent fusional reserves, decompensated near exophoria, and hyperphoria. However, this review noted that the scientific evidence supporting these claims is weak. A study found that people with migraine have a slightly higher than usual prevalence of heterophoria, aligning prism, and impaired stereoacuity (Harle & Evans, 2006). This research indicates decompensated heterophoria is unlikely to be a cause of migraine in all but exceptional cases. Although correcting decompensated heterophoria did not decrease the prevalence of migraine, it was found to decrease symptoms of pain and need for analgesia in some patients with migraine (Harle, 2007). Common sense advice is for practitioners to ask patients about any association between migraine, or other headaches, and visual tasks. It often helps if patients keep a diary of their headaches, including activities before the headache starts, and the diary in Appendix 11 can be issued to patients for this purpose. If specific visual tasks trigger headaches, including migraine, attention should be paid to the refractive and binocular status at the relevant test distance(s).

It has been claimed that a device, SightSync, is effective for prescribing prismatic corrections as a treatment for chronic daily headache, or 'migraine' (Miles, Krall, Thompson, & Colvard, 2015). These authors only presented a single group observational study and it is therefore unclear whether this intervention is more than a placebo.

A double-masked placebo-controlled trial revealed that some patients with migraine experience a visual trigger in the form of lights or patterned stimuli (including lines of text) and that this trigger can be treated with individually prescribed coloured filters, in a condition related to the sensory visual stress described earlier (Wilkins et al., 2002). This subgroup of migraine patients are more prone to binocular vision anomalies (Evans, Patel, & Wilkins, 2002) and can be identified with the headache diary in Appendix 11.

COVER TEST

The method of performing the cover test is described in Chapter 2. Here, we are concerned with evaluating the results. In heterophoria, three things should be noted during the cover test:

1. *Direction of phoria.* The direction of the recovery movement will indicate how the eye was deviated under the cover before its removal, and hence the type of phoria. For distance fixation, most patients show little or no movement. For near fixation, the average patient becomes gradually more exophoric from the mid-twenties and has about 6Δ of **physiological exophoria** by the age of 65 years (Freier & Pickwell, 1983). Obvious departures from this usual state may be decompensated, depending on other factors.

2. *Magnitude of phoria.* The larger the amount of heterophoria present, the more likely it is to be decompensated. However, quite small departures from the normal degree are sometimes decompensated, and sometimes high degrees are compensated.
3. *Quality of recovery.* The speed and ease of recovery are a good guide to the degree of compensation. A quick, smooth recovery is likely to indicate compensated heterophoria, whereas a slow, hesitant or jerking recovery movement usually accompanies decompensation. A schema for grading the quality of cover test recovery movements in heterophoria is given in Table 2.4.

It will be seen that all three of the aforementioned aspects of the recovery movement to the cover test need to be considered in deciding if the heterophoria is compensated.

REFRACTION AND VISUAL ACUITY

Because of the accommodation—convergence relationship, there is an association between esophoria and uncorrected hypermetropia in young patients. When the patient can accommodate to compensate for hypermetropia and thereby achieve clear vision, the extra accommodation brought into play will induce increased convergence. Usually this will show as esophoria and there will be an unusual stress on binocular vision, sometimes resulting in decompensation. This will be exaggerated in near vision when the amount of accommodation required may be a large proportion of the patient's total amplitude. In such cases, the degree of heterophoria is usually less with the refractive correction, and the clinical signs of decompensation will be less apparent. In hypermetropic cases with exophoria, the correction may make the decompensation worse. This is not always the case: in some patients with low uncorrected hypermetropia, correction of the refractive error may sharpen the retinal image which, through aiding sensory fusion, improves the ability to compensate for an exophoria (Fig. 4.1).

In myopia, if exophoria is present, the refractive correction usually assists the compensation. Sometimes the first sign of a refractive change towards myopia is decompensation of an exophoria, often at near. Myopia onset can be associated with a near esophoria and that is discussed in the next section, on myopia development.

The effect of the refractive correction on the heterophoria should always be considered. Correction of refractive errors may reduce blur and so improve sensory fusion (Carter, 1963), even if these refractive errors are relatively small, such as low astigmatism.

Although there are methods of binocular refraction which do not require the use of an occluder, such as the Humphriss immediate contrast method (Humphriss & Woodruff, 1962), many refractive methods occlude each eye in turn. When both the monocular refractions have been completed, the occluder is removed and the eyes are free to resume binocular vision. In compensated heterophoria, this is done promptly, and the binocular acuity is found to be slightly better than the best monocular acuity (Jenkins, Abd-Manan, Pardhan, & Murgatroyd, 1994). The patient will usually report a slight subjective improvement. However, in decompensated heterophoria, the increase in binocular acuity over monocular is less than usual, unless an appropriate prism is prescribed. This effect occurs at distance (Jenkins et al., 1994) and near (Jenkins, Abd-Manan, & Pardhan, 1995).

The removal of the occluder may therefore be regarded as an important part of the assessment of compensation. The patient is asked to look at the best line of Snellen letters which was seen monocularly, the occluder is removed, and the patient is asked if the line is better or worse. In most cases, it will be better, and the binocular acuity can be recorded. Where there are binocular vision problems, the patient may report that the appearance is not quite so good or may hesitate and blink a few times before comfortable binocular vision is restored. In some cases, diplopia may be reported, and the patient may have to make a convergent movement to look at a near object before binocular vision can be obtained. These reactions are subjective correlates of the objective observation of poor recovery during the cover test and suggest decompensated heterophoria. Where binocular difficulties are suggested at this stage, particular attention to this aspect is indicated in the rest of the eye examination.

Myopia Development

Some research has found myopia onset to be associated with increased accommodative lag and one hypothesis is that increased accommodative lag leads to hyperopic defocus resulting in axial length growth (Wildsoet et al., 2019). An interesting finding is that the increased accommodative lag is associated with, and preceded by, an increased AC/A ratio (Mutti et al., 2017). The increased AC/A ratio starts to occur 4 years before the onset of myopia. Mutti and colleagues hypothesised that compromised accommodation requires an increased effort needed per dioptre of accommodative output, which could also explain the finding of increased prevalence of esophoria in children who become myopic (Mutti et al., 2017).

When the onset of myopia is associated with a near esophoria, there is some evidence that myopia progression can be slowed by multifocals and this is discussed further in Chapter 6.

MEASUREMENT OF THE DISSOCIATED HETEROPHORIA

Indications for Measuring the Dissociated Heterophoria

It has long been recognised that dissociation test results do not relate to symptoms (Percival, 1928), except for the case of cyclo vertical heterophoria. Vertical heterophoria, if consistently 1Δ or more, often requires correction (Sheard, 1931). High degrees of heterophoria can be compensated and low degrees decompensated (Yekta, Jenkins, & Pickwell, 1987). As early as 1954, Marton suggested that the size of prism to eliminate a fixation disparity might be more closely related to symptoms than the dissociated heterophoria (Yekta et al., 1987). Tests which use this fixation disparity principle are described later in this chapter and are better uses of clinical time than dissociation tests. However, dissociation tests are sometimes useful to monitor changes in the magnitude of a heterophoria over time. They are also valuable for detecting cyclovertical deviations which are difficult to see on cover testing.

In accommodative esophoria, a hypermetropic correction reduces the magnitude of the esophoria. Measurement in these cases may give an indication of the likely effect of wearing the glasses. If the heterophoria is reduced by the glasses, it is likely that it will become compensated by wearing the glasses without any other treatment. However, other tests for compensation (e.g., Mallett unit) may give similar indications.

One occasion when it may be useful to carry out a dissociation test is to quantify the relationship between the dissociated heterophoria and the opposing fusional reserves (see later). One limitation of dissociation tests is that, with a large slightly paretic heterophoria, the eye may make a secondary movement of elevation in abducting or adducting. This is not likely to be a problem with a fixation disparity test.

Methods of Assessing the Dissociated Heterophoria

Dissociation tests may be carried out at 6 m and at the reading distance and several methods are available. The Maddox rod (multiple groove) consists of a series of very-high-power cylindrical elements which blur a spot of light into a streak. When placed before one eye, the Maddox rod produces this streak, which cannot be fused with the spot seen with the other eye at the same time. The eyes are therefore dissociated and take up the heterophoria position. The amount of the deviation can be noted by the patient subjectively as the separation of the spot and streak judged by a tangent scale (Thorington test), or by the power of prism required to restore the streak to the central position where it appears to pass through the spot. Clear Maddox rods may be preferable to coloured ones, which might influence accommodation.

In another technique (von Graefe's), dissociation is achieved by using a prism that is too large to be fused whose axis is orthogonal to the direction of phoria which is to be measured. For example, to measure the horizontal phoria, a 10Δ base up or down would be placed before one eye which would cause the object of regard to become vertically diplopic. Horizontal prisms would then be introduced and varied until the two diplopic images were vertically aligned: the magnitude of the horizontal prism to achieve this would equal the horizontal phoria. The Howell phoria card is a tangent scale to be used with a vertical prism in a variation of the von Graefe method (Wong, Fricke, & Dinardo, 2002).

For near vision, the same sorts of method may be used, or the phoria measurement made with a Maddox wing test. This employs septa to dissociate one part of the field from that seen by the other eye. The measurement is read by the patient where an arrow seen by one eye points to a tangent scale seen by the other. A disadvantage of the Maddox wing test is the fixed distance the test uses. More stable results are obtained if a smaller than usual print size is used (Pointer, 2005).

When the heterophoria is measured it is not just the degree of phoria that needs to be assessed, but also the stability of the phoria should be noted (Chapter 5). For example, in the Maddox wing test the amplitude of movement can be recorded in addition to the median position of the arrow (e.g., recorded as 4Δ XOP $\pm$ 2Δ).

Most subjective methods of measuring heterophoria have limitations which make them unreliable on some patients. The degree and duration of dissociation and the stimulus to accommodation may vary, so that different techniques produce different results (Schroeder, Rainey, Goss, & Grosvenor, 1996). The 95% confidence limits of most tests are approximately $2-5\Delta$ (Schroeder et al., 1996). A comparison of the interexaminer repeatability of dissociation tests (Rainey et al., 1998) found that the Thorington test was the most reliable with 98% confidence limits of $\pm2.3\Delta$ and compared well with the reliability of the cover test (98% limits $\pm3.3\Delta$). The Howell phoria card interexaminer repeatability is $\pm3.5\Delta$ for continuous presentation, which had better repeatability than flashed presentation (Wong et al., 2002). Less repeatable results are obtained with a refractor head (phoropter) than with a trial frame (Casillas & Rosenfield, 2006).

The measurement obtained with these methods should be taken only as one factor in helping to evaluate the heterophoria. Although dissociation tests are time-honoured procedures, it is doubtful they are the best way of spending time in a routine eye examination.

FUSIONAL RESERVES

The fusional reserves represent the amount of vergence (motor fusion) which can be induced before fusion is compromised leading to blurred and/or double vision. Fusional reserves can be measured with rotary or variable prism devices (ramp stimulus) or, most commonly, with a prism bar (step stimulus; Fig. 4.2). The patient is asked to look at a target (see later) and the prism power introduced and slowly increased until the patient reports that the print blurs or doubles. The prism is then reduced until single vision (not necessarily clear) is recovered. The prism power at which these occur is noted and recorded as the fusional reserve to blur (the relative convergence or divergence), break, and recovery. This may be carried out with prism base-in (divergent reserves), with prism base-out (convergent reserves), or (for vertical fusional reserves) base up and base down. Measurements can be taken for distance and for near vision. In young children, and unreliable patients, the break and recovery points should be checked by observing the eye movements.

Testing Details

The fusional reserve test method and norms are summarised in Table 4.2.

The repeatability of fusional reserve testing is reasonable, but rotary prisms give somewhat different results to prism bars so the two methods should not be used interchangeably (Antona, Barrio, Barra, Gonzalez, & Sanchez, 2008). Indeed, the testing of fusional reserves is strongly influenced by factors such as patient instructions, target design (Stein, Riddell, & Fowler, 1988), and speed of adjustment (Fowler, Riddell, & Stein, 1988), yet there seems to have been very little research on the test parameters that are most appropriate and few textbooks discuss these factors.

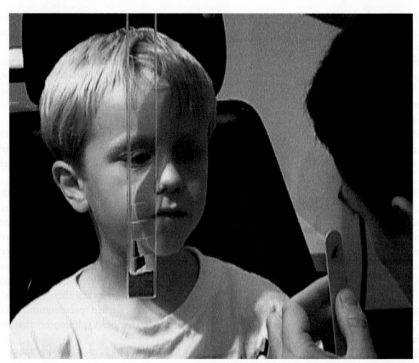

Fig. 4.2 Fusional reserves measured with a prism bar. The child is viewing a small detailed target at his usual reading distance. He has been instructed to report when the target blurs, doubles ('say when there are two pictures or two cards'). Base-out prisms are being introduced to measure the convergent fusional reserve.

Fowler et al. (1988) recommended a rate of adjustment of 0.5Δ per second for subjects with reading difficulties. Griffin and Grisham (1995) recommended 4Δ per second, although they did not cite any published work. Ciuffreda and Tannen (1995) recommended 'slowly' for horizontal and 'very slowly' for vertical measurements.

There are believed to be two components of vergence control: a **fast component** and a **slow component** (Schor, 1979; Ciuffreda & Tannen, 1995). The fast component rapidly adjusts to changes in the stimulus and feeds into the slow component, which gradually adapts to the new situation. For example, if a 5Δ base-out prism is held before one eye whilst a person views a target, most people will make a rapid vergence movement (fast component) to overcome the prism and then, after perhaps 10 seconds, manifest prism adaptation (slow component) so that their heterophoria adapts to the prism and returns to its normal value. It is implicit from this model that the speed of adjustment during fusional reserve testing is important (Sethi & North, 1987). If the prism is changed rapidly, the test will primarily assess the fast component of vergence; if adjusted slowly, the influence of the slow component is likely to predominate. Schor (1979) suggested that slow vergence adaptation takes over from the fast component after about 7 seconds, although there will be a gradual changing of predominance.

In the absence of research on the optimal rate of testing to detect symptomatic patients, it seems sensible to invoke significant degrees of fast and slow fusional vergence during testing. The fast component will respond to rapidly changing stimuli, greater than 1Δ per second (Ciuffreda & Tannen, 1995). The rate of adjustment should not be too much faster than this, or the test may be over before the slow component has had time to adapt. Therefore, it is suggested that the test rate should be between $1-2\Delta$ per second.

TABLE 4.2 ■ Test Method and Norms for Fusional Reserves.

1. The most common method is to use a prism bar, but rotary prisms also can be used.
2. Base-out prisms are used to measure the convergent fusional reserves, and vice versa.
3. The fusional reserve opposing the heterophoria (convergent in exophoria) should be measured first.
4. Introduce the prism at about the rate of $1-2\Delta$ per second.
5. The patient fixates a detailed accommodative target (e.g., vertical line of letters on a fixation stick if testing at near).
6. First, the patient should report when the target goes blurred, which is recorded as the blur point. Sometimes, there is no blur point.
7. The patient should be asked to report when the target goes double: the break point. The practitioner should watch the patient's eyes to confirm this objectively. Some patients suppress and perceive the target moving off to one side rather than diplopia.
8. The prism is then reduced until single vision and ocular alignment is restored.
9. Record the results as blur / break / recovery. For example:
   Fus. Res. N con 12/20/15   div − /10/8 ('−' indicates no blur point)
10. Results can be compared with norms, but the precise norms depend on the test conditions. It is more meaningful to relate the results to the heterophoria.
11. Sheard's criterion says that the fusional reserve (to blur or, if no blur, to break) that opposes the heterophoria should be at least twice the heterophoria. For example, if a patient has 8Δ exophoria at near, their convergent reserve should be at least 16Δ. This criterion works well for exophoria.
12. Percival's criterion says, in essence, the fusional reserves should be balanced so that the smaller fusional reserve is more than half the larger one. For example, if the convergent fusional reserve to break point is 20Δ, then the divergent fusional reserve should be at least 10Δ. Percival's criterion is useful for esophoric patients.

Vergence adaptation will also have an impact on the order of testing, as the reserve that is measured second will be influenced by vergence during measurement of the first reserve (Rosenfield, Ciuffreda, Ong, & Super, 1995). These authors made the sensible suggestion to first measure the fusional reserve that opposes the heterophoria. Ideally, it would also seem sensible to allow $2-3$ minutes between the measurement of opposing reserves.

There is a lack of research on the target design that is most appropriate to detect symptomatic patients. Small targets have been advocated for patients with reading difficulties (Eames, 1934; Stein et al., 1988), which would help with the identification of blur and diplopia. The target should include detail to induce accommodation but should be resolvable by the eye with worst acuity. The author uses a small detailed picture. If the worst eye cannot resolve this then a vertical black line is used, of a width that makes it readily resolvable by each eye.

One reason why fusional reserve test results can be quite variable is the influence of 'mental effort' or encouragement (Lanca & Rowe, 2019). If patients try hard to fuse, they do much better than if they just 'gaze lazily' at the target. Hence, verbal instructions to the patient are crucial, but have not been standardised. The purpose of the test is to detect the fusional reserve that the patient can comfortably use to overcome their heterophoria. So, it would seem inappropriate to ask the patient to uncomfortably force their vergence. The wording the author has found most useful is to ask the patient to 'look at the target normally but continue to look at it throughout the test'. Some patients ask if they should 'really force the eyes', and they are told to 'just look at the target normally'.

Terminology

There are many synonyms that have been used for fusional reserves, and some of these are listed in Table 4.3. No term is perfect, and Table 4.3 gives comments on alternative nomenclature. The phrase **fusional reserves** is used in this book because it is felt to be a clear and commonly used term.

TABLE 4.3 ■ Synonyms of the Term 'Fusional Reserves', Giving Reasons Why Each Term is Felt to be Less Appropriate Than 'Fusional Reserves'.

Term	Criticism
Fusional amplitude	Amplitudes are sometimes used to refer to the difference between positive and negative break or blur points, and at other times to refer to the difference between the phoria position and a fusional reserve. In this book, **fusional amplitude** describes the amplitude between corresponding convergent and divergent reserves
Fusional limits	In most patients, blur and break points do not represent a limit of everyday fusion so much as an amount of fusion which is 'held in reserve'; so, **reserve** may be more appropriate than **limit**
Relative vergences	Sometimes used to refer to the blur point only
Vergence reserves	Sensory fusion can be maintained for some 2 degrees of disconjugate image movement, without any change in vergence angle (Chapter 12)
Prism vergences	The measurement can be made without varying prism (e.g., with a synoptophore)
Binocular ductions	This term no longer seems to be in common use

Evaluation of Results

Several methods have been suggested for the evaluation of fusional reserves and these can be broadly classified into intersubject and intrasubject. Intersubject techniques are based on a comparison of the results with normative values. A simple comparison with norms is of limited use and it is unsafe to diagnose binocular vision anomalies based on a single test result (Harle & Evans, 2006; Karania & Evans, 2006b; Lanca & Rowe, 2019). Fusional reserve data from a normal population are given in Appendix 10, but most norms apply to ramp measurement methods, not step (Lanca & Rowe, 2019). Norms for monocular hand-held rotary prisms were given by Wesson and Amos (1985), who found ocular dominance did not significantly influence the result. The small range of vertical fusional reserves explains why the visual system is so insensitive to vertical prismatic effect, which can be induced by incorrectly centred spectacle lenses. In science, the range of normality is generally considered to be the mean ± 2 standard deviations, which encompasses approximately 95% of a normally distributed population (Whyte & Kelly, 2018). A less stringent criterion, of ± 1 standard deviation, would increase sensitivity but reduce specificity. It is interesting that the oft-cited Morgan norms provide a 'normal range' based on the mean ± 0.5 standard deviations (Morgan, 1944). This means that 30% of the population would fall below the 'normal range', which would seem likely to overdiagnose binocular vision anomalies.

Intrasubject methods compare an individual's fusional reserve with some other measure of that person's binocular function. An early intrasubject technique was that of Percival (1928) who proposed that, for comfort, the working fixation point should lie in the middle third of the total fusional amplitude obtained by adding the divergent to the convergent blur points. That is to say, the opposing fusional reserves should be balanced within the limits that one should not be less than half the other. It should be noted that Percival's criterion does not take account of the phoria. In contrast, Sheard (1930) related the heterophoria to its opposing blur point. Sheard's criterion is often stated thus: the opposing fusional reserve to the blur point should be at least twice the degree of the phoria. In fact, Sheard (1930, 1931) gave several possible criteria based on this principle, with the required amount of opposing reserve ranging from two to four times the phoria, and later settled on his 'middle third' approach (Sheard, 1934). Research evaluating these criteria is discussed at the end of this chapter. Evans and colleagues derived a continuous variable based on Sheard's criterion (Evans, Busby, Jeanes, & Wilkins, 1995) and a similar approach has been followed by other workers (Conway, Thomas, & Subramanian, 2012). This principle has been developed further as **fusional stamina,** calculated by dividing the convergent fusional reserve (to break) by two and then subtracting the heterophoria (Myklebust & Riddell, 2016).

Percival's criterion seems to be appropriate for near vision only as Appendix 10 shows that Percival's middle third rule is inappropriate for normal values for distance vision.

It has been suggested that if the recovery result is not within 4−6Δ of the break result, this can be a sign of decompensated heterophoria (Rowe, 2004).

It should also be noted that the divergent reserve for distance is very small in comparison with other values and there is seldom any blur point when measuring the divergent fusional reserve for distance vision. Perhaps the most significant aspect of this measurement is when it becomes excessively large, e.g., over 9Δ, to break. This is a sign of divergence excess (Chapter 8).

VERGENCE FACILITY

Fusional reserves measure the maximum vergence that can be exerted. A vergence facility prism (Fig. 4.3) can be used to assess the vergence facility, or rate of change of vergence. Because the ability to converge is usually greater than the ability to diverge, the base-out prism is typically three or four times the base-in prism. The best flipper power to discriminate between symptomatic and asymptomatic subjects at near is 3Δ base-in/12Δ base-out (1.5Δ in/6Δ out each eye) and norms, based on 1 standard deviation below the mean of an asymptomatic control group, are 12 cycles per minute (cpm) at distance and 15 cpm at near (Gall, Wick, & Bedell, 1998a). It appears that the target does not need to include a suppression check, so 6/9 equivalent letters can be used with the lenses flipped when the target is clear and single (Gall, Wick, & Bedell, 1998b). Test results appear to be variable in presbyopes (Pellizzer & Siderov, 1998). In pre-presbyopes, the test is useful at detecting symptomatic patients and is a little more sensitive when combined with a test of accommodative facility (Gall & Wick, 2003).

PARTIAL DISSOCIATION TESTS

Methods for measuring the degree of heterophoria require complete dissociation of the two eyes, e.g., the Maddox rod or the wing test. Another approach is to dissociate only part of the visual field by presenting a partial impediment to binocular vision and assessing the disturbance to binocularity this causes. These methods leave part of the visual field common to both eyes, which provides a stimulus to fusion. The term used to describe this is **fusion lock**: it may be the central fixation area, or it can be a peripheral fusion lock. Tests have been used in the past which provide a variable amount of dissociation, so that the amount which just causes a breakdown in binocular vision can be measured, but these tests are no longer in widespread use.

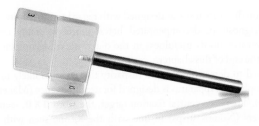

Fig. 4.3 Vergence facility prism. (Courtesy Bernell Inc.)

The dissociation can be achieved by a septum (e.g., Turville infinity balance test), by a method of cross-polarisation, or by coloured filters. One approach combines a septum and polarisation and has been called **parallel testing infinity balance** (Shapiro, 1995, 1998). It is claimed that this can assess horizontal, vertical, and cyclo deviations, although there do not appear to have been any controlled studies.

The principle underlying partial dissociation tests is that, owing to the slight degree of dissociation, in decompensated heterophoria a misalignment of the targets becomes apparent. However, these methods seem to have been superseded by fixation disparity approaches, which more closely replicate the conditions of everyday viewing and are described next.

FIXATION DISPARITY TESTS

In normal binocular vision, the fovea of one eye corresponds with a small area centred on the fovea of the other eye: **Panum's area**. Similarly, each point in the binocular field of one eye corresponds with a small area in the other eye. This point-to-area correspondence means that if there is a very small deviation of one eye, no diplopia will be seen until the eye has deviated enough to move the image out of Panum's area. Panum's areas are small and horizontally oval. Measurements of their size vary depending on the retinal eccentricity and on the spatial and temporal properties of the test stimulus; they should be thought of as a phenomenon of cortical processing rather than an entity of fixed size (Reading, 1988).

Panum's areas allow the eyes to be deviated by a very small amount before any diplopia is noticed. This minute deviation from fixation can occur without diplopia and is called **fixation disparity**. It is very likely to occur when binocular vision is under stress; that is, in decompensated heterophoria (Charnwood, 1950). Tests which detect fixation disparity are therefore very useful in assessing decompensation (Yekta & Pickwell, 1986). The deviation can occur in one eye or in both eyes, but because the magnitude is so small it cannot be seen with the cover test. Research methods of objectively recording eye movements can detect objective fixation disparity, the values of which are different to subjective fixation disparity (Jaschinski, Jainta, & Kloke, 2010). Objective fixation disparity can be categorised as state or trait (Jainta & Jaschinski, 2009) and are different to clinical measurements (Pickwell & Stockley, 1960; Jaschinski et al., 2010). Objective fixation disparity cannot be predicted from subjective measures (Jaschinski, 2018), and objective fixation disparity changes when prisms are introduced, albeit in nonclinical population (Schroth, Joos, & Jaschinski, 2015). Methods of recording eye movements that are affordable for clinical practice lack the accuracy required for reliably detecting fixation disparity.

There is a fundamental distinction between fixation disparity tests and dissociation tests. Dissociation tests are by their very nature disruptive to normal binocular vision, whereas fixation disparity tests aim to mimic everyday vision. From an understanding of this, one can deduce the ideal features of a fixation disparity test (Table 4.4).

The Mallett Fixation Disparity Test

Fixation disparity, like all binocular vision parameters, is not a fixed entity but varies with test conditions. Therefore, two fixation disparity tests with different designs should not be expected to give the same result.

The Mallett fixation disparity test was designed with regard to the features in Table 4.4 and has revolutionised the diagnosis of decompensated heterophoria in many countries. The test is described here and research on its usefulness in the diagnosis of decompensated heterophoria is summarised towards the end of this chapter.

The test is designed to detect the fixation disparity that is most likely to occur when there is decompensated heterophoria. Apparatus is designed for use at distance (Mallett, 1966) and for near vision (Mallett, 1964). There is a central fixation target, the word **0 X 0**, seen with both eyes, and two monocular markers (Nonius strips) in line with the **X**, one seen with each eye (Fig. 4.4). Dissociation of the monocular marks is achieved using cross-polarised filters. In fixation disparity,

TABLE 4.4 ■ Ideal Features of a Fixation Disparity Test.

Feature	Requirement
Fusion lock	To simulate everyday viewing conditions, there should be a detailed foveal and parafoveal fusion lock, and a peripheral fusion lock.
Monocular markers (Nonius markers)	Monocular markers by definition cannot be fusional, and so should be small to minimise the departure from normal viewing conditions. The monocular markers should facilitate judgement of misalignment and should not be easily suppressed.
Visual field	A trial frame is preferable to a phoropter as it allows a more normal head position and field of view. Similarly, full-aperture trial lenses are preferable to reduced-aperture.
Non-dissociative	Care should be taken to avoid any procedures which could interfere with normal fusion: Polarisation is preferable to anaglyph (red/green) for controlling which eye sees each marker. Trial lens prisms should be used instead of rotary prisms or prism bars. The patient should be instructed to read a line of text before a new prism is introduced to renormalise binocular vision.
Lighting	Ambient lighting should mimic that used by the patient at work or when they have symptoms and should be increased to counteract the effect of polarised filters.
Working distance	Should mimic that used by the patient.
Head posture	A natural head posture should be maintained.

Modified from Mallett, R. [1988a]. Techniques of investigation of binocular vision anomalies. In K. Edwards and R. Llewellyn (Eds.), *Optometry* (pp. 238–269). London: Butterworths.

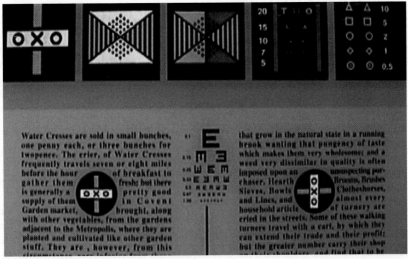

Fig. 4.4 Mallett near vision unit. The tests, starting at the *top left* and working clockwise, are Mallett ARC and suppression test in strabismus (MARCS) or 'large OXO' (Chapter 14); cross cylinder and balance chart; duochrome (bichromatic) test; quantitative test of foveal suppression; stereoacuity test; vertical fixation disparity test; and horizontal fixation disparity test. The fixation disparity tests are embedded in text to more closely simulate normal viewing conditions.

the images will be displaced slightly on the retina. Having no corresponding image in the same place on the other retina, the monocular markers will be given a visual direction associated with the retinal area stimulated, whilst the binocular image **O X O** will be seen centrally. The monocular markers may therefore appear to the patient to be displaced from their alignment with the **X**. Throughout the test, the patient should be instructed to keep looking at the **X**. As well as the target with the vertical Nonius strips to detect horizontal fixation disparity, the unit has a similar target rotated through 90 degrees to detect vertical fixation disparity.

A cyclophoria is indicated by tilting of a Nonius strip. If this occurs in the presence of high astigmatism at an oblique axis, the test should be repeated with the target rotated so that the strips are at right angles to their original orientation. An opposite tilt confirms that the effect is due to astigmatic distortion, whilst a tilt in the same direction confirms that it is due to cyclophoria (Rabbetts, 2007).

The Mallett units do not measure the degree of fixation disparity, that is, the amount by which the eye is misaligned. What is measured is the degree of prism relief required to neutralise the fixation disparity and restore the monocular markers to alignment with the **X**. This has been called the **associated heterophoria**, to distinguish it from the dissociated phoria which is revealed by methods which give complete dissociation such as the cover test, Maddox rod, etc. However, because the term heterophoria implies dissociation, the term associated heterophoria is, in fact, a contradiction. Therefore, the term **aligning prism,** originally suggested by an International Standards Organisation committee but never published, is used throughout this book. The angle of the actual fixation disparity is correlated with the magnitude of the aligning prism (Pickwell, 1984a).

Exceptionally patients are encountered who have a **paradoxical fixation disparity**, typically eso-slip in exophoria. This may represent an overcompensation and can sometimes require (paradoxical) base-in prism to remove the eso-slip, or exercises to increase the convergent fusional reserve. Other tests of compensation are required in these cases, as summarised at the end of this chapter.

There are a few people who, without the polarised visors, perceive a misalignment of the two Nonius strips. This may be a true **alignment error**, which some people experience on vernier tasks (Tomlinson, 1969), or indicate an unreliable patient. If there is a genuine alignment error, the position of the strips with the polarised filters in place should be compared to their position without the filters (Jaschinski, Brode, & Griefahn, 1999).

Mallett (1988a) stated that the aligning prism represents the extent of the **uncompensated** part of the heterophoria. Jenkins, Pickwell, and Yekta (1989) found that an aligning prism of 1Δ or more in pre-presbyopes and 2Δ or more in presbyopes was likely to be associated with symptoms (see later). Fixation disparity, however, increases under the stress of working in inadequate illumination (Pickwell, Yekta et al., 1987), working at too close a reading distance (Pickwell, Jenkins et al., 1987), and at the end of a day's close work (Yekta et al., 1987). As it may be either physiological or the result of binocular stress, the presence of fixation disparity suggests decompensation of the heterophoria which needs to be confirmed by the other methods discussed in this chapter.

The Mallett fixation disparity tests provide a considerable amount of information and, as with many subjective tests, the precise instructions given to the patient are very important. A suggested procedure, with appropriate patient questions and resultant diagnoses, is given in Fig. 4.5, and research evaluating this is described here. This diagram applies to horizontal testing, but an analogous procedure can be used for vertical testing. As an aligning prism of 1Δ is abnormal in pre-presbyopes (Jenkins et al., 1989), it is preferable to use smaller step sizes than this. However, exceptional patients will be encountered with quite large (6Δ or more) aligning prisms (Parmar, Dickinson, & Evans, 2019). It is therefore recommended that when a fixation disparity is detected the practitioner starts with 0.5Δ and if this does not eliminate the fixation disparity increase to 1Δ, then 2Δ, 4Δ, 8Δ. Between changes of prism or lens, patients should be asked to stabilise their binocular vision and accommodation by reading a few words from the surrounding text. During measurements, the patient should be repeatedly reminded to fixate on the **X** (Mallett, 1964; Karania & Evans, 2006a).

MALLETT FD TEST ROUTINE

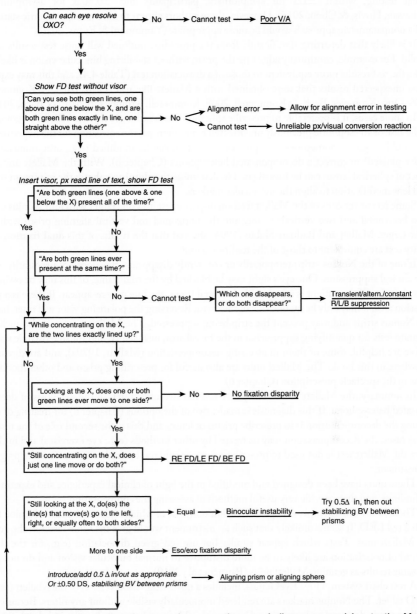

Fig. 4.5 Flow chart illustrating the procedure, questions, and diagnoses applying to the Mallett Fixation Disparity Unit. It should be stressed to patients, before and during testing, that they should keep looking at the central X. The chart applies to horizontal readings, although slight rephrasing of the questions allows it to be used for vertical readings. The actual questions to be asked are in inverted commas and the appropriate diagnoses are underlined. *BE*, both eyes; *BV*, binocular vision; *FD*, fixation disparity; *LE*, left eye; *Px*, patient; *RE*, right eye.

The Mallett fixation disparity test has been found to have good 95% limits of agreement on repeat testing, within ±1Δ for symptomatic participants and ±0.50Δ for asymptomatic (Alhassan, Hovis, & Chou, 2015). However, these authors appear to have used parametric statistics and a nonparametric approach would be more appropriate (Yammouni & Evans, 2020).

It is likely that departing significantly from the procedure outlined will cause test results to be invalid. For example, continually adjusting the prism without stabilising binocular vision is likely to make the test results more equivalent to those of a dissociation test (Table 4.4), and this may explain some unexpected results that were obtained with a Mallett-like test (Otto, Bach, & Kommerell, 2008; Otto, Kromeier, Bach, & Kommerell, 2008; Kommerell, Kromeier, Scharff, & Bach, 2015).

In some cases, it is preferable to prescribe spherical lenses rather than prism relief. For example, in the case of an esophoric previously uncorrected hypermetrope, the correction for the hypermetropia would be given. Sometimes the spherical correction can be modified (e.g., over-minussed or under-plussed) to correct a decompensated heterophoria (Chapter 6). With the Mallett unit, the effect of spherical lenses can be investigated to determine the **aligning sphere**: the minimum spherical lens modification to align the monocular markers.

Some recent versions of the Mallett fixation disparity test uses one target with four Nonius strips (two horizontal and two vertical) to measure the horizontal and vertical aligning prism with the same target. Mallett and Radnan-Skibin (1994) showed that the results of this **dual fixation disparity test** are equivalent to those of the traditional unit.

If one of the Nonius strips temporarily or constantly disappears, this does not necessarily indicate clinical suppression. One eye's sight may be blocked by the trial frame, or this may be owing to retinal rivalry. If the patient is asked to blink several times, the line may re-appear. If there is a suppression area, it may only be on one side of the fovea. Reversing the polarising visor will interchange the Nonius strips and may prevent the strip being suppressed. The Mallett near unit also includes separate tests for quantifying suppression in the foveal area, near acuity, and for stereoscopic vision. These are helpful, some of them in assessing decompensation (Mallett, 1979a), and are discussed elsewhere in this book. The Mallett units are also useful for prescribing prism and other modifications to the spectacle prescription (Chapter 6).

In summary, the Mallett fixation disparity test has two uses. First, in the diagnosis of decompensated heterophoria. If this diagnosis is made, two of the options (Chapter 6) for treating or correcting the decompensation is to prescribe prisms or lenses and this is the second role of the test. In some cases, the decompensation may be treated by other methods (e.g., eye exercises) and in these cases the Mallett test is not used to prescribe prisms or spheres, but rather to monitor the progress of treatment.

These units have been designed and modified in the light of clinical experience and experimental findings, and they provide very useful methods of assessing the compensation.

There have been attempts to copy the Mallett unit, one of which replaced the textual fusion lock with a red LED. It seems unlikely that such an instrument would give the same result as the genuine Mallett unit. Tests which appear similar but use red-green dissociation (e.g., for the iPad) instead of polarisation are likely to be more disruptive to normal binocular vision and do not give the same results as genuine Mallett units (Parmar et al., 2019).

A test chart system, Hoya EyeGenius, includes a novel near vision version of the Mallett test on a 3-D tablet. The Nonius markers are rendered monocularly visible without any filters. Because the Mallett test is designed to be as natural as possible, this would seem to be a logical development, providing the lower resolution of 3-D displays is not associated with any limitations. It will be interesting to see the results of validation studies of this new approach.

The efficacy of the Mallett test at diagnosing symptomatic heterophoria is summarised in the next chapter where it is noted that the test performs well for near vision, but not so well for distance vision. The test method and norms for the Mallett fixation disparity test are summarised in Fig. 4.4 and Table 4.5.

TABLE 4.5 ■ Summary of Test Method and Norms for the Mallett Fixation Disparity Test.

Step	Description	Patient instructions
1	Without the polarised visors, show the patient the horizontal test (green strips vertically placed above and below the **O X O**) and check that the patient perceives both green strips in perfect alignment.	'Do you see both green strips and are they exactly lined up?' See Fig. 4.4
2	Introduce the polarised visor, increase illumination, and normalise vision by reading text. Ask the patient if the two green strips are still exactly aligned, whilst they keep their head still and look at the **X**.	'While you look at the **X**, are the two green strips exactly lined up, or does one or both move a little?'
3	If (2) reveals any misalignment (even transient), introduce prisms in front of the relevant eye(s) or spheres in front of both eyes and repeat step (2). For an exo-slip (right eye's strip moving to the patient's left) add base-in or minus.	After introducing prism or lens: 'Are the two lines perfectly aligned, or does one or both still move a little?'
4	After changing the prism or spheres, have the patient read a line of text to stabilise their binocular vision before re-testing for fixation disparity.	
5	Make a note of the results in (3), remove the aligning prism or sphere, and then repeat for the vertical test.	As above
6	An aligning prism of 1Δ or more in pre-presbyopes or 2Δ or more in presbyopes is very likely to be associated with symptoms.	

Other Fixation Disparity Tests

There is a variety of fixation disparity tests (Brownlee & Goss, 1988; London & Crelier, 2006) and one that is popular in North America is the Sheedy Disparometer (Fig. 4.6). This differs from the Mallett unit in that there is no central binocular lock, just a parafoveal fusion lock which is raised in front of the plane of the Nonius markers (Jaschinski, 2001). The inclusion of only a peripheral lock causes the degree of fixation disparity obtained to be larger and more variable (Ukwade, 2000), because Panum's areas are larger in the periphery. This probably explains why the Sheedy Disparometer has poor repeatability (Alhassan et al., 2015) and is less repeatable than the Mallett test (Pickwell, Gilchrist, & Hesler, 1988). The Sheedy and Wesson (also, lacking a foveal fusion lock) tests produce extreme ranges of values compared with, for example, the Mallett unit (Alhassan, Hovis, & Chou, 2016).

In the patient's everyday vision, a central fixation lock will always be present because objects are fixated with both foveae. Clinical assessment should explore whether the patient's heterophoria is compensated under normal viewing conditions, and therefore a good central and peripheral fusion lock is essential (pp. 11–12).

In some cases, there will be foveal suppression, and in these patients the lock will be provided by the parafoveal regions, and fixation disparity will be larger, hence the importance of knowing if there is suppression. Reading (1992) recommended that clinical tests should allow the monocular components of the fixation disparity to be determined: this is not possible with the Sheedy Disparometer.

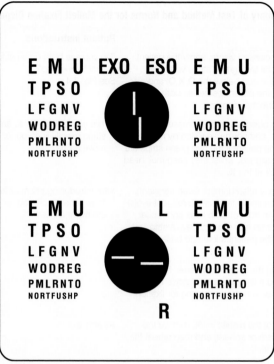

Fig. 4.6 The Sheedy Disparometer. This is an example of a disparity test which has no central fixation lock. This apparatus allows the measurement of the actual disparity as well as the aligning prism.

All methods of detecting or measuring fixation disparity involve slightly abnormal circumstances which do not perfectly coincide with everyday vision. It is therefore important that immediately before investigating disparity the patient should undertake a few moments of binocular vision, such as reading a line of letters binocularly for distance or a few lines of print for near.

The Zeiss Polatest (MKH or method of Hasse) also provides a range of targets designed to analyse the compensation of the heterophoria. Fixation disparity is detected, and the aligning prism measured using more peripheral areas, so the fixation disparity is greater than with tests using parafoveal locks (Brautaset & Jennings, 2001). Both the distance and near Polatests, however, incorporate a wide range of targets, and the designers claim that this allows a greater degree of analysis of binocular vision (Haase, 1962; Pickwell, 1977a, 1979a). Nonetheless, it has been demonstrated that a fixation disparity that is detected with one of the key Polatest subtests (Zeigertest) does not indicate a fixation disparity under natural viewing conditions (Gerling, Ball, Bomer, Bach, & Kommerell, 1998).

Advocates of the Polatest system recommend the prismatic full correction of distance heterophoria (Cagnolati, 1991; Goersch, 1979), which has been associated with a reduction in symptoms (Lie & Opheim, 1985) and an improvement in high spatial frequency contrast sensitivity (Methling & Jaschinski, 1996). However, the Polatest method may cause a heterophoria to progress into strabismus requiring surgery (Lie & Opheim, 1990). The Polatest approach has been criticised for a lack of supporting evidence (Brautaset & Jennings, 2001) and as leading 'to excessive amount of prisms and unnecessary eye muscle surgery' (Lang, 1994).

There is now a plethora of varieties of fixation disparity tests, used clinically and in research. As noted earlier, tests without both a good foveal and peripheral fusion lock are likely to produce spurious results. Even tests that appear quite similar to, for example, the Mallett unit will not necessarily give equivalent results (Parmar et al., 2019), and the wording of the practitioner's instructions is important (Karania & Evans, 2006b). Therefore, research using novel designs of instrument (Lederer, Poltavski, & Biberdorf, 2015) cannot be compared to previous work. It is recommended that genuine Mallett units are used in clinical practice and research.

Further Analysis of Fixation Disparity Results

As the degree of fixation disparity can be changed by prisms, it is possible, with an instrument like the Sheedy Disparometer, to plot the degree of fixation disparity against the power of the prism (Ogle, 1950). Fixation disparity (in minutes of arc) is plotted vertically (y-axis) against the prism power (in prism dioptres) horizontally (x-axis). Several types of curve have been found, of which type I is the most frequent and is illustrated in Fig. 4.7A. It will be noticed that the middle part of this typical sigma-shaped curve has a flatter slope: fixation disparity changes less over the range of lower power prisms, but with the higher powers of prism, it rises steeply. Eventually, diplopia occurs at the limit of the fusional reserves.

It is suggested that if the patient's normal fixation lies in the flatter part of the curve, it is likely that the heterophoria will be compensated (Sheedy & Saladin, 1978). This is the case in Fig. 4.7A, where a small amount of esophoric fixation disparity is present: where the curve cuts the y-axis. The aligning prism is also small: where the curve cuts the x-axis. In Fig. 4.7B, the curve is placed further towards the right-hand (base-out) side of the figure. This illustrates a case of decompensated esophoria. The fixation disparity and the aligning prism are larger, and the base-in prism part of the curve is closer to the y-axis. This means that the base-in fusional reserve must be less, and the base-out relatively greater, which is to say that the fusional reserves are unbalanced. Fig. 4.7C shows a similar plot, but for exophoria.

If a relieving prism were to be prescribed, it would bring the patient's fixation into the flatter part of the curve. For example, in the case illustrated in Fig. 4.7C, for exophoria, 3Δ base-in vergence would mean that the patient would be operating from the position of the dotted line rather than the actual y-axis. Here, the fixation disparity and aligning prism are less.

Fixation disparity can also be changed by using positive or negative spheres to bring about changes in accommodation. This occurs because of the accommodation-convergence relationship. Fig. 4.7D shows an example of plotting the changes in fixation disparity (y-axis) against the changes in spherical lens power.

One problem with the measurement of fixation disparity curves is that the variability of fixation disparity measures increases with larger fixation disparities (Cooper, Feldman, Horn, & Dibble, 1981). Wildsoet and Cameron (1985) showed that clinicians' attempts to classify fixation disparity curves into the different types were very unreliable and the Wesson Fixation Disparity Card produces different results to the Sheedy Disparometer (Goss & Patel, 1995). The Wesson and Saladin Fixation Disparity Cards have also been shown to produce different results (Ngan et al., 2005). Yekta et al. (1989) found that the central slope of the forced vergence disparity curve was not significantly associated with symptoms, but the aligning prism (as measured with the Mallett unit) was useful in detecting symptomatic binocular problems.

Is Fixation Disparity Normal or Abnormal?

There seem to be two schools of thought regarding fixation disparity. One, exemplified by Mallett (1988a), argues that any measurable fixation disparity is undesirable, is a sign of ocular motor stress and decompensated heterophoria, and should be corrected with changes to the workplace, eye exercises, spheres, or prisms. Several lines of evidence support this view:

1. The cortical response is significantly greater when monocular receptive fields are superimposed very precisely (Suter, Bass, & Suter, 1993);
2. Stereoacuity decreases as fixation disparity increases (Abd Manan, Jenkins, & Collinge, 2001; Cole & Boisvert, 1974; Momeni-Moghaddam, Eperjesi, Kundart, & Sabbaghi, 2014a; Ukwade, Bedell, & Harwerth, 2003; Zaroff, Knutelska, & Frumkes, 2003);
3. Stereoacuity improves when fixation disparity is corrected (Abd Manan et al., 2001).

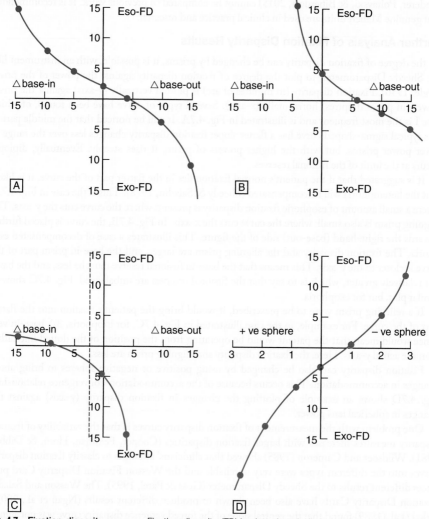

Fig. 4.7 Fixation disparity curves. Fixation disparity *(FD)* is plotted vertically in minutes of arc and, in the first three curves, the prism power before the eyes in prism dioptres is plotted horizontally. (A) Type I, the most usual curve. (B) Type II, curve in esophoria. (C) Type III, curve in exophoria. (D) Fixation disparity plotted against spherical lens power before both eyes (dioptres) for near vision. See also text.

The opposing viewpoint (Saladin, 2005) is based on a model of the vergence system which assumes that a small amount of fixation disparity may be physiological and represents an error in the eyes' alignment, providing feedback to help control vergence (Schor, 1979). There is clinical evidence to support both arguments: researchers in North America typically find that many asymptomatic subjects have a fixation disparity (Sheedy & Saladin, 1978), yet similar studies in the UK find that a fixation disparity is uncommon in asymptomatic subjects (Jenkins et al., 1989).

This controversy probably can be resolved by considering the fusional lock that is present in different fixation disparity tests. Most research in the USA seems to have used the Sheedy Disparometer

(Fig. 4.6), which does not have a central fusional lock. In contrast, research in the UK tends to use the Mallett unit which has a good foveal fusion lock and finds values of fixation disparity and aligning prism that are about half the typical values with the Sheedy Disparometer (Pickwell, 1984). For example, about a quarter of asymptomatic subjects with normal binocular vision demonstrate a vertical fixation disparity on the Sheedy Disparometer (Luu, Green, & Abel, 2000). If a central fusional lock is added to the Sheedy Disparometer, this has a significant effect on all fixation disparity parameters, causing a stabilisation of the Nonius strips (Wildsoet & Cameron, 1985). This agrees with objective data on the effect of a central fusional lock on fixation disparity (Howard, Fang, Allison, & Zacher, 2000; Pickwell & Stockley, 1960). Indeed, the presence of a foveal fusion lock makes subjective fixation disparity not only smaller (Ogle, Mussey, & Prangen, 1949), but also a more accurate indicator of the objective eye position (Brautaset & Jennings, 2006b).

Even with the Mallett unit, experience shows that occasionally patients have small amounts of fixation disparity, but there is no other reason to suspect decompensation. This is not surprising; it is unlikely that any single test will ever be able to infallibly diagnose decompensated heterophoria (Pickwell & Kurtz, 1986). Nevertheless, research suggests that the aligning prism as measured with the Mallett unit is the single best predictor of whether a phoria is associated with symptoms (Jenkins et al., 1989; Yekta et al., 1989). At near vision, patients who require higher base-in aligning prism have significantly lower convergent fusional reserves (Conway et al., 2012), linking Mallett's criterion with Sheard's criterion. Indeed, over 65% of the variance in convergent fusional reserve could be accounted for by the variance in base-in aligning prism.

A small double-masked randomised controlled trial showed that prisms prescribed with the Mallett unit were consistently preferred by patients to spectacles without prism (Payne, Grisham, & Thomas, 1974).

It is not just the presence of a foveal lock that influences the results of fixation disparity tests. As with most other binocular vision tests, different results will be obtained using instruments that appear similar but have slightly different designs (Van Haeringen, McClurg, & Cameron, 1986). Other factors such as lighting levels and the precise instructions given to the patient will also be important. If, for example, a trial frame is used to assess the fixation disparity at the first appointment, then similar equipment should be used at subsequent visits (Frantz & Scharre, 1990).

The role of fixation disparity tests in the diagnosis of decompensated heterophoria is considered further at the end of this chapter and of the next.

FOVEAL SUPPRESSION TESTS

If binocular vision continues under stress, sometimes small suppression areas may occur within the foveal region. Small parts of the central field of one eye are inhibited by the mismatch in the slightly displaced images, although the rest of the binocular field appears to be fused normally. If fixation disparity is not corrected, monocular acuities measured under binocular (haploscopic) conditions may be worse than the true monocular acuities, measured when the other eye is occluded (Sucher, 1991). Foveal suppression may act as a compensatory mechanism to prevent symptoms in decompensated heterophoria. Foveal suppression may vary in different positions of gaze, and this variation may be associated with frequent headaches (Sucher, 1994). Larger areas of suppression are more likely in cases where a decompensated exophoria is breaking down to intermittent exotropia (Holmstrom et al., 2014).

Foveal suppression areas can be detected by the **binocular status** test on the Mallett near vision unit (Figs. 4.4 & 4.8). This is a Snellen-type letter chart where some letters are seen binocularly (the fusion lock) and others are cross-polarised to be seen monocularly. The test is calibrated for 35 cm (Mallett, 1988a) although, using the approach described later (Tang & Evans, 2006), the test can be used at other viewing distances. If there is suppression, some letters will not be read by the patient.

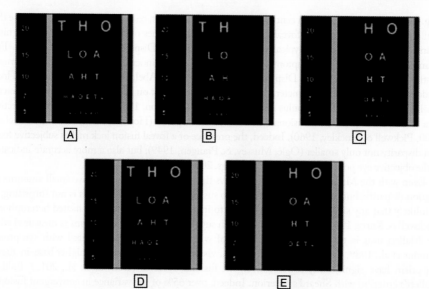

Fig. 4.8 Diagram illustrating the use of the Mallett foveal suppression test. The numbers on the left-hand side of the test represent the acuity in minutes of arc ('). It is recommended that the patient is only shown the test whilst wearing the polarised filter, when (depending on the orientation of the polarisers) the right eye sees the image in (B) and the left eye the image in (C). If, for example, a patient reports seeing the letters illustrated in (D), under binocular conditions the left eye has an acuity of 10′ compared with 5′ for the right eye. The poorer acuity in the left eye might result from a monocular factor (e.g., refractive error) or a binocular sensory adaptation (e.g., foveal suppression). If, whilst the polarised filter is still worn, the better eye (right in this example) is covered, then the best acuity of the left eye under monocular conditions can be determined. In the example, the patient sees the letters illustrated in (E), so the patient has one line of foveal suppression in the left eye and an acuity of 5′ in the right eye and 7′ in the left eye.

Fig. 4.8 details a recommended method of using this test, and this approach was researched by Tang and Evans (2007). This method is based on an intrasubject comparison of the performance at the test under dichoptic but binocularly fused conditions and under monocular conditions. A key component of the test procedure is that the polarised visor is worn for both conditions and the patient should not view the test without the visor in place. Tang and Evans (2007) produced the recommended method of use outlined in Table 4.6. These authors noted limitations of the test, most notably the small number of optotypes on each line, and they found that abnormal results at the test do not invariably indicate the presence of binocular vision anomalies. However, they felt that the test can provide useful information when the results are taken in the context of other clinical tests.

STEREOTESTS

The value of stereoscopic tests (stereotests) in routine examination is twofold. First, they help establish that binocular vision is present and to assess its quality. When a heterophoria is decompensated or is associated with central suppression or amblyopia, the stereoscopic perception may be reduced (Rutstein, Fuhr, & Schaafsma, 1994). The second use is to assess the ability to undertake visual tasks requiring good depth perception. For example, reduced stereoacuity in conjunction with poor visual acuity has been linked to an increased risk of road accidents in older people (Gresset & Meyer, 1994).

TABLE 4.6 ■ **Recommended Method of Use of the Mallett Foveal Suppression (FS) Test. Suggested instructions to the patient are given in the right-hand column.**

Step	Description	Patient instructions
1	The polarising visor is worn by the patient over any refractive correction that is usually worn at near. If the prescribing of a new, significantly different, refractive correction is contemplated, the test can be repeated to investigate the effect of this proposed correction on FS.	
2	The Mallett unit is held at their normal viewing distance and the patient is shown the FS test.	
3	Have the patient read down the chart, continuing until none are seen or all responses are errors. Record the letters seen under these dichoptic but binocularly fused conditions.	'Please read the letters from the top to the lowest line you can read'
4	The left eye should then be occluded. The patient should not close their eye under the occluder. Have the patient read down the chart again. Record these polarised letters seen by the right eye.	'Some letters may have changed now, but please read from the top of the chart to the lowest line you can see again'
5	This is then repeated whilst occluding the right eye. Record these polarised letters seen by the left eye.	'Some letters may have changed now, but please read from the top of the chart to the lowest line you can see again'
6	The degree of FS is abnormal if the patient reads at least one line further under monocular conditions than under dichoptic conditions.	

From Tang S.T.W., Evans B.J.W. [2007]. The Near Mallett Unit Foveal Suppression Test: a cross-sectional study to establish test norms and relationship with other optometric tests. *Ophthalmic and Physiological Optics*, **27**(1), 31–43.

However, clinical methods of testing stereopsis (Fig. 3.3) do not necessarily relate to everyday visual tasks. Indeed, they do not relate strongly to each other, as other factors influence performance in these tests (Hall, 1982; Simons, 1981). Clinical stereotests, therefore, need to be interpreted with caution in respect to their second function of assessing everyday depth perception.

Many clinical stereotests suffer from a ceiling effect, so that the most challenging level of the test is passed easily by most of the population (Coutant & Westheimer, 1993). Other factors which may limit the usefulness of stereotests, particularly for assessing subtle deficits in heterophoria, are a failure to take account of the time the subject takes to carry out the test (Larson & Faubert, 1992), and poor psychophysical techniques.

DIAGNOSTIC PRISMS

Occasionally, prisms can be used to determine if symptoms are due to a heterophoria (Ansons & Davis, 2001), especially if the symptoms are atypical and the results of tests of decompensation are inconclusive. Prisms can be prescribed as described in Chapter 6 and, if they alleviate symptoms, the other management options considered in Chapter 6 can be considered.

THE SKEFFINGTON MODEL AND BEHAVIOURAL OPTOMETRY

Skeffington founded the Optometric Extension Program in 1928 and his teachings have been followed by a group of clinicians who are sometimes called behavioural optometrists (BOs). Although only a very small proportion of UK optometrists follow this discipline, the Skeffington model of binocular vision (Birnbaum, 1993) is rather different to the conventional view and will be briefly described.

Skeffington stressed the interaction between vision, movement, orientation, language, and information processing and he viewed myopia as an adaptation to stress imposed by near work (Birnbaum, 1994). BOs argue that many patients, despite having healthy eyes, good visual acuity, no refractive problems, and no binocular problems according to conventional criteria (Birnbaum, 1994), nonetheless have some form of visual disability that requires treatment with spectacles or vision therapy. BOs' vision therapy is often very different to conventional eye exercises for orthoptic problems. Training may be for pursuit or saccadic eye movements and might, for example, involve doing convergence exercises whilst a patient jumps on a trampoline. Some BOs prescribe reading glasses or multifocal glasses to a high proportion of children in the belief this will prevent or control the progression of myopia. Another BO approach is to prescribe yoked prisms (e.g., 4Δ base-down each eye), although a study reveals only minor effects on binocular vision and accommodation, at least in the short-term (Schmid et al., 2019). A minority of BOs practice syntonics, where patients view a coloured light source for prolonged periods of time in the belief that this might improve visual fields, academic performance, and myopia (Kaplan, 1983).

Jennings (2000) carried out a detailed and balanced review of BO. He concluded that 'The author finds much of the theory unconvincing and notes the lack of controlled clinical trials of behavioural management strategies.' The healthcare professions have gone through a quiet revolution in the last 50 years in their adoption of the **evidence-based approach**. This is necessary because patients and practitioners are subjective and therefore prone to confounding factors, such as the placebo effect. So, research to investigate treatments should use an objective design (e.g., a randomised controlled trial; RCT). Jennings' (2000) finding, that BO lacks any RCTs, must raise serious doubts over the validity of this approach.

A more recent review (Barrett, 2008) reached broadly similar conclusions. It was critical of the lack of evidence relating to: yoked prisms (unless for neurological disorders and neuro-rehabilitation after trauma/stroke); low plus lenses for near vision stress; vision therapy for myopia control; behavioural approaches to managing strabismus and amblyopia; training central and peripheral awareness; syntonics; and sports vision therapy. Three areas were highlighted where evidence is consistent with claims made by behavioural optometrists: the treatment of convergence insufficiency, and yoked prisms for neurological patients and after brain disease/injury.

However, the Barrett review has been criticised for, amongst other things, making inaccurate statements about BO, omitting significant publications, and applying higher standards to the literature on BO than were applied to conventional approaches such as strabismus surgery (Press, Overton, & Leslie, 2016). It is true that many everyday optometric activities lack the high-level evidence that Barrett complained is lacking concerning BO (Rowe & Evans, 2018), but also noteworthy that the paper by Press and colleagues included as evidence many publications that are highly prone to bias (e.g., retrospective case series, uncontrolled trials). There would appear to be a need for advocates of BO to be more self-critical and for the critics to be more proportionate. Another difficulty is in defining the scope of BO, with Press and co-authors considering perceptual learning to be synonymous with vision therapy.

One of the tenets of BO, that a reduction of near motor visual stress (e.g., with bifocals) will slow the rate of myopia progression, is not generally supported by the literature (p. 101). There have also been criticisms of the over-zealous use of 'vision therapy' to treat people with specific learning difficulties (reviewed by Evans, 2001a) and for enhancing sporting performance (Hazel, 1996;

Wood & Abernethy, 1997). Some elements of BO are similar to the Bates method of ocular treatment (Elliott, 2013), which is practised by individuals who are not eyecare professionals (Cullen & Jacques, 1960).

It is important that the controversy surrounding some vision therapies used within BO does not cause validated eye exercises to be brought into disrepute. As noted in Chapter 10, eye exercises to treat decompensated heterophoria by training fusional reserves have been validated by RCTs.

SUMMARY OF THE DIAGNOSIS OF DECOMPENSATED HETEROPHORIA

The evaluation of heterophoria occurs as the routine eye examination proceeds. It is not usually a process that has to be added on to the routine. The symptoms may cause the practitioner to suspect a decompensated heterophoria, which is one of the most common binocular anomalies. The cover test may further suggest this possibility, and the subjective aspect of binocular examination eventually confirms the diagnosis. There is no single test that will provide a conclusive diagnosis in all cases and a summary of the main factors to be considered is given in Table 4.7.

Several research studies have attempted to determine which tests are most useful in diagnosing decompensated heterophoria. Sheedy and Saladin (1978) studied a group of optometry students who, using rather vague criteria, were classified as symptomatic or asymptomatic. Looking only at the near muscle balance the researchers found that, overall, Sheard's criterion was the best predictor

TABLE 4.7 ■ Summary of Main Factors in Assessing Compensation of Heterophoria.

Factor	Heterophoria more likely to be compensated if:	Heterophoria more likely to be decompensated if:
Symptoms	No symptoms attributable to the phoria	Symptoms (Table 4.1)
Visual aspects of working conditions	No recent changes	Recent changes that may place vision under stress
Cover test	Quick, smooth recovery	Slow or hesitant recovery
Aligning prism on Mallett unit (Mallett criterion)	Less than 1Δ for pre-presbyopes Less than 2Δ for presbyopes	1Δ or more for pre-presbyopes 2Δ or more for presbyopes
Uncorrected clinically significant refractive error	None	Present
Fusional reserve opposing phoria (Sheard's criterion)	Fusional reserve to blur at least twice the phoria	Fusional reserve to blur less than twice the phoria
Balanced fusional reserves (Percival's criterion)[a]	Smallest fusional reserve more than half the largest	Smallest fusional reserve less than half the largest
Vergence facility (near)	15 cpm or worse	Better than 15 cpm
Foveal suppression	Less than one line difference between haploscopic and monocular acuities	At least one line difference between haploscopic and monocular acuities
Stereoacuity	Good	Reduced
Binocular acuity	Better than monocular	Not as good as monocular

[a] Percival's criterion does not work for distance vision because the normal fusional reserves (Appendix 10) do not meet the criterion.

of symptoms. Percival's criterion was also useful for esophores and the fixation disparity and type of fixation disparity curve were useful for exophores. However, Wildsoet and Cameron (1985) showed that the classification of fixation disparity curves into different types is unreliable. The fixation disparity instrument that Sheedy and Saladin used, the Sheedy Disparometer, does not have a foveal fusion lock.

Dalziel (1981) found that 83% of 100 patients who failed Sheard's criterion at near had symptoms, but only about half of those who failed Sheard's criterion had an aligning prism of 1Δ or more on the Mallett unit at near. She did not investigate the relationship between the Mallett aligning prism and symptoms. A double-masked study by Worrell, Hirsch, and Morgan (1971) provided some support for using Sheard's criterion to prescribe prism for distance esophores and near presbyopic exophores, but not for other near exophores or near esophores. A recent RCT did not support prescribing prisms based on Sheard's criterion (Scheiman, Cotter et al., 2005). Another double-masked RCT supported the prescribing of prisms based on the Mallett unit but found that there was little correlation between the prism indicated by the Mallett unit and by Sheard's criterion (Payne et al., 1974). Indeed, these authors noted that 'based on our results, one would not expect to find a significant preference for prism prescribed according to Sheard's criterion.'

Jenkins and colleagues, using a modified Mallett unit, found that neither the measurement of the forced vergence disparity curve nor the dissociated heterophoria were useful tests (Yekta et al., 1989). These researchers showed that the best predictor of symptoms was the aligning prism and, if this was measured on an instrument with a good foveal lock, it is not necessary to measure the angular fixation disparity (Jenkins et al., 1989). This study, which looked at near vision symptoms and horizontal heterophoria in a large clinical population, provided strong support for the use of the Mallett unit (Fig. 4.9). The study showed that, under the age of 40 years, 75% of patients with an aligning prism of 1Δ or more on the Mallett unit had symptoms, whilst only 22% of those without symptoms had such a result. For subjects aged 40 years and over, similar results are obtained if the criterion of 2Δ or over are used.

This work was broadly supported by Pickwell and colleagues (1991), but who found that the best cut-off in pre-presbyopes was 2Δ or more, which was manifested in 30% of patients with near vision symptoms and only 1% of those without symptoms. For presbyopes, the best criterion was

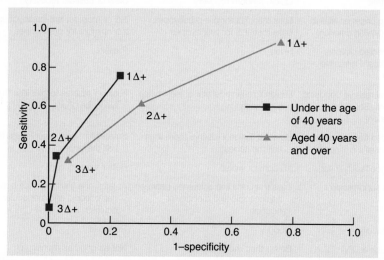

Fig. 4.9 Receiver operator characteristic curve (ROC) of aligning prism for detecting decompensated heterophoria. (Redrawn with permission from Jenkins, T.C.A., Pickwell, L.D., Yekta, A.A. [1989]. Criteria for decompensation in binocular vision. *Ophthalmic and Physiological Optics*, **9**, 121–125.)

3Δ or more which was present in 25% of those with near vision symptoms and only 6% of those without symptoms. This study also looked at the distance vision Mallett fixation disparity test results and symptoms but found no useful relationship. These authors speculated that this may be because of the rarity of distance vision problems (Pickwell et al., 1991).

Another study agreed that the Mallett fixation disparity test is less useful for distance vision than for near (Karania & Evans, 2006b). This research found the precise questions that are asked are important and supported the test method detailed in Fig. 4.5. In particular, it is important to enquire not just whether the Nonius strips are aligned, but also whether they move. These authors demonstrated that people with the highest degrees of aligning prism tend to be those with the most marked symptoms (Fig. 4.10).

The aforementioned research on the Mallett fixation disparity test has been centred on symptoms, which have been shown to be the main factor that optometrists consider when prescribing prisms (O'Leary & Evans, 2003; Shneor et al., 2016). On average, practitioners would consider prescribing a horizontal aligning prism if this was 1.5Δ or more in the presence of symptoms but would not usually prescribe an aligning prism in the absence of symptoms (O'Leary & Evans, 2003). This raises the question of whether there is ever an indication for prescribing prisms in heterophoria in the absence of symptoms, and this was investigated in a double-masked RCT (O'Leary & Evans, 2006). These authors studied the relationship between the near Mallett test aligning prism and speed of reading. For near exophoria, an aligning prism of 2Δ or more was manifested by 67% of participants who showed a significant improvement in visual performance and by only 21% of those who did not. The results were similar for pre-presbyopic and presbyopic exophores, but other types of heterophoria did not exhibit this effect.

The studies described earlier concerning the Mallett aligning prism did not report fusional reserves, so the diagnostic capabilities of the Mallett unit cannot be compared with Sheard's and Percival's criterion. It is quite likely that improved sensitivity and specificity would be obtained by combining these three results. A flow chart summarising the diagnosis of decompensated heterophoria is reproduced in Fig. 4.11 and an algorithm for diagnosing decompensated heterophoria and binocular instability is suggested at the end of the next chapter.

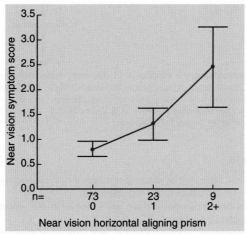

Fig. 4.10 Graph of mean symptom score vs aligning prism (using the testing method in Fig. 4.5) at near. The error bars represent the standard error of the mean (SEM). The number of participants (shown above scale for horizontal axis) is small for higher degrees of aligning prism and this may explain why the SEM increases. (Reproduced with permission from Karania R., Evans B.J. [2006b]. The Mallett Fixation Disparity Test: influence of test instructions & relationship with symptoms. *Ophthalmic and Physiological Optics*, **26**, 507–522.)

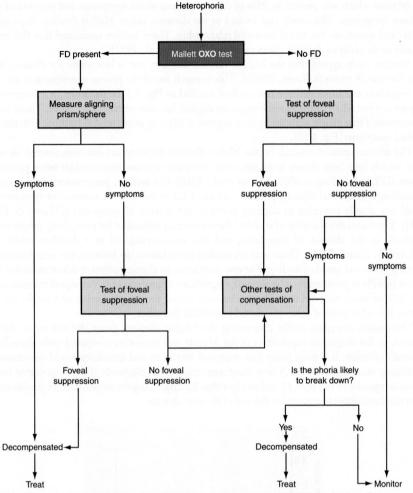

Fig. 4.11   Flow chart summarising the diagnosis of decompensated heterophoria. Symptoms are described in Table 4.1. 'Other tests of compensation' are listed in Table 4.7. (Modified from Evans, B.J.W. [2001b] Decompensated exophoria at near, convergence insufficiency and binocular instability: diagnosis and the development of a new treatment regimen. In B. Evans and S. Doshi (Eds.), *Binocular vision and orthoptics* (pp. 39–49). Oxford: Butterworth-Heinemann.)

CLINICAL KEY POINTS

- Heterophoria requires treatment (is decompensated) if it is causing symptoms, decreased performance, or is likely to deteriorate if left untreated
- A heterophoria can decompensate if there are changes in the working environment, the visual system, or systemic factors
- Symptoms can be nonspecific, and a battery of tests is required to diagnose decompensated heterophoria, including cover test, aligning prism, fusional reserves, and foveal suppression or stereoacuity
- The aligning prism should be assessed with fixation disparity tests that have a good foveal and peripheral fusion lock (e.g., Mallett unit)

CHAPTER 5

Binocular Instability

A heterophoria is compensated when the vergence system can adequately overcome the heterophoria. Yet there are subjects with a negligible heterophoria and whose opposing fusional reserves meet the conventional criteria for compensation discussed in Chapter 4, and yet who have symptoms associated with poor binocular coordination. These patients may be best described by the term **binocular instability**, also known as **fusional vergence dysfunction**.

Binocular instability is characterised by low fusional reserves and an unstable heterophoria. The fusional reserves are usually low in both directions (divergent and convergent), so the fusional amplitude is lower than 20Δ, which is more than 1 standard deviation below normal (Evans et al., 1994). The unstable heterophoria can be detected with a Maddox wing test, but is likely to be more significant if it is present with more naturalistic tests, such as the Mallett fixation disparity test when it will manifest as movement of the Nonius strips. A movement of the arrow in the Maddox wing test of $\pm1\Delta$ is normal, but $\pm2\Delta$ or more is abnormal. Binocular instability may be associated with suppression (possibly, transient) with the Mallett foveal suppression test.

Historical Perspective

Nearly 70 years ago, binocular instability was defined as 'uncertainty in the collaboration of the vision of the two eyes', 'a kind of binocular anarchy' (Cantonnet & Filliozat, 1938). These authors said that the condition was common and often associated with symptoms of asthenopia, blurring, and reversals of letters and numbers. It could be diagnosed using an early precursor of the Maddox wing test (Cantonnet's test of binocular vision), where there was an inability to maintain the arrowhead in a fixed position. Cantonnet stressed that a test for binocular instability should require precise focusing. He looked upon binocular instability as a different condition to the cases of heterophoria and strabismus that required treatment.

Gibson (1947) also considered binocular instability to be a separate entity from strabismus and symptomatic heterophoria. He said binocular instability often caused a maladjustment of letters and numbers, causing complaints of reversals and of the eyes jumping from one line to another when reading. He noted that the condition was sometimes associated with foveal suppression and with anisometropia, unequal acuities, and unequal accommodation. Gibson (1955) stated, binocular instability is often associated with low fusional reserves. He advocated the Turville Infinity Balance test, which was, in this context, a precursor of the Mallett foveal suppression test.

Giles (1960) considered that there were two types of binocular instability. The first, a 'fusion deficiency', was regarded as midway between heterophoria and strabismus. The second was caused by poor general health associated with neurosis, fatigue, debility, or toxaemia. In the latter type, symptoms may be much worse in the evening when the patient is tired.

Mallett (1964) noted that binocular instability was sometimes associated with decompensated heterophoria when there would usually be variation in the amount of prism or sphere required to eliminate a fixation disparity. He advocated his foveal suppression test for detecting suppression in binocular instability, noting that treatment involved correction of refractive error, alleviation of gross decompensated heterophoria, and antisuppression exercises.

More recently, fixation disparity techniques have investigated binocular instability under normal binocular viewing conditions. Jaschinski-Kruza and Schubert-Alshuth (1992) found a range of variability of fixation disparity in different subjects and Cooper et al. (1981) suggested that variability of fixation disparity might be a useful clinical measure. Duwaer (1983) found the stability of fixation disparity to be a useful predictor of symptoms.

Investigation

Binocular instability can co-occur with dyslexia (Evans et al., 1994) and the clinician should always consider this when examining children or adults who report difficulty with reading or spelling. This study found that about 15% of people with dyslexia had a fusional amplitude less than 20Δ, compared with 5% of good readers (Evans, 1991). It seems likely that a test of vergence facility will also detect binocular instability in children with educational difficulties (Dusek, Pierscionek, & McClelland, 2010; Quaid & Simpson, 2013).

It should be noted, however, that nearly all dyslexic people reverse letters and words, probably owing to problems in the higher cortical processes of decoding sequential material stored in short-term memory. Optometrists should not necessarily expect to correct reading difficulties, or even reversals, by treating binocular instability. However, in some cases treatment of binocular instability may help by reducing symptoms and, possibly, by improving the perception of text.

In those with symptoms of asthenopia or perceptual distortions, or in reading disabled children who may be too young to recognise these symptoms, it is advisable to carry out a fixation disparity test even if no movement has been seen on the cover test. When carrying out the fixation disparity test it is not enough to simply ask whether the strips appear to be aligned (Karania & Evans, 2006b). The patient should be asked whether one or both strips ever move (Fig. 4.4). If the patient can discern the movement as being predominantly in one direction, the effect of prisms or spheres can be investigated in the usual way. If there is no aligning prism but there is binocular instability (a movement) on the fixation disparity test, this can be investigated further with the Maddox wing test and by measuring fusional reserves.

DIAGNOSTIC OCCLUSION AND INVESTIGATIVE OCCLUSION

Since the 1920s, it has been suggested that prolonged occlusion (known as 'Marlow occlusion', or diagnostic occlusion) for up to 14 days can be useful in investigating asthenopic symptoms from binocular vision anomalies. It was originally thought that the increase in the deviation that occurred after this time was meaningful, but it is now known that most symptom-free patients show a large increase in horizontal and vertical heterophoria after occlusion (Duke-Elder, 1973; Neikter, 1994a). Diagnostic occlusion has been suggested for cases where symptoms suggest a hyperphoria but one cannot be found on normal testing (Surdacki & Wick, 1991).

An alternative use of occlusion, 'investigative occlusion' can be helpful in rare cases where there are vague signs and symptoms of binocular instability or decompensated heterophoria. In a few cases it can be unclear whether the patient would benefit from treatment of the ocular motor problems, especially when the symptoms have another potential cause, such as sensory visual stress (pp. 64—66) or general fatigue. The patient can be asked to occlude one eye for the tasks when the symptoms occur and report whether this reduces symptoms. If it does help, treatment of the binocular instability is warranted; if not, another cause for the symptoms should be sought.

Caution is necessary, because it is conceivable that investigative occlusion could cause a decompensated heterophoria to break down into a strabismus. This is unlikely, however, and some studies suggest that even prolonged full-time occlusion does not adversely affect ocular motor function (Holmes & Kaz, 1994; Neikter, 1994b). Indeed, it has been suggested that occlusion can be used to treat sensory and motor factors in intermittent exotropia, reducing the frequency of strabismus

(Freeman & Isenberg, 1989; Jin & Son, 1991), possibly because it reduces amblyopia (Santiago, Ing, Kushner, & Rosenbaum, 1999). A randomised controlled trial supports this view, with deterioration of intermittent exotropia in slightly fewer (0.6%) of those undertaking part-time occlusion (3 hours daily) compared with a control group (PEDIG et al., 2014). However, even in the control (observation only) group, only 6.1% deteriorated.

Evaluation

IS BINOCULAR INSTABILITY DIFFERENT FROM DECOMPENSATED HETEROPHORIA?

Decompensated heterophoria and binocular instability are contrasted in Table 5.1. Binocular instability can be present in an orthophoric patient who, by definition, cannot have a decompensated heterophoria. If a patient is orthophoric, they only need negligible fusional reserves to satisfy Sheard's criterion. To take an extreme example, an orthophoric patient with convergent and divergent reserves (to blur and break) of 3Δ and 2Δ respectively, will meet both Sheard's and Percival's criteria. A cover test will not detect any abnormality. In such a case, binocular instability may be detected as a movement of the Nonius strips during the fixation disparity test. The strips may move equally often in either direction, so there is an unstable fixation disparity without there being any aligning prism. Similarly, during the Maddox wing test the arrow may move over a large area, with the mean position orthophoria. Measurement of the fusional reserves would reveal them to be low, confirming the diagnosis of binocular instability.

A patient with a low heterophoria might meet all, or most, of the criteria for their heterophoria being compensated yet still have binocular instability. When binocular instability is combined with a large heterophoria, the heterophoria is likely to be decompensated. Indeed, most patients with a significant aligning prism report some instability of the Nonius strip(s). As the magnitude of the heterophoria increases, the distinction between binocular instability and decompensated heterophoria becomes less clear.

TABLE 5.1 ■ Differential Diagnosis of Binocular Instability and Decompensated Heterophoria.

Sign	Binocular instability	Decompensated heterophoria
Heterophoria	May be present, or may be orthophoric	Heterophoria must be present
Stability of heterophoria	Unstable: movement of arrow in Maddox wing test usually $\pm2\Delta$ or more	May be stable or unstable
Cover test	Recovery may or may not be normal	Recovery usually slow and hesitant
Fusional reserves	Usually both convergent and divergent reserves are low, so fusional amplitude $<20\Delta$. Result may worsen markedly as patient tires	Fusional reserve opposing the heterophoria is usually low. The other fusional reserve may be normal or supra-normal.
Fixation disparity/ aligning prism	One or both Nonius strips move. There may be an aligning prism, or the movement may be similar in both directions	Nonius strips are misaligned; may or may not be moving
Foveal suppression	Often present, likely to be transient, may be alternating	May be present, likely to be constant during binocular viewing, usually unilateral
Correlation with dyslexia: Evans et al. (1994)	Statistically significant association	Not associated with dyslexia

There are both sensory and motor factors that might contribute to difficulties with fusion and lead to binocular instability. Sensory factors include uncorrected refractive errors, anisometropia, aniseikonia, and possibly sensory visual stress.

It is not surprising that motor factors can cause a negligible heterophoria to be associated with symptoms from binocular instability. Julesz (1971) showed that, even when inspecting small targets, vergence errors in excess of 20′ arc occur during saccadic eye movements. For very large saccades (such as when reading, the eyes' return to the beginning of the next line) the vergence error is likely to be greater. Vergence errors of up to 2 degrees also occur during natural vergence eye movements (Cornell, MacDougall, Predebon, & Curthoys, 2003). So, even for an orthophoric patient, significant fusional reserves may be required (both divergent and convergent). Hence, motor demands may result in a significant need for 'vergence in reserve' for patients who are orthophoric or have a low heterophoria.

The distinction between binocular instability and decompensated heterophoria may be an artificial one resulting from the historical way in which we view heterophoria and fusional reserves. The two main methods of assessing fusional reserves (pp. 72–73) are intersubject, comparing values with norms, and intrasubject, comparing the opposing fusional reserve with the heterophoria. The usual intrasubject method (Sheard's criterion) requires that the appropriate fusional reserve is a multiple (2×) of the phoria. If 'P' is the phoria, 'V' is the opposing fusional reserve, and N is the norm for the fusional reserves, then the intersubject method can be summarised as

$$V > N$$

and Sheard's criterion as

$$V > 2P$$

In view of the above argument that orthophoric and low heterophoric patients may need significant fusional reserves, a better arithmetic approach may be

$$V > MP + C$$

where C is a constant minimum amount of vergence that needs to be held in reserve and M is some factor that needs to be multiplied by the heterophoria. This formula would be applied to the opposing fusional reserve; the nonopposing fusional reserve would simply need to exceed C. Hence, for an orthophore, the convergent and divergent reserves would have to exceed C. The author is unaware of any research investigating this hypothesis which must, therefore, remain conjecture at present.

If the above hypothesis is correct, where binocular instability co-exists with a significant heterophoria it may be considered as one aspect of the decompensated heterophoria. In cases where the binocular instability occurs in the absence of a significant heterophoria, it may be appropriate (but inelegant) to consider the binocular instability as a 'decompensating orthophoria'.

Management

If there are sensory factors interfering with fusion, these are likely to be contributing to binocular instability and should be treated. These sensory factors are described in Chapter 4 and may also include significant refractive error. Additionally, sensory visual stress (pp. 64–66) can cause visual perceptual distortions and this unstable perception might impair sensory fusion, which speculatively could be a causal factor in some cases of binocular instability.

Orthoptically, binocular instability can be treated by training the fusional reserves (Chapters 6–8, 10) to exceed the values given in Appendix 10. If binocular instability is caused by poor health,

TABLE 5.2 ■ **Algorithm to Assist in Deciding When to Treat Horizontal Heterophoria and Binocular Instability.**

Sign or symptom	score
Score based on the number of symptoms of decompensated heterophoria (Chapter 4)	+3
Cover test: heterophoria detected	+1
Cover test: absence of rapid and smooth recovery (+1 if quality of recovery 'borderline')	+2
Aligning prism (Mallett): ≥1Δ for under 40 years or ≥2Δ for 40 years and over	+2
Aligning prism (Mallett): <1Δ but unstable	+1
Foveal suppression of one line or more on the Mallett foveal suppression test	+2
If score: ≤3 probably normal, ≥6 treat, 4–5 continue in Table adding to score so far	
Sheard's criterion: failed	+2
Percival's criterion (only use in near vision cases): failed	+1
Dissociated heterophoria unstable so that result is over a range ≥4Δ (i.e., ≥phoria ±2Δ)	+1
Fusional amplitude (divergent break point + convergent break point) <20Δ	+1
If total score: ≤5 unlikely to need treatment, if >5, likely to benefit from treatment	

A patient accumulates a 'score' based on the figures in the right column according to the signs and symptoms listed in the left column. The same procedure should be followed for each working distance.

it can be corrected by using prisms or, if there is adequate accommodation, spheres to correct any aligning prism (Chapter 6).

Summary of the Diagnosis of Decompensated Heterophoria and Binocular Instability

Based on the contents of this and the previous chapter, the algorithm in Table 5.2 is suggested as one approach to the diagnosis of decompensated horizontal heterophoria and binocular instability. This has been used in research studies (Harle & Evans, 2006) and has been shown to be useful at detecting people who are likely to experience symptoms on using 3-D displays (Lambooij et al., 2010). This is reproduced in more detail, as a clinical worksheet, in Appendix 3. When this algorithm is used in clinics or research, it is preferable to complete all tests in the Table and quote the score, which carries more information than summarising the result as pass/fail.

CLINICAL KEY POINTS

- Binocular instability is characterised by an unstable heterophoria and low fusional reserves; the heterophoria may be minimal
- Binocular instability can cause similar symptoms to decompensated heterophoria: asthenopia and visual perceptual distortions
- Binocular instability affects ~15% of people with dyslexia
- Diagnosis, as with decompensated heterophoria, should be made on the basis of a complete clinical picture (Table 5.2)
- Treatment is by correcting significant refractive errors and other impairments to sensory fusion, and fusional reserve exercises

CHAPTER 6

Management of Heterophoria: Basic Principles

Before dealing with the individual heterophoric conditions in the next three chapters, this chapter outlines the basic principles of management. There are two reasons to treat a heterophoria: to alleviate symptoms and to prevent the heterophoria breaking down into a strabismus. It is easier to treat a heterophoria than a strabismus and if a heterophoria breaks down into a strabismus, this can lead to serious problems such as diplopia and amblyopia.

Following the investigation of binocular vision and the total findings to reach a diagnosis, a decision must be made regarding the best course of action to assist the patient: the management of the case. In general, there are five possible lines of action which may help in alleviating symptoms:

1. Remove the cause of decompensation.
2. Refractive correction or modification.
3. Give eye exercises.
4. Prescribe prism relief.
5. Refer to another practitioner.

Although it is logical to consider them in this order, it may be that some are not appropriate or possible in a particular case. Sometimes one course of action is going to comprise the primary or sole treatment of the case. For example, in many cases of decompensated heterophoria, the refractive correction by itself will result in the phoria becoming compensated and no further action will be necessary. In other cases, where there is the possibility of active disease or pathology, or of recent injury, referral will be the first priority and other possibilities may not be pursued until appropriate medical attention has been given.

In the healthcare sciences there are several levels of the type of evidence that may be produced in support of an intervention or treatment (Evans, 1997a). The initial evidence is often in the form of anecdotal clinical observations. These may be supported by open trials (e.g., Dalziel, 1981) but these types of evidence are influenced by the placebo effect. The placebo effect should not be underestimated (Evans, 1997b) and a therapy can only be convincingly proven by double-masked placebo-controlled trials (RCT). In recent years, strong RCT evidence supporting eye exercises to treat convergence insufficiency exophoria syndrome (Chapter 8) has emerged (Chapter 10), but other interventions for decompensated heterophoria still lack a strong evidence base (Rowe & Evans, 2018). If there is an obstacle to fusion, removing that obstacle has face validity. Likewise, providing a patient with optimised vision through refractive correction would seem to be an obviously sensible approach.

Removal of Cause of Decompensation

Consideration must be given to those general factors that put stress on the visual system or on the general well-being of the patient. These factors are discussed in Chapter 4. It will be obvious that all treatments will aim at removing the cause of the decompensation, and therefore the other four options may also contribute to this. However, there are some factors that contribute to binocular anomalies which do not come under the other headings. For example, a patient working long hours at excessively close work in poor illumination will need to give consideration to proper working conditions and should be advised accordingly. In some cases, improving the visual working environment will be all that is required to restore compensation of the heterophoria.

Immediate removal of some of these general factors of decompensation may not be possible, as in some instances of poor general health, in old age, or in some vocations. Greater reliance must then be placed on the other options.

Refractive Correction

The importance of the refractive correction has already been discussed in the section on refraction and visual acuity in Chapter 4. In many cases, decompensated heterophoria and binocular instability become compensated when a refractive correction is given. This may be explained by one or more of the following factors:

1. *Accommodation-convergence relationship.* Uncorrected spherical error may result in an abnormal degree of accommodation. This will be excessive in hypermetropia and, for near vision, it will be less than normal in myopia. Because of the link of accommodation to convergence, this can result in stress on convergence.

   If significant esophoria is found, the practitioner should search carefully for hypermetropia. Significant esophoria in a young patient is an indication for cycloplegia (Table 2.11). Some cases will require multifocal lenses and these types of cases are discussed further in Chapter 7.

   For esophoria with myopia, a myopic correction is required to give clear distance vision, but care must be taken not to give an overcorrection; an undercorrection of 0.50D may be tolerated.

   In cases of decompensated exophoria and myopia, an overcorrection can be considered if the patient's amplitude of accommodation is adequate. The patient should be given the minimum overcorrection ('negative add') for the exophoria to become compensated. The negative add is then gradually reduced over a period of months so that the patient's fusional reserves increasingly compensate for more of the deviation. For exophoric patients with hypermetropia, care must be taken that the correction does not contribute to the phoria becoming decompensated; a partial correction can be considered if this is likely.

2. *Blurring.* If it occurs in one or both eyes, blurring will make binocular vision more difficult. This is particularly important in high astigmatism, and care must be taken to ensure an accurate astigmatic correction. Dwyer and Wick (1995) suggested that the correction of even small refractive errors can dramatically improve binocular function, although other research suggests that this may be unlikely (Ukwade and Bedell, 1993). Dwyer and Wick (1995) argued that, even in low hypermetropia, spectacles might eliminate slight blur and aid the compensation of phorias. It would be interesting for placebo-controlled trials to investigate this hypothesis. In the meantime, this is a matter for professional judgement and reasons for prescribing should be carefully documented in the clinical records (College of Optometrists, 2012).

3. *Anisometropia.* Anisometropia produces interocular differences in blurring. It can be important in making the heterophoria decompensated and in causing binocular instability. This is especially the case in high anisometropia (Chapter 11). In other cases, care must be taken to ensure that the refractive correction is properly balanced, either by a retinoscopic method or subjectively. The methods are described in Chapter 2.

THE EFFECT OF CONTACT LENS WEAR AND REFRACTIVE SURGERY

Theoretically, myopes have to exert more accommodation and convergence when wearing contact lenses than spectacles (Rabbetts, 2007). Research validates this prediction but finds large interindividual variation, with some individuals showing the opposite effect (Hunt, Wolffsohn, & Garcia-Resua, 2006). This is likely to explain why, when myopic children undergo refractive surgery, there is initially (at 1 week and 1 month) a reduction in mean near convergent fusional reserves and then a recovery to normal (Han, Yang, & Hwang, 2014). It also probably explains why, on average, when myopes wear contact lenses the accommodative lag is higher (by about 0.25 to 0.50D) than with spectacles (Jimenez, Martinez-Almeida, Salas, & Ortiz, 2011). These authors speculated that this could contribute to myopia progression.

It is possible that in some cases the improvement in peripheral fusion from the wider field of view with contact lenses improves the binocular status. In practice, if a patient with a binocular vision anomaly is motivated to try contact lenses, it may be sensible to undertake a trial and reassess the ocular motor status when wearing contact lenses.

The fact that hypermetropic spectacles require patients to exert a greater amount of accommodation for near fixation than an emmetrope can exacerbate, or even simulate, a convergence excess type of deviation (Black, 2006). Contact lenses may be helpful in these cases and, as for other issues discussed in this section, the same applies to refractive surgery.

CONDITIONS AMENABLE TO TREATMENT THROUGH REFRACTIVE MODIFICATION

It can be seen from the section above on the accommodation-convergence relationship that, even for an emmetropic patient, a refractive correction can be used to correct a decompensated heterophoria. The principle is to prescribe over-minus or under-plus ('negative add') in exophoria and over-plus or under-minus ('positive add') in esophoria. This form of treatment is sometimes described as refractive modification. The conditions that can be managed using refractive modification are summarised in Table 6.1 and in Chapters 7 and 8.

For a 'negative add' to be effective, the patient must have adequate accommodation and a higher AC/A ratio will make refractive modification more likely to succeed. The only conditions that are not amenable to treatment by refractive modification are cases of esophoria that are producing symptoms with distance vision. This is because, in the absence of latent hypermetropia, there is clearly a limit to how much over-plussing a patient can tolerate before the blur produces problems.

STRENGTH OF EVIDENCE

An understanding of basic physiology of vision provides intuitive support for the approach of providing clear vision and using the accommodative-convergence link to reduce a deviation. However, a narrative review noted a lack of strong evidence (e.g., RCTs) for this approach (Rowe & Evans, 2018). The evidence-based approach indicates that clinicians should integrate the best available

TABLE 6.1 ■ Summary of Refractive Modification as a Treatment for Decompensated Heterophoria.

Condition	Modification to refractive correction
Basic esophoria (problematic esophoria at distance and near)	Maximum plus, bifocals may help at near
Divergence weakness esophoria (problematic esophoria at distance)	Maximum plus at distance
Convergence excess esophoria (problematic esophoria at near)	Bifocals or varifocals
Basic exophoria (problematic exophoria at distance and near)	Over-minus at distance and near
Divergence excess exophoria (problematic exophoria at distance)	Over-minus at distance, maybe bifocals
Convergence weakness exophoria (problematic exophoria at near)	Upside down executive bifocals (p. 122)

external evidence with their own clinical expertise and with the patient's priorities (Rowe & Evans, 2018). Tests, like the Mallett unit, which mimic everyday viewing, are well-suited to investigating whether refractive corrections are likely to improve compensation under natural viewing conditions, as described later. In some cases, glasses can be prescribed as a diagnostic tool (Elliott, 2014), although the clinician should be mindful of the possibility of a placebo effect.

CLINICAL APPROACH TO TREATMENT THROUGH REFRACTIVE MODIFICATION

The clinical technique for this approach is very simple and is summarised in Table 6.2. In most cases, the spherical correction that eliminates any fixation disparity on the Mallett unit, at the relevant distance(s), is determined. The result should be confirmed with a cover test where improved recovery (Table 2.4) indicates the refractive modification is adequate. The required correction is the smallest that will eliminate a slip on the Mallett unit and give good cover test recovery (bearing in mind the effects of tiredness).

This approach, of customising the intervention according to the ocular motor status of the patient, is fundamental to the approach described in this book and would seem to have considerable face validity. Perhaps surprisingly, some authors describe a more generic approach, for example prescribing full cycloplegic plus to every hypermetrope with an esotropia (Wutthiphan, 2005), maximum tolerated over-minus as standard in intermittent exotropia (Bayramlar, Gurturk, Sari, & Karadag, 2016), or 'standard clinical practice' of prescribing +2.50 or +3.00D bifocal power in accommodative esotropia (Whitman, MacNeill, & Hunter, 2016). It seems unlikely that such approaches will be as beneficial as a customised approach, as illustrated in Case Study 6.1.

TABLE 6.2 ■ **Method of Use for Refractive Modification to Treat Decompensated Heterophoria.**

1. Using the Mallett fixation disparity unit (Chapter 4) at the appropriate distance, investigate the minimum refractive modification that is required to bring the Nonius strips into alignment. For example, in exophoria, increase the minus until the strips are aligned.
2. Remove the polarised visor and check the visual acuities at the appropriate distance. In the case of a negative add, this checks that the accommodation is overcoming the minus: negative adds are only appropriate in patients with adequate accommodation.
3. Check the cover test to make sure that the heterophoria recovery movement is adequate (see Chapter 2).
4. Advise that spectacles are to be worn for concentrated visual tasks at the appropriate distance or, if symptoms or the risk of strabismus are severe, constantly.
5. Prescribe the spectacles (or contact lenses), annotating the prescription 'Rx modified as "exercise glasses" to treat decompensated heterophoria'. Explain this to the patient and parent.
6. Advise the patient to return immediately if they have any diplopia or any persistent blurred vision or asthenopia.
7. Check again in 3 months, repeating steps 1–5 and reducing the refractive modification when you can.

CASE STUDY 6.1	**First Appointment (aged 3 years)**

SYMPTOMS & HISTORY

First eye examination. Birth by caesarean but no complications and first year normal. For last year, parents notice right eye occasionally turns in momentarily, about two to three times a week, mostly when eating, not worsening, not linked to any visual tasks. No problems seeing detail at DV or NV, no eye rubbing, no headaches and health good, no medications. Normal performance at pre-school. Family history: nil.

Relevant Clinical Findings
Normal: ocular health, pupil reactions, ocular motility, NPC, Amp. Acc.

Unaided DV (Cardiff):	R 6/9.5	L 6/9.5	B 6/7.5
Unaided NV (Kay):	B 6/12		
'Dry' retinoscopy:	R + 2.00DS	L + 2.00DS	
Stereoacuity (Lang 2):	only 1 picture (car) seen, but star (control target) seen		
Cover test (no Rx):	DV orthophoria	NV 25Δ SOP, Grade 5 recov.	
		(breaks down rapidly to R SOT)	

Follow-up 1 Week Later.

Cover test (no Rx):	DV 25 SOP Grade 5	NV 25Δ SOP, Grade 5 recov.
Cycloplegic retinoscopy:	R + 2.25DS	L + 2.25D
Ophthalmoscopy:	checked through dilated pupils and all normal	

Management. Prescribed full cyclo Rx for constant wear. Explained aim is to try to prevent constant strabismus. No guarantee, and if unsuccessful may develop esotropia and need patching/surgery. Monitor in 2 months, sooner if worsens.

Next Exam (6 months later). Initially, reluctant to wear glasses, now happy and constant wear. Turning eye seen less often, now only when very tired. DV & NV clear and pre-school OK. Findings similar to first appointment, except:

Cover test (Rx):	DV orthophoria	NV 15Δ R SOT

Investigated minimum Add to correct esotropia: + 2.50. Prescribed bifocals.

Subsequent Follow-ups (15 appointments over 10 years). 2 months later, orthophoric with bifocals at DV & NV; 6 months later orthophoric at DV & NV and stereopsis improving. By age 6 years, 6/7.5 in each eye with adult LogMAR chart, orthophoric at DV & NV, stereoacuity 15″, other findings normal. From age 7 years, hypermetropia gradually reducing and Add also reduced, whenever possible for good cover test result and no Mallett aligning prism. At age 9 years, ~ R = L + 1.50 DS Add + 1.50. By age 12 years and age 13 years no Rx required, small (<5Δ) compensated esophoria at near only; good stereoacuity.

Comment. There are two main features in this case.
1. Initial decompensating esophoria that required maximum hypermetropic correction and a near add to prevent esotropia. Constant esotropia was prevented resulting in good stereoacuity and no symptoms to this day.
2. 'Myopic drift', causing the hypermetropia to reduce. At the last appointment (2020), the patient was borderline for becoming myopic. There is an argument for continuing in bifocals to try to prevent/slow myopia progression, but the family are very keen to enjoy no spectacles whilst the child remains asymptomatic.

Amp. Acc, Accommodative amplitude; *B,* both; *D,* dioptre; *DS,* dioptre sphere; *DV,* distance vision; *L,* left; *NPC,* near point of convergence; *NV,* near vision; *R,* right; *Rx,* prescription; *SOP,* esophoria; *SOT,* esotropia.

If bifocals are used with children, the segment should be fitted high, aiming to bisect the pupil. Regular adjustment of the spectacles is necessary as, if they slip down the nose, the bifocal add may become ineffective. An initial follow-up appointment as soon as a month after the spectacles are prescribed may be advisable.

Patients with abnormal binocular vision (Schor & Horner, 1989) and symptoms (Fisher, Ciuffreda, Levine, & Wolf-Kelly, 1987) often do not show the usual adaptation to prisms or refractive corrections, and this may explain why they have a binocular vision anomaly. If a patient does not seem to be responding to treatment by refractive modification then, before increasing the sphere further, it is a sensible precaution to leave the patient with the new correction in place for about 2–3 minutes to ensure that its effectiveness is maintained (North & Henson, 1985).

Some practitioners may be concerned that 'negative adds' might lead to myopia. However, Grosvenor, Perrigin, Perrigin, and Maslivitz (1987) found no convincing evidence that refractive modification influences refractive development over the age of 2 years.

Spectacles designed to treat orthoptic problems by refractive modifications are often described as 'exercise glasses' and this is a useful metaphor. The goal should be to reduce the strength of the overcorrection, if possible, every three or six months. The effect can be conceptualised as slowly increasing the fusional reserves by gradually reducing the strength of the overcorrection. At each appointment, the usual tests of compensation (Chapter 4) are repeated with the proposed new refractive correction, and the minimum refractive modification to render the heterophoria compensated is prescribed.

In intermittent exotropia, minus lens therapy improved the quality of fusion in 46% of cases (Caltrider & Jampolsky, 1983). These authors cautioned that cases with high AC/A ratios could develop an esotropia, which required discontinuation of this treatment. They recommend the first check 3–4 weeks after prescribing. The duration of treatment ranged from 2 months to 13 years with a median of 18 months. They concluded 'We have been impressed by the long-term success in control of the exodeviation after removal of the minus lenses'.

MYOPIA CONTROL

It is sometimes argued that prescribing young myopic or pre-myopic patients with multifocal lenses or low plus reading glasses might reduce the rate of myopic progression (Press, 2000). However, research shows that the effect of multifocal spectacles at controlling myopia is minimal, although modest effects have been achieved in some studies of children with near esophoria (Wildsoet et al., 2019). It has been argued that individually prescribed additions may be more effective (Press, 2000), although there is no universal agreement regarding the criteria for prescribing an addition (Fulk, Cyert, & Parker, 2000). If a child has a symptomatic near esophoria and a myopic shift in prescription, multifocal spectacles would be expected to alleviate symptoms from the esophoria and may have some effect at slowing the progression of myopia. Multifocal contact lenses of a centre-distance design or orthokeratology are likely to have a greater effect at slowing myopia progression (Wildsoet et al., 2019), and might also have some effect at normalising the heterophoria (Kang et al., 2018).

Possible mechanisms for the effect of multifocals at slowing myopia progression have been discussed by several authors (Goss & Rosenfield, 1998; Gwiazda, Grice, & Thorn, 1999). It was noted on p. 68 that myopia onset can be preceded by increases in the AC/A ratio and accommodative lag and if these findings are relevant to myopia progression, they may play a role in the benefit from multifocals in some cases. Binocular and accommodative functions may therefore be one factor in the onset and progression of myopia (Kang et al., 2018; Gifford, Gifford, Hendicott, & Schmid, 2020), but other factors including relative peripheral hyperopic defocus are also known to be relevant in this multifactorial condition (Wildsoet et al., 2019).

Eye Exercises (Vision Therapy)

Usually, the effect of correcting any significant refractive errors on the heterophoria is assessed before eye exercises are considered. The patient is asked to wear any significant refractive correction for about 1 month to see if this will alleviate the symptoms. If there is a negligible refractive error, eye exercises may be considered immediately.

In general, decompensated heterophoria responds well to eye exercises although the response varies from one case to another. Suitable exercises are discussed in Chapter 10. Specific types of heterophoria are discussed in the next three chapters, which indicate the conditions likely to respond to exercises. In brief, exophoria responds best to exercises and hyperphoria is least likely to respond.

Although some authors argue that eye exercises are harder for older patients (Winn, Gilmartin, Sculfor, & Bamford, 1994), they can be effective although further follow-up exercises are quite often necessary (Wick, 1977). Pickwell and Jenkins reported successful results in 100 cases aged 11−19 years who were treated with eye exercises (Pickwell & Jenkins, 1982).

Another factor influencing the success of eye exercises is patient motivation. Where the symptoms are marked, the incentive will usually be high. In conditions where suppression has intervened to lessen the symptoms, the disturbance to binocular vision may be marked, but there may be less incentive for the patient to carry out exercises. Teenage patients may have a great deal of schoolwork and a broad range of other interests competing for their time. Some patients will readily undertake exercises and conscientiously carry them out to the end. Others start enthusiastically but prove to have insufficient patience to complete the course. The practitioner's enthusiasm, however, may prove infectious and regular follow-up appointments can help to encourage compliance.

It is important to understand the nature of eye exercises. Eye exercises are a learning process, in the same way as other motor skills are learned. There are many motor skills which we may require during life. They vary from such things as learning to ride a bicycle to touch-typing. They require practice until the motor and sensory systems are coordinated to undertake them automatically (automaticity). At first, a good deal of thought and concentration is required, but in time they become 'conditioned reflexes'. Exercises involve re-educating the visual reflexes and acquiring proper visual habits. Eye exercises are not concerned with strengthening the power of the individual eye muscles, but re-establishing correct muscle and sensory coordination. Both the fast and slow vergence mechanisms seem to be improved by eye exercises for convergence insufficiency (Brautaset & Jennings, 2006a).

The conventional view that exercises increase the fusional reserves without affecting the size of the heterophoria has been questioned (Jennings, 2001a). This is because research on prism adaptation suggests that exercises may also reduce the heterophoria by enhancing the ability to adapt to prisms (North & Henson, 1982). This view is supported by research which showed that convergent fusional reserve exercises not only increased convergent fusional reserves, but also significantly reduced exophoria (Evans, 2000).

Early evidence suggested that eye exercises for decompensated exophoria might increase the AC/A ratio, although the effect regressed within a year (Flom, 1960). Other research indicates no change in AC/A ratio after eye exercises for convergence insufficiency (Brautaset & Jennings, 2006a).

The patient must be able to understand what is required, and the exercises should be explained simply enough to be understood. The patient does not need to understand the exact nature of the binocular anomaly, only what he or she is required to do. However, it usually helps in maintaining interest and cooperation if the broad aims of the treatment can be explained.

The exact type of eye exercises that may be given will vary with the type of heterophoria, and this is discussed in Chapters 7−9. Specific types of exercises are discussed in detail in Chapter 10.

The literature on the efficacy of fusional reserve exercises is discussed in more detail in Chapter 10. This chapter also discusses the different types of exercises and the features of exercises that are likely to improve their efficacy. A general rule is that intensive exercises for 2−4 months are much more likely to be successful than many months of infrequent exercises (Evans, 2001b; Jennings, 2001a).

Prism Relief

Where eye exercises are inappropriate because of age or ill health, or due to lack of time or incentive on the part of the patient, prism relief may be considered. As mentioned above, some heterophoric conditions are unlikely to respond to exercises (e.g., hyperphoria), and relieving prisms are more appropriate. The prism direction that is required allows the eyes to adopt a position that reflects the type of heterophoria (Fig. 6.1). This is an important point: the prism is not a treatment but provides relief (Appendix 1).

The power of the prism to be prescribed is the minimum which just allows the heterophoria to become compensated, sometimes described as the uncompensated portion of the heterophoria. This is invariably less than the degree of the phoria measured by a dissociation method. It is more likely to be the degree of the aligning prism (Lyons, 1966). Indeed, the Mallett fixation disparity test (Chapter 4) is designed to give an adequate fusional lock, so the weakest prism which neutralises the fixation disparity is the appropriate prism to incorporate in the prescription (Mallett, 1966). The method of this approach is summarised in Table 6.3.

A small double-masked RCT showed that prisms prescribed with the Mallett unit were consistently preferred by patients to spectacles without prism (Payne et al., 1974). The authors

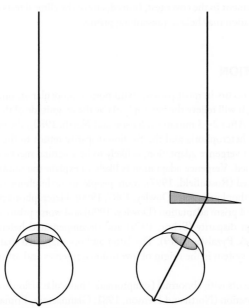

Fig. 6.1   Diagram illustrating the required prism direction. In the example, the patient has an exophoria so relief for the heterophoria is provided using a prism (base-in) which allows the eyes to adopt a more divergent position.

TABLE 6.3 ■ **Method of Use of Prismatic Correction for Decompensated Heterophoria.**

1. Using the Mallett fixation disparity unit (see Chapter 4) at the appropriate distance, investigate the minimum prismatic correction modification that is required to bring the polarised strips into alignment. For example, in exophoria increase the base-in until the strips are aligned.
2. Have the patient read a couple of lines of text through the lenses to stabilise their binocular vision. Then check the cover test to make sure that the recovery movement is adequate (see Chapter 2).
3. Patients with abnormal binocular vision usually do not adapt to prisms, but this can be checked by repeating steps 1–2 after the patient has read for about 3 minutes (p. 104).

commented 'Based on our results, one would not expect to find a significant preference for prism prescribed according to Sheard's criterion'. It is therefore not surprising that RCTs of prisms prescribed based on Sheard's criterion are equivocal, as summarised below.

An RCT of prism for convergence insufficiency exophoria (CIES), which used prisms prescribed by Sheard's method, produced negative results (Scheiman, Cotter et al., 2005). Another study of prisms prescribed based on Sheard's criterion found that these significantly reduced symptoms in CIES (Nabovati, Kamali, Mirzajani, Jafarzadehpur, & Khabazkhoob, 2020). An RCT of low-power base-in prism for decompensated near exophoria showed a marked reduction in symptoms with the prism compared to placebo (Teitelbaum, Pang, & Krall, 2009). An RCT of the immediate effect of the Mallett prism on the speed of reading showed a significant benefit when the prism required was 2Δ or more (O'Leary & Evans, 2006).

When prescribing, Mallett recommended the prism should be given to the eye with the fixation disparity, or split between the two eyes when over 3Δ, with the eye with the disparity receiving a stronger prism (Mallett, 1964).

The prism power can also be assessed by finding the weakest prism which produces a quick and smooth recovery movement to the cover test. Indeed, any of the clinical tests described in Chapter 4 for assessing compensation may help in prescribing prisms.

PRISM ADAPTATION

Adaptation to prisms occurs in most patients with normal binocular vision. When a prism is first placed before the eyes, it will relieve the heterophoria by the magnitude of the prism, and also lessen any fixation disparity. After 2—3 minutes (Henson and North, 1980), the binocular system adapts to the prism, and the heterophoria and the fixation disparity return to the original value (Carter, 1963, 1965). Prism, or vergence adaptation, is likely to be a natural mechanism to keep the visual axes comfortably aligned. Vergence adaptation is likely to explain the finding that heterophoria is not normally distributed (Rosenfield, 1997): more people are orthophoric than would be expected to occur by chance ('orthophorisation'; Dowley, 1987, 1990). Heterophoria probably occurs because of a partial saturation of prism adaptation (Dowley, 1990) and worse prism adaptation is associated with increased fixation disparity (Schor, 1979) and decompensated heterophoria (Przekoracka-Krawczyk, Michalak, & Pyzalska, 2019). The latter authors suggested that an impairment in the slow vergence control system is the origin of low fusional reserves and asthenopia with prolonged viewing.

It appears that patients with abnormal (symptomatic) binocular vision are characterised by poor prism (vergence) adaptation (North and Henson, 1981; Giannaccare, Primavera, & Fresina, 2018) and poor accommodative adaptation (Schor & Horner, 1989). Abnormal vergence adaptation is found in convergence insufficiency and also affects horizontal fusional reserves (convergence and divergence) at other distances (Brautaset & Jennings, 2005a), but not vertical vergence (Brautaset & Jennings, 2005b). Some patients with abnormal adaptation to prisms show an improvement to normal prism adaptation after eye exercises (North & Henson, 1982, 1992). Prism adaptation decreases linearly with age, which may be why older patients do slightly less well with exercises but often respond well to the prescribing of prisms (Winn et al., 1994).

Carter commented that practitioners should only be wary where there are repeated increases in prism (Carter, 1963). In such cases, before increasing the prism further it is a sensible precaution to briefly try the proposed new prism in a **pre-prescribing prism adaptation test**. This term has been used to differentiate this brief test from the more prolonged presurgical prism adaptation test, described at the end of Chapter 17. Research suggests that patients who adapt will show significant signs of this after as little as 2 minutes (North and Henson, 1981, 1982), although some authors have recommended longer (Rosenfield, Chun, & Fischer, 1997). The deviation should then be reassessed to check that adaptation has not occurred (Rosenfield, 1997). If most of the original deviation has returned, the prismatic correction is unlikely to be successful and another mode of treatment should be used. This test is not usually necessary but might be useful in a case where the practitioner is considering prescribing prisms but the patient reports that these have not helped in the past.

Referral

Under some circumstances, a patient must be referred, or a report sent to another practitioner. It is important to be guided in this decision not only by the law or local guidelines, but also by what is in the best interests of each patient. Patients should be referred if:

1. There is a factor contributing to the decompensation of the heterophoria or binocular instability which requires attention by another practitioner: for example, the patient's health may have deteriorated, causing the decompensation.
2. The cause of the binocular anomaly is suspected to be pathological or recent trauma.
3. The binocular anomaly is unlikely to respond, or has not responded, to any of the approaches described in this chapter.

All practitioners need to appreciate the limitations to their own field of expertise, experience, and competence, and to refer appropriately is in their own interest as well as that of the patient.

Summary

The management of heterophoria consists of identifying factors contributing to the decompensation and removing as many of these as possible. In many cases, the correction of the refractive error will achieve this end. Sometimes it is necessary to improve binocular functions by refractive modification, eye exercises, or prism relief. If the patient is suffering from more general stress or poor health, referral to an appropriate practitioner may be required.

Often, symptoms due to heterophoria can be said to be the result of some change in the patient's circumstances which has contributed to stress on the binocular vision; for example, additional close work, or poor health. This change is likely to be recent: long-standing problems either have developed suppression of one eye to alleviate the symptoms or the patient will have been aware of the problem over a long time. Recent changes in the patient's circumstances are easier to identify and the heterophoria can be managed by one of the five lines of action described in this chapter.

CLINICAL KEY POINTS

- Regularly check for active pathology
- Clear retinal images aid fusion, so correct significant refractive errors
- Removing the cause of decompensation, including refractive corrections and changes to the workplace, often eliminates the need for treatment
- Modifying the refractive correction can be an effective treatment
- Exo-deviations are easiest to treat with eye exercises: hyper deviations are hardest

CHAPTER 7

Esophoric Conditions

Most esophoria is 'accommodative', in that it largely results from excessive accommodation due to uncorrected hypermetropia or prolonged close work. As a result of the accommodation/convergence linkage, the overactive accommodation produces excessive convergence. Some eso-deviations do not have this accommodative factor and are then known as 'nonaccommodative' or sometimes as anatomical esophoria.

Esophoria can be classified (Duane-White classification) according to whether the esophoria is greater for distance or for near vision, or if it is the same for both:

1. *Divergence weakness:* shows decompensated esophoria for distance vision. In near vision, the heterophoria will be smaller and compensated.
2. *Convergence excess:* characterised by an increase in the degree of esophoria for near vision. There is usually a small degree of compensated heterophoria for distance vision, and a higher degree of esophoria which is decompensated for near vision. This is in contrast to the normal physiological exophoria.
3. *Basic (or mixed or nonspecific) type:* shows decompensated esophoria of about the same degree in distance and in near vision. The methods of investigation and management that apply to both divergence weakness esophoria and to convergence excess esophoria will apply to basic esophoria. A separate section on basic esophoria is therefore not included.

Divergence Weakness Esophoria

AETIOLOGY

Uncorrected Hypermetropia

This is the most common cause for decompensated esophoria in distance vision. It is usually decreased by the refractive correction to the extent that it becomes compensated.

Anatomical Factors

Factors such as abnormal orbital shape, lengths of check ligaments, muscles insertions, etc., are thought to contribute to esophoria in some patients. There is no evidence to show that these change in adult life, except after injury. If esophoria becomes decompensated, therefore, it is because other factors have intervened: poor health, deteriorated working conditions, etc. The anatomical factors may, however, explain why some patients have a predisposition for their esophoria to decompensate.

Excitable or 'Neurotic' Temperaments

The esophoria in these cases may be variable with the emotional state and level of anxiety, being compensated one day and decompensated the next. It may be aggravated by stimulants.

Pathology

Patients with uncontrolled HIV/AIDS have more esophoria/less exophoria at distance and near than a control group (Espana-Gregori, Montes-Mico, Bueno-Gimeno, Diaz-Llopi, & Menezo-Rozalen, 2001) and may therefore be more likely to suffer from decompensated esophoria.

Pathological disturbances, particularly those affecting the central nervous system, can cause incomitant esophoria which will tend to break down into strabismus in one direction of gaze. A retrospective study found a high correlation between adult onset distance esophoria or esotropia and cerebellar disease (Hufner et al., 2015). It is important to detect lateral rectus palsy, which causes an eso-deviation which is worse for distance vision and when the patient looks to the side of the affected muscle (Chapter 17).

INVESTIGATION

A routine examination of the eye and vision is carried out in each case. In this type of esophoria, particular attention can be given to the undermentioned factors:

1. *Symptoms,* usually associated with distance vision and with prolonged use of the eyes. Symptoms will usually be less or absent in the morning, except headaches which may occur on the day after prolonged use of the eyes (Rabbetts, 2007). The symptoms are likely to be headaches in the frontal area, sometimes intermittent diplopia and blurred near vision if uncorrected hypermetropia is present.
2. *Refraction,* which is very important because of the association with uncorrected hypermetropia. In young patients, significant esophoria is an indication for cycloplegia (Table 2.11).
3. *Decompensation tests,* which will be the most important aspect in the investigation and are fully described in Chapter 4. Measurement of the heterophoria by the cover test or subjective dissociation tests will show a higher degree for distance than for near vision.

MANAGEMENT

Removal of Cause of Decompensation

The factors likely to put stress on the visual system or on the general well-being of the patient should be considered (Chapter 4). Consider particularly the patient's visual working conditions in this type of esophoria.

Refractive Correction

Significant hypermetropia should be corrected and, in many cases, no other form of treatment is required. To encourage emmetropisation in young children (Hung et al., 1995), it is advisable to give the weakest correction that renders the esophoria compensated and which provides good visual acuities. Some patients will require the full refractive correction to prevent decompensation. In children and young adults, a cycloplegic refraction is necessary if variable refractive findings make it difficult to assess the refractive error or if latent hypermetropia is suspected.

Patients should be asked to wear the correction constantly for distance and near vision for about a month, and then tests for compensation repeated if symptoms persist. Where the spectacles or contact lenses resolve the symptoms and the esophoria becomes compensated, the refractive correction should continue to be worn.

In some cases, the esophoria is not changed by a hypermetropic correction or there is found to be no refractive error: the esophoria is nonaccommodative. Consideration should then be given to eye exercises or relieving prisms. Occasionally, myopes have decompensated esophoria for distance vision and in young patients the possibility of latent hypermetropia should be excluded with cycloplegia.

Eye Exercises

If the decompensation of divergence weakness type esophoria persists after consideration has been given to the general decompensating factors and the refractive correction, exercises may be considered.

Teaching an appreciation of physiological diplopia has been found to be useful in this condition (Pickwell & Jenkins, 1982). The patient is asked to look at a small isolated object (not easily confused with background details) at a distance of 3—6 m. A second object, such as a pencil, is held on the median line at about 40 cm from the eyes. The patient is encouraged to notice that this second object is seen in physiological diplopia, providing fixation is maintained on the distance one. When this has been appreciated, fixation is changed to the near object, and physiological diplopia of the distance one is observed. The patient is then encouraged to alternate between fixating the distance object with crossed physiological diplopia of the near one, and fixating the near object with uncrossed physiological diplopia of the distant one. A pause of several seconds must be made with each change of fixation, or confusion results. This exercise in vergence coordination seems to be particularly helpful in young patients. This is a useful first stage in treatment, followed by exercises to increase the divergent amplitude of fusional reserves (the negative fusional reserve) and/or the positive relative accommodation. A range of suitable exercises is described in Chapter 10.

Relieving Prisms

Prism relief in esophoria is required only for a minority of cases. The symptoms in most cases are relieved by refractive correction or by eye exercises. Prisms may be considered when eye exercises have been tried and found not to be successful, or where it is inappropriate because of the patient's age, poor health, unwillingness, or inability to give the time required. The power of the prism required is that which is likely to make the esophoria compensated, as assessed by the methods described in Chapter 6. In general, it will be the lowest prism power which will give no disparity on the fixation disparity test, and/or a smooth prompt recovery on the cover test.

Referral

This will be the first consideration when a pathological cause is suspected, but it is unlikely that surgery will help in other cases. As noted earlier, lateral rectus underaction should be detected and referred (Chapter 17).

Convergence Excess Esophoria

This type of esophoria is low in degree for distance vision but increases for near vision.

AETIOLOGY

Excessive Accommodative Effort

This is usually the main factor, and may be caused by uncorrected hypermetropia, latent hypermetropia, early presbyopia, spasm of the near triad or of accommodation, or by pseudo-myopia. Another cause is prolonged work at an excessively close working distance.

High AC/A Ratio

The accommodative convergence/accommodation, or AC/A, ratio is often a factor in producing convergence excess esophoria. The ratio is a measure of the effect of a change in accommodation on the convergence and is expressed as the change in convergence (Δ) for each dioptre change in accommodation (pp. 42—43). This is normally about $4\Delta/D$ (Appendix 10) and when it is high (over ~6), accommodation for near vision will result in an excess of convergence. Convergence excess rarely occurs with a low AC/A ratio.

Visual Conversion Reaction (pp. 18–19)

Convergence excess can also be present as a visual conversion reaction. This typically occurs in young energetic patients, often accompanied by some psychological stress or anxiety; for example, school examination pressures or relationship difficulties.

Incipient Presbyopia

This can occasionally result in convergence excess, due to the high ciliary muscle effort required to produce adequate accommodation.

Excessive Proximal Convergence

Of the three main cues that cause convergence during near vision (proximity, disparity, and accommodation; p. 3) the proximal cue is the most powerful (Joubert & Bedell, 1990; North, Henson, & Smith, 1993). The magnitude of the proximal cue varies between individuals and it is quite likely that a convergence excess esophoria that is not caused by any of the previously listed causes will result from excessive proximal convergence.

INVESTIGATION

Each case of convergence excess esophoria will require a full routine eye examination and probably a cycloplegic refraction. Particular attention should be given to the following factors:

1. *Symptoms* are usually associated with prolonged use of the eyes in near vision. Sometimes they are so severe as to render close work impossible for more than short periods. Frontal headache, ocular fatigue, and blurred near vision are usual symptoms. Sometimes difficulty is experienced in refocusing the eyes for distance vision after sustained close work.

2. *Refraction*, which may show variable and unreliable results. It may be seen during retinoscopy: neutralisation appearing at one moment and 'with' or 'against' movement the next, without any trial lens change. This is a sign of variable accommodation and may indicate the presence of latent hypermetropia. Another sign of latent error is markedly lower hypermetropia by subjective refraction than that shown in retinoscopy. These are clear indications that a cycloplegic refraction is required to reveal any latent error or spasm of accommodation that may accompany convergence excess esophoria (Table 2.11). Occasionally, the spasm is such that pseudo-myopia occurs (pp. 35–36). This is usually of low degree, but can be as high as 10 D. Where myopia occurs in a young patient with high esophoria, the possibility of spasm should be explored by cycloplegic examination.

3. *A gradient test* gives useful information in convergence excess. It is one way of measuring the AC/A ratio, and is described on p. 42.

4. *A cover test and fixation disparity test* for near vision, which will indicate decompensation of the heterophoria at near (Chapter 4).

5. *Fusional reserves*, especially at near.

6. *Amplitude of accommodation* is relevant for detecting decompensating near esophoria resulting from 'pseudo-accommodative insufficiency' (pp. 32, 35–36).

MANAGEMENT

Removal of Cause of Decompensation

It may be necessary to restrict the patient's close work and/or to increase the working distance. In many cases of convergence excess, the working distance has become unnecessarily close, due to bad visual habits. Patients acquire the habit of working excessively close during childhood, when the amplitude of accommodation was sufficient to permit this without symptoms. On reaching an age when the amplitude is reduced, the working distance causes motor visual stress and becomes the cause of convergence excess. The onset will vary with the amount of close work and the working distance, as well as with the degree of uncorrected refractive error. It may also be brought on by a marked increase in the amount of close work; for example, due to an approaching school examination period, a particularly engrossing computer game, or leaving school for an office job with longer hours of sustained near vision.

In some cases, changing the visual habits to require the patient to employ a more appropriate working distance will resolve the symptoms with no other treatment. A distance of 35—40 cm should be regarded as a minimum and with modern computer use in offices this is usually achievable. It is not always easy for patients to acquire new visual habits when the concentration is on the job in hand. It may be necessary for them to ask someone else to keep reminding them of the required working distance.

Refractive Correction

As noted earlier in this chapter, the minimum correction required to render the esophoria compensated and to allow clear and comfortable vision should be prescribed. Some cases require the full hypermetropic correction, which may initially blur distance vision. If it does not clear after a few days, a cycloplegic can be instilled to help the patient adjust to the glasses. As noted on pp. 97—98, contact lenses should induce less accommodative convergence than spectacles.

In any case, the patient should be seen again after wearing the correction for a few weeks, and the symptoms and decompensation reassessed. If the symptoms have cleared, the correction should continue to be worn for reading and other close work, as required to maintain relief of the symptoms. In cases of high hypermetropia, this may involve continued constant wear.

Multifocals, with a reading addition that relieves the decompensation of the esophoria for near vision, are sometimes prescribed (Case Study 7.1). The addition can be found with the gradient test method, or by adding positive spheres until the cover test and fixation disparity test indicate compensation. This approach to convergence excess is seldom necessary in patients over the age of 14 years. The bifocal design should be large and set with the segment top at the same height as the pupil centre (Chapter 14). Where convergence excess occurs in incipient presbyopia, reading glasses or multifocals are prescribed.

CASE STUDY 7.1	First Appointment (Aged 9 Years)

SYMPTOMS & HISTORY
First eye examination. For 2 months, patient reporting diplopia and mother noticed patient closing one eye, not sure if worse for distance or near or how often. No strabismus observed. Distance (D) and near (N) vision clear. Headaches for the last 2 months with concentrated D & N, once or twice a week. General health good and no medication. Family history of myopia.

RELEVANT CLINICAL FINDINGS
Normal: ocular health, pupil reactions, 25 degree fields, NPC, Ishihara.
Ocular motility: full, smooth, no diplopia.

Distance unaided vision	R 6/15-	L 6/24
'Dry' retinoscopy:	R −0.50/−0.25 × 180	L −1.00DS
Subjective:	R −0.75/−0.25 × 25 6/6+	L −1.25DS 6/6+
Cover test:	D orthophoria	N 8Δ SOP, Grade 2 recov.
Mallett aligning prism:	D nil	N unstable, variable eso-slip
Dissociation tests:	D 4Δ eso	N 10Δ eso; nil vertical

Fusional reserves not measurable as immediate diplopia
Amplitude of accommodation: R = L = 14.00D
Stereoacuity: Randot 2 shapes 250″, circles 30″
[above BV tests with no Rx]
AC/A ratio: 14Δ/D.

N cover test with subjective: 10Δ SOP, Grade 3 recovery,
                                        needs +1.25 add for ortho
                                        when FD aligned & stable.
Cycloplegic refraction: R −0.50/−0.50 × 15 6/7.5   L −1.50DS 6/6−2

MANAGEMENT
Explained myopia, large AC/A ratio, decompensated N SOP with binocular instability. Prescribed bifocals:
                                    R −0.75/−0.25 × 25   L −1.25DS Add +1.25

FOLLOW-UP (3 MONTHS)
Patient voluntarily wears glasses in class, television, near vision. Reports vision is better with glasses
and no longer experiences diplopia or headaches or closes one eye. Rx stable, cover test and FD well-
compensated with glasses.

FOLLOW-UP (OVER NEXT 12 YEARS)
Myopia stable for 2 years, then gradually progressed. N SOP and FD reduced and not keen on myopia
control, so Add reduced until single vision aged 11 years and since.

COMMENT
MEM retinoscopy would have been useful at the first appointment. Although the binocular status
improved, continuing in bifocals (ideally, centre distance contact lenses) may have slowed the myopia
progression which reached −4D in 2016.

BV, Binocular vision; DS, dioptre sphere; FD, fixation disparity; L, left; MEM, monocular estimate method;
NPC, near point of convergence; R, right; Rx, prescription; SOP, esophoria.

Sometimes convergence excess breaks down into a strabismus for near vision. In these cases,
bifocals may be appropriate if binocular vision is restored when the patient looks through the segment (Chapter 14). Patients with bifocals should be checked every 3−6 months, with a view to
reducing the addition, when possible. Bifocals are unlikely to be effective if the AC/A ratio is low.

Myopia Control
Accommodative facility and lag are independent predictors of myopia progression (Allen &
O'Leary, 2006), but the link between inaccurate accommodation and myopia progression is found in
progressing myopes, not stable myopes (Abbott, Schmid, & Strang, 1998). Indeed, myopia is often
preceded by increases in AC/A ratio, accommodative lag, and esophoria (p. 101; Case Study 7.1).

The rapidly increasing prevalence of myopia (Flitcroft, 2012) has increased interest in myopia
control, most commonly (in the UK) with optical interventions (Gifford, Richdale et al., 2019).
The least effective of these seems to be multifocal spectacles (typically, bifocals), with greater success from contact lens approaches that create a centre-distance/peripheral-near effect on the cornea
(orthokeratology) or in soft contact lenses. All these interventions seem to achieve greatest success
for patients with a near esophoria (Goss & Grosvenor, 1990; Aller, Laure, & Wildsoet, 2006),
especially when combined with high accommodative lag (Gwiazda et al., 2004).

Eye Exercises
If symptoms persist after the constant wear of any appropriate refractive correction for several weeks,
exercises may be considered, although there is a lack of high-quality evidence from randomised

controlled trials. Exercises that develop the positive relative accommodation are reported to be useful. The aim of such exercises is to encourage accommodation without convergence; pairs of negative spheres increasing in power can be placed before the eyes whilst the patient maintains clear single vision. Additionally, the divergent amplitude of the fusional reserve can be developed. In this case the accommodation is unchanged while the eyes diverge. Details of these exercises are given in Chapter 10. In the case of convergence excess, the exercises will be carried out for near vision.

Relieving Prisms

These can sometimes help in convergence excess, especially when the AC/A ratio is low (e.g., $2\Delta/D$), which is unusual. In Case Study 7.2, the near esophoria could not be fully compensated by the refractive correction determined by cycloplegia and benefitted from additional prism.

CASE STUDY 7.2   **9-Year-Old Boy**

HISTORY
First eye examination. Has passed vision screening checks.

SYMPTOMS
Frequent diplopia, horizontal, at any distance. Slightly blurred vision at distance and near. Difficulty with literacy and numeracy at school. Headaches, about once a week, occurring at any time.

RELEVANT CLINICAL FINDINGS
Normal: ocular health, pupil reactions, NPC.
Ocular motility: no incomitancy, but transient LE convergent spasm.

Distance unaided vision:	R = L = 6/12.	
'Dry' retinoscopy:	R = L = +0.50DS = 6/9	
Cover test:	D orthophoria	N 5△ SOP, Grade 2 recovery.
Mallett aligning prism:	D 1.5△ out RE	N 2△ out RE.
N aligning prism with + 1.00:		N 1△ out each eye
Dissociation tests:	D 4△ out	N 8△ out; nil vertical
AC/A ratio:	3.5△/D.	
Fusional reserves not measurable as immediate diplopia		
Amplitude of accommodation:	R = L = 11.00D	
Stereoacuity:	normal	
Cycloplegic refraction:	R +1.25/−1.00 × 10	L +1.00/−0.50 × 165

MANAGEMENT
Prescribed cyclo correction with 1△ out each eye

FOLLOW-UP (3 MONTHS)
Patient voluntarily wears glasses most of time, diplopia very rare when wearing glasses, headaches reducing. Clinical findings similar, but VA and orthoptic function improved with spectacles.

FOLLOW-UP (12 APPOINTMENTS OVER 15 YEARS)
Prescription gradually reduced, first reducing prisms. By age 13 years no prisms required, by age 20 years no correction required. At age 24 years: asymptomatic, no headaches, no refractive correction required; cover test orthophoric at distance, 6△ SOP at near, no aligning prism.

COMMENT
In some cases, a relatively low refractive correction with prism can be enough to render a heterophoria compensated.

D, Dioptre or distance; *DS,* dioptre sphere; *L,* left; *LE,* left eye; *N,* near; *NPC,* near point of convergence; *R,* right; *RE,* right eye; *SOP,* esophoria; *VA,* visual acuity.

Referral

Medical attention should be sought if pathology is suspected, or appropriate help can be sought where there is psychological stress.

CLINICAL KEY POINTS

- In decompensated esophoria, always suspect hypermetropia. If hypermetropia is not readily apparent in young patients, undertake a cycloplegic refraction. Significant hypermetropia should be corrected
- Sometimes, quite small hypermetropic corrections can have a large effect on symptoms
- In divergence weakness, carefully look for a lateral rectus palsy
- Convergence excess responds well to treatment with multifocals
- Eye exercises appear to be helpful in some cases

CHAPTER 8

Exophoric Conditions

Although it has been shown that divergence is actively stimulated (Breinin, 1957), exophoria appears to be a much more passive condition than esophoria. There are several potential explanations for this: the position of anatomical rest is relatively divergent (Fig. 1.2), divergence has been thought to be a relaxation of convergence associated with a relaxation of accommodation, and the eyes do not diverge beyond parallel in normal vision. High tonic impulses to the abductors do not seem to be considered such a major factor in most exophoria in the way that high muscle tonus of the adductors contribute to esophoria. For near vision, factors that produce excessive convergence in children can even mask a basic exophoric deviation.

Based on the Duane-White classification, exophoria is usually considered under three headings:

1. *Divergence excess exophoria:* a moderate or large distance exophoria, typically sometimes decompensating to a distance intermittent divergent strabismus, with compensated exophoria for near vision.

2. *Convergence insufficiency exophoria:* shows decompensated exophoria for near vision. For distance vision, there is usually a smaller degree of exophoria which is compensated. The condition is typically diagnosed as a syndrome based on symptoms, larger exophoria at near than distance, low convergent fusional reserves, and remote near point of convergence (pp. 118—123).

3. *Basic (or mixed) exophoria:* where the degree of exophoria does not differ significantly with the fixation distance.

Confusingly, the term convergence insufficiency, often abbreviated to CI, is used by some authors to describe convergence insufficiency exophoria (diagnosed in a variety of ways; pp. 118—123) and by other authors to describe isolated findings of a remote near point of convergence (Cacho-Martinez et al., 2010). To avoid confusion, in this book, two different acronyms will be used, CIES for convergence insufficiency exophoria syndrome and NPCI for near point of convergence insufficiency, an isolated finding of a remote near point of convergence.

The differential diagnosis of decompensated exophoria and intermittent exotropia is not always clear, and this is especially so for divergence excess. Typically, patients with this condition fluctuate from good control (no exotropia or symptoms) to no control (distance exotropia). This contrasts with other forms of exophoria and esophoria, where the patient may have symptomatic decompensated heterophoria with no episodes of intermittent strabismus. It is debatable whether intermittent exotropia should be included in this chapter or in the section of Chapter 15 that deals with exotropia. Topics most relevant to heterophoria will be covered in this chapter and those relating most to strabismus in Chapter 15, but both sections should be read in conjunction with each other.

Intermittent exotropia is more likely to be associated with neurological conditions (e.g., developmental delay, cerebral palsy, attention deficit disorder, history of intracranial haemorrhage) if it is of the convergence weakness type rather than the other types listed below (Phillips, Fray, & Brodsky, 2005); although one study did not find an association between attention deficit disorder and convergence insufficiency (Mezer & Wygnanski-Jaffe, 2012).

Divergence Excess

Divergence excess shows a large degree of exophoria for distance vision, which in many cases will be found to break down into a divergent strabismus. For near vision, the heterophoria is less by at least 7Δ (Duane, 1897), and is compensated. Sometimes it is defined as an exo-deviation of 15Δ greater for distance vision than for near. Most patients with divergence excess are female, and the condition commonly presents itself in the mid-teens (Pickwell, 1979b), often as distance intermittent exotropia.

Approximately 10% of patients with intermittent exotropia have amblyopia (Santiago et al., 1999). A long-term follow-up study of intermittent exotropia found that 36% converted to exophoria or orthophoria (Rutstein & Corliss, 2003). Another study found the deviation only resolved in 4%, and more than half had an increase of at least 10Δ within 20 years of their diagnosis (Nusz, Mohney, & Diehl, 2006). In a heterogeneous group of children (aged 3−10 years) with intermittent exotropia (mostly, divergence excess) who were not considered to require surgery and received no treatment over a 3-year period, progression to constant exotropia was uncommon and binocular control, stereoacuity, and magnitude of deviation typically remained stable or improved slightly (Mohney et al., 2019).

Haggerty and colleagues described a grading system for intermittent exotropia (Haggerty, Richardson, Hrisos, Strong, & Clarke, 2004). Consulting room assessment is problematic because the presentation is sometimes highly variable (Hatt et al., 2007), although in approximately two-thirds of children the condition is stable (Buck et al., 2007).

AETIOLOGY

The causes of divergence excess are uncertain (Cooper, 1977). It has been argued that accommodative convergence is the mechanism that maintains ocular alignment (Ahn, Yang, & Hwang, 2012). A different view is that intermittent distance exotropia is controlled by convergence rather than accommodation, with the convergence inducing accommodation via the AC/A link (Horwood & Riddell, 2012). These authors argued that minus lenses help in this condition not because they induce accommodation which induces convergence, but rather the minus lenses allow more controlling convergence to be recruited by correcting any secondary excessive accommodative (pseudomyopia) blur.

True and Simulated Divergence Excess

A distinction has been made between 'true divergence excess' and 'simulated divergence excess' (Burian & von Noorden, 1974). In simulated divergence excess, unilateral occlusion for 30−45 minutes causes an increase in the near deviation revealing a basic exo-deviation, not divergence excess. It seems likely that in these cases, high tonic, accommodative, or proximal convergence obscures the real nature of the deviation for near vision. The high convergence lessens as the patient reaches adulthood, and simulated divergence excess then reveals itself to be a basic exo-deviation. This may be important where surgery is to be considered, but nonsurgical management may be the same for true and simulated divergence excess in the initial stages. In simulated divergence excess, the management may have to be modified as the patient gets older.

Ansons and Davis (2001) further classified the condition, mainly based on the response to occlusion and on the size of the AC/A ratio. Their classification is summarised in Table 8.1.

TABLE 8.1 ■ A Classification of True and Simulated Divergence Excess, According to Ansons and Davis (2001).

Classification	Response of near deviation to occlusion	AC/A ratio
True divergence excess	No significant increase	Normal or low
Simulated with high AC/A ratio	Increases to be similar to distance deviation	High
Simulated with normal AC/A	Increases to be similar to distance deviation	Normal or low

Ansons, A.M., Davis, H. (2001). *Diagnosis and Management of Ocular Motility Disorders.* Oxford: Blackwell Science.

INVESTIGATION

The investigation of divergence excess should follow the routine eye examination, giving particular attention to the following:

1. *Symptoms:* patients with divergence excess do not usually complain of any marked symptoms. If asked, they may report that intermittent diplopia has been present for as long as they can remember, but often there is established suppression and no diplopia. Some patients learn to control the deviation for distance by accommodating and will report blurred vision. The most usual reason given for presenting for eye examination is that their friends and relatives have noticed the divergence of one eye. This deviation becomes apparent with inattention, tiredness, emotional stress, poor health, and alcohol. Bright sunlight is also reported to produce the deviation (Eustace, Weston, & Druby, 1973). Patients may therefore report that they close one eye in bright light. This is more likely to be related to photophobia (Wiggins and von Noorden, 1990) than to avoiding diplopia and confusion (Wang and Chryssanthou, 1988). Intermittent exotropia in children can be a cause of excessive blinking (Coats, Paysse, & Kim, 2001).

2. *Visual acuity:* In intermittent exotropia, worse binocular than monocular visual acuity can be a sign of diminishing fusional control (Ahn et al., 2012).

3. *A cover test,* which may show decompensated exophoria for distance vision, but sometimes this can appear compensated if the patient is exercising a high level of concentration. If the cover test is repeated, or the alternating cover test carried out, the distance vision deviation increases and the exophoria may break down into a divergent strabismus. Cover test recovery can be graded using a general grading system for all types of heterophoria and intermittent heterotropia (Table 2.4) or using a scale specifically developed for intermittent exotropia (Kim et al., 2017). A V-syndrome often accompanies divergence excess (Chapter 17).

   An important diagnostic sign is the deviation increases for true distance vision, that is fixation distances much greater than 6 m. This can be detected by repeating the cover test when the patient looks through a window.

4. *Refractive error,* which in divergence excess is usually either low hypermetropia or myopia (Pickwell, 1979b).

5. *Fusional reserves,* which are usually highly abnormal in that the divergent reserve for distance vision is very high: instead of the average value of 6–9Δ, it may exceed 20Δ. The very divergent position produced by measuring the base-in fusional reserve for distance vision is usually accompanied by suppression. This means that in some cases, when the limit of the divergent amplitude is reached, no diplopia is reported and this may give the appearance of a very much higher amplitude, unless the practitioner watches the patient's eyes to note the point at which the divergence of one eye ceases. The very high divergent fusional reserve for distance vision is a major diagnostic feature.

MANAGEMENT

Removal of Cause of Decompensation

This is not usually possible in divergence excess.

Refractive Correction

Correction of any myopia assists by clearing the blurred distance vision and inducing accommodative convergence. In some cases, a negative distance addition can be used to correct the distance deviation and bifocals may be necessary to prevent excess accommodative convergence at near (Percival, 1928). A prospective trial (nonrandomised) found 52% of patients with divergence excess intermittent exotropia achieve a good outcome with over-minus lenses alone and those who cannot be weaned out of lenses and ultimately require surgery also have a good outcome (Rowe, Noonan, Freeman, & DeBell, 2009). These authors recommend over-minus lenses as the primary treatment and note they do not appear to induce myopia. Another study confirmed over-minus lens therapy for intermittent exotropia does not induce refractive errors (Paula, Ibrahim, Martins, Bicas, & Velasco e Cruz, 2009).

In mild cases of divergence excess, a small adjustment to the prescription may be all that is required to alleviate symptoms. Case Study 8.1 is such a case.

CASE STUDY 8.1	First Appointment (Aged 13 Years)

SYMPTOMS & HISTORY
Previous eye examination with local optometrist 6 months ago. Birth and first year normal; adenoidectomy at age 3 years. Spectacles for myopia since age 9 years, currently wearing MiSight contact lenses most of the time. Referred to the author because for the last 6 months reports transient diplopia with distance vision. Turning eye not seen by parents but noted by optometrist. The diplopia occurs three to four times a day and resolves immediately when the patient concentrates on his vision, but this often leads to a headache. Headaches are two to four times a week and patient believes result from straining to avoid diplopia. Diplopia is slightly less common with contact lenses. School progress good, spends a lot of time playing computer games. General health good and no medication. Family history: grandfather glaucoma and type 2 diabetes.

RELEVANT CLINICAL FINDINGS
Normal: ocular health, pupil reactions, ocular motility, Amp. Acc., 25 degree visual fields, OCT scans, Ishihara.

Spectacles & VA:	R −2.75DS 6/6+	L −2.00/−0.75 × 35 6/6+
		B 6/5
Retinoscopy:	R −2.25/−0.75 × 175	L −2.00/−0.25 × 180
Subjective:	R −3.00/−0.25 × 5 6/6+	L −2.25/−0.50 × 35 6/6
+1.00 blurring test:	R 6/12	L 6/12+
Stereoacuity (Randot, glasses):shapes − 250″ circles −16″		
Cover test (glasses):	D 10Δ XOP Grade 4	N 5Δ XOP Grade 2 recovery
NPC (glasses):	8 cm	
Mallett aligning prism (glas.):	D 1Δ in L, nil vertical	N 0.5Δ in, nil vertical
Mallett aligning sphere (gla.):	D −0.75 in addition to subjective findings D cover test with this ' −ve Add': D 6Δ XOP Grade 1	
Dissociation tests (glasses):	D 16 exo 0.5Δ down R	N 7Δ exo nil vertical/cyclo
AC/A (gradient, −1):	4Δ /D	
D fusional reserves (glasses):	convergent −/4/2	divergent −/18/16

COMMENT
The cover test recovery at D (Table 2.4) supports decompensating distance exophoria from mild divergence excess. The aligning sphere and cover test indicate this will be compensated by a 'negative add' of −0.75 and this was prescribed. A letter was sent to the family optometrist explaining the management and asking them to increase the contact lens Rx similarly.

FOLLOW-UP 9 MONTHS LATER
No problems. Diplopia now rare, just when exceptionally tired and not a problem as easy to control. No turning eye seen. Distance and near vison clear. Headaches now once a week or fewer, when too much computer gaming. Findings similar to before, except improved cover test and aligning prism:

Cover test (glasses):	D 8Δ XOP Grade 2	N 3Δ XOP Grade 1 recovery
Mallett aligning prism (glass.)	D 0.5Δ in R, nil vertical	N 0.5Δ in R, 0.5Δ up L

MANAGEMENT
No change recommended.

COMMENT
This case only required a small over-minus to render the divergence excess compensated.

Amp. Acc, Accommodative amplitude; *D,* distance/dioptre; *DS,* dioptre sphere; *L,* left; *N,* near; *OCT,* optical coherence tomography; *R,* right; *Rx,* prescription; *VA,* visual acuity; *XOP,* exophoria.

Where there is a low degree of hypermetropia, the correction of this is unlikely to assist, unless it is required to equalise the acuities. Sunglasses or tinted prescription lenses sometimes assist compensation (Eustace et al., 1973).

Eye Exercises

With teenage patients, eye exercises can be helpful for divergence excess. The incentive of the patient may not be very high, as there are often no marked symptoms, but where there is a reasonable level of cooperation, exercises may be an appropriate form of management. Exercises are less likely to work in cases where there is a vertical deviation, high AC/A ratio, or large angle (Daum, 1984).

Where eye exercises are given, the three main aims are to: treat any suppression; develop the convergent fusional reserves and/or negative relative accommodation; and develop a correct appreciation of physiological diplopia. These aims may be achieved by some of the exercises described in Chapter 10. They may be taken in the preceding order, or an exercise used which incorporates more than one aim. For example, physiological diplopia can be used in such a way that it develops convergence and relative accommodation, and at the same time will, by its nature, help in checking suppression. This type of exercise has been found particularly useful in divergence excess (Pickwell, 1979b).

Relieving Prisms

These are seldom satisfactory in divergence excess, as they disturb near vision.

Referral

Surgery may be considered in cases of simulated divergence excess as the patient ages, particularly if an exo-deviation occurs at all distances of fixation.

Convergence Insufficiency Exophoria Syndrome (CIES)

Convergence insufficiency exophoria syndrome (CIES) is found relatively infrequently in children aged under 6 years, but in approximately 5% of those aged 6−18 years (Scheiman et al., 1996).

A borderline result across a variety of tests may be as indicative of a disorder as one definitely abnormal result (Rae, 2015). A sensible approach is to combine different test results in a diagnostic algorithm and this approach for CIES is described later, and more generally for decompensated heterophoria in Chapter 5.

AETIOLOGY

Anatomical and Physiological Factors

Anatomical factors seem to play a large part in most cases of exophoria. When uncorrected, myopia may build up a false accommodation-convergence relationship for near vision.

Age

The average phoria for near vision increases with age from the early twenties, in a steady progression, becoming on average about 6Δ exophoria by the age of about 60 years. With normal patients, this increasing physiological exophoria for near vision does not seem to be caused by the reading addition (Freier and Pickwell, 1983). Elderly patients often have decompensated exophoria for near vision.

INVESTIGATION

A routine eye examination should be carried out in each case, as described in Chapter 2. In addition to appropriate tests of binocular function, three points should be noted, particularly, in this type of exophoria:

1. *Symptoms*, which are not usually as marked in exophoria as in esophoria. Suppression is more likely to be associated with exophoria, which exists to lessen the symptoms. It is unclear whether this is why, in old age, there is often a high degree of exophoria for near vision which is not accompanied by symptoms. The symptoms are likely to include frontal headache associated with prolonged use of the eyes (Rabbetts, 2007), ocular fatigue, and sometimes intermittent diplopia for near vision.

   A prototype symptom questionnaire was developed (Borsting, Rouse, & De Land, 1999) and later modified (Fig. 8.1) into the Convergence Insufficiency Symptom Survey (CISS) questionnaire (Rouse, Borsting et al., 2004). The questionnaire has been criticised because 5 of the 15 items could relate to non-ocular difficulties (Horwood, Toor, & Riddell, 2014) and its emphasis on reading leads to overdiagnosis of NPCI (Clark & Clark, 2015). This questionnaire was not designed as a screening tool and, not surprisingly, used in isolation it has a low sensitivity for detecting CIES (Horwood et al., 2014). The overlap between the symptoms measured by CISS and those of dry eye was noted on p. 16.

   CIES may be more common in children with attention deficit/hyperactivity disorder and the presence of both conditions may have a greater influence on parents' perceptions of problem behaviours at school (Rouse et al., 2009). Successful treatment of CIES is associated with a reduction in the frequency of adverse school behaviours and parental concern about school performance (Wakayama, Nakada, Abe, Matsumoto, & Shimomura, 2013).

2. *A cover test* is likely to reveal the near exophoria early in the routine examination. Particular attention must then be paid to the recovery movement (Table 2.4).

3. *Tests of compensation*, as described in Chapter 4. An alternative approach to diagnosis is discussed next.

4. *Near point of convergence* is often (but not always) unusually remote in CIES (p. 30).

5. *Accommodative function* should be assessed since CIES is sometimes associated with accommodative insufficiency (Rouse et al., 1999).

	'Please answer the following questions about how your eyes feel when reading or doing close work'	Never	Infrequently	Sometimes	Fairly often	Always
1	Do your eyes feel tired when reading or doing close work?					
2	Do your eyes feel uncomfortable when reading or doing close work?					
3	Do you have headaches when reading or doing close work?					
4	Do you feel sleepy when reading or doing close work?					
5	Do you lose concentration when reading or doing close work?					
6	Do you have trouble remembering what you have read?					
7	Do you have double vision when reading or doing close work?					
8	Do you see the words move, jump, swim or appear to float on the page when reading or doing close work?					
9	Do you feel like you read slowly?					
10	Do your eyes ever hurt when reading or doing close work?					
11	Do your eyes ever feel sore when reading or doing close work?					
12	Do you feel a 'pulling' feeling around your eyes when reading or doing close work?					
13	Do you notice the words blurring or coming in and out of focus when reading or doing close work?					
14	Do you lose your place while reading or doing close work?					
15	Do you have to re-read the same line of words when reading?					
	Total the number of ticks in each column:					
	Multiply by the column value	× 0 =	× 1 =	× 2 =	× 3 =	× 4 =
	Sum the five values (from multiplication)	Sum =				

Fig. 8.1 CISS questionnaire. The clinician should read the patient instructions in the top row and then read each question exactly as written. If the patient responds 'yes', qualify with frequency choices. Do not give examples.

Two Approaches to Diagnosis

The first diagnostic approach, typically followed in the UK, is to use a test of compensation (usually, the Mallett unit). A decompensated near exophoria is usually diagnosed as a near exophoria that is associated with symptoms and clinically significant aligning prism ($\geq1\Delta$ in pre-presbyopes and $\geq2\Delta$ in presbyopes), as discussed in Chapters 4 and 5.

In North America, where fixation disparity tests often do not have a good central fusion lock and therefore give less useful diagnostic information, a lengthier approach to diagnosis is followed. The Convergence Insufficiency Treatment Trial (CITT) study group have done a great deal to standardise this and defined CIES as follows (Scheiman, Mitchell, Cotter, Cooper et al., 2005):

1. *Symptom score* on the CISS of >8 (Scheiman, Mitchell, Cotter, Cooper et al., 2005) or >15 (CITT-ART Investigator Group, 2019).
2. *Exophoria* at near at least 4Δ greater that at distance.
3. *Low convergent fusional reserve*, defined as failing Sheard's criterion or <15Δ (Scheiman, Mitchell, Cotter, Cooper et al., 2005) (or $\leq15\Delta$ (CITT-ART Investigator Group, 2019)) to break.
4. *Receded near point of convergence (NPCI)*, defined as ≥ 6 cm break.

The UK approach has the advantages of simplicity and brevity. With this approach, a decompensated exophoria at near may or may not be associated with NPCI, and this would influence the type of eye exercises that might be used. Clinicians will encounter occasional cases where there is a near decompensated exophoria with a normal near point of convergence, possibly because of an unusually strong proximal cue to convergence close to. Such cases may have symptoms and yet not be diagnosed by the North American model.

With the North American method, the number of signs does not correlate significantly with the number of symptoms (Bade et al., 2013). In contrast, the severity of symptoms does correlate significantly (Karania & Evans, 2006b) with the Mallett aligning prism (Fig. 4.10).

There has been no research directly comparing the two approaches, but research showing the convergent fusional reserves are strongly inversely correlated with aligning prism (Conway et al., 2012) may indicate both approaches will reach the same diagnostic outcome in many cases.

A disadvantage of the UK approach is that although the sensitivity and specificity of the Mallett unit are good (Jenkins et al., 1989), the test is not perfect (Fig. 4.9). An algorithmic approach is therefore advocated, which includes elements of both approaches. This was discussed in Chapter 5.

MANAGEMENT

Removal of Cause of Decompensation

Attention should be given to the patient's working conditions, adequate illumination and the possibility of a visual task involving monocular vision and causing extrinsic suppression. The patient's general health and any medication (Thomson, 2020) should also be considered.

Refractive Correction

In myopia or in absolute hypermetropia, the refractive correction can assist in making the exophoria compensated. In hypermetropic cases, care needs to be exercised in prescribing, as sometimes the correction increases the symptoms and difficulties. In other cases, low refractive errors (e.g., astigmatism or absolute hypermetropia) might cause blur and impair sensory fusion. In these cases, refractive correction may help to make a decompensated heterophoria become compensated.

The exophoria should be assessed for compensation with the proposed refractive correction in place. Sometimes it can be demonstrated quickly that the degree of exophoria is increased by the correction, and the binocular vision has become less stable. It should be noted, however, that the patient's exophoria may adapt to the lenses if they are left in place for 2–3 minutes. In those cases where the hypermetropic correction results in the exophoria becoming decompensated, or if it is likely to so do, a partial correction is given. In the case of a patient who has had no previous refractive correction, the correction should be reduced by about one-third of the mean spherical error, and the assessment of the exophoria repeated. The correction required is the highest correction that will maintain a compensated exophoria and which will at the same time relieve symptoms associated with the hypermetropia. In a few cases, this may not be possible, and for these, prism relief or eye exercises are required in addition to correction of the hypermetropia.

In presbyopic patients with CIES, the reading addition should be kept as low as is compatible with adequate near vision.

Modification of the refractive error can be used to treat some cases of decompensated exophoria, particularly when the patient does not have the time or inclination for eye exercises or when exercises are unsuccessful (Case Study 8.2). A 'negative addition' can be used: over-minussing or underplussing the refractive correction (Chapter 6). For example, in an emmetrope the effect of negative lenses on the deviation at the appropriate distance(s) can be investigated using the cover test and fixation disparity test. If a power of lens (**aligning lens**) is found through which the patient can comfortably accommodate and which renders the heterophoria compensated, this is prescribed. The aim, as with all treatments based on modification of the refractive error, is to reduce the correction over a period of months, and possibly years, as the patient becomes more able to compensate for the heterophoria themselves.

A patient with CIES might require a negative add for near, but not for distance. Such cases can be prescribed with executive bifocals fitted upside down. For example, an emmetropic patient could have executive bifocals made of the following prescription: -2.00DS add $+2.00$. If these were glazed upside down into a spectacle frame, the top portion would be plano and the bottom -2.00.

CASE STUDY 8.2

BACKGROUND
Girl, aged 12, previously given eye exercises for decompensated exophoria, but abandoned these (motivation poor).

SYMPTOMS
Near vision blurs. Headaches, about twice a week, at school.

RELEVANT CLINICAL FINDINGS
Normal: ocular health, visual acuities, refractive error (low long-sightedness), accommodative function.
  Cover test: D orthophoria N 10Δ XOP, poor recovery.
  Convergent fusional reserve (Δ) at near $-$ /7/2.
  Mallett aligning prism at near 2Δ in each eye or aligning sphere -1.75D each eye. With this 'negative add' near cover test recovery and near visual acuity good.

MANAGEMENT
Patient not keen on more eye exercises, so given negative add 'exercise glasses' for near vision.

FOLLOW-UP
Glasses used for most close work and in class, virtually eliminate symptoms. Negative add gradually reduced every 3 months (each time, minimum prescription to give alignment on Mallett fixation disparity test and good cover test recovery). After 18 months, patient asymptomatic and compensated without glasses.

D, Distance/dioptre; *N*, near; *XOP*, exophoria.

Eye Exercises

In patients who are old enough to understand the instructions, eye exercises may be appropriate, depending on the motivation of the patient, the time available, etc. (Chapter 6). Exercises may be successful if the exophoria has been compensated but due to stress has become decompensated. In such cases, a short course of exercises aids the restoration of compensation when the factors of stress have been dealt with.

Where treatment is given, the general plan should be:

1. Develop the convergent fusional reserves and/or the negative relative accommodation.
2. Develop a correct appreciation of physiological diplopia.
3. Treat any suppression that has been demonstrated.

Examples of exercises appropriate to these objectives are described in Chapter 10, which includes a review of research on their effectiveness.

Relieving Prisms

Prism relief in CIES often proves a simple and effective method of management. It is frequently more appropriate than eye exercises in adult patients. The efficacy of prisms was reviewed in Chapter 6.

The power of the prism required is the lowest that ensures compensation of the exophoria. This can be estimated by repeating the near cover test and Mallett fixation disparity test with prism relief in place. Typically, the smallest prism which restores the monocular markers to their central position is prescribed. There is often a subjective improvement reported by the patient when reading the near-test types with the prism in place, and it may be noticeably worse if the prism is removed.

If there is a small degree of comitant hyperphoria in addition to the exophoria, then an appropriate vertical prism will help the compensation of the exophoria (London and Wick, 1987).

Referral

Where other methods of treatment fail, surgical relief is sometimes considered, but the degree of exophoria needs to be large enough to exceed the accuracy of surgery.

Near Point of Convergence Insufficiency (NPCI)

As noted on p. 115, NPCI is used here to refer simply to a remote near point of convergence, which may or may not be associated with CIES. NPCI has been recognised as a common condition since it was described by von Graefe (1862). It may be defined as a weakness in the ability to converge or to maintain convergence (Millodot, 2009).

AETIOLOGY

1. *Disuse of accommodative convergence* can be a cause of NPCI. Uncorrected myopes, presbyopes wearing their reading glasses and absolute hypermetropes may all make reduced accommodative effort, which can result in insufficient convergence because of the accommodation/convergence relationship.

2. *Accommodative insufficiency.* Approximately half of cases with accommodative insufficiency also have NPCI (Francis, Rabbetts, & Stone, 1979). It is not always clear whether the accommodative or convergence anomaly is the primary dysfunction.

3. *Prolonged use of digital displays* can cause the near points of convergence and of accommodation to become more remote (Gur et al., 1994). This might cause a borderline NPCI to become symptomatic.

4. *Anatomical factors,* such as a large pupillary distance or a divergent position of anatomical rest, may contribute.

5. *Developmental (or phylogenetic) factors* may also play a part. Convergence is said to be the most recently developed aspect of binocular vision and may most readily break down under stress.

6. *Disuse of an eye* for any length of time (e.g., from amblyopia or a blurred image) can also induce NPCI.

7. *Hyperphoria or cyclophoria* may contribute to NPCI. The cyclovertical heterophoria may be comitant in some cases, or it may be found to be incomitant and break down into a strabismus in some direction of gaze or under adverse visual conditions. In the latter case, surgery is suggested before treatment of the convergence inadequacy (Lyle & Wybar, 1967).

8. *General debility and pathology.* Poor general health has been shown to be a factor (Pickwell & Hampshire, 1984). Independent of health, there is a greater prevalence with age (Pickwell, 1985), and in urban populations compared to rural (Pickwell, Viggars, & Jenkins, 1986). Metabolic disorders, toxic conditions and local infections or endocrine disorders are important factors. For example, convergence weakness can accompany thyrotoxicosis as an early sign (Moebius' sign) and poor convergence often accompanies Parkinson disease (Almer, Klein, Marsh, Gerstenhaber, & Repka, 2011), improving with treatment. In very rare cases, NPCI can be associated with pineal gland tumours (Ainsworth, 1999) and combined convergence and accommodative palsy can result from lesions in the superior colliculus (Ohtsuka, Maeda, & Oguri, 2002). NPCI is a common finding postconcussion (Trbovich, Sherry, Henley, Emami, & Kontos, 2019). The effect of any medication should also be considered (Thomson, 2020).

9. *Paralysis of convergence* can also rarely occur in conditions affecting the brain stem, in multiple sclerosis, tabes dorsalis, and in some traumatic conditions. In these cases, there is a sudden onset of diplopia for near vision, and usually other signs and symptoms of the primary condition. Convergence paralysis may be associated with reduced accommodation (Bishop, 2001).

10. *Paralysis of the near vision triad* is rare and requires referral to exclude pathology, but can be idiopathic (Kothari, Mody, Walinjkar, Madia, & Kaul, 2009). These authors reported a case study managed with +3.00DS 5Δ base-in each eye, in half-eye spectacles.

Classification: Primary and Secondary NPCI

Some authors differentiate between primary NPCI, resulting from a primary deficit of convergence, and secondary NPCI, where the poor convergence results from some other anomaly, such as intermittent exotropia, heterophoria, neurological disease, and mechanical and paralytic strabismus (Ansons & Davis, 2001). Some authors classify NPCI that is associated with monocularly decreased amplitudes of accommodation as primary (Ansons & Davis, 2001) and others as secondary (Bishop, 2001).

INVESTIGATION

In the investigation of NPCI, particular attention should be paid to the following points.

Symptoms

Symptoms are typically associated with near vision and consist of tired or sore eyes, intermittent blurring and double vision, and headache. The headache is often said to be frontal (Bishop, 2001). Sometimes patients report the symptoms are relieved if one eye is closed or covered. The symptoms are worse if the patient is suffering from tiredness, ill health, overwork, anxiety, etc.

Convergence Tests

Two clinical tests are of particular value and are simple and brief enough to include in a standard routine examination. The methods of application of these tests are described in Chapter 2.

Near Point of Convergence
The near point of convergence was discussed in detail on p. 30.

Jump Convergence
This test was introduced on p. 30. The patient is asked to look at a distance object, and then to change fixation to one held at about 15 cm from the eyes and on the median line (Pickwell and Stephens, 1975). The eyes are observed to see if the change of convergence is performed satisfactorily. Normally, a prompt and smooth convergence movement from distance fixation to near is seen. There are four types of abnormal response which may be observed:

1. Over-convergence, which may be followed by a corrective movement. This is not significant in the context of NPCI.
2. Versional movement: both eyes move an equal amount to allow the motor dominant eye to take up fixation. The non-motor-dominant eye then converges to restore binocular fixation.
3. Slow or hesitant movement.
4. No movement of either eye or of only one eye.

The last three of these responses indicate a failure of normal convergence, and it is likely that there will be trouble in maintaining convergence for near vision. If the patient has a near point of convergence of 8–15 cm, and the jump convergence is normal, it is unlikely that there will be symptoms. Failure on the jump convergence test occurs more often than a poor near point and appears to be associated with symptoms more frequently (Pickwell & Hampshire, 1981a). Some patients can perform well on the near point test by exercising excessive effort but cannot maintain this degree of convergence for sustained near vision.

Heterophoria Tests for Near Vision

These tests usually show compensated exophoria at typical near test distances. In about one-third of the patients with NPCI there is decompensated exophoria for near vision (Pickwell & Hampshire, 1981a), and these cases are better described as CIES. This is more likely to occur in elderly patients. Fixation disparity tests for near vision show suppression of one of the monocular markers in about one-fifth of NPCI cases. In the absence of strabismus, this suppression for near vision can be taken as a possible indication of the presence of convergence inadequacy.

It can also be useful to carry out tests of compensation, particularly the Mallett fixation disparity test, at an unusually close working distance. Reading at 20 cm usually results in an increased exo-slip (Pickwell, Jenkins, & Yekta, 1987) and this effect is likely to be greater in NPCI.

Tests of Accommodation (Chapter 2)

The amplitude of accommodation will be found to be low in some patients with NPCI. Indeed, it has been suggested that the symptoms of CIES are attributable to accommodative insufficiency (Marran, De Land, & Nguyen, 2006). Cases of combined convergence and accommodation insufficiency are distinguished from ophthalmoplegia (Chapter 17), as the latter condition has a sudden onset of symptoms. The effect of any medication that the patient is taking should also be considered

(Thomson, 2020). Convergence insufficiency with accommodation insufficiency usually starts to give trouble in the teenage years, and sometimes improves after several years. The AC/A ratio is very low in these cases.

A useful objective measure of accommodative function is accommodative lag which can be assessed by monocular estimate method (MEM) retinoscopy (pp. 33−34). Some patients with poor convergence maximise their accommodation to induce accommodative-convergence in order to augment poor convergence (Jennings, 2001a). These patients will have an accommodative lag that is lower (less plus) than the usual +0.50D.

MANAGEMENT

Treatment of NPCI is usually by eye exercises and is nearly always successful, even with older patients. The management will be considered under the five general headings given in Chapter 6 on the basic principles of management. Many cases of NPCI are associated with accommodative insufficiency and these cases are considered separately towards the end of this section.

Removal of Cause of Decompensation

The factors that create decompensation of heterophoria may also aggravate NPCI so that thought should be given to the working conditions, to the general health, and to the general well-being of the patient.

Refractive Correction

A refractive correction should be given where necessary. Patients with previously uncorrected myopia may find that correction of the myopia relieves the NPCI. Very rarely, a negative add can be useful to induce accommodative convergence.

Eye Exercises

Convergence insufficiency is easier to treat than CIES. In CIES, simple push-up (ramp) convergence exercises are not an adequate treatment (Chapter 10), probably because the deficiency is not simply a remote NPC. In NPCI, the deficit is solely of the NPC, and therefore 'pencil-to-nose' type exercises appear to be quite successful for NPCI (although there is a lack of evidence from randomised controlled trials). Some practitioners prefer 'jump' (step) convergence exercises in which the patient alternates their fixation between distance and near targets (Case Study 8.3). It is likely that a combination of both approaches will be more successful than either in isolation. Slightly more sophisticated exercises that include an appreciation of physiological diplopia can be very successful if properly understood by the patient. All these types of exercises are discussed in more detail in Chapter 10.

CASE STUDY 8.3

BACKGROUND
10-year-old boy, first eye examination.

SYMPTOMS
Near vision blurs and occasionally appears to change size. Rare horizontal diplopia when reading: after a blink, text returns to single. Sore and tired eyes when reading and headaches, but details of headaches vague.

RELEVANT CLINICAL FINDINGS
Normal: ocular health, visual acuities, refractive error (low long-sightedness).
    Amp. Acc.: slightly low (R = L = 8.0D)

Acc. lag: R = L = 0.75D, accommodative facility (±2.00D) 7 cpm. Orthophoric at distance with small exophoria at reading distance, adequate fusional reserves, no aligning prism on D or N Mallett units. Ocular motility, foveal suppression test, and stereoacuity all normal. Push up near point of convergence breaks at 14 cm, recovery at 17 cm.

MANAGEMENT
Given eye exercises to train 'jump' convergence (and accommodation) between distance and near accommodative targets, whilst trying to bring the near target in closer, with parent watching eyes to ensure correct convergence. These are a combination of ramp and step exercises.

FOLLOW-UP 3 WEEKS LATER
Exercises found to be 'fairly easy', can now converge to nose. Symptoms greatly improved: only one headache since last appointment. Clinical findings similar to before, except amplitude of accommodation improved (R = L = 11D), near point of convergence break 7 cm, recovery 8 cm. Exercises stopped.

FOLLOW-UP 6 MONTHS LATER
Improvement in signs and symptoms sustained.

Amp. Acc, Accommodative amplitude; *cpm*, cycles per minute; *D*, distance/dioptre; *L*, left; *N*, near; *R*, right.

Patients will usually be able to teach themselves to develop a near point of convergence of less than 8 cm, and to perform jump convergence test quite quickly: usually in several weeks. Some authors argue that the exercise should be continued for 2 weeks after this, else the NPCI may recur. However, this is certainly not always the case (Case Study 8.3). Regardless of the approach, with some patients it may be necessary to repeat the exercises at intervals of a few months to maintain adequate convergence. If the NPCI does recur after a few months, more thought should be given to the possibility of aggravating factors such as poor general health, inadequate lighting, etc.

It is sometimes stated that voluntary convergence should be trained as the final stage of the treatment of NPCI (Bishop, 2001). One approach is for the patient to try to maintain convergence at their near point of convergence once the near fixation target has been removed. Free-space stereogram exercises usually involve an element of training voluntary convergence, when the patient reaches a stage when a pencil is not needed for fixation (Chapter 10).

In fact, any of the exercises that can be used to train convergent fusional reserves (Chapter 10) can be used to treat NPCI and Bishop (2001) recommended that convergent fusional reserve exercises should be part of the treatment plan for NPCI. Research indicates that an intensive programme of exercises is much more likely to be effective than simple pencil push-ups (Scheiman, Mitchell, Cotter, Kulp et al., 2005). Indeed, this research found that for CIES, more sophisticated exercises are necessary. The Institute Free-space Stereograms (pp. 152–156) have been used to successfully treat NPCI (Evans, 2000).

Relieving Prisms

These are not usually appropriate for NPCI, except when it is combined with accommodative insufficiency, as described below.

Combined Convergence and Accommodative Insufficiency

When NPCI is combined with accommodative insufficiency, it is sometimes necessary to give a reading addition. The power can be estimated as that which allows the patient to use about two-thirds of the amplitude of accommodation for the normal near working distances, the rest being made up by the reading addition. Base-in prism may also help, sometimes combined with the near correction (Francis et al., 1979). The prism power can be determined by giving the weakest prism which will allow the patient to show prompt and smooth convergence on the jump convergence test, or (in CIES) to eliminate any fixation disparity at the appropriate distance. These reading glasses relieve the symptoms in convergence and accommodative insufficiency and are usually discarded by the patient when the condition becomes less problematic, typically within 2 or 3 years.

Convergence exercises can treat combined convergence and accommodative insufficiency (Francis et al., 1979), although this can be challenging (Pickwell and Jenkins, 1982). A randomised controlled trial shows that eye exercises can be effective at improving accommodative amplitude and facility in children with CIES and accommodative dysfunction (Scheiman et al., 2011).

Referral

Usually, NPCI is treated by eye exercises and does not require referral. Where primary spasm of convergence is suspected, or where it is combined with the signs of a pathological cause, the patient will require medical investigation. For example, NPCI will require referral where it appears with other indications of thyroid problems: Moebius' sign (see Chapter 17 for thyroid eye disease).

Basic Exophoria

In basic exophoria, the deviation is of similar magnitude for distance and near vision. The assessment and management of this condition has much in common with CIES. In decompensated basic exophoria, the management will depend on whether the condition is decompensated at distance, near, or both.

AETIOLOGY

Anatomical and Physiological Factors

Anatomical factors seem to play a large part in most cases of exophoria, and hypertonicity of the abductors may be a contributory factor.

Absolute Hypermetropia

This may be a factor in the cause of exophoria. Patients whose hypermetropia is high in comparison with their amplitude of accommodation reach an age when they are no longer able to compensate for their refractive error by accommodating. They allow their accommodation and convergence to flag, which can result in decompensated exophoria. This can happen in high hypermetropia in children, and commonly in low degrees of hypermetropia in incipient presbyopes, particularly in people who do not have to undertake a lot of near visual tasks. If the hypermetropia is fully or partially corrected, the patient may recommence using their accommodation and convergence for near vision, reducing the exophoria. It should be noted that this is counter-intuitive: a plus correction can in these cases reduce an exophoria.

INVESTIGATION

A routine eye examination should be carried out in each case, as described in Chapter 2. The investigation should concentrate on the distance(s) at which the patient has symptoms, following the advice in earlier sections of this chapter.

Concluding Remarks on Patient Selection for Management Options

For most of the cases of decompensated exophoria that optometrists encounter, all that is required is to choose between spectacles (with a 'negative add') or exercises. Practitioners should not be too dogmatic about their personal treatment preferences; it is best to reach a joint decision with the patient and, for children, with their parents. The commitment required for eye exercises and opinions about wearing glasses should be discussed. If the parent/child team have made a voluntary commitment to exercises, they are far more likely to do them than if they have been persuaded by the practitioner. If they choose glasses, they are told they can always come back later for exercises.

It is important that patients with a refractive modification to treat a heterophoria fully understand that their glasses are not for a refractive error but are to improve their binocular coordination. If the patient moves to another practitioner, they may need to explain to this practitioner why the spectacle prescription differs from their refractive error. A useful phrase to describe these glasses is 'exercise glasses'. The optical prescription should be annotated to this effect.

CLINICAL KEY POINTS

- Exophoria can be classified as basic (mixed), divergence excess, and convergence insufficiency exophoria syndrome (CIES), which may be associated with near point of convergence insufficiency (NPCI)
- The effect of correcting the refractive error should be investigated, particularly with uncorrected myopia or astigmatism
- Eye exercises are usually an effective treatment, particularly for CIES and NPCI
- Refractive modification (negative adds) or base-in prism can be effective treatments in some cases

CHAPTER 9

Hyperphoria and Cyclophoria

Hyperphoria is a potential deviation of one eye upwards which becomes an actual deviation when the two eyes are dissociated, and which recovers when the dissociating factors are removed. In hypophoria, the deviation is downwards and, as hypophoria of one eye may be regarded as the same as hyperphoria of the other, the term 'hypophoria' is not in general use. Right hyperphoria is the same as left hypophoria. Occasionally, vertical heterophoria occurs in one eye only which is usually found to be amblyopic.

Secondary Hyperphoria

AETIOLOGY

Hyperphoria is often present as a secondary condition, and the first step is to treat the primary cause. Any residual hyperphoria can then be managed as discussed in the next section. First, the main causes of secondary hyperphoria are summarised.

Horizontal Heterophoria

High degrees of comitant esophoria or exophoria are often accompanied by a small vertical component. In these cases, the treatment will be that which is appropriate to the primary condition, but prism relief of the hyperphoria may help.

Incomitant Deviations

Paretic conditions involving the elevator or depressor muscles may begin as hyperphoria and develop later into strabismus. It is important that this early sign of pathology is detected. The sudden onset of intermittent vertical diplopia and/or other symptoms, and the incomitant nature of the deviation, are the main diagnostic features. The most common cyclovertical incomitancy is superior oblique underaction, so it is important to look carefully for cyclophoria in all cases of hyperphoria and skew deviation is another differential diagnosis (Chapter 17). Congenital incomitant deviations are frequently accompanied by a vertical element, but symptoms are usually absent.

Unilateral High Myopia (Heavy Eye Syndrome)

Heavy eye syndrome involves anisometropia, usually with high myopia, and hyperphoria or hypertropia. The more myopic eye is hypotropic or hypophoric. The notion that the disorder results from a 'heavy' myopic eye is incorrect: the cause is an abnormally low muscle path of the lateral rectus in the involved eye (Yanoff & Duker, 1999). The vertical deviation ranges from $2-25\Delta$, although there is no correlation between the amount of anisometropia and the amount of hypotropia. Elevation of the low eye may be limited. Frequently, the head tilts to the side of the hypotropic eye.

Tilted Spectacles, Unilateral Toric Contact Lenses, and Anisometropia

If spectacles are incorrectly fitted or the frame becomes bent, a vertical prism element may be introduced which initially shows as hyperphoria. Usually, the patient adapts quite quickly to this abnormal prism and the hyperphoria reduces. When this occurs, hyperphoria will be present when the glasses are removed, or the spectacle frame straightened. This will disappear after a few days.

Toric contact lenses, most commonly disposable soft lenses, often contain a vertical prism to aid lens orientation. The strength of prism ranges from 0.52Δ to 1.15Δ which, in patients who only require monocular correction of astigmatism, might cause symptoms in sensitive patients (Sulley, Hawke, Lorenz, Toubouti, & Olivares, 2015).

Corrections for anisometropia may also produce hyperphoria when the eyes are not looking through the lens optical centres. Again, adaptation to this variable prismatic effect usually occurs after a few days of using the anisometropic correction, but difficulties can arise with a correction for marked anisometropia particularly where no glasses have been worn before (Chapter 11). Similarly, problems may arise if a refractive correction has changed markedly (e.g., after a cataract extraction operation). A near hyperphoria can result when multifocal spectacles are prescribed to a patient with significant anisometropia (Chapter 11).

A spectacle correction which has not been correctly balanced between the two eyes may also cause hyperphoria. The same applies to uncorrected anisometropia.

Primary Hyperphoria

Primary hyperphoria is usually considered attributable to slight anatomical misalignments of the eyes and/or orbits or muscle insertions for which there is a physiological compensation. Usually, this type of hyperphoria is less than 3Δ, and it seldom causes symptoms. It has been shown that about 98% of symptom-free people will show some degree of hyperphoria after a period of prolonged occlusion of one eye, but this disappears after a few hours when the binocular vision is restored (Duke-Elder, 1973). Vertical heterophoria is not associated with the convergence system in the way that applies to horizontal heterophoria, and this further suggests that anatomical factors play a larger part in its aetiology.

However, hyperphoria can decompensate due to stress on the visual system or on the general well-being of the patient (Chapter 4).

INVESTIGATION

A routine eye examination should be carried out. The following points may be particularly useful in hyperphoria:

1. *Symptoms*, which can sometimes be very marked in hyperphoria, even where the degree of the heterophoria is low. They seem to occur more frequently in middle age. Frontal headache and ocular discomfort or pain are the most common symptoms. Sometimes, there is an anomalous head position, and other patients may report that vision is more comfortable if one eye is closed or occluded. An association has been suggested between hyperphoria, lower back pain, and postural stability (Matheron & Kapoula, 2011), although this requires further research with larger sample sizes.
2. *History* should include questions about the history of traumatic brain injury as hyperphoria is a common finding in such cases (Doble et al., 2010).
3. *Motility test* for incomitancy. The test method is described in Chapter 2 and interpretation in Chapter 17. If the clinical results suggest an incomitancy of recent onset, the patient should be referred.
4. *Refraction*, particularly attending to the binocular balance of the spherical error between the two eyes. An unbalanced correction can sometimes be the cause of hyperphoria.
5. *Compensation assessment*, as described in Chapter 4. The cover test and fixation disparity tests are likely to be useful.

MANAGEMENT

Removal of Cause of Decompensation

Care must be taken to explore the visual working conditions and any stress or ill health that may be the cause of the decompensation. These should receive attention before other aspects of management.

Refractive Correction

In some cases, the provision of a correction for previously uncorrected refractive error will alleviate the hyperphoria without any other treatment. Balancing the refractive correction is very important in hyperphoria.

In the case of marked anisometropia where no previous correction has been worn, a partial correction of the more hypermetropic eye may prevent disturbance by vertical prismatic effects when the patient is not looking through the optical centres of the lenses. The correction is reduced in the more hypermetropic eye until the vertical heterophoria is compensated when looking through the lenses a little above or below the optical centres. This can be judged by Turville's 'nodding test'. Traditionally the infinity balance septum is used, and the patient asked to raise and lower their head in a slight nodding motion until the reduced sphere does not create a change of level in the two letters. Nowadays, it is more common to carry out a version of this test with the patient slowly nodding whilst viewing the vertical Mallett fixation disparity test. This correction may be increased to a fuller prescription with subsequent glasses (see also Chapter 11).

Eye Exercises

Eye exercises to improve the vertical fusional reserves very seldom prove successful, and do not seem to help in making the hyperphoria compensated. This is not surprising as vertical vergence may not be disparity driven (Ygge, 2000) and, unlike horizontal vergence, is not influenced by emphasising the need for accuracy during vergence changes (Stevenson, Lott, & Yang, 1997). However, one study (a non-controlled trial) indicated that it might be possible to change vertical fusional reserves with exercises (Luu et al., 2000). When the hyperphoria is associated with horizontal heterophoria, exercises to increase the horizontal fusional reserves will often result in the vertical heterophoria becoming compensated (Cooper, 1988a).

Relieving Prisms

Most primary hyperphoria can be readily relieved by weak vertical prisms, although randomised controlled trials are lacking (Doble et al., 2010). As explained earlier, the smallest prism that will neutralise the fixation disparity with a Mallett unit can be prescribed. As noted in Chapter 8, such vertical prism relief may also help any decompensated horizontal heterophoria (Sheard, 1923; London and Wick, 1987).

Referral

Incomitant hyperphoria with intermittent diplopia of recent onset indicates the need for medical investigation. When there is a high degree of hyperphoria and congenital incomitancy which gives rise to intolerable symptoms, surgical relief is sometimes considered. Medical advice should be sought.

Dissociated Vertical Deviation (DVD)

This is a comparatively unusual anomaly which is also known as 'alternating sursumduction'. Although it could be mistaken for hyperphoria, the clinical appearance is not the same. It is usually seen during the cover test. When one eye is covered with an occluder or a dark filter it slowly deviates upwards, possibly by as much as 40Δ. This differs from hyperphoria in that, whichever eye is covered, there is an upward movement of the eye behind the cover. When the cover is removed, the eye slowly recovers to the fixation position. The upward movement is not always equal in the two eyes, and sometimes it can be absent in one eye, giving the appearance of a 'unilateral hyperphoria'. In all cases, if a neutral density filter bar is placed before the uncovered eye and the density of the filter increased, the eye under the cover will slowly move down. When the density of filter is reduced, the covered eye moves slowly up again. This is called the Bielschowsky phenomenon.

DVD is usually associated with a history of infantile esotropia syndrome (p. 227). There is sometimes a cyclorotation of the occluded eye (Burian & von Noorden, 1974). Various surgical approaches have been used for DVD, but the evidence-base for these is weak (Hatt, Wang, & Holmes, 2015).

When DVD exists without any other deviation or anomaly, there are usually no symptoms and no independent treatment is required. If it exists with other conditions, treatment appropriate to the primary condition can be considered. Occasionally, patients with DVD complain that one eye deviates spontaneously and this is noticed by other people. The condition rarely produces symptoms (Mallett, 1988a), but if the condition is cosmetically unacceptable surgery is indicated (Kanski, 1994).

Cyclophoria

Many patients with long-standing cyclodeviations are asymptomatic because of sensory adaptations (Von Noorden, 1996). Dissociation tests reveal that it is normal to have a small degree of excyclophoria, typically 0.7—1.5 degrees (Flodin, Pansell, Rydberg, & Andersson Grönlund, 2019). Clinically, cyclophoria can be readily detected with the Maddox wing test.

In heterophoric patients, a double Maddox rod test (p. 259), which dissociates the eyes, will reveal more cyclodeviation than an associated test (e.g., Mallett fixation disparity test or double Bagolini lenses; p. 259). Patients with cyclodeviations that had an onset in the first 6 years of life may develop torsional harmonious anomalous retinal correspondence (HARC) (Chapter 12), and it has been suggested that this might prevent subjective torsion from being detectable even on dissociation tests, like the double Maddox rod test (Phillips & Hunter, 1999).

However, the double Maddox rod test is generally accepted as the most thorough way of assessing cyclodeviations. The example shown in Fig. 9.1 indicates 10 degrees incyclophoria in the left eye. The patient is viewing (in darkness, not as shown) a spotlight and sees two horizontal red lines. If the lines are not separated (i.e., there is no hyperdeviation) a vertical prism is introduced. When the Maddox rods are both orientated at 90 degrees (not as shown), this patient reports the line seen by the left eye as tilted. The left Maddox rod had to be rotated, top inwards (in the

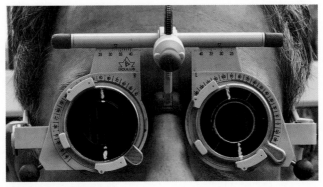

Fig. 9.1   Double Maddox rod test (see text).

opposite direction to the apparent tilt), to make the left eye's image parallel with that of the right. The angle of the left rod, as seen on the trial frame axis (100 degrees), indicates the dissociated position of the left eye is 10 degrees intorted (i.e., 10 degrees incyclodeviation). As with all dissociation tests, this test gives little indication of compensation, but this can be determined with the Mallett fixation disparity test (Chapter 4).

When measured with large field stimuli, 8 degrees of motor cyclovergence have been demonstrated in normal subjects, who can also exhibit 8 degrees of sensory cyclofusion, allowing them to fuse up to 16 degrees of cyclodisparity (Phillips & Hunter, 1999). Another study of cyclofusion showed a total mean amplitude of 16 degrees, with a fusion range from +7 degrees of incyclotorsion to −9 degrees of excyclotorsion.

CLINICAL KEY POINTS

- Vertical heterophoria is very rarely unilateral: right hyperphoria is usually the same as left hypophoria
- Significant hyperphoria is likely to produce symptoms, particularly if there is a recent onset when vertical diplopia is likely
- Recent onset hyperphoria often results from an incomitancy which may indicate active pathology and requires referral
- The most common pathological cause of hyperphoria is superior oblique muscle palsy, so cyclotorsional tests should be carried out
- Other causes of decompensated hyperphoria include an old hyperphoria decompensating and inappropriately prescribed or fitted spectacles
- Hyperphoria responds well to vertical prisms, but not to eye exercises
- Significant cyclophoria is probably always associated with incomitant deviations, and if these are long-standing, there may be sensory adaptations

CHAPTER 10

Eye Exercises for Heterophoria

The preceding chapters on various heterophoric anomalies have described the general outlines for the management of these conditions. This chapter gives details of particular exercises which may be fitted into the aims outlined. For example, the treatment of central suppression is appropriate to several different anomalies. The details of exercises for the treatment of suppression are given later rather than repeating them in each of the previous chapters.

The general principles of eye exercises and the factors to be considered in the selection of patients are described in Chapter 6. A distinction can be made between exercises that provide a smooth, gradual, stimulus (ramp) and those that employ a sudden, step-like, stimulus (Fig. 10.1). An example of the former is push-up, 'pen-to-nose' near point of convergence exercises. Ramp exercises are exemplified by flipper exercises where the patient rapidly alternates accommodation between plus and minus lenses. Although a few studies support the argument that one of these types is more effective than another, most authors nowadays accept that eye exercises are more likely to be effective if they employ a variety of approaches.

Exercises in this chapter will be considered under three main headings: (1) development of fusional reserves and relative accommodation; (2) exercises that train accommodation and convergence in their usual relationship; (3) exercises for the treatment of central suppression. The treatment of central suppression has been left until last because, in many cases, this does not require treatment. Sensory adaptations to heterophoria often spontaneously resolve when motor factors have been treated.

A study, somewhat limited by excluding participants with binocular vision anomalies, found that methods that exercise convergence and accommodation independently are most effective (Horwood & Toor, 2014). The study found that an enthusiastic therapist and the patient trying harder was a major factor on the outcome. Fusional reserves can be used to assess the outcome, but the reserves to blur point were so inconsistent they were unusable (Horwood & Toor, 2014).

Development of Fusional Reserves and Relative Accommodation

The aim of the exercise appropriate to each kind of anomaly has been described in the previous chapters, but the general principles can be summarised as follows:

1. In esophoric conditions: develop **divergent** reserves and/or positive relative accommodation.

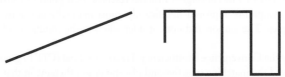

Fig. 10.1 Schematic illustration of ramp-type of exercise (on *left*; e.g., push-up NPC exercises) and step-type (on *right*; e.g., flippers). *NPC*, Near point of convergence.

2. In exophoric conditions: develop **convergent** reserves and/or negative relative accommodation.

In general, the object of this type of exercise is to exert the fusional reserve while keeping the accommodation unchanged: or, the other way round, induce changes in the accommodation while maintaining fixed vergence. Some methods exercise both, but one function is changed in excess of the other. The intention is to strengthen and increase the function which opposes the troublesome heterophoria, and to extend the range, or to 'loosen up' the accommodation-convergence relationship.

ARE FUSIONAL RESERVE EXERCISES EFFECTIVE?

Exercises to increase the fusional reserves are essentially visual feedback-based neuro-motor conditioning or enhancement therapies. On a very simple level, repeating a vergence task results in an improvement in performance, assessed by objective eye movement recording (Jainta, Bucci, Wiener-Vacher, & Kapoula, 2011), although this study was not a randomised controlled trial (RCT). Indeed, most research in this field has significant limitations, but four thorough RCTs have been carried out and provide mixed results.

The first two RCTs, of 46 adults (Scheiman, Mitchell, Cotter, Kulp et al., 2005) and 221 children (CITT, 2008) with convergence insufficiency exophoria (CIES; p. 118) produced similar results, replicating a smaller pilot study of children (Scheiman, Mitchell, Cotter, Cooper et al., 2005). Intensive exercises were found to be more effective at treating CIES than simple pen-to-nose exercises. Indeed, the pen-to-nose exercises, which have been criticised as very basic (Kushner, 2005), were not found to be effective at improving the near point of convergence and convergent fusional reserves. This is perhaps not surprising because the participants were selected as having the syndrome of CIES. As they had low convergent fusional reserves in addition to a remote near point of convergence, it is not surprising that push-up exercises were ineffective because these would only be expected to address the near point of convergence. Second, the treatment dose in each group was not matched. The intensive vision therapy group and placebo therapy group received a 60 minute clinic session weekly, in addition to 15 minutes a day home therapy, whereas the push-up group received only 15 minutes a day (CITT, 2008). So, the placebo therapy group received more hours of treatment and are likely to have received a greater placebo effect than the push-up group.

Using the Convergence Insufficiency Symptom Survey (CISS) questionnaire, in children symptoms improved most in the group receiving intensive exercises (CITT, 2008). With adults, symptoms improved significantly in all groups and the groups receiving push-up exercises or more intensive exercises did not improve symptomatically better than the group receiving placebo exercises (Scheiman, Mitchell, Cotter, Kulp et al., 2005). It is interesting that in the group that received the most intensive vision therapy, at the end of the trial 56% of children and 58% of adults were still symptomatic (see pp. 64—65).

A smaller RCT in 2018 compared three approaches for treating CIES: simple home push-up exercises; office-based vision therapy with a synoptophore (120 min/week) and additional home exercises; and augmented office-based vision therapy involving synoptophore and near vision tasks through minus lenses and base-out prism (120 min/week). There were 28 participants in each group, aged 15—35 years, and the study was single-masked (Aletaha, Daneshvar, Mosallaei, Bagheri, & Khalili, 2018). The convergent fusional reserves, near point of convergence, near exophoria, and CISS symptoms improved significantly, most markedly in the two groups receiving office-based therapies. The authors did not consider whether the results could be explained by a simple dose effect.

A later study by the Convergence Insufficiency Treatment Trial (CITT) group in children aged 9—14 years improved the matching of active and placebo vision therapy, in that the therapist contact time and treatment time was matched in both groups (Scheiman et al., 2019). This research showed an improvement in convergent fusional reserves and near point of convergence in the experimental group, but no significant improvement in symptoms (CITT-ART Investigator Group, 2019) or reading performance compared with the control group (Scheiman et al., 2019). The lack of a significant improvement in symptoms could be explained by inadequacies of the CISS tool for measuring symptoms (Horwood et al., 2014; Horan, Ticho, Khammar, Allen, & Shah, 2015), and it is noted that the CISS questionnaire is not well-suited to the digital age (CITT-ART Investigator Group, 2019). An alternative explanation is that much of the positive effect of eye exercises on symptoms is attributable to placebo effects or response bias, as active and control treatments were better matched in the CITT-Attention & Reading Trial (ART) study than in previous research by this group.

Overall, these studies support the conclusion that patients with CIES experience an improvement in convergent fusional reserves and near point of convergence following intensive vision therapy. Some evidence indicates that this can be associated with an improvement in symptoms, but this finding is equivocal.

There is some evidence from objective recordings of eye movements and functional magnetic resonance imaging (fMRI) that these parameters improve when CIES is treated. As well as improving the appropriate fusional reserve, the exercises train proximal vergence (Hokoda & Ciuffreda, 1983) and may (Bobier & McRae, 1996; Singh, Mani, & Hussaindeen, 2017), or may not (Hung, Ciuffreda, & Semmlow, 1986; Brautaset & Jennings, 2006a) increase the AC/A ratio.

Most research relates to horizontal fusional reserves, particularly convergent reserves which most often require treatment. There is a suggestion, from a noncontrolled trial, that vertical fusional reserves could possibly be improved (Luu et al., 2000), although the evidence base is weak for vision therapy to train any motor function other than convergent fusional reserves and near point of convergence.

WHAT ARE THE ESSENTIAL FEATURES OF SUCCESSFUL EXERCISES?

The evidence reviewed earlier, provides some support for eye exercises to train convergent fusional reserves, especially in patients whose exophoria is at risk of breaking down to a strabismus. This raises the question of how best to provide this vision training.

Fusional reserve exercises can employ a variety of methods of dissociating the eyes, including red/green filters (anaglyph), polarisation (vectograms), and haploscopic devices (e.g., stereoscopes). An alternative method used since 1940 (Revell, 1971) is to employ free-space fusion. This has several advantages, including that no specialist equipment is needed. Additionally, research indicates that vergence latencies are much shorter, equivalent to saccades, under free-space conditions, but not when viewing through artificial instruments (Hung, 1998). This may support the clinical observation that when exercises are carried out under more natural free-space conditions, improvements in visual function are more likely to translate into everyday life.

Notwithstanding the method of dissociation, there appear to be two schools of thought regarding the most effective type of exercise. One viewpoint, typified by Vaegan (1979), is that the details of the exercises are relatively unimportant, and the key feature is to maintain an overconverged posture for as long as possible. If this hypothesis is correct, the benefit some clinicians report from combining varied approaches may simply be that they keep the patient interested during potentially boring periods of overconvergence.

An alternative viewpoint is that the use of more than one technique may help the effect transfer into everyday vision (Cooper et al., 1983), as may the use of different stimulus parameters (Feldman, Cooper, & Eichler, 1993). Stimulus parameters can be varied, for example, by using different target types and sizes. Another important factor may be whether the vergence is changed gradually (ramp) or in jumps (step). Some studies have found that steps of disparity yield greater improvements than ramps, although another study found slow stimulus changes to be optimal (Daum, Rutstein, & Eskridge, 1978). It may be ideal to use both step and ramp stimuli

(Ciuffreda & Tannen, 1995). A range of different instruments for eye exercises are available from the American company, Bernell (Appendix 12).

In the CITT study, the group that benefitted most from treatment had a longer duration of treatment and included procedures (Table 10.2) designed to target fusional vergence and others aimed at overall convergence, with the therapist able to freely manipulate vergence and accommodative demand using multiple procedures (Scheiman et al., 2010). These authors found that 4 weeks is an appropriate time for a progress evaluation.

VIRTUAL REALITY SYSTEMS

An exciting development in this field is the use of three-dimensional (3-D) displays for eye exercises. In particular, the immersive nature of virtual reality headsets has great potential for creating a game environment, to engage patients in vision therapy. One device that is currently available has been described in the literature (Backus, Dornbos, Tran, Blaha, & Gupta, 2018; Fortenbacher, Bartolini, Dornbos, & Tran, 2018), but it is likely that other devices will be available in due course.

POLARISED VECTOGRAM AND ANAGLYPH TECHNIQUES

With polarised vectograms (Fig. 10.2) the eyes are dissociated by means of cross polarisation. The targets are transparent plastic sheets with a picture on each sheet of the same scene but taken from slightly different angles. The sheets are polarised in different directions and the patient wears appropriately polarised glasses. The sheets are back-illuminated by a uniform source and are placed so that the two pictures are directly on top of one another. A nonstrabismic patient should report seeing one picture, in 3-D relief. To treat an esophoric condition, the sheet that the right eye sees is slowly moved to the right of the left eye's sheet. If the patient continues to perceive a stereoscopic image, the right eye must have moved to the right to follow the target, i.e., divergence has occurred. The sheet is moved further until the patient reports blur, diplopia, or suppression (loss of stereopsis) when the sheet is moved back until binocularity is restored. The procedure is repeated, encouraging the patient to try and maintain binocularity for as long as possible. To train convergence (to overcome an exophoria) the right eye's image would be crossed over to the left of the left eye's image.

A similar technique can be used with anaglyphs, where the eyes are dissociated by means of red and green targets and goggles instead of polarisation. Because wearing different coloured lenses in front of each eye is unnatural, anaglyph techniques are more 'artificial' than polarised vectogram methods. However, dissociation by red/green lenses allows the targets to be generated on television or basic computer screens (Cooper, 1988a). This type of eye exercise is available on the internet in a system called Orthoweb (Field, 2002).

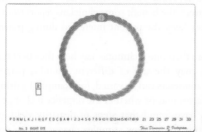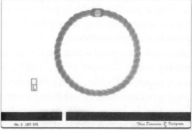

Fig. 10.2   A typical polarised vectogram, Quoits Vectogram. (Courtesy Bernell, a division of Vision Training, Inc.)

HAPLOSCOPIC EQUIPMENT

Variable Prism Stereoscopes

A variable prism device, such as a rotary prism, prism bar, or variable prism stereoscope, is used in the same way as described for the measurement of fusional reserves in Chapter 4. The patient looks at targets small enough to require precise convergence and accommodation while the power of the prism is gradually increased to change vergence in the direction opposing the phoria. The patient is asked to maintain clear single vision as long as possible, but when blurring or doubling occurs, the prism power is reduced, and the patient asked to recover clear single vision as soon as possible. The procedure is repeated for periods of about 5 minutes. The exercise is carried out for near vision, distance vision, or both, as the patient's difficulties suggest is appropriate.

If a variable prism stereoscope is used for distance vision, the card holder is removed, and the patient looks across the room. For near vision, this instrument can be used either with a single line of letters in the card holder and the septum removed or using a stereoscope card with separate right and left eye pictures and with the septum in place. In the latter case, 9Δ base-out in each eye will be required. The stereoscope cards appropriate for this should have most of the picture common to both eyes, so 'fusion' can take place, but have small parts of each eye's picture presented to only one eye to act as 'monocular markers'. In those cases where suppression is particularly marked, this type of card should be used in the early stages of treatment. Note that in all cases the patient should be asked to report that doubling has been observed, in the sense that the target is seen to break into two and the images drift apart. In some cases, double vision may not occur until one of the images has moved outside a fairly large suppression area. In these cases, the target is not seen to double, but a second peripheral image suddenly appears; this is most likely in divergence excess exophoria.

A simple variable prism method is to use a prism bar with a target placed at the appropriate distance. This can be loaned to the patient to use at home.

Lens (Holmes) Stereoscope

It will be seen from Fig. 10.3 that a lens (Holmes) stereoscope can be considered to have two 'orthophoria lines' from the focal point of each of the lenses to a point mid-way between the lenses themselves. In most stereoscopes, these are purely imaginary lines, but are useful in deciding which exercise is appropriate to esophoria or to exophoria. If the two pictures on the stereoscope card are of such a separation and at such a distance that they fall one on each of these orthophoria lines, their images will coincide with each other on the mid-line of the instrument. This will mean that, ignoring any proximal convergence, the eyes will have to converge and accommodate according to the normal accommodation-convergence relationship for the distance of the images. To use a card with a greater picture separation, but at the same card distance, would require the eyes to diverge in order to 'fuse', and a card with less picture separation would induce convergence. No change in accommodation would be required.

The diagram in Fig. 10.3 also shows that if the card distance is increased without changing the separation of the pictures, i.e., the card holder is drawn away from the patient's eyes, the picture separation will now be narrow for the new card distance and therefore convergence will be required to maintain 'fusion'. In this new position, the card's picture will lie inside the orthophoria lines. At the same time, the image distance will have increased, so that less accommodation is required. This means that when the card distance is increased, convergence and negative relative accommodation will be exercised which will help patients with exophoric conditions. In summary, when using the Holmes stereoscope:

1. In esophoric conditions: use cards of increasing picture separation and/or move the card holder **towards** the patient's eyes.
2. In exophoric conditions: use cards of decreasing picture separation and/or move the card holder **away from** the patient's eyes.

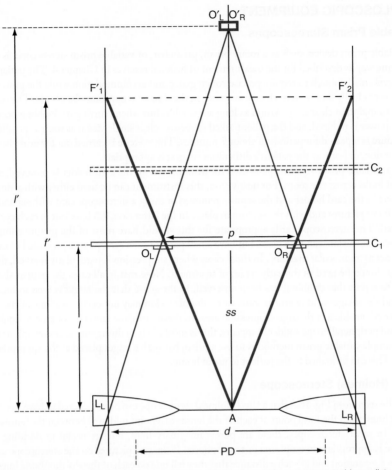

Fig. 10.3 The principle of the Holmes stereoscope. Two lenses, L_R and L_L, are separated by a distance, d, which is greater than the patient's pupillary distance, so that a base-out prism effect is produced. A septum at ss prevents the right eye from seeing the left image, and the left eye from seeing the right image. The pictures, O_R and O_L, on the card C_1, are held at a distance, 1. If these pictures are separated by a distance, p, such that they lie on the two lines joining the focal points of the lenses, F'_1 and F'_2, with the mid-point between the lenses, A (the 'orthophoria' lines), the images of the pictures, O'_L and O'_R, will coincide on the mid-line at a distance, I'. The eyes should then have to exert accommodation and convergence in the normal relationship for looking at an object at $1'$ (ignoring proximal convergence). If the pictures lie outside the orthophoria lines, forced divergence will be required for single vision. Such forced divergence, which is required as an exercise in esophoric conditions, can be achieved by either increasing the picture separation, p, or by decreasing the card distance, I. Similarly, the forced convergence required in exercises for exophoric conditions can be produced by decreasing the picture separation or by increasing the card distance, e.g., moving the card to C_2. (After Lyle, T.K., & Wybar, K.C. (1967). *Lyle and Jackson's Practical Orthoptics in the Treatment of Squint (and Other Anomalies of Binocular Vision)*. London: Lewis.)

Other Stereoscopic Devices

There are many different designs of stereoscope. A well-known one is the Brewster stereoscope, which is fairly similar to the Holmes design. A currently available Brewster stereoscope is the Bernell-O-Scope (Appendix 12).

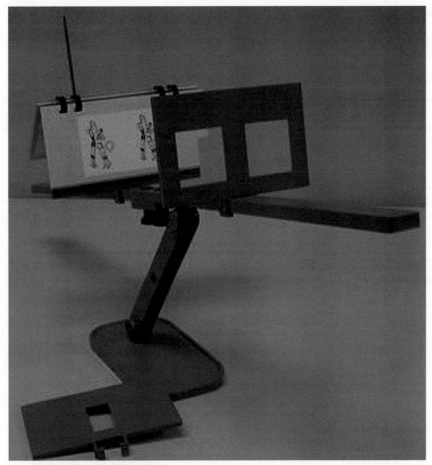

Fig. 10.4 Bernell Aperture Rule, with the double aperture used to train relative divergence (see text for description). (Reproduced with permission from Vision Training Products, Inc. (Bernell Division)).

A slightly different approach is to use apertures rather than lenses to achieve dissociation, as in the Bernell Aperture Rule (Fig. 10.4). A single aperture is used to train relative convergence and two apertures are used to train relative divergence.

Mirrors can also be used to dissociate the eyes, as in the single mirror haploscope, which is consulting-room equipment. A new version of the Pigeon-Cantonnet stereoscope, which is a portable instrument employing mirrors, is available as the Bernell Mirror Stereoscope (Appendix 12).

Synoptophore

Exercises of the fusional reserve type can also be carried out with a major haploscope (synoptophore) using 'fusion slides'. The restricted field, stimulation of proximal convergence and other disadvantages of this type of instrument do not seem to affect its use for training fusional reserves. However, this major instrument is hardly necessary for heterophoria problems.

FREE-SPACE TECHNIQUES

Free-space techniques do not require a stereoscope but involve the fusion of two stereo-pairs by overconverging or underconverging in 'free-space'.

Physiological Diplopia

One feature of free-space techniques is the use of physiological diplopia and it will be seen that there are many ways in which physiological diplopia can be useful in the treatment of heterophoria. The first step with any of these exercises is to demonstrate physiological diplopia and the easiest method is to use two fairly large and obvious objects as targets, for example, two pencils. These objects are held on the median line against a plain background (Fig. 10.5). The demonstration should include the patient fixating the nearer pencil and noticing the far pencil in uncrossed physiological diplopia, and then fixating the far pencil and being aware of the near one in crossed diplopia. Difficulty in seeing both the diplopic images indicates a gross degree of suppression, which is usually overcome quite quickly in heterophoria. Patients may have difficulty in alternating between uncrossed and crossed diplopia. In these cases, it is useful to ask the patient to practise doing this alternation as an exercise (p. 147). Once the patient has mastered the principle of physiological diplopia with pencils, then they can progress to other free-space techniques, such as the 'three cats' exercise.

'Three Cats' Exercise

The equipment for this exercise is simply a piece of card with two line drawings of cats, side by side and separated by about 5 cm from centre to centre. Each cat is incomplete in some way: an ear, an eye, or the tail is missing, so only when the two are fused is a complete cat formed (Fig. 10.6). This method does not require a stereoscope and is particularly useful for exophoric conditions, using the procedure in Table 10.1. The process of converging to achieve fusion of two laterally separated

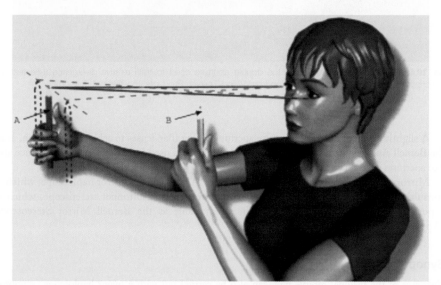

Fig. 10.5 Physiological diplopia. The patient fixates the further pencil, *A*, and notices that the nearer pencil, *B*, is seen in crossed physiological diplopia: the right eye's image on the left and the left eye's image on the right. A change of fixation to the nearer pencil should result in the farther one being seen in uncrossed physiological diplopia. For details of exercises, see text.

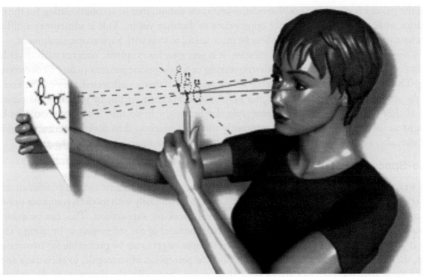

Fig. 10.6 'Three cats' exercise (see Table 10.1).

TABLE 10.1 ■ **Method for the 'Three Cats' Exercise.**

1. The card with drawings of two incomplete cats is held at about 40 cm.
2. The patient fixates on a pencil held between the card and the eyes.
3. Physiological diplopic images of the cats will be seen as four blurred images.
4. The pencil distance is adjusted until the middle two cats fuse into a complete cat with two incomplete cats, one each side (the resultant percept is of three cats).
5. The patient is asked to try to see the cats clearly. This involves maintaining convergence for the pencil distance and relaxing accommodation (exercising negative relative accommodation).
6. Encourage the patient, if they can, to exercise voluntary convergence, or 'go cross-eyed', to obtain three cats without the pencil.
7. Typically, the exercise is carried out for 10 minutes twice a day.
8. The patient should be checked again soon, typically after about 3 weeks.

targets, such that the right eye fixates the left target and the left eye the right target, is sometimes called **chiastopic fusion** (Goss, 1995).

This exercise can also be used for esophoric conditions, but patients tend to have more difficulties initially. It is easier if the card is cut between the cats and the exercise is started with the cats very close together. With esophoria, the patient is asked to fixate a distant object just over the top of the card, with the card held at about 30 cm from the eyes. When physiological diplopia of the two pictures on the card is appreciated, the card distance is adjusted to obtain fusion of the middle two picture designs. Fusion is maintained as the card is moved upwards slightly and thus obscures the initial fixation object. An alternative method is to photocopy the card onto a plastic transparency and instruct the patient to literally look through the cats at a distance object. It is likely that the cats will appear very blurred at first, but the patient should concentrate on maintaining fusion with underconvergence rather than clear vision at this stage. When this can be done, it is useful in obtaining clear vision if the card is moved away from the eyes to about 40 cm, where clear vision may be easier. When the patient can clearly see a fused middle picture with an incomplete one each side, the patient is exercising positive relative accommodation; that is, accommodating for the card distance while maintaining vergence appropriate to distance vision. This is sometimes a difficult exercise to use with esophoria, and it may be more useful to start with haploscopic equipment.

When undertaking the three cats exercise, it is very easy for exophoric patients to discover how to obtain fusion into three cats by underconverging or for esophoric patients to fuse by overconverging. That is, patients do the exercise the wrong way, and if this is undetected, they can be exercising the wrong function. The practitioner may be able to check for this by watching the patients' eyes as they do the exercise, and parents can also be taught to do this. The card should be held straight as, if the two cats are at significantly different heights, then fusion will be impossible. Occasionally, a card may need to be moved slightly to keep the images at the same height.

Free-Space Stereograms

Any stereoscope card can be used in a similar way to the three cats exercise to train positive or negative relative accommodation, or suitable targets can be drawn easily with modern computer drawing programs. Targets should be chosen which allow a check for suppression. This can be achieved either by having detail which is unique to each half (picture) of the stereo-pair or by using a target which gives stereoscopic relief (Fig. 10.7). Stereoscopic targets may be preferable for two reasons. First, they give the patient some feedback, a positive perception of stereopsis, to encourage and to assure them that the exercises are helping their vision. Secondly, the direction of the perceived stereopsis can be used to check that the patient is converging or diverging as appropriate.

The patient's perception can be checked by monitoring their perception of the size of the targets, using the mnemonic 'SILO' (small in, large out). This refers to the movement of the eyes ('in' during convergence): if a patient is exercising their convergent fusional reserve, as they converge the target should appear to be smaller and closer. The opposite effect should be seen if patients are exercising their divergent reserves. However, occasionally patients are encountered who demonstrate the opposite perception to that expected (Hokoda & Ciuffreda, 1983).

Once patients have mastered free-space stereograms using simple line targets, the exercises can be further developed using autostereograms. These were developed from the work of Julesz (1971) with random dot stereograms. Care should be taken to ensure that the correct type of vergence movement is being used and all patients should be closely monitored to confirm an improvement in their binocular status.

A series of free-space stereogram exercises for training convergent fusional reserves have been developed at the Institute of Optometry and these include simple targets and free-space stereograms. These are described next.

An advantage of many free-space techniques is that they utilise physiological diplopia: the two outside pictures (e.g., the two outside cats in the 'three cats' exercise) are seen in physiological diplopia. By maintaining an awareness of these images during the exercises some of the benefits described later from physiological diplopia exercises will be produced.

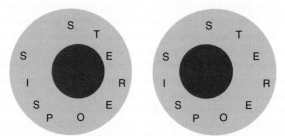

Fig. 10.7 An example of a free-space stereogram. The exercise is carried out in the same way as the 'three cats' exercise, but the patient enjoys stereoscopic vision as feedback that the exercises are being performed correctly. The reader can appreciate this by over-converging until they obtain a middle pair of circles, when they will appreciate the letters stereoscopically.

Prisms in Free-Space

Prisms can be used in free-space, for example with a prism bar.

FACILITY TRAINING

Vergence Facility (Prism Flippers)

The 'flip prisms', or prism flippers, consist of two pairs of prisms mounted on a horizontal bar, one pair (base-in) on the top of the bar and the other pair (base-out) below the bar (Fig. 2.6). One pair of prisms can be held before the eyes, and then quickly changed to the other pair by a simple flip.

Patients should be able to change their vergence and maintain accommodation as the prism is changed from base-in to base-out and back again; a monocular vergence facility flipper can also be used (p. 73). Exercising with flip prisms is carried out by asking the patient to look at a card with letters printed on it and held at about 40 cm, while the prisms are flipped from base-in to base-out and back. Patients should practice with 3Δ base-in and 12Δ base-out total prisms until they can execute 20 complete cycles per minute. This is known as training the vergence facility.

Accommodative Facility (Lens Flippers)

Accommodative facility can be tested (p. 32) and exercised by flip lenses of, for example, $+2.00DS$ / $-2.00DS$ (Fig. 2.6). As a home exercise, it is adequate to use the flipper with a normal page of print at the usual reading distance, and to check for suppression at follow-up visits to the practice (Table 2.9). This 'flipper' exercise should be carried out for a few minutes several times a day. Patients usually respond in 1 or 2 weeks. Patients with accommodative problems (e.g., insufficiency, infacility, fatigue; p. 35) may also benefit from this type of exercise.

If a young patient is suspected of having an accommodative anomaly, a cycloplegic refraction is usually required and correction of any significant hypermetropia before eye exercises for accommodative dysfunction. Active pathology as a cause of the accommodative problem should also be ruled out, as should the antimuscarinic effects of some systemic medications (Thomson & Lawrenson, 2006). Patients who will respond to the flip lenses type of exercise are usually aged $10-25$ years and this type of exercise has been validated by controlled trials (Rouse, 1987; Sterner, Abrahamsson, & Sjostrom, 2001). The exercise can also be preceded by a 'push-up' exercise, carried out as if repeating the measurement of amplitude of accommodation.

A study of patients with accommodative insufficiency compared the effect of $+1.00$ reading addition with ±1.50 flippers (Brautaset, Wahlberg, Abdi, & Pansell, 2008). Improvement was similar in both groups, but not normalised by the end of 8 weeks. Other possible explanations for the improvement in both groups is a regression to the mean, natural improvement over time, or placebo effects.

As with all exercises, a systematic programme involving different approaches is more likely to be effective. For example, the accommodative element of treatment in the CITT-ART trial (Table 10.2, Accommodative section) combines near-far exercises with flipper and other approaches to changing accommodative facility. As already noted, it is unclear whether the inclusion of different approaches is beneficial for therapeutic reasons, because it keeps the patient entertained for longer periods, or for both reasons.

Exercises That Train Accommodation and Convergence in Their Usual Relationship

It is sometimes useful to use procedures that exercise the accommodation and convergence in their normal relationship. It seems that decompensated heterophoria may be associated with difficulty interpreting the cues which stimulate the appropriate degree of vergence change. In these cases, the

TABLE 10.2 ■ Treatment Protocol Used in the CITT-ART Trial.

Exercise	Phase 1 P	Phase 1 H	Phase 2 P	Phase 2 H	Phase 3 P	Phase 3 H	Phase 4 P	Phase 4 H
Gross convergence								
Bead on string	✓	✓						
Convergence cards	✓			✓				
Voluntary convergence				✓				
Fusional vergence								
Polarised vectograms	C		R		J		J	
Computer orthoptics (RDS)	C	C	R	R	J	J	J	J
Free-space stereogram cards			C	C	C	C	J	J
Aperture rule					R		J	
Accommodative								
Monocular loose lens facility	✓		✓					
Distance-near facility	✓	✓	✓					
Viewing through minus lenses	✓	✓	✓					
Stereoscope biocular facility					✓			
Prism dissociation binocular facility					✓			
Computer orthoptics accommodative rock	✓			✓	✓	✓		✓
Binocular ± 2.00D flipper facility							✓	✓

C, Techniques that emphasise convergent fusional reserves only; H, home therapy; J, jump vergence (some with added prism); P, in-practice procedures; R, ramp/smooth convergent & divergent fusional reserve training; RDS, random dot stereopsis. The various exercises that make up this protocol are described in various places in this chapter.

Modified after CITT-ART Investigator Group. (2019). Treatment of symptomatic convergence insufficiency in children enrolled in the Convergence Insufficiency Treatment Trial-Attention & Reading Trial: a randomized clinical trial. *Optometry and Vision Science* **96**(11), 825–835.

disparate images of an object not at the fixation distance (in physiological diplopia) are misinterpreted. A patient with convergence excess esophoria, for example, when asked to change fixation from a near object to one slightly further away, will make a divergent movement only with one eye. This will leave the eyes in the position of a temporary convergent strabismus. Suppression and abnormal correspondence may be produced, leading to a more permanent strabismus (Gillie & Lindsay, 1969). This occurs mainly in young children before the binocular reflexes are firmly established, i.e., earlier than the age of 7 years. Such patients may benefit from general coordination exercises, which are based largely on teaching a correct interpretation of physiological diplopia.

Older patients may also benefit from procedures which exercise the accommodation and convergence in the normal relationship. These are cases in which both the convergence and the accommodation amplitudes are low and may be improved by 'push-up' type exercises, or near-far 'jump' exercises (described later).

The exercises described in this section are probably insufficient in isolation for training CIES (CITT, 2008), but may be useful for this condition when used in conjunction with other approaches as described later. It is also possible that the exercises in this section are adequate for training NPCI, when this occurs in isolation without the other features of CIES.

PHYSIOLOGICAL DIPLOPIA

The patient is taught a proper appreciation of physiological diplopia by using two objects held on the median line against a plain background (Fig. 10.5). The exercise consists of fixating one pencil, pausing long enough to be sure that it is single while the other is in physiological diplopia, and then changing fixation to establish single vision of the other with diplopia of the first. This alternation of fixation can cause confusion if carried out too fast; there should be a 3-second pause at each change to ensure the correct interpretation has been made. At first, the patient's eyes should be observed to see the steady and regular change of vergence of both eyes.

When this can be carried out successfully using isolated objects like the two pencils or two knitting needles against a plain background, the patient can be taught to appreciate physiological diplopia at any time by holding up a pencil or a finger and noticing the doubling of objects beyond. A change of fixation to the distant object will produce diplopia of the pencil.

In cases of NPCI, the nearer object initially is held at 40 cm from the eyes, but gradually moved closer as the patient is able to alternate between near fixation with uncrossed physiological diplopia and distance fixation with crossed diplopia. By this procedure, the patient is encouraged to perform the jump convergence test, with the nearer fixation object starting at 40 cm and gradually moving closer to the eyes to the 10 cm position.

The bead-on-string exercise, described later in the chapter, is also useful as a home exercise, and is an extension of the physiological diplopia principle (Fig. 10.11).

PENCIL-TO-NOSE (PUSH-UP) EXERCISES

This type of exercise can be a variant on the physiological diplopia exercise previously. The patient is asked to look at a pencil placed at about 50 cm or well outside the range of the near point convergence. It is then moved towards the eyes until it appears double, or the practitioner (or parent) sees that one eye has ceased to converge. This is repeated until the amplitude of convergence is closer than 10 cm. The patient is urged to 'make the eyes pull' to keep them converged on the near target as it approaches. If diplopia is not appreciated as soon as the practitioner notices that one eye has ceased to converge, then the patient should be taught to perceive physiological diplopia of some distant object. They should monitor the increased separation of these images as the pencil is brought closer to the nose and start moving the target back out when one of the diplopic images disappears. Sometimes preliminary exercises for suppression are required before the pencil-to-nose exercises.

NEAR-FAR 'JUMP' EXERCISES

Pencil-to-nose exercises are a 'ramp' type of exercise and should be complemented by a 'step' type of vergence (and accommodative) exercise. The patient moves a small, detailed, target in as close as they can towards their nose before it goes blurred, double, or one eye diverges (observed by the practitioner or a parent). They hold the near object still but relax their accommodation and convergence by looking at a distance object, until this distance object has become clear and single. They then look at the near target and, once this is clear and single, back at the distance target. This 'near-far' cycle is repeated as quickly as possible (but only when the targets are clear and single) for about 10 minutes, at least twice a day. Typically, the near target will be some small print which should be regularly changed so that it is not memorised. As with pencil-to-nose exercises, this exercise can be combined with an appreciation of physiological diplopia.

Exercises for Treatment of Central Suppression or Stereopsis

In heterophoria, suppression is mostly confined to a small foveal area and is usually intermittent. Only where there is a long-standing intermittent strabismus, as in divergence excess, will a larger suppression area be present. Where suppression is demonstrated in heterophoria, it is treated first or at the same time as any vergence treatment. As will be seen, some of the techniques described earlier for treating fusional reserves and general coordination can also be used simultaneously to treat foveal suppression. In many cases the suppression will resolve spontaneously when the motor deviation is treated. Where it does not, all or some of the following exercises may be appropriate.

STEREOSCOPE CARDS

Several stereoscope cards have been designed for the treatment of suppression in heterophoria. These usually consist of 'fusion' cards, in which most of the design is common to both eyes, but some of the detail is presented to one eye only. The patient is asked to look at the fused design and ensure that the part of the total picture presented only to the eye with a tendency to suppress is seen and is retained without intermittently disappearing.

PHYSIOLOGICAL DIPLOPIA

It has already been seen that there are many ways in which physiological diplopia can be useful in the treatment of heterophoria. First, it should be demonstrated that the patient can appreciate physiological diplopia as described in the first section of this chapter.

When the patient has appreciated physiological diplopia with the pencils, foveal suppression can be treated by using thinner targets such as a straightened length (about 15 cm) of wire. This is interposed between the eyes and a page of print (Fig. 10.8). This is the **wire reading** method. Initially, it is placed at the mid-distance from the eyes to the page, so that it is seen in physiological diplopia with two images apparently separated by 1—2 cm.

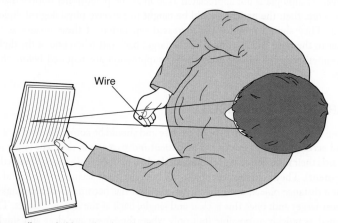

Fig. 10.8 Wire reading. A thin rod or length of wire is held on the median line between the printed page and the eyes. When fixating a letter on the page, the wire is seen in crossed physiological diplopia unless there is suppression. As the patient reads, the wire is moved across the page to maintain the two images at equal distance on each side of the point of fixation.

The patient is asked to read the page, slowly moving the wire along to keep the word being read mid-way between the two diplopic images and being conscious of both images all the time. When this is done, the wire is moved slightly nearer to the page so that its images appear closer together and more into the central suppression area. The patient should be asked to practise this exercise for several 10-minute periods each day for 1 or 2 weeks (Earnshaw, 1960). In the case of children, the exercise needs to be supervised by a parent to ensure that they do not forget to maintain a check that both diplopic images are there, otherwise interest in the book may absorb all their attention.

Bar reading is a further extension of this exercise (Fig. 10.9). In this case, the patient uses a thicker object, such as a pencil or even broader object. If a pencil is interposed between the eyes and the book, it should be about one-third of the distance from the eyes. This will ensure that it acts like a septum, occluding a vertical strip of the print from each eye. In this exercise, the pencil is held still on the median line, and is not moved along the line as in the previous method. As the patient's eyes cross the page during reading, the beginning of the line is seen by both eyes. There is then a strip occluded from the right eye by the pencil, but visible to the left if there is no suppression. Then there is a strip of the page seen by both eyes before the pencil occludes the left eye. The end of each line of print may be seen by both eyes.

Unless there is suppression, the patient should be able to read across the page without being aware of the pencil occluding either eye. At first, the patient may have to make a conscious effort to 'see through' the pencil in the position where it occludes the dominant eye. It is important that during the exercise the head is held quite still. If patients experience difficulty, small movements of the head will be noted as they try to look round the pencil. A parent may need to watch that this does not happen. An anaglyph (red green) bar reading approach is also available (see later).

If the suppression is present mainly for distance vision, the **septum test** (Fig. 10.10) can be modified to provide an exercise. The patient holds a finger or other object of about the same width, 10–20 cm from the eyes, while looking across the room or out of a window for distance vision. It is noticed that the 'septum' occludes objects in the visual field from each eye. The patient is asked to identify these objects by closing each eye in turn or by occluding each with the other hand, e.g., the tree and the man in Fig. 10.10. Then, with both eyes open, they are asked to look first at one of the

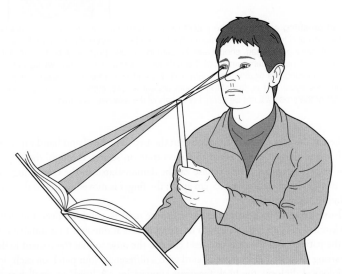

Fig. 10.9 Bar reading. A slightly wider septum is held a little closer than mid-way between the page and the eyes. It is kept still on the median line so that it occludes a different part of the page from each eye. The patient must use both eyes to be able to read across the page.

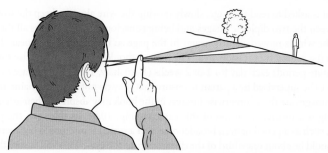

Fig. 10.10 A septum for exercising simultaneous vision for distance vision. The finger (or a septum) is held about 10 cm from the eyes while the patient looks at a distant scene. The patient should be aware of physiological diplopia of the finger and that both images are apparently transparent, that is, an object can be seen 'through' each finger, e.g., the tree and the man. The patient alternates fixation from one subject to the other, pausing at each to ensure that both objects and images of the finger are still visible.

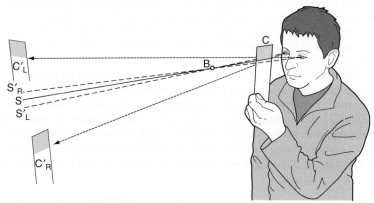

Fig. 10.11 Bead-on-string exercise. The patent holds a card, C, close to the nose. A length of string, SBC, tied to the card and to some more distant object, stretches horizontally. A bead, B, acts as a fixation object. The patient, fixating the bead, should see the card in crossed physiological diplopia: if it is a different colour on each side, it helps identification of the crossed diplopia. The string will be seen in increasing uncrossed diplopia beyond the fixation point, S'_R and S'_L, and in increasing crossed diplopia between the fixation bead and the eyes; that is, the string should appear as two strings crossing through the bead. In suppression, part of the cross will not be seen. For details of the exercise, see text.

objects and then at the other, alternating between the two. The head and hand must be kept quite still during this, and the patient is asked to concentrate on seeing 'through' the finger each time there is a tendency to suppress. The exercise can be demonstrated in the consulting room using a distance of 6 m and two objects about 75 cm apart: the finger is moved nearer to the eyes or further away to obtain the best position.

The **bead-on-string** (Brock string) exercise can be used to combine near and distance vision exercises (Pickwell, 1971, 1979b). A length of string is tied at one end to a suitable object several metres from the patient, and the near end held close to the nose so that the patient looks down the length of the string (Fig. 10.11). A piece of card with a different colour patch on each side is seen in crossed physiological diplopia to check for gross suppression. A bead, or small hexagonal metal nut, is threaded on the string and serves as a movable fixation target. The string should be seen in continuous physiological diplopia, with the 'two strings' appearing to cross at the fixation point, i.e., through the bead or nut. Any suppression is indicated by the absence of part of one of the two strings: closer than fixation in the case of exophoria, and beyond fixation in esophoria. The fixation bead or nut can be moved along the string to check for suppression at all distances. With a little practice, the patient can move fixation along the string without having to move the bead or nut and can maintain a continuous check on suppression at all distances.

Note that this procedure does not exercise relative convergence or accommodation, as the accommodation and convergence are changed together. It may, however, assist in heterophoria cases where the patient has difficulty in appreciating physiological diplopia correctly: this was discussed earlier in the chapter. The bead-on-string exercises can also be useful as a first stage of treatment in severe cases of convergence insufficiency, when the near point of convergence is greater than 20 cm.

Some forms of free-space stereograms include features that are designed to detect and treat suppression. Fine detail, some of which is specific to each eye's image, will aid the treatment of foveal suppression. This feature of the Institute Free-space Stereogram (IFS) exercises is described later.

RED AND GREEN FILTERS

If the eyes are dissociated by placing before one eye a red filter and before the other a green one, while the patient looks at a small spot of light any suppression will show as an absence of one colour. Normal patients will see one light which is a mixture of red and green in retinal rivalry. In unstable heterophoria, two lights may be seen and, where there is suppression, one of these may be present only intermittently. A prism of 6Δ, base downwards before one eye, will produce vertical diplopia, and suppression is more easily overcome.

In this exercise, the prism is rotated slowly toward the base direction in which it relieves the heterophoria: base-in for exophoria or base-out for esophoria. The patient will see the two lights rotate round each other and move closer together as they become level and the prism relieves the phoria. As the images move into the central foveal suppression area, one colour will disappear. The prism base-apex line is turned back towards its original base-down position and the patient tries to see the missing colour. The patient can have red and green filters and a prism on loan to practise this at home. This exercise is particularly useful in divergence excess cases.

Another approach that uses dissociation achieved by red and green filters is anaglyph bar reading. A coloured overlay which has alternating vertical strips coloured red and green is placed over the page. The patient wears red/green glasses and as they read along a line some of the text is only visible to each eye, so that suppression must be overcome.

PERCEPTUAL LEARNING

A small randomised controlled trial of successfully treated amblyopes suggests it may be possible to train stereopsis by perceptual learning (Portela-Camino, Martin-Gonzalez, Ruiz-Alcocer, Illarramendi-Mendicute, & Garrido-Mercado, 2018). Perceptual learning techniques are described in more detail in Chapter 13.

An Example of a Programme of Combined Clinic and Home Exercises

The best evidence for the efficacy of eye exercises, at least for improving clinical signs in CIES, is the exercise protocol used in the CITT-ART RCT (CITT-ART Investigator Group, 2019). This was adapted from therapy protocols used in earlier CITT trials. This procedure combined a range of in-practice and at-home exercises in four phases, summarised in Table 10.2. At some stages, similar procedures are carried out with different targets. For example, the free-space stereogram cards used in the CITT-ART trial involved some that are coloured and have text (known as lifesaver cards) and some with eccentric circles. The accommodative facility training starts with monocular, then biocular (both eyes open and uncovered, but minus lenses introduced only in front of one eye, then to the other), and finally to binocular (same powered lenses presented to both eyes that maintain binocular single vision).

An Example of Combined at Home Exercises: The IFS Exercises

INTRODUCTION

The Institute Free-space Stereogram (IFS) exercises were developed at the Institute of Optometry (see ethical declaration in Appendix 12) to train convergent fusional reserves, negative relative accommodation, and to treat foveal suppression in heterophoria (Evans, 2001b). The exercises were designed to keep the patient in an overconverged posture for as long as possible while keeping them occupied with a variety of tasks and different stimuli (Table 10.3). The various targets and types of stimulation (step and ramp) may help the benefit translate into everyday life. An open trial of over 20 consecutive patients produced encouraging results (Evans, 2000), as has a single-masked RCT of another 20 participants (Neuenschwander et al., 2018). The exercises are designed to be used at home, employing a parent and child team. They can be used by adults or older children by themselves, when it should be explained that some of the instructions are phrased in 'child friendly' language.

The principle of free-space stereograms dates back to 1940, although the IFS exercises have been designed with recent research in mind. A key feature of the exercises is very detailed instructions to make the parent, or older patient, the 'vision therapist'. The instructions are arranged in a series of stages to enhance a sense of progress for both the patient and parent. Usually, several stages are progressed through each day and this encourages participants.

Patients are asked to do the exercises for 10 minutes twice a day. It is best to have a short period (e.g., 3 weeks) of concentrated exercises before a review appointment. Even 3 weeks is

TABLE 10.3 ■ Details of Goals and Design of IFS Exercises.

Goal	Design feature
Affordable	Printed home exercises
Easy to understand	Comprehensive instructions
Fun to do	Novel 3-D images Varied tasks
Motivating	Encourage parent/child team One or two 10 min. sessions daily Check in 3–4 weeks
Checks on progress	10 self-test questions
Variety of stimuli	18 targets with step and ramp Different size stimuli Different shape stimuli Vergence angles: 3–30Δ
Control/treat suppression	Physiological diplopic images Monocular markers Stereopsis

quite a long time for a child and it helps if, when the exercises are issued, the child is aware that a follow-up appointment has been booked in 3 weeks so that they have a clear date to work towards.

DESIGN OF THE IFS EXERCISES

The IFS exercises comprise four cards, which the patient views, and detailed instructions which are read out by the parent or by the patient if old enough. Practitioner instructions are also included.

Card 1

Card 1 introduces the patient to the concept of physiological diplopia, starting with a simple target of two dots. The instructions train the patient to fixate a pencil above the page to create overconvergence. They are taught to appreciate the page as being doubled, so they see four dots. The distance of the pencil is then adjusted, and they are taught to be aware of the two pairs of dots moving, until the innermost dots become superimposed. Once they have practised this they progress to a similar exercise, but with rings. At this stage, the patients experience depth perception, and this tends to rejuvenate interest. They progress to more dramatic stereopsis, although the separation of targets on this card is small so that only a mild degree of overconvergence is required.

Quite early on in Card 1 the patient experiences the first of 10 self-test questions. These ask the patient about their stereoscopic perception, to confirm that they are making appropriate vergence movements. If not, then they are instructed to stop the exercises and to consult their eyecare practitioner.

Card 2

Card 2 uses targets with a very marked stereoscopic relief. In addition to the conventional 'ring' targets, there are also several shapes which are seen to 'float in 3-D space' (Fig. 10.12). Throughout this card, the need to keep the targets clear is stressed, which exercises negative relative accommodation.

A variety of different techniques are used on Card 2 and there are again regular self-checks to ensure that the patient is overconverging and not over-diverging. The awareness of physiological diplopia and stereopsis should help reduce any suppression, but there are also special targets which are designed to treat foveal suppression. With these small targets, the patient sees a four limbed star (✱), but with some of the limbs seen only by each eye. This reveals any suppression, and the patient is taught to overcome this. The patients then progressively 'jump' down to the lower set of rings and repeat the exercises with those. Because these become further apart, they require greater degrees of positive relative convergence.

After spending some time concentrating on the stereoperception of each target, patients are then instructed to rapidly track down the page, overconverging as appropriate for each successive target. This represents a form of 'step' (phasic) exercises, rather like using prism flippers. In the final stage for Card 2 patients are taught to gradually move the page towards them whilst maintaining an overconverged posture. This represents a form of 'ramp' (tonic) exercises.

Cards 3 and 4

To maintain patient interest, Card 3 employs a different approach. It uses an autostereogram, which has been specially created for the exercises (Fig. 10.13). Autostereograms are pictures based on random dot stereograms and the principle and history of the development of these has been summarised by Thimbleby and Neesham (1993).

Autostereograms can be viewed by converging or by diverging, so great care is taken in the IFS instructions to ensure that only convergence is used by patients during the exercises. Patients are taught to first exert positive relative convergence to obtain a stereoperception and then exert negative relative accommodation to make the elements of the stereogram clear. When the stereograms are viewed appropriately, patients perceive a series of steps, leading up towards them. As 'their eyes

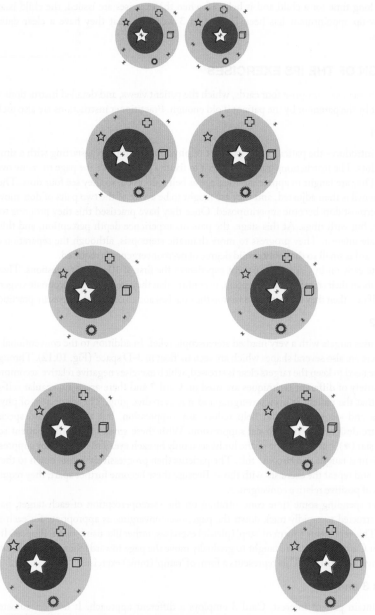

Fig. 10.12   IFS Card 2. The actual card is A4 size, larger than that shown.

walk up each step' they converge by increasing degrees. On each step is a letter for the patient to identify. There are the usual 'self-checks' to ensure that the exercises are being performed correctly, and the result is recorded for the practitioner to check at follow-up appointments. As with the rest of the exercises, the instructions clearly guide the patient through the stages of this phase of the exercises.

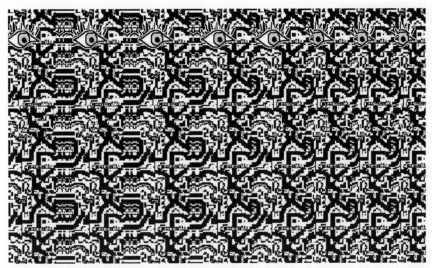

Fig. 10.13 IFS Card 3. The actual card is A4 size, larger than that shown. The autostereogram was created by Altered States, a developer of custom-designed autostereogram images.

Card 4 is another autostereogram and follows a similar principle to that used in Card 3.

PATIENT SELECTION

The most common use of the IFS exercises is to treat decompensated exophoria at near (Case Study 10.1). They can also be used to treat NPCI, some cases of decompensated basic exophoria, intermittent near exotropia, and (for more experienced practitioners) constant exotropia at near. For many patients, IFS exercises are the only treatment that is required. With other patients, particularly those with strabismus, the IFS exercises can be used as part of a complete treatment regimen, supplementing other exercises described elsewhere in this chapter.

As with any form of eye exercises, patient selection is crucial. If the patient or parent lack enthusiasm for exercises, they are unlikely to work, and other options should be considered, such as refractive modification (Chapter 6). The IFS exercises are most likely to be effective in patients over the age of 10 years (Evans, 2000), and can be effective in older patients (Case Study 10.1).

ISSUING THE EXERCISES TO THE PATIENT

One of the main objectives of IFS exercises is to allow home orthoptic therapy, with minimal input from the eyecare practitioner. The exercise booklet can usually be dispensed to the patient without lengthy explanations. Parents need to be told that the exercises require teamwork and a quiet time and place for the parent to read the instructions and for the child to view the cards. The diverse treatment approaches contained in the IFS exercises are designed to stimulate similar functions to clinic (office)-based vision therapy, with the detailed instructions replacing the therapist.

Patients are told that there are self-checks and they can telephone the practitioner if they are concerned. They are also warned that the exercises will be hard work so that a few minor symptoms of sore, tired, or aching eyes are to be expected for the first few days. The instructions warn that if these symptoms persist, or if any blurring or diplopia occur, the patient should stop the exercises and consult the practitioner. Typically, a follow-up appointment is booked in 3 weeks.

CASE STUDY 10.1

BACKGROUND
Insurance broker aged 61 years, wearing bifocals with minimal distance correction and +2.00 add. General health good, no medication.

SYMPTOMS
Last few months when reading eyes feel sore and tired and non-localised headache about twice a week after day in office.

RELEVANT CLINICAL FINDINGS
Normal: visual acuities, refractive error (minimal hypermetropia for distance, +2.25 add), visual fields, pupil reactions, ophthalmoscopic findings, intraocular pressures, anterior segment, D ocular motor balance, NPC (4 cm).
   N cover test 6Δ XOP with poor recovery.
   N aligning prism (with correction) 2.5Δ in LE.
   N convergent fusional reserve − /8/6Δ.

MANAGEMENT
Discussed decompensated exophoria and possibility of prism in glasses or eye exercises. Patient preferred to have eye exercises and given IFS exercises. Reexamination advised in 4 weeks.

FOLLOW-UP
Found exercises easy, done for 20 mins a day. Symptoms 'cleared up' and no headaches.
   N cover test 4Δ XOP with good recovery.
   N aligning prism (with correction) 0.5Δ in LE.
   Convergent fusional reserve 26/34/18.
   Exercises stopped, to return if more symptoms.

FOLLOW-UP 18 MONTHS LATER
No symptoms (broken glasses), results as at last appointment except for aligning prism now zero.

D, Distance; *IFS*, Institute Free-space Stereogram; *LE*, left eye; *N*, near; *NPC*, near point of convergence; *XOP*, exophoria.

FOLLOW-UP

Very rarely patients telephone the practitioner to report a problem with the exercises. The problems they might report and solutions to these are given in the practitioner instructions.

At the follow-up appointment, after 3−4 weeks, the practitioner should enquire about how easy or difficult the exercises have been, how often they been done, and for how long on average each day (Case Study 10.1). The patient should be asked about any change in their initial symptoms and asked whether any new symptoms have occurred.

The relevant clinical tests should be repeated, and the results compared with those obtained before giving the exercises. If the symptoms and clinical signs have improved, the exercises can be stopped (Case Study 10.1). Occasionally, the exercises need to be continued for longer. If there has been no or very little improvement, alternative approaches need to be considered, as discussed elsewhere in this chapter and in Chapter 6. If the exercises have been successful, the patient is asked to keep the booklet in case further 'top-up' exercises are required. Most older patients recognise the return of their symptoms and initiate a further session of exercises themselves. Of course, patients should be warned that if symptoms persist, they should return. Younger patients may need to be reexamined, perhaps in 3 months, to check the clinical signs. Patients can be re-assured that top-up exercises are usually easier and briefer.

CLINICAL KEY POINTS

- Exophoric conditions are treated by training convergent fusional reserves and/or negative relative accommodation
- This generic type of exercise has been validated by randomised controlled trials
- Fusional reserve eye exercises are most likely to be effective if they
  - are interesting for the patient
  - use a wide range of targets and types of exercise, with both step and ramp stimuli
  - teach an appreciation of physiological diplopia
  - employ feedback (e.g., stereopsis)
  - allow simultaneous training of any foveal suppression
  - are carried out intensively with follow-up every 3—4 weeks
- Various methods of dissociation can be used, including stereoscopic devices, red/green filters, polarisation, free-space methods, and virtual reality
- Facility training can also be helpful

CHAPTER 11

Anisometropia and Aniseikonia

Binocular vision can be disturbed by large differences in the refractive error between the two eyes: **anisometropia**. When this is left uncorrected, central suppression areas can develop in the eye with the more blurred vision. Anisometropia over 1.50D results in a significant increase in the risk of amblyopia and decrease of binocular function (Weakley, 2001) and higher anisometropia is likely to be associated with worse amblyopia and stereoacuity (Rutstein & Corliss, 1999). Poorer stereoacuity is associated with reduced performance at motor tasks (Hrisos, Clarke, Kelly, Henderson, & Wright, 2006) and at driving (Bauer, Kolling, Dietz, Zrenner, & Schiefer, 2000; Gresset & Meyer, 1994). A surprising finding is that approximately a quarter of hypermetropic anisometropic patients exhibit, in their amblyopic eye, less accommodation at near than at distance (Toor, Horwood, & Riddell, 2018). This was resolved with spectacle correction, emphasising the importance of optometric care for these patients. These authors noted that aniso-accommodation is more common than previously suggested, even in a normal control group.

Anisometropia over 1.00D occurs in 0.7% of preschool children (Donahue, 2006). Anisometropia in children is an indication for cycloplegic refraction (Table 2.11). If anisometropia occurs in young patients, and particularly before the age of 6 years when the visual system is still not firmly established, amblyopia may also be present. Often in these cases, the vision is very good in one eye, so that the anisometropia and reduced vision in the other eye is not discovered. The older the child, the more difficult it is to treat the amblyopia and restore full acuity (Chapter 13). The importance of early eye examination is obvious, and the procedures for the examination of young children are dealt with in Chapter 3. There is no doubt that many cases of anisometropic amblyopia are preventable by early examination and correction by spectacles. The treatment of anisometropic amblyopia is covered in Chapter 13, together with other types of functional amblyopia.

With patients of any age, prescribing glasses to correct anisometropia may present two additional problems:

1. *Prismatic effects:* when the patient is not looking through the optical centres of the lenses, a difference in prismatic effect between the two lenses can make binocular vision difficult or impossible. These prismatic effects present more difficulties when the patient looks above or below the centres, as the vertical tolerance to prisms is very much less than the horizontal. For some patients, a vertical prismatic effect of 0.5Δ can impair stereopsis (Jimenez, J.R., Rubino, M., Diaz, J.A., Hita, E., & Jimenez-del Barco, L., 2000).
2. *Aniseikonia:* when the lenses are of different powers, there will be a larger retinal image in one eye than the other owing to the difference in spectacle magnification.

These two problems are discussed in more detail later. In both cases, these difficulties will cause more problems in older patients, with previously uncorrected patients, or where a large change in prescription is given.

Prismatic Effects

DIAGNOSIS

The main factor in recognising a difficulty due to prismatic effects is the presence of the anisometropia itself. It may also be found that older children and teenage patients with anisometropia have spasm of accommodation, and cycloplegic refraction is especially important in these cases. The symptoms of anisometropia are typically those due to the type of refractive error in the better eye: asthenopia for near vision in hypermetropia and blurred distance vision in myopia. Some patients may be hypermetropic in one eye and myopic in the other. In these cases, they may use one eye for distance vision and the other for close work. If there is no significant refractive error in one eye, the patient may have no symptoms. This may also be true in cases where no glasses have been worn and suppression has developed.

Many patients will experience no problems when spectacles are prescribed; the younger the patient when glasses are first worn, the more likely that trouble can be avoided. This is probably because patients with stable binocular vision or compensated heterophoria can usually adapt to prismatic effects in a very short time (Carter, 1963). The symptoms that occur when the patient does not adapt to the correction for anisometropia consist of difficulties in adjusting to the new glasses: typically, headache or intermittent diplopia. Troubles seldom occur when the anisometropia is less than 2D. If spectacles that fully correct the anisometropia can be tolerated in childhood, the prognosis for successful spectacle wear in adult (pre-presbyopic) life is good, as anisometropia usually gradually reduces over the years (Ohlsson, Baumann, Sjostrand, & Abrahamsson, 2002).

INVESTIGATION AND EVALUATION

Often, the difficulties described above can be avoided by anticipation. A partial correction is given in the more hypermetropic eye in those cases where there has been no previous correction or where there is a large difference between the previous correction and the new one (Howell-Duffy, Umar, Ruparelia, & Elliott, 2010). The extent of this modification to the prescription can be determined by the Mallett fixation disparity test (Chapter 9). The patient looks at the fixation disparity vertical target through the full correction and is asked to move the head vertically up and down in a nodding movement, so the eyes look through the lenses above and then below the optical centres. If a vertical fixation disparity is induced, the prescription is modified until this does not occur.

As a rough guide, the prescription for the more hypermetropic eye is reduced by one-third of the change in the anisometropia (the difference between the two eyes) compared with the previous prescription. This will mean that it is reduced by one-third of the anisometropia in the case of a patient who has worn no previous glasses. However, it must not be assumed that all patients with anisometropia will experience difficulties with their new glasses. Some patients with marked anisometropia will settle very readily to a new prescription, whereas others with low degrees will experience symptoms.

Patients often learn very quickly to turn the head rather than the eyes, so that they always look through the optical centres of the lenses. It sometimes helps to encourage patients to do this. If the patient needs bifocals, round top segments of different sizes in each lens can be used to control the vertical prismatic power in the reading portion. A more detailed coverage of this subject can be found in Rabbetts (2007). Optically, the best approach is to fit contact lenses, which move with the eyes, so no prismatic effect is induced, and which also reduce aniseikonia (Evans, 2006a). Refractive surgery has been advocated for similar reasons (Paysse, Coats, Hussein, Hamill, & Koch, 2006).

Aniseikonia Due to Spectacle Magnification Differences

Most aniseikonia arises from the difference in spectacle magnification that accompanies anisometropic corrections, **acquired optical aniseikonia**. Other types will be considered separately later in this chapter. Interestingly, everyone experiences aniseikonia in asymmetrical convergence of the eyes, for example, when converging to an object in our peripheral vision which will be closer to one eye than the other, and this may become of the order of 5%–10% or more. This **physiological aniseikonia** appears to be automatically compensated and gives rise to no symptoms (Romano, 1999).

INVESTIGATION

The possibility of an aniseikonic problem occurring can be foreseen largely from the presence of anisometropia, and particularly when there is a difference in spectacle magnification of more than 2% (some authors say 5%). This means that anisometropia of as little as 1.25D may cause clinically significant aniseikonia, although the precise value will depend on the prescription, back vertex distance, and relative ocular dimensions (Rabbetts, 2007). Typically, 1D of anisometropia causes between 1% and 1.5% of aniseikonia (Borish, 1975).

There is a large variation between people in the amount of aniseikonia they can tolerate (Romano, 1999). Again, symptoms can lead to nontolerance of new glasses, and sometimes headache and intermittent diplopia. A symptom more characteristic of aniseikonia is a disturbance in spatial perception: the floor appears to slope, or other horizontal objects appear tilted when looking through the new glasses. Induced aniseikonia (using size lenses) of 3%–5% causes a reduction in stereoacuity (Jimenez, Ponce, Jimenez-del Barco, Diaz, & Perez-Ocon, 2002) and of 5% or more significantly reduces binocular contrast sensitivity and binocular summation (Jimenez, Ponce, & Anera, 2004).

Aniseikonia can be investigated with an eikonometer (Morrison, 1993), although this apparatus is uncommon. There are two types of eikonometer:

1. *Ames eikonometer*, which presents a separate image to each eye, so the patient can make a direct comparison of the image sizes. Polarising filters can be used (Romano, 1999).
2. *Space eikonometer*, which allows the patient to recognise distortions of space perception, such as a tilting of the frontoparallel plane.

In both cases, measurements of image size differences are made by an afocal optical system of variable magnification which is adjusted until a normal appearance is reported. Neither of these instruments gives very consistent results. Several readings are taken, and if the spread of readings is less than the mean value, this mean value may be taken as the size difference. Its use may be more necessary in types of aniseikonia other than acquired optical.

Most eyecare practitioners do not have an eikonometer, and a software package called the Aniseikonia Inspector was developed for the investigation and management of aniseikonia (de Wit, 2003). This produces more accurate results in the vertical direction than the horizontal, but underestimates aniseikonia (Rutstein, Corliss, & Fullard, 2006; Antona, Barra, Barrio, Gonzalez, & Sanchez, 2007). A later version of the test may overestimate aniseikonia induced by size lenses (Fullard, Rutstein, & Corliss, 2007).

It is possible to obtain a diagnosis and qualitative estimate of aniseikonia using commonly available refracting equipment which dissociate the right eye from the left eye images. For example, many projector charts have a muscle balance test comprising a pair of 'square brackets', one of which is seen by the right and the other by the left eye. Patients can directly compare the size of these to give an estimate of aniseikonia. A similar technique can be used with letter charts having cross-polarised letters or targets. A more accurate measure can be obtained if a tangent screen is available. The two eyes are dissociated with a vertical prism that is too great to be fused (e.g., 8Δ) and the position of numbers on the smaller image of the tangent scale is compared to the position of the same numbers on the larger to calculate the magnification difference. This approach can be improvised using a line of Snellen letters for distance vision or a centimetre rule for near vision.

MANAGEMENT

Anticipation of the difficulties is again very important. The following should be considered:

1. Warn the patient that difficulties in space perception may occur during the first few days of wearing the new glasses. It is usually adequate to say that the patient's prescription is of the type that may require a few days to settle to the new glasses. In most cases, these problems will disappear after a short time, particularly if some of the factors mentioned next have been considered. Warn the patient not to drive or operate machinery until they have adapted.

   Some strabismic patients may be less able to tolerate optically induced aniseikonia than patients with normal binocular vision (Bucci, Kapoula, Bernotas, & Zamfirescu, 1999), so they may be less able to tolerate large refractive changes.

2. Reduce the difference in spectacle magnification by considering the factors that contribute to it (Fig. 11.1):

   a. *Lens power:* the higher the power, the higher the spectacle magnification. A partial correction for one eye can be considered, again reducing by about one-third of the change in the anisometropia. In some cases, a partial correction in both eyes may be

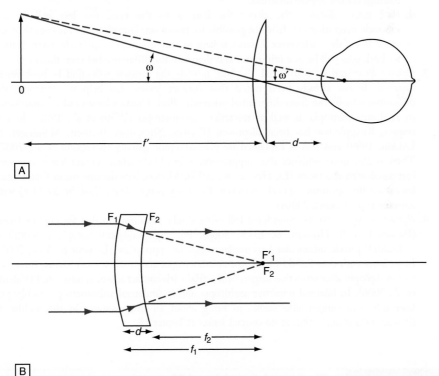

Fig. 11.1 (A) The spectacle magnification (SM) is the ratio of the angle subtended at the eye by the object to the angle subtended at the spectacle lens. This can be shown to be SM = $1/(1-dF)$, where d is the back vertex distance, and F the power of the lens. As the lens is moved closer to the eye (d decreases), spectacle magnification will become unity. As the power of the lens (F) increases, the spectacle magnification will increase. (B) The magnification of a 'thick' lens is the ratio between the focal lengths of the surface powers. This can be shown to be $1/(1+tF')$, where F' is the power of the front surface, and t is the reduced thickness of the lens (d/n).

appropriate, as this will leave the patient to exert the same accommodative effort in both eyes. With young patients, such a binocular reduction will give sufficient correction to relieve any symptoms of hypermetropia, but because both lenses are less powerful, the difference in spectacle magnification will be less.

   b. *Lens form:* the deeper the meniscus (i.e., the higher the base curve), the greater the spectacle magnification. The lenses should be dispensed with the more positive lens in a 'flatter' form than the other (e.g., aspheric front surface). This will reduce the spectacle magnification a little, and it will also result in the front surfaces of the lenses being more similar in appearance. The lenses can be made to an aspheric design, which is thinner, flatter, and lighter.

   c. *Lens thickness:* the thicker the lens, the greater the spectacle magnification. The least powerful positive lens can be thicker than normal, so that its spectacle magnification is increased slightly. This will also have the effect of helping to balance the weight of the two lenses. Clearly, the more powerful lens needs to be kept as thin as is consistent with the type of frame or mount used. This will maintain the spectacle magnification and the weight at a minimum. One possibility is to use a higher refractive index material for the thicker lens, although care should be taken to ensure the antireflection coatings do not appear different.

   d. *Back vertex distance:* the closer the lens is to the eyes, the less will be the spectacle magnification. It is not possible to mount one lens closer to the eyes than the other, but if the back vertex distance is kept to a minimum, the spectacle magnification for both eyes will be at a minimum and therefore the difference between them less.

3. *Contact lenses* can be considered, as these provide the greatest reduction in back vertex distance. It has already been noted that contact lenses also help to overcome the difficulties which arise from differential prismatic effect. Contact lenses reduce aniseikonia in axial anisometropia as well as refractive anisometropia (Winn et al., 1988). In this respect, Knapp's law has been disproven (Kramer, Shippman, Bennett, Meininger, & Lubkin, 1999) and this is explained by photoreceptor spacing (Kitaguchi et al., 2007). There is also some evidence that suppression is less likely when contact lenses are worn compared with spectacles (Li, Hess et al., 2013). Modern lens designs mean that contact lenses are the optimum optical correction for many people (e.g., Case Study 11.1) with anisometropia (Evans, 2006a).

4. *Refractive surgery* can be considered following similar reasoning to that for contact lenses (Paysse, Hamill, Hussein, & Koch, 2004). For high unilateral myopia ($-8.00D$ to $-18.00D$) phakic intraocular lens implants may be appropriate (Lesueur & Arne, 2002). In patients with over 3.00D of myopic anisometropia and weak sensory status, there is a risk of diplopia after refractive surgery and a trial with contact lenses is advocated (Valente et al., 2006). In bilateral refractive amblyopia and in unilateral anisometropic amblyopia, laser refractive surgery also seems to bring about an improvement in the amblyopia (Roszkowska et al., 2006), as do contact lenses (Chapter 13).

CASE STUDY 11.1	**First appointment (aged 36 years)**

SYMPTOMS & HISTORY

Last eye examination 10 years ago. First eye examination at age 7 years when hypermetropia discovered, L>R. Wore spectacles until late 20s, not worn since. In recent months, has gradually noticed LE seems worse and this bothers px. Binocularly, vision OK and no other symptoms. No relevant family history.

RELEVANT CLINICAL FINDINGS

Normal: ocular health, pupil reactions, 25-degree fields, IOP, motility, NPC.

Unaided vision:	R 6/5−1	L 6/6
Retinoscopy:	R +1.75DS	L +3.50/−0.50 × 90
Subjective:	R +1.75/−0.25 × 85 6/5	L +3.75/−0.75 × 110 6/5
Cover test:	D orthophoria	N 8Δ R SOP, Grade 1 rec.
Mallett aligning prism:	D nil	N nil
Amp. Acc. (no Rx):	R 13D	L 7D
Stereoacuity (Randot 2):	no Rx	shapes 500″, circles 20″
	subjective Rx	shapes 250″, circles 20″

MANAGEMENT

Explained − anisometropia, effect of age on ability to overcome hypermetropia, best optical correction likely from contact lenses. Patient would like to have clear vision in both eyes so fitted with monthly disposable daily wear contact lenses. Recommended spectacles as backup, but patient feels can cope with no correction if unable to wear contact lenses.

FOLLOW-UP (1−10 YEARS)

Patient happily wearing contact lenses and no problems.

COMMENT

The interesting feature in this case is the lack of amblyopia, despite only starting refractive correction at age 7 years. Speculatively, this could be explained by the anisometropia being less in early childhood, aniso-accommodation, or adequate cortical plasticity at age 7 years.

Amp. Acc, Accommodative amplitude; *D*, dioptre/distance; *DS*, dioptre sphere; *IOP*, intraocular pressure; *L*, left; *LE*, left eye; *N*, near; *NPC*, near point of convergence; *px*, patient; *R*, right; *Rx*, prescription; *SOP*, esophoria.

ASTIGMATIC CORRECTIONS

The aforementioned factors can reduce the difference in spectacle magnification to a degree where it is unlikely to cause problems in those cases where the anisometropia is mainly spherical. Where the anisometropia is astigmatic, requiring a higher cylindrical correction in one eye than the other, or where there are high cylinders in both eyes, it is much more likely that there will be disturbances in space perception due to the meridional magnification. The factors mentioned above will assist in these cases, too. Warn the patient of the likely disturbances during the first few days of wearing the new glasses. Consider a partial astigmatic correction and keep the back vertex distance to a minimum.

Lens thickness and form can be employed to overcome the problems in astigmatic corrections by prescribing **isogonal lenses** (Halass, 1959). These are lenses whose thickness and surface powers are calculated to produce the same spectacle magnification in both meridians of both lenses: there is no difference in spectacle magnification to create aniseikonia. Usually, isogonal lenses need to be made with a toric surface on both surfaces of each lens, with the principal meridians parallel on each side. This is a difficult and expensive process, and therefore isogonal lenses are only prescribed where other methods of relieving the symptoms of the aniseikonia have failed. An eikonometer is not required for prescribing isogonal lenses.

Contact lenses are effective in reducing the problems with astigmatic aniseikonia. When other factors make the patient suitable for contact lens wear, this is the most satisfactory method (Evans, 2006a).

Other Types of Aniseikonia

It is also possible that aniseikonia can be the result of differences that are inherent in the visual system; a difference in the optical components or length of the eyes, or due to an anomaly in the arrangement of the neurons of the two eyes: **anatomical aniseikonia**. These differences are likely to be present at birth, from an early age, or to come on very gradually. In many cases, the visual system adapts to the difference, and either tolerates it or suppresses one eye. Where suppression occurs, no method of detecting the aniseikonia is available, unless the suppression is treated.

Where the aniseikonia is of a degree that is tolerated, it is possible that some change can result in it becoming intolerable and symptoms occur. Diagnosis in these cases requires an eikonometer. A **size lens** (or aniseikonic lens) can be prescribed to give the magnification specified by the eikonometer. As with isogonal lenses, the thickness and surface curves are calculated to give the required magnification. Again, if there is an astigmatic element or if a meridional magnification is required, a size lens will require two toric surfaces.

Because of the cost of making a size lens to a patient's individual prescription, and also because of the indefinite nature of eikonometer readings, trial periods of wearing afocal size lenses are sometimes undertaken. A stock size lens of approximately the magnification required is worn for several days clipped on the patient's normal glasses. It is tried so that it equalises the image sizes, and also for a brief period before the other eye so that it increases the size difference. In the first case it should alleviate the symptoms, and in the second make them temporarily worse. This will verify that it is the aniseikonia which is causing the problems and that a size lens is appropriate to alleviate them. Patients should not drive or operate machinery if their spatial perception is significantly altered.

CLINICAL KEY POINTS

- Anisometropia over about 1–2D can cause problems from prismatic effects and/or aniseikonia
- Many patients adapt to their anisometropia, others can be helped by a partial correction
- Problems from vertical prismatic effects are particularly likely with multifocal lenses
- Aniseikonic problems can be reduced by keeping the back vertex distance as low as possible and by careful choice of lens form and material
- Contact lenses or refractive surgery provide the best optical solution in anisometropia

PART 3

Strabismus

CHAPTER 12

Overview of Sensory Changes in Strabismus

Binocular Sensory Changes in Strabismus

DIPLOPIA AND CONFUSION

Diplopia occurs when a patient sees two images of one object. Fig. 12.1A represents an adult with recent onset left esotropia. The patient is viewing an isolated letter 'A', with no other objects present in the field of view. The letter is imaged on the right fovea (f) but, because the left eye is convergent, it is imaged on a nasal region of the left retina (p) which is not the fovea. In other words, the object is imaged on noncorresponding retinal points. Therefore, the object is perceived in two different visual directions, causing diplopia.

Everyday visual scenes are usually more complicated than the single object in Fig. 12.1A. Fig. 12.1B illustrates the situation, for the same patient, when there are two isolated objects in the visual field (of course, this is still an unrealistically straightforward example). The letter A is imaged on the fovea of the right eye and the letter B is imaged on the fovea of the left eye. As the case is a recent onset strabismus in an adult patient, the patient is likely to have normal retinal correspondence (NRC). This means that both foveae share the same visual direction, so the patient will see the two letters as being superimposed. The visual perception is described as **confusion**. Of course, the diplopia illustrated in Fig. 12.1A would also be present in the situation illustrated in Fig. 12.1B, so in everyday scenes, both diplopia and confusion will coexist. Depending on the visual scene and the magnitude of the separation of the images, diplopia may be more troublesome than confusion.

SUPPRESSION OF THE BINOCULAR FIELD OF THE STRABISMIC EYE

Clearly, diplopia and confusion are undesirable, so the visual system may develop sensory adaptations to avoid them. In young patients, this is what happens. Hypothetically, one method of avoiding symptoms in strabismus might be to suppress the whole of the binocular field of the strabismic eye. This sometimes occurs (Joosse et al., 2005), particularly in divergent strabismus (Ansons & Spencer, 2001), and in decompensated exophoria, suppression is more likely in cases exhibiting intermittent exotropia (Wakayama et al., 2013). The investigation and treatment of suppression is detailed in Chapter 14. However, the visual system usually does not adopt such wasteful measures. Instead of having a large area of suppression, a strabismic patient who is young enough to have a reasonable degree of sensory plasticity usually will develop harmonious anomalous retinal correspondence (HARC). Suppression and HARC are fundamentally different, and elicit different steady state visual evoked potentials (Bagolini, Falsini, Cermola, & Porciatti, 1994).

ANOMALOUS (ABNORMAL) RETINAL CORRESPONDENCE (ARC)

The classical views on Panum's fusional areas and retinal correspondence have, as a result of research over the last 20 years, undergone much revision. The phrase 'corresponding retinal points' is something of a misnomer: a point image on one retina actually corresponds with point images

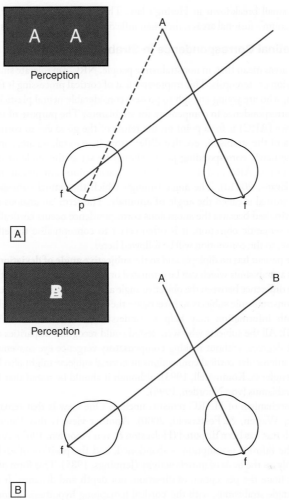

Fig. 12.1 Illustration of (A) diplopia and (B) confusion in left convergent strabismus (see text).

falling in a Panum's area in the other eye. Several researchers have shown that Panum's area is not a fixated entity, but its size varies according to the parameters of the target. What remains unclear is whether, at a given retinal eccentricity, the size of Panum's area really changes or whether apparent changes are experimental artefacts.

Several studies have obtained data indicating that retinal correspondence can change in normal, nonstrabismic, observers (Fender & Julesz, 1967; Hyson, Julesz, & Fender, 1983; Erkelens & Collewijn, 1985; Brautaset & Jennings, 2006a; Fogt & Jones, 1998), or that Panum's fusional areas are much larger than previously believed (Collewijn, Steinman, Erkelens, & Regan, 1991). However, one very thorough paper has concluded from two experiments that retinal correspondence is fixed in nonstrabismic observers (Hillis & Banks, 2001).

There is certainly the need for some flexibility in the vergence system as, during everyday vision and head movements, small errors in vergence occur. This is particularly likely after a large saccade and represents a small breakdown in Hering's law. This is probably why our visual system has evolved to have Panum's fusional areas rather than inflexible point to point correspondence.

Anomalous Retinal Correspondence in Strabismus

Panum's fusional areas mean that, in nonstrabismic people, NRC can tolerate small vergence errors, without losing fusion or stereopsis. This impressive feat of cortical processing is far surpassed by the ability of children, who are young enough to possess considerable neural plasticity, to exhibit large shifts in retinal correspondence to compensate for strabismus. The purpose of this anomalous retinal correspondence (ARC) is for a point on the retina of the good eye to correspond with a new point in the retina of the strabismic eye that differs from its natural, innate, corresponding retinal point. Clearly, the newly corresponding points should be set at the angle of strabismus. This is nearly always the case in ARC and there is said to be **harmonious anomalous retinal correspondence** (HARC; Evans, 2001d). The angle through which the retinal correspondence has been shifted from the normal is called the **angle of anomaly**. The term 'anomalous **retinal** correspondence' has been criticised because the anomalous correspondence occurs cortically, not on the retinae. Despite this semantic objection, it is often easier to conceptualise the effect of HARC by considering retinae, so the convention will be followed here.

In HARC, the patient has no diplopia and so the **subjective angle of deviation** is zero. The cover test usually shows a strabismus which can be estimated or measured (p. 20) to be the **objective angle of deviation**. The difference between the objective angle and subjective angle is the angle of anomaly.

Research in nonstrabismic subjects to investigate the largest amount of visual disparity that can still provide depth information may help to understand the basis for HARC (Dengler & Kommerell, 1993). All the subjects who were tested could recognise disparities of up to 6 degrees, and one up to 21 degrees, without making compensatory vergence eye movements. It is possible that far-reaching interocular cortical connections in normal subjects might also be utilised in cases of strabismus (Dengler & Kommerell, 1993), although it should be noted that HARC is uncommon in vertical strabismus (von Noorden, 1996).

The precise mechanism of HARC remains unclear. One view is that remapping of Panum's areas occurs (Lie, Watten, & Fostervold, 2000). Another view is that Panum's areas become enlarged, although this has been disputed (Helveston & von Noorden, 1967). A third hypothesis is that in HARC the bifoveal assumption is abandoned, and the position of each eye is registered separately, probably on the basis of muscle activity (Jennings, 1985). This form of HARC would be most likely to facilitate the perception of direction, not depth and distance. It might account for HARC in large angle strabismus, with the 'cortical remapping hypothesis' accounting for HARC in cases of small-angle strabismus (Jennings, personal communication).

To summarise, there are three types of binocular sensory status in strabismus. First, there may be no adaptation, resulting in diplopia and confusion. Second, all the binocular field of the strabismic eye may be suppressed. Third, HARC may occur. The third option allows some rudimentary form of 'pseudobinocular vision' and is clearly the preferable outcome, so the question arises, why does this not always occur? This, and some limitations and consequences of ARC, will now be considered.

Factors Influencing the Development of HARC

Although the precise neurophysiological basis of HARC is not known, the main theories all accept that this 'stunning feat of cortical processing' (Nelson, 1988b) must, inevitably, have limitations. One of these limitations relates to the requirement for the visual system to be plastic for HARC to develop. It is therefore not surprising that a younger age of onset of strabismus is associated with a greater likelihood of HARC being present. Von Noorden (1996) states that HARC, albeit superficial (see later), can develop as late as the early teenage years. A survey of 195 patients by Stidwill (1998) found that 97% of cases of HARC had developed in strabismus with an onset before the age of 6 years, although the condition was occasionally present in strabismus developing up to the age of 15 years.

In cases of intermittent strabismus, the visual axes will sometimes be straight, and the patient will have NRC; yet at other times there will be a strabismus and the patient will have HARC. The change from NRC to HARC can be sudden or gradual. The term covariation describes the angle of anomaly covarying with the objective angle of strabismus. Covariation is likely to place additional neural demands on the visual system and hence constant strabismus will be more likely to develop HARC than intermittent or variable strabismus. For similar reasons, unilateral strabismus is more likely to develop HARC than alternating strabismus.

Von Noorden (1996) stated that the rate of occurrence of HARC 'is high in infantile esotropia, less common in exotropia, and uncommon in vertical strabismus'. Other authors have noted that suppression is more common in exotropia and in anisometropia.

Photoreceptor types, receptive field sizes, and ganglion cell types, vary across the retina. An area of retina near the fovea of 1 mm^2 has a much greater cortical representation than 1 mm^2 of retina in the periphery: this has been termed **cortical magnification**. The cortical processing task of remapping anomalously corresponding points must be easier if these points are at similar eccentricities from the fovea. Hence, small angle strabismus is more likely to develop HARC than large angle strabismus (Wong, Lueder, Burkhalter, & Tychsen, 2000).

Depth of HARC

Most patients who exhibit HARC can, under certain circumstances, be made to exhibit NRC. In other words, the neural substrate for innate NRC is still present. The difficulty in eliciting NRC is termed the 'depth of anomaly' (Nelson, 1988b). The factors that make it easier for the visual system to develop HARC are also likely to make the HARC deeper. Therefore, it follows from the previous section that patients are more likely to have deeper (c.f., shallow) HARC in cases where there is a younger onset (Kora, Awaya, & Sato, 1997), a stable angle of strabismus, unilateral strabismus, and a small angle.

The Detection and Treatment of HARC

HARC can be thought of as 'pseudobinocular vision'. It was noted in Chapter 2 that a patient with weak normal binocular vision (e.g., a decompensating heterophoria) could, by using tests which tend to dissociate the eyes, be 'broken down' so the heterophoria degenerates into a strabismus. An analogous phenomenon can occur with shallow HARC. If a patient with shallow HARC is tested with unnatural stimuli, such as after-images or the synoptophore, the pseudobinocular vision may be broken down into NRC, with resulting diplopia or compensatory suppression. If more natural, 'associating', tests are used, such as Bagolini lenses (Chapter 14), HARC may be detected. This is why, if the practitioner is to discover whether HARC is truly present under normal everyday viewing conditions, naturalistic tests should be used. The factors which are particularly important in simulating normal visual conditions are listed in Chapter 14.

The likelihood of treatment succeeding is influenced by the depth of HARC and the age at which treatment is commenced. The shorter the interval between the age of onset of HARC and age at commencement of treatment, the better the prognosis. This highlights the importance of regular professional eyecare for pre-school children, especially if the child is at risk of strabismus.

Sensory Function and Localised Suppression in HARC

In HARC, a point in the peripheral retina of the strabismic eye is said to acquire, during everyday binocular viewing, the same visual direction as the fovea of the fixating eye: this point is directed towards the object of regard and is sometimes referred to as the **zero point**, zero point measure, or diplopia point (Serrano-Pedraza, Clarke, & Read, 2011). The zero point has also been referred to as the pseudofovea, but this can be confusing because 'pseudofovea' is also used to describe the eccentrically fixating area in eccentric fixation. When the good eye is occluded, the patient fixates with the eccentrically fixating point or, if there is no eccentric fixation, with the fovea and this why the cover test works (for an exception, see Chapter 16).

The issue of the exceptionally small receptive field sizes at the fovea was mentioned earlier and this makes HARC difficult in two regions of the strabismic visual field. These areas are the fovea and the zero point. If HARC is not possible in these two areas, the alternative is suppression, and suppression at these two areas is a very common finding in the strabismic eye. These small suppression areas that occur **in the presence of HARC** are quite different to the complete suppression of the binocular field of the strabismic eye that occurs as an **alternative to HARC** (Serrano-Pedraza et al., 2011). The central suppression areas in HARC are of the order of 1 degree (Mallett, 1988a) and often cause, in the Bagolini lens test, the central part of the streak to be absent (Chapter 14). The central suppression areas are also why the modified (large) **OXO** test should be used instead of the smaller **OXO** test to assess HARC (Chapter 14). The cortical task of 'remapping' will be increasingly difficult as the angle of the strabismus increases, because larger peripheral receptive fields will have to be 'remapped' to anomalously correspond with smaller central receptive fields in the other eye. Therefore, if all other factors are constant, it seems likely that with larger angles of strabismus the suppression areas will be larger and pseudostereopsis and pseudomotor fusion (see later) will generally be worse.

The purpose of HARC is to compensate for the strabismus: to provide 'pseudobinocular vision'. Some pseudostereoacuity is possible with HARC (Mallett, 1977). This is more likely to be present and to be better with deeply-ingrained HARC, particularly with small angled strabismus (Henson & Williams, 1980). Stereoacuity can be better than 100″ with the Howard-Dolman or Titmus circles tests (Jennings, 1985) which measure contoured stereopsis, but it has been argued that random dot stereopsis cannot be demonstrated in a patient with strabismus (Cooper & Feldman, 1978; Hatch & Laudon, 1993). Rutstein and Eskridge (1984) argued that some patients with small-angle strabismus have demonstrable stereopsis with random dot tests which is indicative of normal correspondence. Yet another view is that stereopsis is not possible in any form of constant strabismus, even microtropia, and findings to the contrary are attributable to monocular cues in stereotests (Cooper, 1979).

The locus of the horopter and anomalous fusional space in HARC is much larger than in normal binocular vision (Jennings, 1985). A great many questions remain unanswered about the physiological basis for the antidiplopic strategies of suppression and HARC (Serrano-Pedraza et al., 2011).

Motor Function in HARC

In cases of NRC the objective angle will equal the subjective angle. In HARC, the patient will have single vision, so their subjective angle is zero. The angle of anomaly is equal to the difference between the subjective and objective angles. So, in HARC the angle of anomaly is equal to the objective angle: the HARC fully corrects the subjective angle of strabismus.

The objective angle normally exhibited by the patient under undisturbed conditions is called the **habitual angle of strabismus**, and the objective angle following prolonged or repeated dissociation is the **total angle of strabismus**. As the habitual angle changes to the total angle, the angle of anomaly usually remains constant: the difference between the new total objective and subjective angles is the same as that between the habitual objective and subjective angles (Table 12.1, first 3 columns). The fact that the total angle is reduced to the habitual angle during everyday viewing implies that the HARC may induce some motor fusion to maintain the habitual angle. Indeed, vergence movements can occur in HARC and the patient can be seen to 'converge' to follow an approaching target, yet a cover test will reveal that the strabismus is present. Similarly, 'pseudo' fusional reserves can often be measured.

Unharmonious Anomalous Retinal Correspondence (UARC)

The obvious alternative to HARC is NRC with diplopia or suppression of the binocular field of the strabismic eye. Another option, UARC, is exceedingly rare and is best understood with an example. Imagine a young child who develops a small stable strabismus and associated HARC. The purpose of the HARC is to prevent diplopia and confusion and to allow some rudimentary binocular vision

TABLE 12.1 ■ Example of Calculation of Angle of Anomaly in HARC and in (Very Rare) UARC.

Angle	HARC: habitual angle	HARC: total angle	UARC
Objective angle	15Δ R SOT	20Δ R SOT	40Δ R SOT
Subjective angle	0	5	25
Angle of anomaly	15	15	15

HARC, Harmonious anomalous retinal correspondence; R, right, SOT, esotropia; UARC, unharmonious anomalous retinal correspondence. All units are prism dioptres.

in the presence of strabismus. As mentioned earlier, the angle of anomaly will be equal to the objective angle of strabismus. Now, assume that after many years in his adapted state the adult patient suffers, for example, trauma and an extraocular muscle paresis resulting in a change to the angle of the strabismus, with consequent diplopia. If the HARC was shallow, the patient would revert to NRC. In this case, the subjective angle (angle of diplopia) would be equal to the new objective angle and the angle of anomaly would be zero.

However, if the HARC associated with the old strabismus was very deep, the patient may continue with this HARC in the presence of the new strabismus. It is unlikely that a long-standing stable HARC could covary with a new change in the angle of strabismus in an adult. Instead, the patient may develop a 'strabismus on top of a strabismus'. The objective angle will be the angle of the new strabismus, the subjective angle will be the difference between the angle of the old strabismus and the new strabismus, and the angle of anomaly will be neither zero nor equal to either of the subjective angles (Table 12.1).

Clearly, this sequence of events is extremely unlikely (although UARC can also occur secondary to surgery), so why is UARC given such prominence in some textbooks? The reason is that many early methods of investigating retinal correspondence created highly artificial conditions which tend to cause HARC to break down. It was sometimes concluded that these techniques were detecting UARC. Of course, if the patient really has UARC, they would complain of constant diplopia. It would not make sense for the visual system to undergo extensive remapping only to leave constant diplopia.

There are different theories on the aetiology of ARC, reviewed by Jennings (1985). Another detailed description of this condition was given by Nelson (1988b). Chapter 14 includes details of the investigation and treatment of HARC.

Monocular Sensory Changes in Strabismus

There are two other sensory changes that may be present in strabismus, and these are monocular. They occur in the strabismic eye of a patient with unilateral strabismus, and remain when the fellow eye is covered. Indeed, the dominant eye needs to be covered to detect and investigate them. They are amblyopia and eccentric fixation. These sensory changes, which occur in strabismus developing at an early age, are more fully described in Chapter 13, but will be introduced here.

AMBLYOPIA

Amblyopia is an impairment of form vision with no obvious organic cause. In strabismus, amblyopia may assist in lessening the effects of confusion, but there are other types of amblyopia which do not necessarily accompany strabismus (Chapter 13).

ECCENTRIC FIXATION

This is a failure of an eye in monocular vision to take up fixation with the fovea. There are several theories, but little consensus, on its aetiology. These theories are discussed in Chapter 13. Usually, there are no accompanying changes to the localisation system in the monocular vision of an eccentrically fixating eye (Chapter 13).

CLINICAL KEY POINTS

- Diplopia, usually accompanied by confusion, is the obvious consequence of strabismus but can be avoided in young patients by suppression or HARC
- The precise mechanism for HARC is unclear, but it allows for 'pseudobinocular vision', 'pseudobinocular' motor function, and possibly 'pseudostereopsis'
- The factors favouring HARC are: esotropia, small angle, stable angle, and early onset. These factors also increase the likelihood of the HARC being deeply ingrained
- UARC is very rare, and its prevalence is exaggerated by artificial test conditions
- HARC and suppression are binocular sensory adaptations to strabismus: amblyopia and eccentric fixation are monocular sensory consequences of strabismus

CHAPTER 13

Amblyopia and Eccentric Fixation

Amblyopia

DEFINITION

Hippocrates in 400 BCE described amblyopia as 'when the doctor and patient see nothing' (Day, 1997). Lyle and Wybar (1967) defined amblyopia as 'a condition of diminished visual form sense which is not associated with any structural abnormality or disease of the media, fundi or visual pathways, and which is not overcome by correction of the refractive error.' The problem with the 'no structural abnormality' clause is that it depends on the depth of the clinical investigations. This may be why many definitions replace this phrase with alternatives such as 'apparent lesion' (Wingate, 1976; Millodot, 1993) or 'ophthalmoscopically detectable' lesion (Gibson, 1947; Spalton et al., 1984; Nelson, 1988a). Another problem with this definition is that in 22% of cases, amblyopia is cured simply by wearing spectacles, albeit over several months (p. 187). Accordingly, some studies have changed the last clause in the aforementioned definition to 'not directly correctable with glasses' (Cordonnier & de Maertelaer, 2005).

In view of these problems with the definition of amblyopia, the following broad definition is proposed: **a visual loss resulting from an impediment or disturbance to the normal development of vision**.

Two quantitative approaches are commonly used to diagnose amblyopia: a difference between the acuity of the two eyes of two lines or more (Papageorgiou, Asproudis, Maconachie, Tsironi, & Gottlob, 2019) and/or acuity in the amblyopic eye of worse than 6/9 (Jennings, 2001b). It is implicit in this definition that the child is old enough for the visual acuity norms to be 6/6 (Table 3.1). Stewart and colleagues described two more sophisticated approaches to defining amblyopia, and of measuring the outcome of treatment (Stewart, Moseley, & Fielder, 2003). The first is the difference in final visual acuity of amblyopic and fellow eye (**residual amblyopia**) and the second is the proportion of the deficit corrected. Residual amblyopia is similar in principle to a function previously called the **acuity ratio** (Fulton & Mayer, 1988).

Amblyopia can be graded as mild (6/9 to 6/12), moderate (6/12 to 6/36), or severe (worse than 6/36) (Papageorgiou et al., 2019).

CLASSIFICATION

Amblyopia can be classified as follows:

1. *Organic amblyopia* from pathological or anatomical abnormalities of the retina (Spalton et al., 1984). The organic amblyopias can be further subdivided as follows:
   (a) From retinal eye disease, e.g., receptor dystrophy, neonatal macular haemorrhage.
   (b) *Nutritional amblyopia* from nutritional deficiencies.
   (c) *Toxic amblyopia* from poisoning (e.g., arsenic, lead, or quinine). **Alcohol amblyopia** and **tobacco amblyopia** are usually considered to be toxic amblyopias, although they are sometimes classified as nutritional amblyopias. The terms tobacco–alcohol amblyopia/neuropathy have been criticised and it has been argued that these are

not amblyopia but rather nutritional optic neuropathy (Grzybowski & Brona, 2017).

(d) *Idiopathic or congenital* which is amblyopia of unknown aetiology. It may be that, with modern electrophysiological testing and imaging techniques, many of these cases would be found to have subtle pathological causes, cortical or subcortical.

2. *Functional amblyopia* in which no organic lesion exists. The functional amblyopias can be further subdivided into:

(a) *Stimulus (or visual) deprivation amblyopia* from opacities or occlusion of the ocular media (e.g., congenital cataracts or ptosis). A systematic review found no high level (randomised controlled trial; RCT) evidence concerning the treatment of stimulus deprivation amblyopia (Antonio-Santos, Vedula, Hatt, & Powell, 2020). **Occlusion amblyopia** is an iatrogenic visual loss of the 'good' eye from excessive occlusion of this eye to treat primary amblyopia in the other eye (p. 191).

(b) *Strabismic amblyopia* as a result of neural changes in strabismus. Strabismic amblyopia and stimulus deprivation amblyopia used to be called **amblyopia ex anopsia**.

(c) *Anisometropic amblyopia* resulting from a blurred image in the more ametropic eye in uncorrected anisometropia, usually hypermetropia. A unidirectional causal relationship is likely to be an over-simplification (Barrett, Bradley, & Candy, 2013). Anisometropic amblyopia often occurs in association with microtropia (Hardman Lea, Loades, & Rubinstein, 1991), when it is best classified as mixed strabismic/anisometropic amblyopia.

(d) *Refractive amblyopia (isometropic amblyopia)* from blurred images in bilateral uncorrected refractive errors, usually hypermetropia. Visual acuity generally improves with spectacle correction (Wallace et al., 2007; Ziylan, Yabas, Zorlutuna, & Serin, 2007). Refractive amblyopia includes **meridional amblyopia**, which occurs in high uncorrected astigmatism.

(e) *Psychogenic amblyopia (hysterical amblyopia)*, a visual conversion reaction (p. 18) where the amblyopia is of psychological origin.

It is very important to detect any organic cause, so that appropriate medical treatment can be considered. This chapter is principally concerned with functional amblyopia and will concentrate on the two most common types, strabismic amblyopia and anisometropic amblyopia. Differential diagnosis between organic and functional amblyopia also will be discussed and is summarised in Table 13.1.

PREVALENCE

Amblyopia occurs in about 3% of the population (Attebo et al., 1998; Jennings, 2001b). A population-based study (Attebo et al., 1998) found that the relative prevalence of different types of amblyopia is anisometropic (50%), strabismic (19%), mixed strabismic and anisometropic (27%), and visual deprivation (4%). Hospital eye clinics in the UK receive many more referrals with strabismic than orthotropic anisometropic amblyopia, (Woodruff, Hiscox, Thompson, & Smith, 1994b), probably because strabismic amblyopia is more visible to parents and anisometropic amblyopia is often cured by community optometrists.

Seventy-five percent of children attending the hospital eye service do so for amblyopia-related reasons (Stewart, Shah, Wren, & Roberts, 2016). Of the children with anisometropic amblyopia who present to the hospital eye service, those from socially deprived backgrounds present on average about 2 years later than other cases (Smith, Thompson, Woodruff, & Hiscox, 1994). Amblyopia is less likely to be successfully treated in children from poorer socioeconomic groups (Hudak & Magoon, 1997).

Amblyopia is more likely to be present in the left eye, and this asymmetry is exaggerated for anisometropic amblyopia (Woodruff et al., 1994b). In another study, this asymmetry was found in the presence of anisometropia, but not in strabismic-only amblyopia (Repka, Simons, & Kraker, 2010).

DETECTION OF AMBLYOPIA AND VISION SCREENING

Second only to refractive error, amblyopia is a leading cause of visual loss in the age group 20—70 years. Amblyopia can preclude some vocations, mostly related to military or transport (Adams & Karas, 1999). Amblyopia is associated with adverse psychosocial effects, even in nonstrabismic cases (Packwood, Cruz, Rychwalski, & Keech, 1999). The treatment of amblyopia is cost-effective (Konig & Barry, 2004; Membreno, Brown, Brown, Sharma, & Beauchamp, 2002). There is some evidence that occlusion therapy is distressing for children (Parkes, 2001), although two studies found that amblyopia treatment does not have an adverse psychosocial impact (Choong, Lukman, Martin, & Laws, 2004; Hrisos, Clarke, & Wright, 2004).

It is important to discover amblyopia, or the 'amblyogenic' factors which may cause it, at as early an age as possible. Children are at risk if their parents or siblings have amblyopia and/or strabismus. Any adult with amblyopia should be cautioned about the need for professional eyecare in relatives who are children.

Most young children in the UK do not routinely visit community optometrists (Guggenheim & Farbrother, 2005) and screening of children at school entry has been advocated (Hall, 1996). Parents sometimes assume that proper eye examinations are unnecessary because their children have had vision screening. However, the standards of screening programmes are variable (Woodruff et al., 1994b) and have been criticised (Wright, Colville, & Oberklaid, 1995). The evidence for vision screening in preschool children will now be briefly reviewed.

A thorough screening programme at age 37 months significantly improves the visual outcome in the population at age 7.5 years (Williams, Harrad, Harvey, Sparrow, & ALSPAC Study Team, 2001; Williams et al. 2003). The prevalence of amblyopia is almost halved and visual acuity is improved. The problems of vision screening are exemplified by the fact that only 69% of the intervention group attended any of the vision screening appointments and the authors caution that parents must be told that passing vision screening does not guarantee that no abnormality is present.

Inevitably, there is a trade-off between the desirability of early screening (Williams et al., 2002) and the practical issue of the age at which useful screening results can be obtained (Williams et al., 2001). This, together with changing visual status, makes a powerful argument for screening on more than one occasion, so it is surprising that this approach was discontinued in the UK (Hall, 1996). A study highlighted the inaccuracies in screening children aged 4—5 years: over a third of cases thought to require treatment after repeat screening did not actually have acuity loss (Clarke et al., 2003). Conversely, another study argued that screening, at least by photorefraction, should occur at age 9 months (Anker, Atkinson, Braddick, Nardini, & Ehrlich, 2004).

Evidence from other countries supports the benefit of vision screening for reducing the prevalence of amblyopia (Hoeg et al., 2014). The choice in the UK to only screen vision once at school entry (Hall, 1996) seems impossible to justify on any scientific grounds. By comparison, a highly successful screening programme in Sweden which has reduced the prevalence of deep amblyopia from 2% to 0.2%, repeats screening at five different ages, with visual acuity being tested on four of these occasions (Kvarnstrom, Jakobsson, & Lennerstrand, 2001).

A classic study found that 72% of cases of esotropia and/or amblyopia had a refractive error of +2.00DS or more spherical hypermetropia in the more emmetropic eye, or +1.00D or more spherical or cylindrical anisometropia (Ingram, 1977). Infants (mean age 9 months) who are not refractively corrected for significant hypermetropia (more than +4.00D) are four times more likely to have poor acuity at 5.5 years than infants who wore their hypermetropic correction (Anker et al., 2004). Oblique astigmatism significantly increases the risk of developing amblyopia (Abrahamsson & Sjostrand, 2003).

The effect of early correction (before the age of 2.5 years) of significant degrees of hypermetropia (+3.00D or more) and hypermetropic astigmatism (1.00DC or more) was investigated in a retrospective study of the records of 103 strabismic children (Freidburg & Kloppel, 1996). Early refractive correction was associated with significantly better visual acuities at age 8 years or later. Vision screening is only effective if it is followed up with comprehensive eyecare, preferably state-funded. A North American study found that a year after visual screening had detected visual problems, only 30% of cases detected were complying with recommended treatment (Preslan & Novak, 1998).

Recent publications on vision screening in the UK continue to concentrate on amblyopia, with minimal consideration of other conditions (Solebo & Rahi, 2013; Solebo, 2019). Children from less advantaged backgrounds have an increased risk of hypermetropia, which could cause inequity in access to care (Williams et al., 2008). Although not directly related to binocular vision anomalies, the rate of myopia in 10–16-year-olds in the UK has doubled in the last 50 years (McCullough, O'Donoghue, & Saunders, 2016) and most university students are now myopic (Logan, Davies, Mallen, & Gilmartin, 2005). Schoolchildren with visual symptoms often do not self-present for eyecare (Thomson & Evans, 1999; Thomson, 2002) and in the absence of repeated vision screening it seems advisable for schoolchildren to have regular eye examinations with community optometrists.

A promising development is a computerised vision screener (Thomson & Evans, 1999) that takes about 3 minutes per child and has a sensitivity of 97% and a specificity of 96% (Thomson, 2002). Recently, an iPhone App using photorefraction has shown promising results at detecting the risk factors for amblyopia (Walker et al., 2020). However, earlier evidence indicates video-autorefractors fail to detect about one in five cases of amblyogenic ametropia (Schimitzek & Haase, 2002).

Vernier acuity is probably cortically-mediated and has good potential to detect amblyopia (Drover, Morale, Wang, Stager, & Birch, 2010). Vernier acuity can be tested by preferential looking and seems to have potential for vision screening (Drover et al., 2010).

PREVENTION OF FURTHER VISUAL LOSS IN AMBLYOPIA

Another important role for eyecare practitioners is to advise amblyopic patients of ways they can minimise the risk of visual loss in the future. People with amblyopia have almost three times the risk of visual impairment in their better seeing eye compared with people without amblyopia (Chua & Mitchell, 2004). Although amblyopes who lose sight in their nonamblyopic eye often experience an improvement in their amblyopic eye, this is only of a significant degree (two lines or more) in 10% of cases (Rahi, Logan, Borja et al., 2002). Indeed, the lifetime risk of serious visual loss for an individual with amblyopia is at least 1.2%–3.3% (Rahi, Logan, Timms, Russell-Eggitt, & Taylor, 2002b).

Another study calculated the lifetime risk of bilateral visual impairment is 18% for amblyopes, compared with 10% for nonamblyopes (van Leeuwen et al., 2007). Therefore, eyecare practitioners should advise amblyopic patients about wearing eye protection when appropriate. It often helps to bring this message home if practitioners cover the patient's good eye and point out the level of vision in the amblyopic eye.

DEVELOPMENT

The most critical period for loss of binocularity and for the development of functional amblyopia is the first 18 months of life (Levi, 1994). After this, the plasticity of the visual system seems to decrease rapidly at first, and then gradually. The conventional view is that it remains sensitive up to the age of about 6 years (Keech & Kutschke, 1995), 6 to 7 years (Simons & Preslan, 1999), 8 years (Nelson, 1988a; Levi, 1994; Daw, 1997), or possibly 10 years (Vaegan & Taylor, 1979). Different visual functions have different sensitive periods: the sensitive periods for cortical visual functions are longer than for retinal functions (Harwerth, Smith, Duncan, Crawford, & Von Noorden, 1986). Data from monkeys suggests that an earlier onset of strabismus tends to be associated with deeper amblyopia (Kiorpes, Carlson, & Alfi, 1989).

It is sometimes assumed that the upper age limit for the onset of amblyopia is the same as the upper age limit for the treatment of amblyopia, but this is not necessarily the case. It is noted later in this chapter that there is strong evidence for considerable plasticity in the visual system, with even adults responding to intensive amblyopia treatment.

THE IMPACT OF STRABISMIC AND ANISOMETROPIC AMBLYOPIA

Basic Visual Functions

Colour vision is normal but the pupillary function of eyes with strabismic amblyopia is subtly different to that of eyes with anisometropic amblyopia (Barbur, Hess, & Pinney, 1994). The spatial contrast sensitivity of amblyopic eyes is close to normal for low spatial frequencies (coarse detail), but there is a marked loss of contrast sensitivity at high spatial frequencies (fine detail). This loss increases with severity of amblyopia and does not result from optical factors, unsteady fixational eye movements, or eccentric fixation (Flynn, 1991). Ocular pursuit is abnormal in strabismic amblyopia (Bedell, Lee Yap, & Flom, 1990).

Visual processing occurs in inter-linked parallel pathways and the two principal systems are the P-system (parvocellular, sustained) and the M-system (magnocellular, transient). The type of visual deficit in amblyopia has led many to suggest that the P-system is affected, and the M-system relatively unaffected (e.g., Nelson, 1988a), although this is likely to be an over-simplification (Kelly & Buckingham, 1998). Hess and Pointer (1985) showed that in anisome-tropic amblyopia there is reduced sensitivity centrally and peripherally, whereas in strabismic (and mixed strabismic and anisometropic) amblyopia, the loss of acuity is predominantly restricted to the foveal region.

Fahle and Bachmann (1996) found that a small heterogeneous sample of amblyopes had **better than normal** function in their amblyopic eyes at a specific task of spatiotemporal integration at high velocities. One explanation for this might be if amblyopes have a P-deficit and normal or supranormal M-function. An electrophysiological study of anisometropic amblyopes found reduced P- but normal M-function (Shan, Moster, Roemer, & Siegfried, 2000). A psychophysical study of strabismic amblyopia found deficits in both channels, but a relatively greater P-deficit (Davis et al., 2006). The reduction in P- relative to M-sensitivity was significantly greater in the late-onset group and there were more subtle but complex deficits in the fellow eye.

An analysis of sensory processing in amblyopia highlights fundamental differences between strabismic and anisometropic amblyopia (Hess, 2002). In additional to the contrast sensitivity deficit in amblyopic eyes, there is a milder deficit in the fellow eye (Leguire, Rogers, & Bremer, 1990). This may relate to a finding of bilateral changes in foveal structure in individuals with amblyopia (Bruce, Pacey, Bradbury, Scally, & Barrett, 2013).

Amblyopic eyes make misperceptions of spatial structures (Sireteanu, Baumer, & Iftime, 2008) and this has been attributed to errors in the neural coding of orientation in the primary visual cortex (Barrett, Pacey, Bradley, Thibos, & Morrill, 2003). Despite normal visual acuity, reading is impaired in the nonamblyopic eye and binocularly (Kanonidou, Proudlock, & Gottlob, 2010). Other dysfunctions associated with amblyopia include impaired perception of mirror symmetry (Levi & Saarinen, 2004), poor fine motor skills (Webber, Wood, Gole, & Brown, 2008), and temporally unstable perception (Sireteanu et al., 2008). The perception of images of real-world scenes is impaired in amblyopic eyes and binocularly (Mirabella, Hay, & Wong, 2011).

Visual Acuity

Visual acuity can be classified as follows:
1. *Minimum resolvable*, the smallest angular separation between targets that can be recognised; e.g., grating acuity in preferential looking acuity cards (Fig. 3.1). Electrophysiological techniques of measuring visual acuity may also use grating stimuli.

2. *Minimum recognisable*, the capacity to recognise a form and its orientation; e.g., Snellen letters.

3. *Hyperacuity*, the judgement of relative positions; e.g., vernier acuity.

Under ideal conditions, minimum resolvable and minimum recognisable acuity can approach the limit of 0.5−1 minute of arc, which is predicted from the optics of the eye and spacing of foveal cones. Hyperacuity can exceed this anatomical limit by 5−10 times, with optimal thresholds in the order of 3−6 seconds of arc.

Three basic principles can be used to characterise the visual acuity loss in functional amblyopia. First, the types of visual acuity listed previously reflect an increasing degree of cortical processing. Second, amblyopia can be described as a neural deficit and there is a failure in amblyopia to coordinate information from different parts of the spatial frequency spectrum (Jennings, 2001b). Third, it seems that the neural deficit is more complex in strabismic amblyopia than in anisometropic amblyopia. The following statements follow from these three principles. Compared with other measures of acuity, grating acuity is relatively unaffected in functional amblyopia. For a given level of grating acuity, strabismic amblyopes have a relatively greater loss of Snellen acuity than do anisometropic amblyopes. For a given level of grating acuity, strabismic amblyopes have a much greater loss of vernier acuity than anisometropic amblyopes.

Considering minimum recognisable acuity, reading letters in a line (morphoscopic acuity) is a more complex neural task than reading letters individually (angular acuity). It is therefore not surprising that most people perform a little worse when reading crowded as opposed to single letters, and this crowding phenomenon is more pronounced in strabismic amblyopia (Levi, 2008). Real passages of text contain a greater degree of crowding than letter charts, and this may explain why amblyopes who have been successfully treated in terms of Snellen acuity may still have impaired capacity for reading passages of text (Zurcher & Lang, 1980).

It should not be concluded from the aforementioned that **all** strabismic amblyopes show a much greater crowding phenomenon than anisometropic amblyopes; there is probably a continuum between the groups (Giaschi, Regan, Kraft, & Kothe, 1993).

Accommodative Function

Amblyopia is associated with abnormal accommodative function (Ciuffreda, Hokoda, Hung, Semmlow, & Selenow, 1983), which is clinically detected as a reduced amplitude of accommodation. Without refractive correction, about 80% of anisometropic amblyopes exhibit asymmetric accommodation, about half of whom show aniso-accommodation and a quarter of whom fail to accommodate at near, which has been described as anti-accommodation (Toor et al., 2018). The anti-accommodation resolved with spectacle correction, although these were the cases whose amblyopia required patching in addition to refractive correction (Toor, Horwood, & Riddell, 2019).

Other Deficits in Amblyopia

The visual deficit in amblyopia extends beyond the basic functions processed in V1 and involves extensive regions of extrastriate cortex (above), meaning there are likely to be significant suprathreshold processing deficits (Li, Dumoulin, Mansouri, & Hess, 2007). Hand−eye coordination (prehension) is impacted in amblyopia and improvement in these functions is likely to require treatments that restore binocularity (Grant, Melmoth, Morgan, & Finlay, 2007).

INVESTIGATION OF AMBLYOPIA

When a patient reports the symptom of reduced vision, a full routine eye examination should be carried out. This is outlined in Chapters 2 and 3. The present chapter covers the particular procedures in the investigation of amblyopia as a part of that routine, and with supplementary tests that aid a diagnosis with respect to the amblyopia. As a part of this investigation, tests for the presence of eccentric fixation may also be required, and these are described later in this chapter. After the section on eccentric fixation, the differential diagnosis of amblyopia and detection of pathology is discussed.

The worksheet in Appendix 6 summarises a clinical approach to the investigation of amblyopia. One aim of this is to differentially diagnose the type of amblyopia, summarised in Table 13.1. Compared with nonamblyopic eyes, eyes with strabismic amblyopia experience a significant improvement in visual acuity when viewing through a low-density neutral density filter (Habeeb, Arthur, & ten Hove, 2012).

An interesting study found many amblyopic eyes may have a subtle form of optic nerve hypoplasia (Lempert, 2000, 2004). Lempert suggests optic nerve hypoplasia may be the primary reason for the reduced acuity, although he notes it is also possible the reduced size of the optic nerve is the result of the amblyopia. Optical coherence tomography studies indicate increased macular thickness in anisometropic amblyopia but not strabismic amblyopia (Al-Haddad, Mollayess, Cherfan, Jaafar, & Bashshur, 2011). The macular thickness reduces (becomes more normal) after amblyopia treatment (Kavitha et al., 2019). The retinal nerve fibre layer thickness appears normal in amblyopia (Bandyopadhyay, Chatterjee, & Banerjee, 2012; Kavitha et al., 2019).

History and Symptoms

It might seem surprising that so few researchers have paid any attention to the age of onset of amblyopia, but this may be because it can be difficult to determine this with any certainty. There is electrophysiological and psychophysical evidence of differences between patients with early onset (before 18 months) and late onset amblyopia (Davis et al., 2003). As a general rule, the longer the strabismus has been present, the less likely it is to respond to treatment. In strabismic amblyopia, the age at which the strabismus was first noticed (e.g., in photos) can be used as a proxy for the onset of the amblyopia.

It is important to note any previous treatment in the form of glasses, occlusion, or other therapy: when was this given, what was its effect, and why was it discontinued? In the case of spectacles, the prescription should be known and the extent to which they have been worn. Most children are frightened of criticism and overestimate the amount they have worn their glasses. This should be countered by being noncritical and encouraging candour.

Visual Acuity Measurement

Assessment of the unaided vision should be made, but an evaluation of amblyopia can only be made with the optimum refractive correction in place. Acuity will vary with illumination, contrast, and the type of test used (Table 13.1), and every effort should be made to standardise the apparatus and the procedure used. This may need to vary to some extent with the age of the patient, as young children require a different approach. The method used should then be recorded along with the test distance and acuity measurement.

Line (Morphoscopic or Crowded) Acuity

In testing visual acuity, patients with unilateral amblyopia often give up reading when the letters are too small to read easily. If pressed, these patients typically read lower down the chart, and sometimes this can reveal much better acuity than would otherwise have been obtained. It is important to ask the patient to read until the limit of acuity is reached, otherwise no real starting point for any treatment is known and any improvement may be illusory. Modern letter chart designs utilising principles detailed by Bailey and Lovie (1976) are most suitable for accurate visual acuity measurements (Chapter 3 and Appendix 10). The sensitivity to visual acuity changes in amblyopia is increased by decreasing letter spacing (Laidlaw, Abbott, & Rosser, 2003). The chart that these authors recommended has, like most charts, less crowding for letters at the end of the line than for those in the centre of the line. This is undesirable and crowding is perhaps better controlled with individual optotypes in a crowding box (see next section). Great care must be taken to ensure that

TABLE 13.1 ■ Clinical Characteristics of Various Types of Amblyopia to Aid in Differential Diagnosis.

Type of amblyopia	Morphoscopic visual acuity (MVA)	Angular visual acuity	Visual acuity with 2.0 ND filter	Cover test	Fixation	Visual field	Amsler charts	Other
Strabismic	Reduced, usually unilateral, better with letters at end of line	>MVA	≥MVA	Constant strabismus if not microtropia (rarely, intermittent exotropia)	Eccentric, sometimes variable	Normal, except where suppression is very dense	Lang's one-sided scotoma in microtropia (see below)	–
Stimulus deprivation	Reduced, usually unilateral	>MVA	≥MVA	Usually no strabismus, may be unsteady fixation	Central, may be unsteady	Normal	–	Likely to report relevant history (e.g., cataract or ptosis)
Anisometropic and refractive	Reduced, unilateral if anisometropic	=MVA, or very slightly better	Slightly <MVA	Normal, or may show anisophoria if high anisometropia	Central, often unsteady in high refractive errors	Normal	May show large central blur	High refractive error present in one or both eyes
Retinal eye disease, idiopathic or congenital	Reduced, sometimes bilateral	=MVA	<MVA	Normal	Central, often unsteady	Depends on organic cause, sometimes central scotoma	Depends on organic cause, sometimes central scotoma	Often history of ocular pathology & poor or absent foveal reflex
Toxic and nutritional	Reduced bilateral, not always equal	=MVA	<MVA	Normal	Central, sometimes eccentric if advanced	Central scotoma, especially for red	Central scotoma, especially with red chart	Possibly systemic signs, symptoms, or history
Psychogenic (visual conversion reaction; hysterical)	Reduced, variable, inconsistent at different distances, prone to suggestion	Variable	Variable and unpredictable	Normal	Central, may be unsteady	Static perimetry: illogical response kinetic perimetry: star or spiral field	Normal, or illogical response	May have other signs of visual conversion reaction (p. 18)

<, Worse than; ≥, better than or the same; MVA, morphoscopic (linear) visual acuity; ND, neutral density.

Modified after Mallett, R. (1988a). Techniques of investigation of binocular vision anomalies. In K. Edwards & R. Llewellyn (Eds.), *Optometry* (pp. 238–269). London: Butterworths.

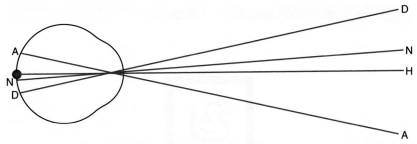

Fig. 13.1   Reading Snellen letters with an eccentrically fixating eye.   The patient is fixating the letter N in a line of Snellen letters. The image of the next letter on the right of N, which is H, will fall on the foveal scotoma and not be seen easily by the patient, who may therefore miss it and read the following letter, A. If the patient reads from right to left instead of beginning at the left as normal, the difficulty does not occur; the image of the letter D, for example, does not fall on the scotoma.

the patient does not 'peep' around the occluder. These precautions are particularly important with children, but also apply to adults. Computerised test charts are preferable because the optotypes can be randomised; if not available, the acuity of the amblyopic eye should be measured first.

Where there is eccentric fixation, a small foveal scotoma may result in patients missing out letters or reading the line backwards more easily than in the normal way from left to right. This may be particularly true of left convergent strabismus (Fig. 13.1). Other factors that may contribute to missequencing of letters are confusion over the visual direction and monocular fixation instability associated with eccentric fixation.

Single Letter (Angular) Acuity

Historically, isolated single letters or other characters were used instead of a line of letters, as with the E-cube or the original Sheridan-Gardner test. These tests should be avoided because they underestimate the visual deficit in strabismic amblyopia. As described in the earlier section on sensory function, this is because single optotypes avoid the 'crowding phenomenon' from adjacent letters. If a patient can only cope with single optotypes, these should be presented in a crowded box. This is possible with many computerised letter charts (Thomson, 2000), and is illustrated in Fig. 13.2.

Neutral Density Filters

Remeasuring the acuity through a neutral density filter can assist in differentiating between strabismic amblyopia and other types of amblyopia (Table 13.1). A neutral density filter, ND 2, is used and a goggle arrangement is required to effectively control the illumination level. In eyes with normal acuity, dark adaptation reduces the acuity by about one LogMAR line and a similar effect occurs in anisometropic or organic amblyopia. In strabismic amblyopia, however, the amblyopic eye's acuity is not affected by the filter.

Stereopsis

Many studies have suggested that strabismic amblyopia may be detected with tests assessing random dot stereopsis (Walraven & Janzen, 1993; Hatch & Laudon, 1993; Schweers & Baker, 1992; Cooper & Feldman, 1978). Contoured stereopsis tests (e.g., Titmus circles) are probably less sensitive for detecting strabismic amblyopia (Schweers & Baker, 1992). The outcome of occlusion treatment is typically defined as improvement in visual acuity, but this is usually accompanied by improvement in stereoacuity, both in small angle or intermittent strabismus and in anisometropic cases (Lee & Isenberg, 2003).

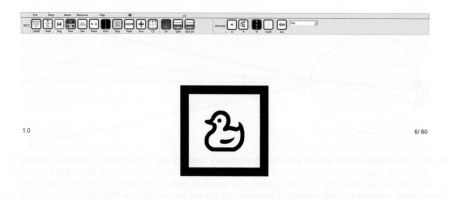

1.0   6/ 60

Eccentric Fixation

Eccentric fixation is a monocular condition in which a point on the retina other than the fovea is used for fixation. Fixation is usually eccentric in patients whose amblyopia is strabismic and the acuity tends to be worse in higher degrees of eccentric fixation (Hess, 1977). A study found eccentric fixation in none of 20 cases of orthotropic anisometropic amblyopia, 19% of cases of strabismic amblyopia, and in 58% of cases of mixed amblyopia (Stewart, Fielder, Stephens, & Moseley, 2005). Of the cases with eccentric fixation, 76% had mixed and 24% had strabismic amblyopia. The presence of eccentric fixation worsened the prognosis for successful treatment of the amblyopia.

The rate of reduction in visual acuity with increasing eccentric fixation is, in most cases of strabismic amblyopia, more rapid than the normal decline in visual acuity in the peripheral retina (Hess, 1977). It is important to know the degree and the stability of the eccentricity as this aids differential diagnosis of the amblyopia (Table 13.1) and can be used to monitor the effect of treatment. However, Cleary and Thompson (2001) noted that instability was common, so precise measurement is often not possible.

There is some controversy about why eccentric fixation occurs (Jennings, 2001b). The initial 'sensory theory' was that there is a central scotoma and the patient fixates with the area giving best acuity rather than the fovea (Worth, 1903). There has also been a suggestion that it arises from a change of the central area of localisation as a central scotoma develops in the amblyopic eye (Duke-Elder, 1973).

A more recent and likely theory is that the habitually strabismic position of the amblyopic eye leads to an error in localising 'straight ahead' when it is required to fixate monocularly (Schor, 1978). This 'motor theory' suggests the eccentric fixation results from an adaptive after-effect. Support for this theory comes from the observation that larger ocular deviations tend to be associated with greater degrees of eccentric fixation (Garcia-Garcia et al., 2018).

In some cases, eccentric fixation may be a sequel to an enlargement of Panum's fusional area which follows decompensated heterophoria at an early age and leads eventually to microtropia (Pickwell, 1981).

These different theories on the aetiology of eccentric fixation are not mutually exclusive. One or more may apply to one patient, and the others in other patients. As far as management is concerned, it does not really matter which theory is correct. Both theories and experimental data disconfirm the notion that occlusion might worsen eccentric fixation (Jennings, 2001b). The presence of eccentric fixation may make it more likely that recidivism will occur (see below).

INVESTIGATION OF ECCENTRIC FIXATION

No method of assessing the fixation seems to be satisfactory for all patients (Cleary & Thompson, 2001) and the clinical worksheet in Appendix 6 can be used for a detailed workup. Ophthalmoscopic methods are most widely used and are therefore described in detail below.

Ophthalmoscopic Methods

Investigation of fixation can be carried out with an ophthalmoscope which will project a target on the retina so that it can be seen by the practitioner and its position judged in relation to retinal details. This is the method of choice for assessing eccentric fixation, and ideally should be carried out with white light (Mallett, 1988a), although with some ophthalmoscopes a filter is associated with the fixation target. It is best to test the nonstrabismic eye first, for training and to check the patient's response. The eye that is not being assessed is occluded. As the target is focused on the retina, it can be seen by the patient and, when the patient is asked to look straight at the centre of the target, it will be seen by the practitioner to be centred on the fovea in the nonamblyopic eye (this serves as a check on the patient's response). It may also be central in an amblyopic eye if the fixation is central. If it appears on any other part of the retina, usually slightly nasally in convergent strabismus, eccentric fixation is demonstrated. Its position is recorded by a clearly labelled diagram, usually representing the fovea with a dot or circle and the fixation target with a cross (Fig. 13.3). The method is summarised in Table 13.2.

A dilated pupil is sometimes necessary for this type of examination. Also, young patients usually accommodate when asked to look at the target, and this blurs the practitioner's view of the fundus. The test is therefore easier to carry out during a cycloplegic refraction, when the large pupil will also increase the field of view for the practitioner and enable better location of the target on the fundus.

Sometimes it is possible to place the target on the fovea, and to ask the patient what can be seen of it with the eccentrically fixating eye. Some patients report that nothing can be seen of the middle of the target, which indicates a central scotoma. Occasionally, patients can give an indication of the visual direction associated with the fovea; that is, whether there is still central localisation or not. The difficulty with this aspect of the investigation is maintaining the amblyopic eye's position when the target is moved from the eccentric area to the fovea.

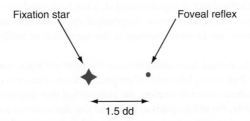

Fixation star   Foveal reflex

1.5 dd

Fixation slightly unstable compared with dominant eye

Fig. 13.3 Suggested method of recording eccentric fixation. It is important to label the foveal reflex and the fixation target. The degree of eccentric fixation can be recorded, using a disc diameter *(dd)* or drawing the ophthalmoscope graticule (if present) as the unit of measurement. If the ophthalmoscope graticule is used, record the make and model of ophthalmoscope. There may be a slight vertical element to the eccentric fixation.

TABLE 13.2 ■ Method of Using the Direct Ophthalmoscope to Test for Eccentric Fixation.

1. If the consulting room is not completely dark, the eye that is not being tested should be occluded.
2. First, test the eye with **better** visual acuity. This serves to train the patient and check their response.
3. Select the ophthalmoscope fixation target (usually a star, sometimes with a measuring graticule).
4. With the room lights turned out or dimmed, project this target onto a surface (e.g., the consulting room ceiling) and point out the fixation target. Explain to the patient that they will see this projected into their eye and, when so instructed, they must fixate the star very precisely, without looking away.
5. Initially, instruct the patient to look straight ahead, and not at the fixation star. Look in their eye, find the optic disc, and focus the ophthalmoscope in the usual way.
6. Once the ophthalmoscope is focussed, ask the patient to look at the star as precisely and steadily as possible.
7. Note if the fixation is central and steady, as expected in this, the nonamblyopic eye. Record the results.
8. Now, repeat steps 5–7 but in the eye with **worse** acuity. Record the result as illustrated in Fig. 13.3.

Other Methods of Assessing Eccentric Fixation

For cooperative children, optical coherent tomography (OCT) can be used to detect and measure eccentric fixation (Garcia-Garcia et al., 2018). Other methods have become primarily of historical interest and will not be described in detail. Previous editions of this book can be consulted if more information is sought on the following approaches: after-image transfer method, entoptic phenomena (Haidinger's brushes and Maxwell's spot), perimetry method, and Amsler charts.

Past Pointing Test and Anomalous Foveal Localisation

This gives an indication if the localisation of objects in space has been disturbed with the amblyopic eye. The procedure is first tried with the patient's good eye, so the practitioner can see the normal ability of the patient to perform the test and can train the patient. The amblyopic eye is covered, and the patient is asked to place a finger on the forehead just above the uncovered eye. A pen torch is held before the eye at a distance of about 25 cm. The practitioner explains that on the word 'Go' the patient moves the finger to touch the light. The patient is allowed to practise if there is any difficulty. The occluder is then changed to the good eye and the test is repeated with the amblyopic eye, the patient being required to touch the light with the tip of the finger. If this cannot be done, but the finger goes a few centimetres to one side, past pointing is demonstrated. This indicates that the eccentric area, upon which the object of regard is imaged, is not being used to estimate the principal visual direction. The innate association between the principal visual direction and the fovea is maintained (see next). The patient may be more uncertain in this test with their amblyopic eye (Fronius & Sireteanu, 1994).

The maintenance of the normal relationship between the principal visual direction and the fovea in most cases of eccentric fixation explains why, when patients fixate a target in the ophthalmoscope light and the examiner detects eccentric fixation, the patients feel that they are looking to one side of the fixation target. Rarely, the amblyopia is so profound that the eccentric area usurps the origin of the principal visual direction and patients perceive the ophthalmoscope fixation target as being 'straight ahead', although they are viewing it eccentrically. This is 'eccentric fixation with anomalous foveal localization' (Mallett, 1988a), and these patients are unlikely to exhibit past pointing. In anomalous foveal localisation the visual acuity is usually worse than 6/60 and the prognosis for treatment is poor.

Past pointing can also occur in an incomitant deviation of recent onset (Chapter 17). This is usually of a greater degree than past pointing in eccentric fixation.

Evaluation, Prognosis, and Management of Amblyopia

The first and most important stage in the evaluation of amblyopia is to confirm that the correct diagnosis is amblyopia; in particular, to exclude the possibility of pathology (Table 13.3). Look for negative signs of pathology (e.g., normal: ophthalmoscopy, pupil reactions, visual fields) and positive signs of an amblyogenic factor (e.g., anisometropia and/or strabismus).

In strabismus, there are three aspects that sometimes require treatment. These are the motor deviation, binocular sensory adaptations to the strabismus, and monocular sensory consequences of the strabismus.

Treatment of reduced acuity in amblyopia has been the subject of considerable controversy, triggered partly by a sceptical review by Snowdon and Stewart-Brown in 1997. Since then, there have been many thorough studies and a consensus has emerged. The management of amblyopia is one of the major roles for eyecare practitioners who examine children, so this is covered in some detail later. The main treatments are refractive correction and occlusion. Alternative or complementary treatment approaches are also reviewed, together with important practical issues such as the duration of occlusion, and recidivism (regression of a benefit from treatment). Key conclusions concerning the treatment of amblyopia are drawn at the end of this chapter.

TABLE 13.3 ▪ **The Differential Diagnosis of Amblyopia.**

Step	What to do
Detect any ocular pathology	• Check pupil reactions, particularly looking for an APD. • Carry out careful ophthalmoscopy. In younger children, dilated fundoscopy might be necessary to obtain a good view, commonly after cycloplegic refraction. At follow-up, check ophthalmoscopy at regular intervals. Fundus imaging is often useful. • As soon as the child is old enough, check visual fields.
Look for neurological problems	• Carefully check pupil reactions. • Assess and record optic disc appearance in both eyes, if possible with photographs. • Look for incomitancy and/or strabismus (which may be a sign of neurological problems). • As soon as the child is old enough, check visual fields. • Enquire about general health (e.g., neurological signs, including headache).
Look for amblyogenic factors	• Look for a cause of the amblyopia: strabismus, anisometropia, high ametropia (cycloplegic may be necessary). • The lack of an amblyogenic factor greatly increases the odds of pathology being present. • The presence of an amblyogenic factor does not exclude the possibility of pathology, but makes it less likely.
Is the amblyopia responding to treatment?	• Treat the amblyopia decisively, so you can be sure that if the patient is not responding to treatment this is not due to lack of effort. • If amblyopia does not respond to treatment, review the diagnosis. • Failure to respond to treatment might indicate a pathological cause, so refer for a second opinion. • If the visual acuity in a presumed amblyopic eye worsens, it is probably something other than amblyopia and requires early referral for further investigation.

APD, Afferent pupillary defect.

Adapted after Evans, B.J.W. (2005a). *Eye Essentials: Binocular Vision*. Oxford: Elsevier.

PROGNOSIS

In evaluating the prognosis for the treatment of amblyopia and eccentric fixation, consideration should be given to the following factors:

1. *Type of amblyopia.* Where the amblyopia appears to be the consequence of uncorrected refractive error, refractive correction is the obvious first step. In strabismic amblyopia, patients are most likely to benefit from improvement of the acuity if the strabismus is eliminated, by glasses in an accommodative deviation (Chapter 15). If the amblyopia is treated but the strabismus remains, recidivism (regression of acuity) after treatment is more likely. One study suggests that even patients whose amblyopia results from structural lesions (media opacities, macular lesions, optic nerve abnormalities) can benefit from full-time occlusion, in about 50% of cases (Bradford, Kutschke, & Scott, 1992). In functional amblyopia, the prognosis is best for pure anisometropic amblyopia (Beardsell, Clarke, & Hill, 1999) and worst for mixed anisometropic and strabismic amblyopia (Woodruff, Hiscox, Thompson, & Smith, 1994a). The effect of type of amblyopia is discussed further later.

2. *Age of the patient.* This is discussed on p. 189.

3. *Age of onset of the amblyopia.* The shorter the time since the onset of factors causing the amblyopia, the more likely it is that the acuity can be restored. Nonetheless, there is evidence that at least some human amblyopes retain cortical plasticity into adulthood (see later).

4. *Acuity.* Not surprisingly, patients who start with worse acuity have a worse prognosis for achieving good acuities (Levartovsky, Oliver, Gottesman, & Shimshoni, 1995; Woodruff et al., 1994a), and lower acuities usually require long periods of occlusion. Acuities worse than 6/36 in patients over the age of 6 years are unlikely to respond to treatment. In young children, visual acuity of 6/9 or 6/12 is unlikely to benefit from occlusion (Clarke et al., 2003).

5. *Cooperation and interest.* Active exercises are only appropriate if the patient's and the parent's interest can be held. In cases where occlusion is being considered, patient cooperation is the most critical factor in predicting success (Lithander & Sjostrand, 1991). Amblyopia, strabismus, and patching have an impact on patients' perspective of visual function and on psychological function (Sabri, Knapp, Thompson, & Gottlob, 2006). The impact of amblyopia and cosmetically disadvantageous interventions such as patching on psychosocial well-being should be considered (Koklanis, Abel, & Aroni, 2006).

It can be difficult to persuade teenage patients to wear an occluder. On the other hand, active stimulation (see later) and physiological diplopia methods seem more acceptable and it is easier for these to be understood and applied by teenagers (Pickwell & Jenkins, 1982). With any treatment, the patient (and parent) need to understand what is required. The importance of compliance in occlusion treatment is considered further later.

WHO CAN TREAT AMBLYOPIA?

Amblyopia is treated in secondary care hospitals, usually by orthoptists, or in primary eyecare practice, typically by community optometrists. As with any area of professional activity, practitioners should only engage in procedures that are within the limits of their competence (College of Optometrists, 2017). This is particularly relevant for children's eyecare, where not all practitioners have the experience required for dealing with young children (Shah, Edgar, & Evans, 2007). Some community optometrists are comfortable treating amblyopia; others choose to refer to the hospital eye service or to paediatric optometrists. Even when cases are to be referred, it is important for the community optometrist to carry out careful ophthalmoscopy and refraction. Ophthalmoscopy may detect pathology and help prioritise the referral. Many cases of amblyopia are cured with refractive correction alone and this can be started by any community optometrist, even if they are referring the patient.

When patients with amblyopia are being treated, 3-monthly follow-up appointments are the minimum, with some authors recommending reviews every 5—6 weeks in the early stages of treatment (Simmers & Dulley, 2014). These authors cautioned that if there is a deterioration of acuity during treatment which cannot be explained by an ocular cause, urgent referral for neuroimaging should be considered.

CHOICE OF METHOD OF TREATMENT

Although several approaches are available, no one method is likely to be appropriate for every patient, and some patients may require more than one type of therapy at some stage in the total management. The factors outlined earlier should be considered in each case. Sometimes it will be obvious where to start, for example with refractive correction if there is a significant refractive error. Sequential management is the key: if one approach does not work then another should be tried, or the patient should be referred for a second opinion. Be candid with the patient; not all cases will respond to treatment and there is no reward for anyone in unsuccessful treatment. The clinical worksheet in Appendix 7 and Fig. 13.4 summarises an approach to the treatment of functional amblyopia. It is helpful to endorse verbal instructions with written information (Newsham, 2002).

REFRACTIVE CORRECTION AND OPTICAL TREATMENT

The prescribing of glasses and contact lenses for strabismus is described in Chapters 14 & 15. Refractive errors are clinically significant when their correction improves the clarity of the retinal images, balances the accommodative effort between the two eyes, or reduces the angle or risk of strabismus.

Anisometropia over 1.50D usually requires correction (Weakley, 2001) and higher anisometropia is likely to be associated with worse amblyopia (Townshend, Holmes, & Evans, 1993) and worse binocularity (Rutstein & Corliss, 1999). As discussed in Chapter 11, contact lenses (Evans, 2006a) are a better optical solution than spectacles for anisometropia, if the child is suitable for safe contact lens wear. Anisometropic amblyopia responds less well to treatment when it is associated with astigmatism (Kutschke, Scott, & Keech, 1991), particularly against-the-rule astigmatism (Somer, Budak, Demirci, & Duman, 2002). Many patients with amblyopia do not have accurate optical correction (Scheiman, Hertle et al., 2005) and this may reflect a tendency for clinicians to sometimes 'write off' the amblyopic eye. This is undesirable for reasons that will now be discussed.

It has been known for many years that the accurate correction of clinically significant refractive errors is an essential feature of treatment for amblyopia (Gibson, 1955). Many authors have noted that visual acuity can improve with spectacles alone (Pickwell, 1976) and have recommended a period of spectacle wear before occlusion is commenced (Asper, Watt, & Khuu, 2018). This effect has been quantified and used to recommend an initial period of treatment solely by refractive correction, sometimes called **optical treatment** or **refractive adaptation**. For approximately one-third of cases of all types of amblyopia, the improvement is so marked with refractive correction that after a few months they no longer meet the criteria for amblyopia and require no patching (Asper et al., 2018).

A systematic review and metaanalysis found optical treatment of amblyopia has a large positive effect size on visual acuity (Asper et al., 2018), and an improvement of two or more LogMAR lines is not uncommon. Asper et al.'s review found large effect sizes, whether the aetiology was refractive, or strabismus or participants were younger or older, although effect sizes were greatest in the youngest and those with less severe amblyopia. The effect size of optical treatment is similar to occlusion.

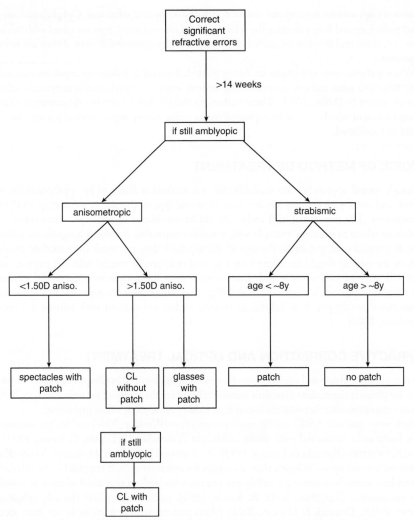

Fig. 13.4 Schematic simplified flow chart illustrating general treatment approach for functional amblyopia. *CL*, Contact lenses.

The authors concluded that optical treatment of amblyopia should be considered prior to other treatment in those with refractive error. Improved acuity before initiating other treatment is likely to make occlusion or penalisation less onerous and may improve compliance with further treatment.

Where there is a significant refractive error, optical treatment should be tried for a minimum of 14 weeks and continue until visual acuity ceases to improve (Asper et al., 2018), which is usually within 30 weeks (Papageorgiou et al., 2019). The usual modality is full-time wear (West & Williams, 2016), with follow-up recommended after 6 and 14 weeks of spectacle wear (Papageorgiou et al., 2019).

As noted previously, many of these anisometropic cases would benefit from contact lenses. In anisometropic amblyopia, there is less likelihood of suppression with contact lenses than spectacles (Li, Hess, et al., 2013). Contact lenses (possibly, with optical penalisation; see later) will avoid problems of bullying that can be associated with spectacles and patches (Horwood et al., 2005). Refractive surgery can also treat amblyopia in adults with bilateral refractive amblyopia and anisometropic amblyopia (Roszkowska et al., 2006), and anisometropic amblyopia in children (Utine, Cakir, Egemenoglu, & Perente, 2008; Pirouzian & Ip, 2010).

It is known that refractive correction can enhance binocularity, but binocularity can also influence refractive error. Children aged under 10 years with amblyopia experience significantly greater reduction in their hypermetropia over time if they are orthotropic (Kulp et al., 2012).

A cycloplegic refraction is required and the usual approach is to fully correct all anisometropia and astigmatism and undercorrect hypermetropia by 0.50 to 1.50D (Asper et al., 2018). The overall priority is to maintain ocular alignment, and some cases require full cycloplegic findings to achieve orthotropia. If there is no eso-deviation, one approach is **postcycloplegic refraction undercorrection** (Chang, 2017). In this method, 1-week postcycloplegic, the patient is seen again and the full cycloplegic refraction is reduced in 0.25D binocular steps until there is no additional improvement in distance visual acuity. This has been shown to be effective for treating amblyopia and promoting emmetropisation (Chang, 2017).

It is important to encourage good compliance with wear of refractive corrections. This will optimise the chances for a good visual acuity outcome (Maconachie et al., 2016).

OCCLUSION

Since c.900 (von Noorden, 1996) the principal treatment for amblyopia has been to patch the non-amblyopic eye (direct occlusion; Pickwell, 1977b) and occlusion is an accepted evidence-based treatment for strabismic amblyopia (Taylor & Elliott, 2014). The conventional view among eyecare practitioners is that if patching is carried out within the sensitive period, some improvement in visual acuity of the amblyopic eye is likely to occur (Snowdon & Stewart-Brown, 1997). This sensitive period during which treatment is thought to be possible was said to end at 6−7 years (Fells & Lee, 1984) or by about 8 years (Snowdon & Stewart-Brown, 1997). Others argue that the visual system is still 'plastic' and can respond to treatment up to (Day, 1997) and beyond (Levi, 1994) the age of 12 years. The evidence concerning occlusion and the effect of age on treatment will now be considered.

Is Occlusion Treatment Effective and, if so, at What Age?

In previous editions of this book, this section presented a comprehensive review of the literature on the efficacy of occlusion. In recent years there has been a large volume of research, summarised in some excellent systematic reviews. The present edition concentrates on these reviews.

As noted earlier in this chapter, when there is a significant refractive error, optical treatment is the first priority. Occlusion is only considered if, after optical treatment for an appropriate interval, there is still a difference of two LogMAR lines. A review that only considered children aged 7 years or less concluded that in cases not cured with glasses alone, occlusion may be more effective than glasses alone (West & Williams, 2016). The review found considerable variability between cases. A broader review concluded that the efficacy of spectacles and patching in the treatment of amblyopia is proven (Papageorgiou et al., 2019).

When considering the efficacy of occlusion, it is important to consider age and type of amblyopia. Much research on amblyopia concentrates on strabismic amblyopia, yet there are many differences between this and anisometropic amblyopia (Mallett, 1988a; Birch & Swanson, 2000).

It is nowadays recommended that treatment should be offered to all amblyopic children regardless of age (Papageorgiou et al., 2019). This review cited research demonstrating functional amblyopia can respond to occlusion throughout life, but improvement is greatest in those younger than 7 years. The older literature, reviewed in previous editions of this book, indicates that occlusion can produce improvements in adults, especially those with anisometropic amblyopia (Evans, 2007b). If strabismus is present, the chances of improvement are reduced and the risk of intractable diplopia, although slight, increases beyond the age of 7−10 years. Therefore, strabismic amblyopia is not usually treated over the age of 7—10 years. In all cases, the greatest improvement of acuity with occlusion is likely when the child is younger (Papageorgiou et al., 2019), so clinicians should not unduly delay treatment.

Types of Occluder and Occlusion

Different types of occluder are listed in the next chapter when considering their use for intractable diplopia (Fig. 14.4), although the more invasive forms (e.g., eyelid occlusion) are not appropriate to amblyopia treatment. In nonamblyopic normal subjects, different types of occluder (e.g., frosted, +1.50 fogging lens, opaque occluder) have different effects on visual function in the unoccluded eye (Wildsoet, Wood, Maag, & Sabdia, 1998), so it is possible that the type of occluder will influence the outcome of patching in amblyopia. However, the most important aspect of an occluder is that it must occlude! Children are resourceful and will seek to achieve the best vision they can, which involves removing or peeping around the patch. Practitioners and parents must be alert to this possibility and continuous monitoring (typically, by parents) and reinforcement of instructions (El Ghrably, Longville, & Gnanaraj, 2007) is required.

The usual method is total occlusion, which tries to ensure that no light enters the eye and the amblyopic eye is brought into use. The traditional device is an adhesive patch which covers the eye and extends a little over the orbit margins. A smaller piece of gauze or lint in the centre of the patch prevents adhesion to the lids. Plastic, rubber, or felt cup devices are also available that fit between the eye and spectacles. These require close supervision as a child can soon learn to peep over them. Alternatives, which may be more cosmetically acceptable and can be used if the child can be trusted to maintain occlusion, include the use of a frosted lens, in glasses. The simple use of translucent tape to occlude the spectacle lens has been shown to achieve good results and possibly better compliance than a stick-on patch (Beneish, Polomeno, Flanders, & Koenekoop, 2009).

Bangerter foils (Appendix 12) are translucent press-on films which are adhered onto a lens, in a similar way to Fresnel lenses. Bangerter foils are 'frosted' in a series of increasing degrees of opacification. They were developed for amblyopia therapy and are graded according to the typical level of decimal visual acuity obtained through the foil. Bangerter foils perform similarly to conventional occlusion in moderate amblyopes (Rutstein et al., 2010) and have the advantage in anisometropia of allowing coarse stereopsis (Iacobucci, Archer, Furr, Beyst Martonyi, & Del Monte, 2001). A review indicates positive results, but the filters degrade and need to be replaced periodically (Papageorgiou et al., 2019). Bangerter filters have some disadvantages, including unequal steps between progressive filters and a greater effect on stereopsis than visual acuity, which might mean that optical defocus is a preferable approach for amblyopia treatment (Li et al., 2012).

Neutral density filters have been suggested for occlusion (Ding & Levi, 2014). Liquid crystal glasses have been described as a promising alternative to occlusion, but more research is required (Papageorgiou et al., 2019). Occlusive contact lenses can achieve success in some cases (Joslin, McMahon, & Kaurman, 2002; Anderson, Brown, Mathews, & Mathews, 2006).

Compliance

Several studies have used objective dose monitoring devices to investigate compliance with patching. On average, patching is carried out by families less than 50% of the prescribed time (Papageorgiou et al., 2019). Success rates increase in proportion to objectively measured hours of patch use (West & Williams, 2016), so practitioners should emphasise the importance of compliance and ask open questions to assess this.

Adverse Events Associated with Occlusion

Some authors advise that prolonged occlusion is contraindicated in strabismic patients after the sensitive period because of the risk of inducing intractable diplopia. However, this complication appears to be very rare and the diplopia disappears if it is detected early and occlusion discontinued (Stankovic & Milenkovic, 2007). In contrast, intermittent **monocular** diplopia in the amblyopic eye during patching is not a contraindication to continued occlusion therapy (Cackett, Weir, & Houston, 2003). Part-time occlusion has been advocated by some as a strategy to reduce the risk of intractable diplopia, as discussed in the next section.

Occlusion amblyopia (reverse amblyopia) occasionally develops in a previously good eye that has been occluded and uncommonly the strabismus can transfer to the previously good eye (Assaf, 1982). This is most likely when children under the age of 3 years are patched aggressively (Assaf, 1982). In the unlikely event that occlusion amblyopia occurs, this can be managed with alternate or inverse occlusion, as discussed below.

Full-Time or Part-Time Occlusion?

Occlusion may carry the greatest risk of causing intractable diplopia in teenagers and adults. This has led some authors to advocate active visual stimulation (see later) for brief periods (e.g., 30 minutes once a week), or for longer periods if the binocular sensory adaptations are monitored (Chapter 14) to ensure the depth of suppression (Ansons & Davis, 2001) or harmonious anomalous retinal correspondence is not reduced. Recent evidence supports the view that in most cases part-time occlusion is as effective as full-time. For moderate amblyopia (6/12 to 6/30), 2 hours of daily patching is as effective as 6 hours and for severe amblyopia (6/30 to 6/120), 6 hours of daily patching is as effective as full-time (Papageorgiou et al., 2019). Full-time occlusion is reserved as a last resort for intractable cases before abandoning treatment. Case Study 13.1 is an example of a typical case who was patched by their community optometrist.

If the child has anisometropic amblyopia, constant occlusion could interfere with binocularity and in these cases it is advisable to allow the child at least 2 hours a day of binocular vision. If there is a significant heterophoria, the patient should be monitored very closely throughout occlusion to ensure that the heterophoria does not break down into a strabismus.

CASE STUDY 13.1	First appointment (aged nearly 4 years)

SYMPTOMS & HISTORY
Birth and first year normal; no history of strabismus. A few months ago, vision screening detected problem in LE and parents noticed tendency to close LE for concentrated tasks. Local optometrist prescribed R +1.00DS L +4.00DS, worn at pre-school and for concentrated visual tasks. Optometrist told parents acuity in amblyopic eye improved by one line but has not improved further over several weeks, so recommended occlusion. Unsure for how long each day, so referred to the author. No problems at school. No headaches and health good, no medications. Family history: aunt amblyopia.

RELEVANT CLINICAL FINDINGS
Normal ocular health, pupil reactions, ocular motility, NPC, Amp. Acc. Child mature for age, cooperative, able to cope with adult LogMAR.

Unaided acuities:	R 6/7.5	L 6/24+	B 6/7.5
'Dry' retinoscopy:	R +1.75/−0.50 × 180	L +4.75/−0.50 × 180 6/24+	
Stereoacuity (Rx):	Randot 2 shapes nil, circles nil		
Cover test (no Rx):	D orthophoria		
(same with Rx)	N orthophoria		
Cycloplegic retinosc.:	R +1.75/−0.25 × 180	L +4.75DS	
Eccentric fixation:	present in amblyopic eye		
Polarised letters:	foveal suppression LE		

COMMENT
The stereoacuity result (tested with refractive correction) and eccentric fixation indicate that the case is likely to be microtropia, with combined anisometropic/strabismic amblyopia. It is unlikely that a stronger refractive correction would be tolerated and highly unlikely that it would improve the binocularity. The parents were not keen on vision therapy as the child is happy with glasses.

MANAGEMENT
Explained that with 6/24 in the amblyopic eye, it is advisable to start with 2 h occlusion a day. Wrote to local optometrist who is planning to undertake occlusion.

NEXT EXAM (AGE 6 YEARS)
Local optometrist is considering ceasing occlusion and referred to the author for second opinion. Still undertaking 2 hours occlusion a day. Sent printout of prescriptions and acuities over the last 2 years. RE stable at 6/6; LE improved 1.5 years ago to 6/12, 1 year ago to 6/9, 9 months ago to 6/7.5 and stable since. Author's findings confirmed improvement in VA, and also in stereopsis with contoured target (Randot circles) to 100″. Confirmed OK to taper occlusion.

Amp. Acc, Accommodative amplitude; *B*, both; *D*, distance; *DS*, dioptre sphere; *h*, hours; *L*, left; *LE*, left eye; *N*, near; *NPC*, near point of convergence; *R*, right; *Rx*, prescription; *VA*, visual acuity.

Alternate and Inverse Occlusion

Historically, it was argued that under age 3 years, the occluder should be worn over the nonamblyopic eye for 3 days and then changed to the amblyopic eye for 1 day to allow the development of the nonamblyopic eye. This practice, **inverse occlusion**, was advocated to reduce the risk of reverse amblyopia. This approach seems to be rarely followed nowadays and a Cochrane review found that reverse amblyopia is rare (West & Williams, 2016).

Duration of Occlusion

Not all cases of amblyopia improve with occlusion, and failure to respond to treatment may in some cases be attributable to subtle optic nerve hypoplasia (Lempert, 2000). The studies described in this section are of occlusion in children, typically after refractive treatment.

Within 3 months, most compliant children are cured (Lithander & Sjostrand, 1991) or at least have undergone most of the improvement that is likely (Oliver, Neumann, Chaimovitch, Gotesman, & Shimshoni, 1986). In contrast, a study found 52% of cases achieved maximum improvement by 4 months (Pediatric Eye Disease Investigator Group (PEDIG), 2003), and another study found that 80% of the improvement with occlusion occurred within 6 weeks (Stewart, Moseley, Stephens, & Fielder, 2004).

When the acuity ceases to improve, the occluder may be removed in the case of the refractive amblyopes. Where there is a strabismus, the next step in the total treatment needs to be considered (Chapter 14). Sometimes, patients with cosmetically acceptable and asymptomatic strabismic amblyopia wish to have the acuity in their amblyopic eye improved, but do not desire any further treatment of their strabismus. They may simply wish to have a better 'eye in reserve'. These cases require monitoring in case there is a regression of their acuity (see below).

Follow-Up Appointments

When a patient is being treated, improvement is expected and if this does not occur, an alternative treatment or referral is required. This means that patients need to be monitored closely, so if they are not responding to treatment an alternative management strategy can be started without delay. Younger patients should be reviewed more frequently. Opinions vary, but typical intervals initially are 4—6 weeks.

Recidivism (Recurrence)

Recidivism refers to a relapse of acuity following apparently successful treatment and this occurs in approximately one-quarter of cases (Papageorgiou et al., 2019). Some consider, if treatment is gradually tapered rather than abruptly stopped, recidivism is less likely.

Recidivism is more likely to be exhibited by patients with worse initial acuities (Levartovsky et al., 1995), and by those with mixed strabismic and anisometropic amblyopia (Tacagni, Stewart, Moseley, & Fielder, 2007). Patients with age-related macular degeneration often showed an improvement in the acuity of an amblyopic eye, typically of two to three lines (El Mallah, Chakravarthy, & Hart, 2000). This improvement is stable over time, suggesting that recidivism might not occur if the amblyopic eye remains in constant use.

Some authors recommend **maintenance occlusion,** part-time occlusion after the cessation of treatment with lengthier periods of occlusion, in the belief this will prevent acuity loss. However, when 32 children who had been treated with occlusion at age 11—15 years were followed up for a mean of 18 months, recidivism was rare and just as likely in those who had received maintenance occlusion (Mohan, Saroha, & Sharma, 2004).

Recidivism still occurs even in cases whose treatment is highly successful (e.g., good acuity, stereoacuity, orthotropia), so monitoring for recurrence of amblyopia is essential (Holmes, Melia, Bradfield, Cruz, & Forbes, 2007). As these authors state, plasticity in the visual system appears to be a double-edged sword.

ACTIVE AMBLYOPIA THERAPY

It has long been argued (Francois & James, 1955) that occlusion treatment is more effective if the patient undertakes a detailed visual task, to interest the patient and stimulate vision. Gould and colleagues used the term **active visual stimulation** to describe these detailed visual tasks, and recommended such treatments for periods of 45—60 minutes, reducing as acuity improves (Gould, Fishkoff, & Galin, 1970).

Care must be taken to ensure the patient is working at the limit of acuity by maintaining an appropriate working distance. The distance should also be monitored when the patient is watching television. With video games, parents can help children keep a record of their scores. One game can be played without occlusion ('with the good eye') and then several games are played, at the same distance, with the better eye covered ('with the bad eye'). The child's goal is to improve the score with their amblyopic eye. The keeping of scores not only acts as an incentive, but also helps children to understand the purpose of the treatment and to monitor improvement. Treatment will be more successful if parents and children can monitor progress and, not surprisingly, prohibiting children's activities is associated with poor compliance (Searle, Norman, Harrad, & Vedhara, 2002). So, if parents can encourage a child to watch their favourite videos, or play their favourite computer games, during occlusion, this is likely to improve compliance.

Some studies have investigated whether near vision tasks enhance occlusion, with mixed results (Papageorgiou et al., 2019). It seems unlikely that the viewing distance is important, but rather the resolution required.

Special techniques and instruments for the active treatment of amblyopia have also been developed and will now be described. Active amblyopia therapies may be effective in treating strabismic (Mallett, 1977) and anisometropic (Wick, Wingard, Cotter, & Scheiman, 1992) amblyopia in patients of any age, beyond the sensitive period. It seems that brief periods of occlusion in adults for active amblyopia therapy does not have any adverse effects on their binocular sensory adaptations to the strabismus (Mallett, 1988b).

INTERMITTENT PHOTIC STIMULATION (IPS)

Mallett (1985) described a unit for the treatment of amblyopia by active stimulation, with the non-amblyopic eye occluded. There are three components to the treatment: detailed targets to stimulate different types of receptive fields, illuminated by red light to encourage central fixation that flashes at 3–5 Hz. Mallett (1985) argued that patients of any age can be treated in periods of 30 minutes once or twice weekly. A small RCT of amblyopes over the age of 10 years found a modest (one line) but statistically significant improvement in visual acuity, but regression to pretreatment levels after 1 year (Evans, Yu, Massa, & Mathews, 2011).

Suppression Treatment and Binocular Therapies

It has long been argued that suppression treatment is an alternative to occlusion as a means of improving acuity in anisometropic amblyopia. One approach is to investigate the depth and extent of the suppression, and to give treatment for significant suppression. Exercises described in Chapter 14 may be required, but often the simpler treatment outlined for suppression in hetero-phoria in Chapter 10 may be effective. Most teenage patients would prefer this approach to wearing an occluder (Pickwell & Jenkins, 1983).

In recent years, binocular therapies for the treatment of amblyopia have been advocated, often using computer 'games', which typically include an element of suppression treatment (Li, Thompson, et al., 2013). Recent reviews note the lack of high-level evidence for these therapies (Papageorgiou et al., 2019; Pineles et al., 2020). More research is required, but one RCT of a bino-cular iPad game found this produced less improvement than conventional part-time patching, pos-sibly because the game was boring (Holmes et al., 2016).

Physiological Diplopia

In some cases of convergent strabismus, physiological diplopia methods can be used as an alterna-tive to occlusion (Pickwell, 1976), sometimes in combination with other treatments and in teenage as well as younger children (Pickwell & Jenkins, 1983). The physiological diplopia method is sim-ple to understand, but in practice it may require considerable supervision. A near vision fixation dis-tance is found where the visual axes cross in convergent strabismus, and an appreciation of physiological diplopia is used to encourage the use of binocular vision. This brings the amblyopic eye into use with the other eye at one fixation distance, and results in an improvement in acuity over several weeks.

The difficulty in applying this method is usually in the early stages. In theory, it is not difficult to see that there is a point in front of the eyes of a patient with convergent strabismus where the visual axes cross and that an object placed there ought to have a foveal image in both eyes; the object is being fixated binocularly. In practice, this can be found by using the cover test and moving the object closer or further away until no strabismus movement is seen. Where the patient increases the angle of deviation as the object is moved towards the eyes (the convergence excess element), this can sometimes be inhibited by explaining to the patient that the eye is turning inwards too much and encouraging less convergence. This may take time.

With some patients, convergence needs to be inhibited by positive spherical additions. When bino-cular fixation of the object has been achieved, the patient is encouraged to see a second object in physio-logical diplopia. This should be introduced at a greater distance than the fixation object. Its image will then fall on the nasal retina in the area where there are likely to be binocular sensory adaptations (Fig. 10.5). With further encouragement, appreciation of physiological diplopia of the second object can be seen, while fixation of the first is maintained. A week of home exercise supervised by a parent should consolidate this. The parent may be taught how to apply the cover test to check that fixation has been maintained. The patient then progresses to wire reading, which is described on p. 148.

This method is appropriate only to angles of strabismus less than 12Δ or when it can be reduced to this by refractive correction. It requires a high degree of interest and cooperation. The starting acuity should be 6/24 or better, and in some cases can go on improving for several months if the method is successful in establishing binocular vision for close work. The method is further described in Chapter 14 in relation to its use in the treatment of binocular sensory adaptations.

Binocular Treatment of Amblyopia

An interesting development is the use of virtual reality systems in amblyopia treatment for children, using interactive two- and three-dimensional games and videos (Eastgate et al., 2006). Preliminary results are promising (Waddingham et al., 2006). Virtual reality headsets allow binocular treatment of amblyopia (Fortenbacher et al., 2018) and there is some evidence this can improve motion-defined form (MDF) perception in the fellow eye, which often has deficits of MDF after occlusion therapy (Birch, Jost, Wang, Kelly, & Giaschi, 2019). However, although the results of preliminary cohort studies appear promising (Tailor, Bossi, Bunce, Greenwood, & Dahlmann-Noor, 2015), further research with RCTs is required (Pineles et al., 2020).

Perceptual Learning

Perceptual learning involves practising certain visual tasks to train amblyopic eyes to better recognise low level features of simple visual stimuli (Polat, Mizobe, Pettet, Kasamatsu, & Norcia, 1998). A review noted that research to date involves low participant numbers and RCTs with long-term follow up are required (Papageorgiou et al., 2019).

Other Approaches

The after-image transfer method is not commonly used nowadays and is mainly of historical interest (Caloroso, 1972; Mallett, 1975; Jenkins, Pickwell, & Sheridan, 1979). Another historic approach is to use a deep red filter placed over the unoccluded eye to reduce eccentric fixation, although a neutral density filter is as good as a red filter (Matilla, Pickwell, & Gilchrist, 1995). Indeed, a recent RCT suggests that occlusion whilst a blue filter is worn over the amblyopic eye may be an effective treatment (Metzler et al., 1998).

The Euthyscope is a special ophthalmoscope that was used in a pleoptic technique to create a ring after-image centred on the fovea of the amblyopic eye, to encourage foveal fixation (Schmidt & Stapp, 1977). Modern views on the risks of excessive exposure to light (Young, 1994) may be a cause for concern with this type of treatment.

One early active stimulation technique required the patient to look at a rotating grating of black and white lines for a few minutes, and to maintain clear vision of the lines: the CAM disc method (Banks, Campbell, Hess, & Watson, 1978). Despite some promising results (Watson, Sanac, & Pickering, 1985), in most studies this method has not been shown to produce good results (Douthwaite, Jenkins, Pickwell, & Sheridan, 1981). Several studies indicate that it produces the same results as occlusion (Nyman, Singh, Rydberg, & Fordander, 1983), which may also be required (Tytla & Labow-Daily, 1981). It may be a little more effective in anisometropic amblyopia than in strabismic amblyopia (Lennerstrand & Samuelson, 1983), although there is little evidence to suggest that the presence of the rotating grating has any effect other than a placebo.

Certain neurotransmitters have been implicated in neuronal plasticity, most notably, levodopa. A review and metaanalysis of research investigating levodopa combined with occlusion concludes levodopa is effective. Corticosteroids may also have a beneficial effect on amblyopia, although this hypothesis requires more investigation (Constantinescu & Gottlob, 2001). Two other interesting approaches, acupuncture and repetitive transcranial magnetic stimulation, require further research (Papageorgiou et al., 2019).

PENALISATION AND FOGGING METHODS

A slightly different approach to occlusion (Fig. 14.4) is to blur the nonamblyopic eye, sometimes called **penalisation**. The blurring can be achieved optically or by a cycloplegic agent. It has been argued that lens blur, because it reduces the contrast in a spatial frequency dependent fashion, is the best form of partial occlusion as it still supports stereopsis for low spatial frequencies (Hess, Thompson, & Baker, 2014).

Cycloplegia can be used for penalisation in a variety of ways. For example, in an emmetrope both eyes can receive a weekly application of 1% atropine ointment, and the nonamblyopic eye provided with a reading addition of +3.00DS. This provokes use of the amblyopic eye for distance vision, and the other eye for near work. It is claimed that the cooperation of the patient is assured, because there is no occluder to peep round, no exercises to be skipped, and the glasses must be worn if the patient wishes to see clearly. However, if the acuity in the amblyopic eye is worse than 6/36, the patient may have better acuity with the other eye by looking over the glasses or by taking them off, depending on the refractive error (Gregorson et al., 1974). An alternative method is to have the reading addition in the amblyopic eye and a normal correction in the other (Dale, 1982).

North (1986) described a variation of this method in which the nonamblyopic eye is penalised with the daily instillation of 0.5% or 1% atropine sulphate. She felt that the best improvement was usually obtained by giving the amblyopic eye a +3.00 overcorrection causing it to be used for all near vision: this is called near vision penalisation. A retrospective study indicated that an intermittent atropine regimen (1–3 days a week) is as effective as full-time atropine (Simons, Stein, Sener, Vitale, & Guyton, 1997).

Another fogging method is to blur the nonamblyopic eye for distance vision by an extra positive sphere, +2D or +3D, which serves as a reading addition for near. This is a less dramatic way of producing a similar situation to drug penalisation: clear distance vision in the amblyopic eye and near vision with the other. The glasses or contact lens may be worn all the time, or as a second pair of glasses which are worn in the evenings each day while watching television. In partially accommodative strabismus, this method assists in further reducing the angle. Alternatively, a spectacle lens

TABLE 13.4 ■ **Method for Treating Functional Amblyopia.**

1. Carry out cycloplegic refraction.
2. Correct refractive error, fully correcting anisometropia and astigmatism.
3. If high anisometropia, consider contact lenses.
4. Check the patient after about 4–6 weeks. If vision is improving, continue with refractive correction alone until the amblyopic eye either (a) stops improving or (b) the acuity of the amblyopic eye is within a line of the better eye.
5. If, after treating for at least 14 weeks, (a) occurs before (b), proceed to occlusion, depending on type of amblyopia and age (Fig. 13.4).
6. Occlusion requires a clear image, so use appropriate refractive correction.
7. Choose an occluder that will be effective and the child will tolerate.
8. In anisometropic amblyopia, avoid full-time occlusion: there should be at least 2 hours a day without the occluder. Typically, the occlusion is started for 2 hours a day in moderate and 6 hours a day in severe amblyopia.
9. If patients have a heterophoria that may decompensate (Chapter 4), occlude for brief periods, starting with 1 hour, gradually increasing if the heterophoria remains compensated.
10. Explain to the parent how the child might 'cheat' (e.g., lifting edge of patch and turning head). It is natural for children to try to use their better eye, but patching will only work if the parent detects and stops cheating.
11. Patients should be warned to monitor for diplopia and look for a turning eye. If this occurs, stop patching and return for binocularity to be checked.
12. Careful monitoring is required, typically 4–6 weeks after treatment starts and regularly thereafter. Monitor parental observations, acuities (both eyes), cover test, stereopsis. Periodically repeat motility, ophthalmoscopy, and retinoscopy.
13. If the acuity does not improve significantly (e.g., by a line), re-evaluate the diagnosis (see Table 14.1).
14. If there is no evidence of pathology and part-time is not working, try full-time occlusion (except in anisometropia or borderline heterophoria).
15. If the patient does not respond to full-time occlusion, refer for second opinion.
16. If the acuity improves with occlusion, continue until no further improvement over 5–6 weeks.
17. The patient is then monitored every few months for recidivism.

or contact lens of a very large and completely inappropriate refractive power (e.g., high oblique cylinder) can be worn in front of the nonamblyopic eye. As with any amblyopia treatment, careful monitoring is required: patients may look over the spectacles or may deliberately displace a contact lens.

Several research studies have evaluated atropine penalisation and a systematic review and meta-analysis concluded that atropine penalisation appears to be as effective as conventional occlusion for treating amblyopia (Osborne, Greenhalgh, Evans, & Self, 2018; Li, Qureshi, & Taylor, 2019).

CONCLUSIONS CONCERNING TREATMENT OF AMBLYOPIA

Refractive error correction and occlusion are validated treatments for functional amblyopia. The type of case that is most amenable to treatment in community optometric practice is anisometropic amblyopia. A typical approach to the treatment of functional amblyopia is summarised in Table 13.4 and Fig. 13.4.

Not all cases respond to treatment, sometimes because of undetected pathology or a structural defect (Barrett, Candy, McGraw, & Bradley, 2005). 'Success' is a relative term: successfully treated eyes may still be on average two lines behind the nonamblyopic eye (Repka et al., 2005).

CLINICAL KEY POINTS

- Regularly look for active pathology: if present refer
- If treatment is not having a significant effect, look again for pathology and refer
- To children, patching is boring and visually impairing. Do whatever you can to motivate them (e.g., TV, videos, computer games, etc.)
- Children are resourceful and often find ways of 'cheating' if you let them. A realistic approach to compliance is essential, with clear instructions for the parent and child
- Don't underestimate the effect of refractive errors. About one-quarter of amblyopic children can be cured with spectacles alone
- In high anisometropia, contact lenses are the preferred optical correction
- Try refractive correction for 14 weeks before occlusion
- Start with low 'doses': occlusion for 2 hours a day if better than 6/30
- Review every 4–6 weeks
- Do not prescribe constant occlusion to orthotropic patients
- Treatment may work over the age of 7–8 years, BUT...
- Prolonged periods of patching in older strabismic patients is contraindicated as it may interfere with binocular sensory adaptations

CHAPTER 14

Techniques in the Investigation and Management of Comitant Strabismus

When to Treat Comitant Strabismus

The first stage in the investigation of strabismus is to discover whether there is any pathological cause for the strabismus. If pathology is present, the patient should be referred for medical investigation and treatment. The detection of pathology is described elsewhere in this book and is summarised in Table 14.1.

There are three good reasons for treating orthoptic anomalies: if they are causing problems; if they are likely to deteriorate if left untreated; or if treatment may be required but less effective when the patient is older. Cosmetically apparent strabismus is associated with social alienation in children as young as 5−6 years (Lukman et al., 2010) and after surgery most cases have an improvement in appearance, self-esteem, and self-confidence (Menon, Saha, Tandon, Mehta, & Khokhar, 2002). The minimum size of strabismus that is cosmetically apparent varies (Larson, Keech, & Verdick, 2003), but is less for exotropia (typically, 8Δ) than esotropia (typically, 14.5Δ) (Wiessberg, Suckow, & Thorn, 2004).

Some cases of strabismus do not result in any overt problems (e.g., symptoms, poor cosmesis), and are unlikely to deteriorate or to be harder to treat later. However, strabismic patients are likely to have a marked reduction in stereoacuity and this is undesirable, even though the patient may not be aware of the deficit. Reduced stereoacuity can impair performance in everyday activities, such as driving (Bauer et al., 2000) and motor tasks (Hrisos et al., 2006), and binocular reaction times are faster than monocular (Justo, Bermudez, Perez, & Gonzalez, 2004). There are reports of individuals with no history of stereopsis (e.g., from strabismus) developing stereoperception in adult life, sometimes with dramatic perceptual gains (Barry & Bridgeman, 2017). This study was of individual's self-report by questionnaire and so is subject to bias. Some of the reported improvements followed vision therapy, but some were reported spontaneously and despite the eyes remaining misaligned. In some cases, these reports could be psychogenic effects and further research is required.

Binocular reading speed is impaired in amblyopia, even when binocular visual acuity is normal (Stifter, Burggasser, Hirmann, Thaler, & Radner, 2005). So, if the strabismus can be treated, this deserves consideration. It should be stressed that these benefits of stereopsis are subtle: people do not report a sudden drop in the quality of their vision when they cover one eye. Even for driving, the loss of stereopsis only affects some tasks and there is evidence that at far distances (e.g., >40 m), where stereopsis ceases to be effective, patients with long-standing strabismus make better use of monocular cues than nonstrabismic people (Bauer et al., 2001). However, this view is controversial as other research indicates that strabismic patients do not have an enhanced ability to use monocular cues (Nuzzi & Cantu, 2003).

Strabismus with a small stable angle is often associated with deep harmonious anomalous retinal correspondence (HARC) and this can give the patient quite good 'pseudo-binocular vision', sometimes with a reasonable degree of stereopsis. If these cases are asymptomatic, have a good cosmesis, and have good visual function, it is hard to justify the disruption to the child and family that accompanies treatment with exercises. Although successful treatment might increase career possibilities, it must be acknowledged that the vast majority of cases would gain little benefit from treatment. Additionally, these well-adapted cases will be difficult to treat and there is always a possibility

TABLE 14.1 ■ **Summary of Steps in Determining if Pathology is Present in Strabismus.**

Step	Rationale	What to do
Detect incomitancy	Any new or changing incomitancy requires prompt referral	• Carry out a careful motility test, including questions about diplopia (p. 26). • A cover test in peripheral gaze is helpful. If in doubt, a Hess screen test is very useful (see Chapter 17). • If there is a new or changing incomitancy, refer.
Look for orbital pathology	Orbital pathology can cause strabismus, although this is rare.	• Is proptosis present? • Are the eye movements restricted? • Is there pain on eye movements?
Detect ocular pathology	Pathology that destroys or diminishes the vision in a significant part of the visual field of one eye can dissociate the eyes and cause strabismus.	• Check pupil reactions, particularly looking for an afferent pupillary defect (APD). • Carry out careful ophthalmoscopy. In younger children, dilated fundoscopy might be necessary to obtain a good view, commonly after cycloplegic refraction. Keep checking ophthalmoscopy at regular intervals. • As soon as the child is old enough, check visual fields.
Look for neurological problems	Pathology in the brain can cause comitant as well as incomitant deviations.	• Carefully check pupil reactions. • Assess and record optic disc appearance in both eyes, ideally with imaging. • Monitor reports of general health (see text).
Look for obvious causes of the strabismus	There will be a reason why a patient develops a strabismus. If you find a nonpathological reason, a pathological reason is less likely.	• E.g., if a child has an esotropia, look for hypermetropia. • E.g., if an older patient is developing an exotropia, have they always had an exophoria which is gradually decompensating with worsening cataract. • In every case, still look for pathology. But if you have found an obvious cause, it is probably **the** cause.
Monitor the size of the deviation	If the deviation is increasing, there must be a reason.	• If you cannot find the reason why a deviation is increasing, then refer so that someone else can give a second opinion.
Is the strabismus responding to treatment?	If you believe you are treating the cause of the strabismus (e.g., correcting hypermetropia), the situation should improve.	• If a strabismus does not respond to treatment (e.g., giving postcycloplegic plus for hypermetropia), review your diagnosis (e.g., accommodative esotropia). • Failure to respond to treatment might indicate a pathological cause, so refer for a second opinion.

that treatment might make the situation worse. Some parents are keen to eliminate a strabismus at any cost, but they should be fully informed of the likely risks and benefits and few practitioners would take on the treatment of this type of case, other than treating amblyopia in children of a suitable age.

The investigation and management of comitant strabismus can be broadly divided into two parts: sensory and motor. Patients who have not managed to achieve a sensory adaptation to their strabismus (usually, this is because they are too old) will have diplopia and this is discussed next. Suppression and HARC are adaptations in the visual sensory mechanisms which occur in strabismus. These adaptations have been reviewed in Chapter 12 and are further described in this chapter with particular reference to the clinical investigation and treatment. As explained in Chapter 12, small suppression areas can coexist with HARC, especially in small-angle strabismus. In strabismus over 25Δ, suppression seems to dominate.

In cases of strabismus where treatment is appropriate, sensory factors (suppression, HARC) are generally treated first. Throughout this period some form of occlusion is maintained during the intervals between treatment to prevent diplopia and confusion. In cases where the patient is diplopic, treatment of the motor deviation can be started straight away. The motor deviation sometimes spontaneously resolves when sensory factors have been corrected. When this does not occur, refractive correction or fusional reserve exercises are required to treat the motor component. Treatment of sensory factors should only be attempted in cases where the practitioner is sure the motor deviation will respond to treatment (see later).

Diplopia

It has already been noted that most patients with strabismus develop a sensory adaptation (HARC or suppression) to avoid diplopia and confusion. In some cases, this is not possible, usually because the patient is too old, and the patient develops diplopia and confusion (Chapter 12). The distinction between diplopia and confusion is illustrated in Fig. 12.1, and both phenomena usually occur together (p. 166). Throughout this section, the word diplopia is used to describe the problems of diplopia and confusion.

INVESTIGATION OF DIPLOPIA

Diagnosis: the Worth Four Dot Test

In most cases, diplopia is detected from the symptom of double vision in everyday life. Occasionally, it may be necessary to formally test for diplopia (e.g., patients who may be denying diplopia to enter certain vocations). In these cases, the Worth Four Dot Test can be used. The test is carried out in room illumination and the patient should not be shown the test targets until they are wearing red-green glasses and should be told not to close or cover one eye. The patient is asked to describe what they see, and the possible responses are illustrated in Fig. 14.1. The figure illustrates a stable situation, but often patients experience a dynamic perception: the monocular inputs may move or disappear.

The red-green glasses create an artificial viewing condition, so it is possible that a patient reports diplopia with the Worth test but does not usually experience diplopia in everyday life (Bagolini, 1999). The test is also sometimes used to investigate HARC and suppression, but there are better tests (Bagolini, 1999) which use more natural viewing conditions (see later).

Investigation

In addition to strabismus, other conditions can lead to reports of 'double vision' and the investigation of diplopia is summarised in Fig. 14.2. The investigation of diplopia is simplifying by asking the patient to view an isolated target. Covering each eye is essential to determine whether the diplopia is monocular or binocular, and a pinhole will further help to determine the aetiology (Finlay, 2000). Monocular diplopia accounts for one-quarter of cases of diplopia presenting to an eye hospital (Morris, 1991). For nearly all these cases a genuine cause can be found, usually lenticular or corneal pathology. Monocular diplopia can result from an epiretinal membrane (Veverka et al., 2017),

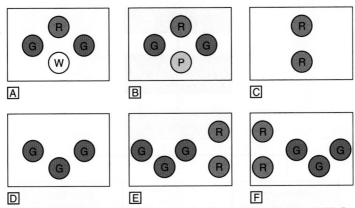

Fig. 14.1   The Worth Four Dot Test. The test, as seen by the practitioner, is shown in (A). Panels (B) to (F) show the possible appearances of the test to patients, who should always view the test through red-green glasses (red in front of right eye). Patients with binocular single vision will perceive (B). Patients who suppress their left eye will describe (C), and those who suppress their right eye will describe (D). Patients with uncrossed diplopia (esotropia) will describe (E) and those with crossed diplopia (F). The effect of vertical diplopia is not shown but is analogous to (E) and (F). *G*, green; *P*, pink; *R*, red; *W*, white.

for example after cataract surgery (Foroozan & Arnold, 2005). Monocular diplopia in children can be due to refractive errors, cataracts, corneal disease, or occasionally retinal disease (Taylor, 1997). Sensory causes of monocular diplopia and polyopia (more than two images) include brain trauma, cerebrovascular accidents, and migraine.

When diplopia is binocular, orthoptic tests should be used to detect the presence of strabismus. The direction of the diplopia (horizontal, vertical, oblique, torsional) should be determined by questioning the patient. By introducing a red filter in front of one eye, or by covering an eye, the practitioner can determine whether horizontal diplopia is crossed (heteronymous, suggesting an exotropia) or uncrossed (homonymous, suggesting an esotropia). If diplopia occurs after surgery, it should be determined whether it is in accordance with the postoperative deviation or **paradoxical** (crossed with esotropia and uncrossed with exotropia), in which case there is a persistence of the preoperative sensory adaptation (von Noorden, 1996). The practitioner should detect and investigate incomitancy as outlined in Chapter 17 and any comitant deviation as outlined elsewhere in this chapter and in Chapters 15 and 16.

Monocular diplopia or binocular triplopia can occur through a persistence of the sensory state preceding a surgical intervention. The strabismic eye sees two images of a fixation point, as a result of competition between the innate normal retinal correspondence (NRC) and long-standing anomalous retinal correspondence (ARC) that existed before surgery. During binocular viewing, the NRC in the dominant eye can cause triplopia (von Noorden, 1996). Rarely, binocular diplopia can result when a previously dominant eye becomes the more myopic causing a change in ocular dominance. Such cases are resolved by correction of the myopia.

Intractable diplopia (see later) from strabismus suggests that either the patient was unable to develop sensory adaptations (e.g., because they were too old when the strabismus occurred) or that there has been a change in their sensory or motor status.

A particularly troublesome form of binocular sensory diplopia occurs in nonstrabismic patients who have developed a macular or retinal lesion (e.g., epiretinal membrane) causing metamorphopsia. Bifoveal fusion may be impossible, yet peripheral fusion is likely to be normal. This is sometimes called central-peripheral rivalry (CPR)-type diplopia (Hatt et al., 2019). A useful way of investigating this **dragged fovea syndrome** is with the **lights on-off** test (de Pool, Campbell,

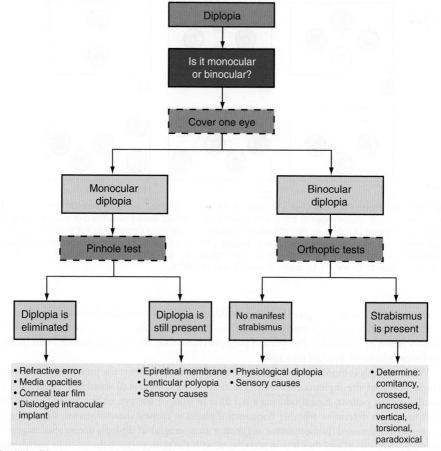

Fig. 14.2   Diagram summarising the investigation of diplopia. Investigative tests are in boxes with dashed outlines, diagnoses are in boxes with bold outlines. (Modified after von Noorden, G.K. (1996). *Binocular vision and ocular motility* (5th ed.). St. Louis: Mosby.)

Broome, & Guyton, 2005). The patient fixates a small isolated target (e.g., dot or single 6/18 letter) that should be white in the centre of a black computer screen. With the room lights on, this will be seen doubled. When the room lights are suddenly extinguished, then within 2−10 seconds the letter should become single. Occasionally, patients need a partial prism correction to achieve this central fusion. There is no complete cure, but some cases benefit from monovision and others require occlusion (De Pool et al., 2005). These authors cautioned that surgery for the epiretinal membrane should not be thought of as a cure, as this can trigger or worsen the problem. A low density Bangerter foil (p. 190) sometimes helps (Silverberg et al., 1999).

It is possible that sensory diplopia might also occur as one of the anomalous visual effects that can accompany sensory visual stress (p. 64). These visual perceptual distortions probably result from hyperexcitability of the visual cortex (Wilkins, 1995). Covering one eye halves the sensory input to the visual cortex and thus reduces the probability of these effects (Wilkins, 1995). Hence, sensory diplopia from this source could conceivably present as binocular diplopia which resolves on covering one eye, although the diplopia is not likely to occur with isolated targets. The treatment of the non-binocular types of diplopia classified in Fig. 14.2 was summarised by Evans (2001c) and the treatment of binocular cases is now described.

Can the Patient Achieve Binocular Single Vision?

In most cases, the complaint of binocular diplopia suggests that there is the potential for binocular single vision, especially if the patient can consciously control the diplopia by adopting a compensatory head posture. Exceptions are the intractable cases described next. In every case, prisms should be used to establish whether the diplopia can be eliminated before surgery is considered. Loose prisms, rotary prisms (e.g., in a phoropter), or prism bars can be used. Errors can occur when prisms are stacked (e.g., several loose prisms placed in a trial frame; Firth & Whittle, 1994).

The effect of prisms on diplopia from comitant strabismus can be investigated using the Mallett **OXO** test (Fig. 14.3). If the diplopia is predominantly horizontal, the horizontal **OXO** should be

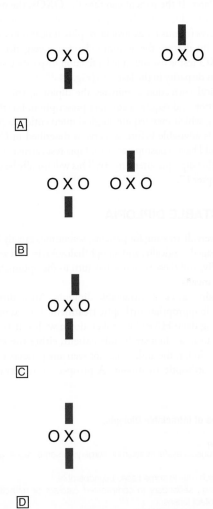

Fig. 14.3   Diagram showing the use of a Mallett unit to investigate the effect of prisms on horizontal diplopia. Patients with predominantly horizontal diplopia are asked to view the OXO target that has vertical Nonius strips. Patients with poor acuity in one or both eyes can view the 'large OXO' (Mallett ARC and suppression test). Patients with horizontal diplopia will describe the perception illustrated in (A). Prisms are adjusted to bring the diplopic images closer together (B) and when superimposition occurs (C), the prisms are further refined to eliminate any fixation disparity (D). See text for more details. *ARC*, Anomalous retinal correspondence.

used. Even incomitant cases, if the incomitancy is subtle, sometimes benefit from the prism suggested by testing with the Mallett unit in the primary position (Chapter 17). For patients with good visual acuity, the usual small OXO can be used. Patients with poor acuity can use the large OXO which is included on modern near Mallett units.

If a patient with horizontal diplopia views the test whilst wearing the polarised visors, they should report seeing two OXOs, one with a line above the X and another with a line below the X (Fig. 14.3A). The position of the OXOs reveals the type of diplopia (e.g., horizontal in Fig. 14.3A). Prisms are introduced and adjusted to bring the OXOs closer together (Fig. 14.3B). It should be determined whether the patient can fuse the diplopic OXOs (as in Fig. 14.3C). If they cannot fuse the two OXOs, then there may be **sensory fusion disruption syndrome** or **horror fusionis**, described later. If the patient can fuse the OXOs, the prism should be refined to eliminate any fixation disparity (Fig. 14.3D). In patients with horizontal diplopia and with adequate accommodation, spheres (minus for exotropia, or plus at near for esotropia) can be used to try and eliminate the diplopia by altering the accommodative convergence. It should be noted that whilst the normal sized OXO test is usually called a fixation disparity test, its use for diplopia correction only involves fixation disparity in the last step (Fig. 14.3C,D).

If a prismatic or spherical correction eliminates the diplopia, this can be prescribed. Some patients adapt to the correction and require a stronger prescription, but this is not usually the case (p. 104). With larger angles, which may require surgical intervention, a prism adaptation test or a trial with botulinum toxin is advisable before surgery, as described in Chapter 17. Patients with diplopia or suppression should have a postoperative diplopia test carried out before surgery, to assess the risk of inducing intractable diplopia after surgery. This will usually be carried out at the hospital and is also described in Chapter 17.

CAUSES OF INTRACTABLE DIPLOPIA

Intractable diplopia can be very distressing for patients, sometimes greatly impairing their quality of life. Some cases can be managed surgically, and an ophthalmologist will advise on this. Other cases cannot be managed surgically, and these patients may turn to the optometrist to manage the diplopia through optical or other means.

Table 14.2 lists the main causes of intractable diplopia. An additional category might be patients who have received inappropriate orthoptic treatment. For example, intractable diplopia might occur if long-standing deep HARC is broken down with full-time occlusion in an adult or if an attempt was made to treat, in a strabismic patient, either the sensory adaptation or the motor deviation in isolation. So far, the author has not seen any patients whose intractable diplopia results from inappropriate orthoptic treatment. A prospective observational study in the UK

TABLE 14.2 ■ **Main Causes of Intractable Diplopia.**

Causes of Intractable Diplopia
- Secondary deviation from unsuccessful strabismus surgery; in some cases, a surgeon advises against further surgery
- Late onset strabismus, which may in some cases be inoperable
- Acquired anisometropia (e.g., secondary to complicated cataract or refractive surgery); some cases may not be suitable for contact lenses
- Retinal distortion following epiretinal membrane, macular lesion, or detachment (central-peripheral rivalry (CPR)-type) diplopia (Hatt et al., 2019)
- Refractive surgery and (rarely) cataract surgery (Gunton & Armstrong, 2010)
- Sensory fusion disruption syndrome (see below)
- Horror fusionis (see below)

(Newsham, O'Connor, & Harrad, 2018) found the commonest cause of intractable diplopia is strabismus surgery (32%), with other main causes being spontaneous (25%), severe head trauma (8%), cataract surgery (6%), and vitrectomy (6%).

The risk of intractable diplopia for people undergoing strabismus surgery has been estimated to be between 0.2% (Newsham et al., 2018) and 0.8% of cases (Kushner, 2002). Intractable diplopia from refractive surgery can be traced to one of five mechanisms (Kushner & Kowal, 2003): technical problems, prior need for prisms, aniseikonia, iatrogenic monovision, and improper control of accommodation in patients with strabismus. Screening methods to detect these problems have been advocated for patients considering refractive surgery (Kowal, Battu, & Kushner, 2005, Kushner & Kowal, 2003). Attempts to induce monovision in a patient with long-standing strabismus or incomitancy is another possible cause of diplopia (Godts, Tassignon, & Gobin, 2004; Evans, 2007a). Indeed, it seems unwise to prescribe monovision with refractive surgery before a temporary trial of monovision with contact lenses (Vogt, 2003), although this will not detect all cases at risk of strabismus (Pollard, Greenberg, Bordenca, Elliott, & Hsu, 2011). The cause of diplopia in these cases has been attributed to **fixation switch diplopia**, when the patient is forced to fixate with a previously strabismic eye (Kushner, 1995).

One uncommon risk factor for intractable diplopia is when patients with unilateral aphakia are fitted with a secondary posterior chamber intraocular lens (Khan, 2008). Pre-surgical prism testing is useful in these cases (Khan, 2007).

Horror Fusionis and Sensory Fusion Disruption Syndrome

Heterotropic patients with **horror fusionis** cannot demonstrate fusion, even when the deviation is corrected with prisms or in a haploscopic instrument. These patients report a 'jumping over' phenomenon: as the prism is increased and the diplopic images move together, they suddenly 'jump' and, for example, crossed diplopia suddenly changes to uncrossed diplopia. The same phenomenon occurs when the prisms are changed in the other direction. It appears that the patient is unable to achieve motor fusion. Caloroso and Rouse (1993) advise the condition should be differentially diagnosed from aniseikonia, undetected small-angle HARC, and deep foveal suppression (when horror fusionis would not be present for large targets). Many affected patients are congenital esotropes and Kirschen (1999) stated that horror fusionis is only seen in occasional patients who have had a strabismus since early childhood. Treatment is usually aimed at alleviating any intractable diplopia, and this may require occlusion (see later).

Heterotropic patients with **sensory fusion disruption syndrome** (Case Study 14.1) can achieve motor superimposition of their diplopic images, but sensory fusion cannot be attained. If appropriate prisms are placed before the eyes, the patient reports the targets are 'on top of each other, but not together'. One of the images is often seen in constant motion (Kirschen, 1999). The condition usually follows closed head trauma, sometimes associated with coma (Case Study 14.1). Treatment includes monovision (London, cited by Evans, 1994) occlusion (full or central; Kirschen, 1999), or hypnosis.

CASE STUDY 14.1	**25-year-old male with intractable diplopia from sensory fusion disruption syndrome**

SYMPTOMS & HISTORY

Head injury 6 years ago resulting in coma for 10 months. Since then has recovered quite well, with rehabilitation. Physically good (takes antiepileptic medication), mentally agile (some memory problems), but intractable diplopia. Referred by ophthalmologist to see if hypnosis can help the diplopia. The diplopia is present all the time, oblique, same for D and N, worse when concentrates, at night, and when tired. The right eye's image stays still, but the left eye's image constantly moves.

INITIAL RESULTS & MANAGEMENT
Low myope and corrected visual acuities 6/6 in each eye. Variable angle strabismus at distance and near, but no marked incomitancy seen on motility testing. Prisms were adjusted in a trial frame and with these the diplopic images could be brought together but the patient never obtained fusion. The left eye's image oscillated and was never stationary. No stereoacuity could be demonstrated with any prismatic correction.

OUTCOME
Hypnosis was tried, but in this case, was unsuccessful. Patient was referred for an occlusive contact lens.

_____

D, distance; *N*, near.

It is essential that horror fusionis and sensory fusion disruption syndrome are identified before surgery, which would not be able to eliminate the diplopia. Indeed, it has been suggested that some patients may find it easier to ignore diplopic images that are far apart, so surgery might make the symptoms worse through reducing the angle of the deviation. However, each patient is different, and it should not be concluded that patients will necessarily be helped by increasing the separation of the two images (Case Study 14.2). In summary, if the diplopia cannot be eliminated, it is best to only change the angle if testing has indicated the patient will be more comfortable with a new angle or equally tolerant of a cosmetically improved angle of deviation.

MANAGEMENT OF INTRACTABLE DIPLOPIA

The management options for intractable diplopia are limited and include occlusion, monovision, and hypnosis. These options are discussed here.

Occasionally, patients with long-standing diplopia are encountered who seem to have 'grown used' to the diplopic image and are happy to tolerate this. Although they can appreciate the diplopia at any time, they seem to have adapted by concentrating their attention on the dominant image, and the diplopic image seems not to interfere with their everyday perception. Even patients with horror fusionis may use the input from each eye in a rudimentary way to maintain a controlled angle of strabismus (Bucci et al., 1999). Such patients can become symptomatic if, for example, prism in their glasses is changed (Case Study 14.2).

CASE STUDY 14.2.	**73-year-old man with intractable diplopia who benefitted from a Bangerter foil**

SYMPTOMS & HISTORY
Strabismus operation age 4 years and diplopia since. For many years, the diplopia was corrected with a prismatic correction in spectacles. At age 62 years, Parkinson disease diagnosed which now produces noticeable tremor and gait problems. Since age 70 years, constant diplopia that cannot be eliminated with spectacles, despite trying several prismatic corrections. Local optometrist referred to HES who tried convergence exercises and Fresnel prisms to no avail. Neurologist opines diplopia unlikely to be related to Parkinson disease. Age 71 years saw strabismus specialist and orthoptist who considered 'vergence eye movements appeared to be absent', but saccades, smooth pursuit, pupils all normal, as are spatial skills and face recognition. Recommended occlusion, but patient disturbed by cosmesis, so is unhappily living with diplopia. Situation has not changed since saw strabismus specialist and patient often closes right eye to eliminate diplopia. Local optometrist referred patient to the author.

RESULTS & MANAGEMENT

Moderate hypermetropia and astigmatism with normal ocular health (including fields) except moderate cataracts in both eyes, worse in right, with commensurate acuities, R6/12 L6/9. Motility difficult to interpret owing to head tremor but appears to be moderate underaction right medial rectus. Vergence movements present but limited (NPC at times 20 cm, at other times exotropic at near). Ocular motor tests with current glasses reveal large variable exophoria/exotropia at distance and near, with variable small vertical deviation and 7.5-degree excyclotorsion. Tested with rotary prisms, but variable nature of ocular motor imbalance means no prismatic strength gives single vision for more than a few seconds.

OUTCOME

Discussed options. The cataract is worse in the right eye but surgery to this eye could make the diplopia more noticeable. Tested with Bangerter filters (p. 190) RE and no diplopia with filter of 0.1. Started with this and after a month progressed to 0.2, but unable to lighten filter further without diplopia recurring. Patient much happier with this than full occlusion. In view of the quite deep filter, at change of spectacles removed prism from spectacles, but continued with Bangerter filter. Interestingly, patient noticed more diplopia so remade with prism. This indicates some perception is occurring through the filter, even though it reduces the acuity to worse than 6/30.

PROGNOSIS

Consider early cataract surgery in the left eye as cataract in right eye progresses, which may present a 'natural' equivalent of the Bangerter filter.

HES, Hospital eye services; *L*, left; *NPC*, near point of convergence; *R*, right; *RE*, right eye.

Occlusion

Occlusion is the simplest method to alleviate intractable diplopia resulting from binocular anomalies. There are various types of occluder, listed in Fig. 14.4.

Tarsorraphy and botulinum toxin are invasive, associated with a higher risk than other methods, and achieve a very poor cosmetic outcome. They are a last resort and corneal tattooing (Stone, Somner, & Jay, 2008; Laria, Alio, & Pinero, 2010) and opaque intraocular lenses are alternatives (Hadid, Wride, Griffiths, Strong, & Clarke, 2008). If a simple eye patch fits well, this method is virtually guaranteed to achieve a satisfactory outcome, in terms of completely blocking out the image from the unwanted eye. However, the method is unsightly and is best considered a temporary measure.

Similarly, the use of a blackened spectacle lens achieves a poor cosmetic outcome. However, this approach can be helpful, for example, with elderly patients with diplopia from a recent onset deviation who are waiting for a hospital appointment.

For reasons of safety, glass Chavasse lenses have been superseded by CR39 or polycarbonate lenses which can be frosted. An inexpensive translucent occluder can be made with Favlon or with sticky tape (e.g., Scotch tape) stuck onto a normal spectacle lens. A few diplopic patients who are particularly sensitive to any image in their nonpreferred eye can still be bothered by the image from translucent occlusion.

Bangerter foils (Appendix 12) are a form of translucent occlusion, described on p. 190. The filters are graded according, approximately, to the level of acuity (using the continental decimal scale) to which a normal eye would be reduced when viewing through the filter. They were originally developed for amblyopia therapy, but can be used in cases of intractable diplopia, when the goal is to gradually reduce the density of the required filter until the patient is asymptomatic with no filter or with an almost clear filter. An open trial (McIntyre & Fells, 1996) suggests that this goal can occasionally be achieved with children, and some adults can end up with only a fairly light, cosmetically good, filter. Other cases continue to need quite a heavily 'frosted' filter (Case Study 14.2).

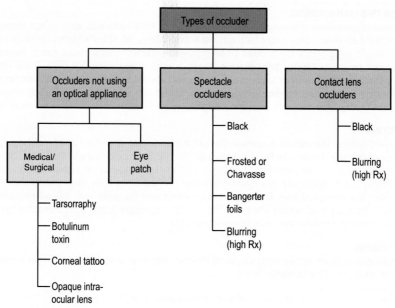

Fig. 14.4 Types of occluder.

Compared with occlusive spectacles, occlusive contact lenses have an improved cosmetic appearance and can have a wider field of occlusion (Astin, 1998). Various designs of occlusive contact lens are available and the best type for a given patient needs to be carefully selected. Factors that need to be considered are how absolute the occlusion needs to be, eye colour, the desired cosmetic appearance, and corneal health and physiological requirements (Astin, 1998; Gasson & Morris, 1998). Astin (1998) recommended that conventional occlusion methods be tried before contact lenses are fitted.

Spectacle or contact lenses of a high and/or inappropriate power can be used to blur, or 'fog' the nonpreferred eye and this may make it easier for the patient to suppress a diplopic image. This approach is particularly suitable for cases where the nonpreferred eye already has a high refractive error. In presbyopic patients, monovision (typically, with contact lenses) can be a successful form of correction, especially if the degree of diplopia is not too large and there is good acuity in each eye. This is discussed further in Chapter 17 and Case Study 17.2. Monovision is contraindicated in cases with long-standing unilateral strabismus, when it could cause fixation switch diplopia (Kushner, 1995). Not all cases are able to suppress a blurred image and, occasionally, patients may prefer relatively clear diplopic images, at a 'familiar' degree of separation, to diplopia where one of the images is deliberately blurred (Case Study 14.3). In this type of case, called CPR-type diplopia, a Fresnel prism or Bangerter foil can be useful (Hatt et al., 2019). These authors found that, in CPR-type diplopia resulting from epiretinal membrane (ERM), vitrectomy with ERM peel may eliminate the diplopia, but this is not always the case (p. 202).

CASE STUDY 14.3.	**73-year-old man with intractable diplopia who did not benefit from blurring of the weaker image**

SYMPTOMS & HISTORY

High myope, right macular haemorrhage 15 years ago. Patient has had constant oblique diplopia associated with strabismus for over 10 years (initially fully investigated), particularly problematic with television. The diplopia is not changing, and the patient does not drive. He has tried various prismatic corrections, none of which have eliminated the diplopia. Wearing: R −13.00DS L −9.50/−0.50 × 135 with 4Δ down L and 5Δ out L effective prism at pupil centres (patient said RE is partial correction).

INITIAL RESULTS & MANAGEMENT
VA with glasses: R3/60 L6/9. Refractive error: R −18.00DS = 6/60 L− 9.00/−0.50 × 95 = 6/9+. Distance cover test with usual glasses 6Δ esotropia. Unable to eliminate diplopia with prisms. Dilated fundoscopy, fields, pressures, etc, all OK. Explained to patient that RE is blurred and already only partially corrected. Suggested trial with reduced RE prescription to a −8.00DS (to balance L) in the hope he will find the RE easier to ignore, so decentring/prism may not be required. Patient agreed to try this.

OUTCOME
Patient reported that diplopia was worse with new glasses, images are further apart, and he finds that this makes it harder to ignore the diplopia. R lens was changed back to −13.00 and fine-tuned prism for maximum comfort. With the final glasses, the patient reported, the double vision was easier to tolerate than he could remember it ever being in the past.

DS, Dioptre sphere; *L*, left; *R*, right; *RE*, right eye; *VA*, visual acuity.

Hypnosis

Hypnosis is a procedure during which a practitioner suggests that the subject experience changes in sensations, perceptions, thoughts, or behaviour (Fellows, 1995). Optometric uses of hypnosis were reviewed by Evans, Barnard, et al. (1996) and its use for treating intractable diplopia was discussed by Evans (2001c). The author found the most common use of hypnosis in optometric practice is for intractable diplopia (Case Study 14.4). Typically, adults with acquired diplopia following trauma or unsuccessful strabismus surgery try hypnosis as a last resort. A moderate or marked degree of success is observed in 50%−72% of cases (Evans, 2000b).

CASE STUDY 14.4	**13-year-old boy with intractable diplopia successfully treated by hypnosis**

SYMPTOMS & HISTORY
Squint surgery at age 5 and 6 years, which was unsuccessful at eliminating strabismus. Patient has experienced constant diplopia (horizontal for distance vision, oblique for near) 'for as long as can remember'. Discharged from HES some years ago when patient was told that nothing more can be done. Patient reports the diplopia has not changed over the years but is worse when he is tired. He closes his right eye with some sports, television, and reading.

INITIAL RESULTS & MANAGEMENT
Moderate myope with VA: R6/9 L6/9. Esotropic at distance and near, with small vertical deviation. Images 'come almost together' with 26Δ base out at distance and 15Δ base out at near, but even with optimum prism still drifts in and out of diplopia. Hypnosis discussed and patient and mother agreed to try this. Mother attended throughout all sessions.

OUTCOME
Patient good hypnotic subject. Given posthypnotic suggestion that he will be able to ignore the 'doubled part' of the image in the right eye. At his third visit he reported that he no longer experienced diplopia unless someone asks him about it. If this happens, he can still notice the diplopia until he starts thinking about something else, when the diplopia disappears.

HES, Hospital eye service; *L*, left; *R*, right; *VA*, visual acuity.

Advising Diplopic Patients About Driving

In the UK, the DVLA make the following recommendations (Driver & Vehicle Licensing Authority (DVLA), 2020).

Group 1 (ordinary driving, cars and motorcycles)

Cease driving on diagnosis of diplopia. Resume driving on confirmation to the DVLA that it is controlled by glasses or a patch which the licence holder undertakes to wear while driving. Exceptionally, a stable uncorrected diplopia of 6 months' duration or more may be compatible with driving if there is consultant support indicating satisfactory functional adaptation.

If a patch is used, the advice concerning monocular vision applies which is that the DVLA must be notified. The person may drive when clinically advised that they have adapted to the disability and are able to meet the visual acuity standard.

Group 2 (lorries and buses)

Recommended permanent refusal or revocation if insuperable diplopia. Patching is not acceptable.

The Investigation of Binocular Sensory Adaptations to Strabismus

Most people with strabismus have developed a sensory adaptation (HARC or suppression) to avoid diplopia and confusion. The investigation of these sensory adaptations will now be described in more detail. The clinical worksheet in Appendix 5 summarises the clinical investigation of sensory status in strabismus. Table 14.3 summarises the visual conditions that influence retinal correspondence. These conditions vary from one test to another, and therefore determine the likelihood of a given test detecting HARC or causing a patient who might normally have HARC to revert to NRC.

TABLE 14.3 ■ Visual Conditions That Influence Retinal Correspondence.

Visual condition	Influence on retinal correspondence (likelihood of test breaking down sensory adaptations and causing the patient to revert to NRC)
Degree of dissociation	If the conditions of everyday vision are disturbed by dissociating the eyes, it is likely that NRC will return while the dissociation is present. The more complete the dissociation, the more likely it is that NRC will be present.
Retinal areas stimulated	NRC is most likely to occur with bifoveal images. HARC is more likely when the fovea of one eye is stimulated simultaneously with a peripheral image in the other eye.
Eye used for fixation	HARC is likely when the dominant eye is used for fixation, but NRC is likely to return if the usually strabismic eye takes up fixation.
Constancy of deviation	If the angle of the strabismus is variable, HARC is less likely to be firmly established (Chapter 12). In intermittent strabismus, NRC will return when the eyes are straight. The same is true of patients with fully accommodative strabismus when wearing their refractive correction; and in long-standing incomitant strabismus in the position of no deviation.
Relative illuminance of retinal images	NRC is more likely to occur if the illuminance of the image in the strabismic eye is less than that of the fixating eye.

HARC, Harmonious anomalous retinal correspondence; *NRC,* normal retinal correspondence.

DIFFERENTIAL DIAGNOSIS OF HARC AND SUPPRESSION

The correction of significant refractive errors can influence the sensory status as well as the motor deviation. For example, a clear retinal image may help to overcome suppression. If the patient has a significant uncorrected refractive error, or change in refractive error, the practitioner should assess the sensory status with and without the new correction.

There are two main approaches to differentially diagnosing HARC from suppression:

1. *Battery of tests* (Pickwell & Sheridan, 1973). A sensitive test such as the Mallett ARC and suppression test in strabismus (MARCS) test or Bagolini test is used to determine the sensory adaptation (ARC or suppression) under natural conditions. Additional tests, of increasing degrees of invasiveness (less naturalistic) are then used to evaluate when the sensory adaptation breaks down and thus to estimate the depth of the adaptation. These tests are described later, in increasing order of invasiveness, after the sections on the Bagolini and MARCS tests.

2. *Degrading the image* (Mallett, 1970). A sensitive test (e.g., MARCS test or Bagolini test) is used to determine the sensory adaptation under natural conditions. Then, still using this test, the patient's perception is degraded until the sensory adaptation breaks down. Historically, a red filter bar was used to degrade the image, but neutral density filters are the preferred method (Mallett, 1988a; Bagolini, 1999), and neutral density filter bars are available (Appendix 12). Alternatives to this are to use two counter-rotated polarised filters, Bangerter foils, or to decrease the illuminance of the Nonius strips on the MARCS test.

The first of these two techniques, using a battery of tests, is time-consuming and uses equipment that is not available in most eyecare practices. Hence, only the latter method will be described in detail.

Bagolini Striated Lenses

This test, combined with the cover test, can be used to differentially diagnose the four possibilities for binocular sensory status in strabismus (Chapter 12): NRC, HARC, suppression, or unharmonious anomalous retinal correspondence (UARC). The Bagolini striated lens is a plano trial-case lens which has a fine grating of lines ruled on it (Bagolini, 1967). When the patient views a spotlight through a Bagolini lens, a faint streak is seen crossing the spot, but the lens does not significantly disrupt vision (Cheng, Woo, Irving, Charman, & Murray, 1998). In unilateral strabismus, one lens can be used before the deviated eye to produce a vertical streak rather like a 'see-through' Maddox rod, while the patient looks at a spot of light with both eyes open. In alternating deviations, it is usually necessary to use a striated lens before both eyes, so that they produce streaks at 45 degrees in one eye and 135 degrees in the other. Some authors recommend using both striated lenses in all cases, but in unilateral cases this is more dissociative than is necessary.

If the streak (or streaks in alternating cases) appears to pass through the spot of light, HARC is demonstrated. A central suppression area (Chapter 12) may result in a gap in the central part of the streak, but the patient may be able to report that the ends of it can be seen in line with the spot (Fig. 14.5). If the streak and the spotlight are not perfectly aligned (but within about 0.5Δ of one another) this does not necessarily indicate UARC but can result from an imperfection in the new anomalous sensory relationship. The diagnosis of UARC (which is very rare: see Chapter 12) or NRC is confirmed by the presence of diplopia and confusion (Fig. 14.5).

Occasionally, patients may change fixation to the normally deviating eye and hence see the streak passing through the light. Close observation of any eye movements during the test and a confirmatory cover test should be used to verify that the eye behind the lens is still deviating. Unnecessary repeated covering should be avoided because this could cause HARC to break down to apparent UARC or suppression.

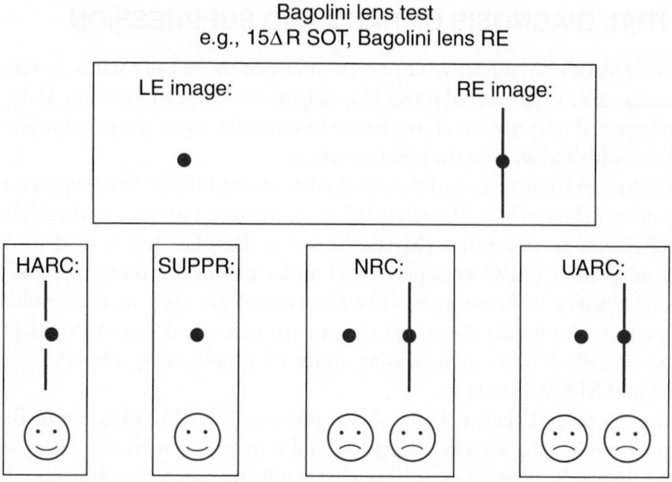

Bagolini lens test
e.g., 15△ R SOT, Bagolini lens RE

Fig. 14.5 Schematic illustration of Bagolini test. Underneath the patient's binocular perception, the faces illustrate whether they have single vision (usually asymptomatic) or diplopia (usually symptomatic). *HARC*, Harmonious anomalous retinal correspondence; *LE*, left eye; *NRC*, normal retinal correspondence; *R*, right; *RE*, right eye; *SOT*, esotropia; *SUPPR*, suppression; *UARC*, unharmonious anomalous retinal correspondence.

If the streak is misaligned and the patient is diplopic, either NRC or UARC is present, depending on whether the angular separation of the spot and the streak is the same as the angle of the deviation. With UARC, the angle of separation between the spot and the streak, the angle of diplopia, is different to the angle of strabismus. If the patient reports diplopia during the Bagolini lens test but does not during everyday viewing, this indicates they have HARC which has 'broken down' under the very slightly abnormal viewing conditions of the Bagolini test. Such cases are rare and careful questioning may reveal that the HARC also breaks down when the patient is fatigued, or in dim illumination. In these cases, the 'pseudobinocular vision' of HARC breaks down in an analogous way to the breaking down of binocularity in a decompensated heterophoria. If the patient reports an unstable perception of the streak in the Bagolini test, this can indicate an instability in the HARC. Again, this can be associated with symptoms (analogous to those of binocular instability) and such cases may require treatment (see later).

The depth of HARC can be quantified by introducing filters in front of the strabismic eye. The filters are used in the form of a filter bar or ladder: this is a series of filters of increasing absorption mounted in a continuous strip so that they can be introduced before the eye one after the other (Fig. 14.6, lower figure). In the past, a red filter bar was used, but a neutral density filter bar is preferable (Mallett, 1988a; Bagolini, 1999). The depth of the filter is gradually increased (usually in 0.3 neutral density (ND) steps) until suppression of the streak occurs or diplopia. If a deep filter is required, this suggests the HARC is deeply-ingrained, which is associated with a worse prognosis for treatment.

If the complete binocular field of the strabismic eye is suppressed, the streak will not be seen. The depth of suppression can be measured by using a filter bar placed in front of the nondeviated eye. The filter depth is increased until the patient sees the streak. If a deep filter is required, this suggests the suppression is deeply ingrained, and the prognosis for treatment is poor.

An approximation to a Bagolini lens can be made by using a plano (or −0.12D) trial lens with a spot of grease (e.g., from the skin) lightly smeared across it. The fainter the streak produced, the more likely it is that HARC will be detected, as there is very little disturbance of the patient's habitual vision.

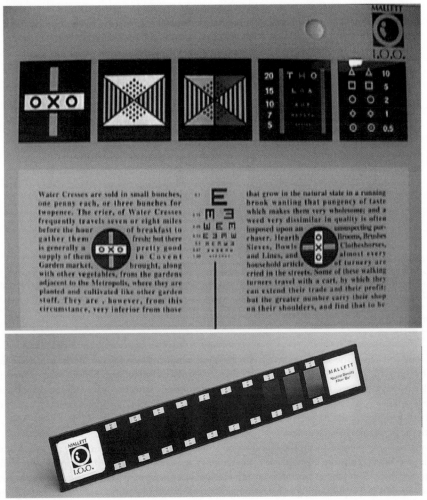

Fig. 14.6 Mallett near vision unit showing the Mallett ARC and suppression in strabismus (MARCS) test ('large OXO test'; top left of top figure) and neutral density filter bar (lower figure). *ARC*, Anomalous retinal correspondence.

Mallett ARC and Suppression in Strabismus (MARCS) Test

The Mallett near vision unit employs naturalistic viewing conditions and monocular markers (equivalent to the streak in the Bagolini test). The standard Mallett fixation disparity test cannot be used to assess sensory status in strabismus because the monocular markers are small and may fall into the small suppression area at the zero point (Chapter 12). This problem can be avoided by using the distance Mallett fixation disparity unit at a viewing distance of 1.5 m or by using the special Mallett ARC and suppression in strabismus (MARCS) test (the 'large OXO test') on modern versions of the near Mallett unit (Fig. 14.6). With the MARCS tests, the presence of approximately aligned Nonius markers in a strabismic patient confirms the presence of HARC (Fig. 14.7). The Nonius marker in the strabismic eye may appear to be a different size, dimmer, and slightly misaligned with the other marker. This is because of inherent imperfections in the anomalous alliance of receptive fields of unequal dimensions and properties.

Modified OXO test
e.g., 15 pd R SOT, large OXO on Mallett near unit

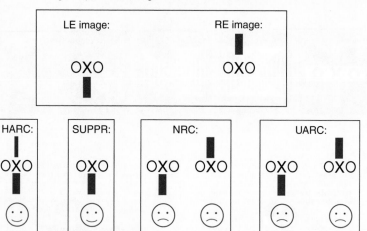

Fig. 14.7 Schematic illustration of MARCS test. Underneath the patients' binocular perception, the faces illustrate whether they have single vision (usually asymptomatic) or diplopia (usually symptomatic). *HARC*, Harmonious anomalous retinal correspondence; *LE*, left eye; *NRC*, normal retinal correspondence; *R*, right; *RE*, right eye; *SOT*, esotropia; *SUPPR*, suppression; *UARC*, unharmonious anomalous retinal correspondence.

The absence of the strabismic eye's Nonius marker indicates suppression of the binocular field of that eye (Fig. 14.7). A neutral density filter bar (Fig. 14.6) can be used between the eye and the polarised visor to assess the depth of HARC or of suppression, in a similar way to that described for the Bagolini striated lens test earlier. The response should be checked with the cover test and, if the patient is diplopic, the degree of diplopia can be investigated to diagnose UHARC or NRC, as with the Bagolini striated lens test.

As with any polarised test, the illumination should be increased to counteract the effect of the polarised filters. Like the Bagolini test, the patient's response should be monitored to determine whether their 'pseudobinocularity' from the HARC has a tendency to break down or to become unstable. If it does, questioning may reveal that symptoms occur in everyday life and treatment may be required (see later).

Both the Bagolini and MARCS tests closely approximate normal viewing conditions and these tests are very likely to reveal the sensory status that normally exists. They will detect HARC in about 80% of cases of strabismus seen in optometric practice (Mallett, 1988a). For the reasons explained in the preceding section, the tests described later create artificial viewing conditions, and their results are therefore unlikely to reflect the normal situation.

Other Methods of Differentially Diagnosing HARC and Suppression

Four after-image tests have been discussed in detail by Mallett (1975) and summarised by Mallett (1988a). A synoptophore or stereoscope can be used to investigate correspondence (Pickwell, 1989) but, owing to the artificial nature of the instrument, can produce spurious results. The single mirror haploscope (Earnshaw, 1962) provided a versatile alternative to the synoptophore, with slightly more natural viewing conditions, but is not commonly found nowadays. Various other haploscopic instruments have been devised but are not in regular use in the UK. Personal computers can be used with LCD shutter goggles or, less usefully, red/green dissociation. Another technique which creates abnormal (dissociating) viewing conditions is the red filter method (Siderov, 2001).

ADDITIONAL TECHNIQUES FOR THE INVESTIGATION OF SUPPRESSION

Many polarised stereo tests (e.g., Titmus and Randot tests) include tests of suppression. Additional tests that are described elsewhere in this book are the four base-out prism test (Chapter 16) and Mallett polarised letters test (p. 83).

The Worth four dot test can be used to assess suppression, as described on p. 200, with the inclusion of a cover test to check the motor status during the test. However, this test creates unnatural viewing conditions, overestimates the prevalence of diplopia and suppression (Bagolini, 1999) and is of limited value (von Noorden, 1996). Nonetheless, the four dot test result can be combined with clinical stereoacuity measures to provide a **composite binocular function score** in patients with strabismus and amblyopia which may be useful to extend stereoacuity measures in cases with no stereopsis (Webber, Wood, Thompson, & Birch, 2019).

Depth of Suppression

Usually, it is most convenient for the practitioner to use the test which detected the suppression to assess its depth and several suitable techniques have already been described. One very simple additional technique is to find the depth of filter held before the nonsuppressing eye which will overcome the suppression. The method is to ask the patient to look at a detailed scene (to create normal viewing conditions) and to introduce the filter bar before the nonsuppressing eye, beginning with the lightest filter. As the darker filters are introduced, the retinal illuminance decreases until the patient reports diplopia, or the strabismic eye moves to take up fixation. The filter then in place indicates the depth of suppression.

Extent of Suppression Scotoma

Almost all strabismic patients have either 'total' suppression or HARC. For suppression to successfully prevent diplopia and confusion, there must be suppression of all the binocular field of the strabismic eye. This suppression is very different to the small areas (about 1 degree) of central suppression which occur at the fovea and at the zero point of the strabismic eye in HARC. Although these suppression areas may not be of major clinical significance (Mallett, 1988a), it used to be fairly common practice to measure their size, using a form of binocular haploscopic perimetry. As with other aspects of the investigation of sensory status, test procedures which interfere more with normal binocular vision tend to produce artefactual results.

The situation is confused further by attempts to plot the extent of the suppression area in patients with large angle strabismus who do not have HARC or diplopia. Clearly, these patients must be suppressing all the binocular field of their strabismic eye, yet some investigative techniques only detect an elliptical or D-shaped suppression area around the fovea and zero point in such cases. These measurements are probably explained by deeper suppression in this region, which is detected by a test which creates artificial viewing conditions and does not detect the shallower suppression elsewhere (Mallett, 1988a). In view of the doubtful clinical usefulness of plotting suppression areas, methods will not be described.

The Evaluation and Management of Suppression

EVALUATION

Some ability to suppress seems innate to the visual system. Most people need be taught to appreciate physiological diplopia, and yet the constraints of Panum's areas mean the physiologically diplopic image must be present all the time. It could be argued, the observation that very few patients spontaneously notice 'physiological diplopia' means that term is a misnomer and in fact there must be everyday 'physiological suppression' of physiological diplopia images in normal observers. Suppression also occurs in normal, nonstrabismic, subjects under conditions of retinal rivalry. However, the suppression in strabismus (Freeman & Jolly, 1994; Smith, Fern et al., 1994) or at least large angle strabismus (Harrad, 1996) has different characteristics to this rivalry suppression.

Suppression in strabismus should be considered together with the assessment of all the other factors present. If factors such as the patient's age, time since strabismus onset, degree of cooperation likely and other factors are favourable, treatment of the suppression will be more likely to succeed. The deeper the suppression, the more difficult it will be to treat.

Suppression is an adaptation to the strabismus, and it should not be treated unless the deviation can also be eliminated. If the sensory adaptations to the strabismus are treated but the strabismus remains, the patient will be troubled by diplopia and confusion.

It should be remembered that there are two types of suppression in strabismus. First, there is suppression of all the binocular field of the strabismic eye, which occurs as an alternative to HARC to prevent diplopia and confusion. Second, there is suppression of the fovea and zero point which occurs in HARC because of the difficulties inherent in 'remapping' large receptive fields with small receptive fields (Chapter 12). It usually seems that, if the HARC and motor deviation are treated, suppression at the fovea and zero point of the strabismic eye resolve without treatment.

Treatment of suppression, therefore, is usually confined to cases where there is complete suppression of the binocular field of the strabismic eye. If this suppression is very superficial, it will probably not require treatment but will resolve spontaneously when the motor deviation is corrected. If the suppression is deeper, it will need to be treated as outlined later before the motor deviation can be treated.

MANAGEMENT

This section is mostly concerned with treating suppression, but cases will be encountered where suppression is preventing symptoms and patients benefit from measures that favour suppression. It should be remembered that suppression is a natural adaptation to avoid the symptoms of diplopia and confusion and some individuals prefer to maintain suppression.

The general aim of treating suppression is to encourage the patient to become aware of the suppressed image, and then to integrate it correctly with the image from the other eye. Both aspects of this are essential for normal binocular vision. It is important that the method of treatment ensures simultaneous stimulation of the foveal areas of both eyes, or of other pairs of normally corresponding points. For normally corresponding points to be simultaneously stimulated, the angle of the strabismus must be relieved during treatment. This can be done by the refractive correction in fully accommodative strabismus, and in other strabismus by prisms, or the use of a haploscopic device set at the angle of the strabismus. In some convergent strabismus, a position in front of the eyes where the visual axes intersect may be found; bifoveal images of an object placed at this position can be a good starting point.

It must be emphasised that it is not sufficient to obtain simultaneous vision of any kind, but the aim is simultaneous vision of normally corresponding areas. The successful treatment of suppression could result in diplopia occurring, until the motor deviation has been treated. If binocular single vision cannot be restored at once (e.g., by correcting the motor deviation with spectacles), occlusion will be required. Occlusion of the nonstrabismic eye may, in any event, be desirable to treat amblyopia (Chapter 13).

The basic principle behind eye exercises for suppression is to change the stimulus parameters of the target before the suppressing eye. Since the suppression will be deeper for the more 'cortically significant' foveal area, the suppression is often attacked with larger, more peripheral targets initially, and smaller targets are used as the treatment progresses. One or more of the following methods may be useful in the management of suppression in strabismic patients.

Synoptophore and Other Stereoscope Devices

At one time this was the principal instrument used in the treatment of strabismus, but it has become increasingly rare to use this equipment. Nowadays, even in hospital clinics less artificial methods are more commonly used. The use of the synoptophore for treating suppression will therefore not be described here, and more details on this can be found in Pickwell (1989).

In strabismus over 10Δ, a variable prism stereoscope can be used, and the prism power adjusted to compensate for the angle of the strabismus. For smaller angle strabismus, it may be possible to obtain superimposition of the pictures with a Holmes stereoscope by adjusting the card distance. The difficulty with either type of stereoscope is being sure that bifoveal vision is being stimulated. More details on this approach can be found in Pickwell (1989). A single-mirror haploscope can also be used, rather like a synoptophore.

Coloured Filter Methods

With the red filter method, the patient has a red filter before the dominant eye and is asked to trace a picture on tracing paper using a red pencil or ballpoint pen. Through the red filter, the page will appear to be red, so the patient's own drawing in red cannot be seen against it with the dominant eye and the suppressing eye has to be used. Younger patients can be encouraged to sort coloured beads, and to do this the suppressing eye must be used, as the true colours cannot be seen through the red filter. Another version of this approach is for the patient to wear red and green glasses whilst reading through a coloured overlay consisting of alternate strips of red and green film (available from Bernell; see Appendix 12). Before using this method, it is necessary to ensure there is good monocular acuity, to assess colour vision, and ensure that the possibility of anomalous correspondence has been eliminated.

Physiological Diplopia

This method is appropriate in cases of convergent strabismus when a point can be found where the visual axes cross in front of the eyes. The details of the method are described in Chapter 13 and are further developed in a later section of this chapter on the management of HARC. An advantage of the method is that the cover test can be undertaken at any time to ensure bifoveal fixation.

Prisms

Mallett (1979b) suggested that some cases of suppression could be treated with prisms. These are cases where there is no HARC, and where the prism adaptation test (described later) demonstrates that the motor component of the strabismus can be corrected with prisms. He felt that if normally corresponding receptive fields are stimulated by nearly identical images, suppression will be eliminated. He stressed that this type of treatment should not be attempted if there is any question of HARC. This approach may be most likely to work if shallow suppression is present.

Additional Comments on the Treatment of Suppression

It will be apparent that the possibility of stimulating noncorresponding points is present with all these methods, and great care has to be exercised to ensure this does not happen. To begin with, most of the binocular treatment should be given in the consulting room where it can be overseen by the practitioner. Home treatment in the early stages should be confined to the monocular types of treatment for amblyopia. As the case progresses, some home treatment can be given by carefully instructing the parent on how to check for simultaneous macular vision; a simple explanation of the cover test check may suffice. Patients should, however, be seen at very frequent intervals (every few days) at this stage.

The Evaluation and Management of HARC

EVALUATION

HARC is an adaptation, or solution, to a problem and often does not require treatment. Treatment should be undertaken cautiously, and practitioners and patients should have fully discussed the risks and benefits before treatment is started.

In the management of HARC, we are concerned mainly with the group of patients showing moderately deeply ingrained HARC. Patients with very lightly ingrained HARC may require no treatment other than correction of the motor deviation. Those with very deeply ingrained HARC usually have a poor prognosis; typically, these patients have long-standing strabismus of early onset. Using Bagolini lenses, a very dark neutral density filter is required to break down the HARC and there is then suppression rather than NRC.

Occasionally, patients are encountered who have an unstable HARC. The 'pseudobinocular vision' can break down in an analogous way to the breaking down of binocularity in a decompensated heterophoria. The sensory status of these patients may alternate between HARC and NRC with diplopia and/or suppression. This is likely to be associated with symptoms (analogous to those of binocular instability) and such cases may require treatment.

MANAGEMENT

Accurate correction of the refractive error is the first essential step. Its effect is twofold: in accommodative strabismus the angle is reduced, and in all strabismus, it ensures that each eye has a sharp retinal image which also aids normal correspondence.

Again, it needs to be emphasised that the HARC should not be treated at all if the motor deviation may not be successfully treated. To do so would leave the patient with diplopia. In strabismus with a deviation over 20Δ, the best approach is to refer for a surgeon's opinion on an operation. It must be remembered, however, that surgery in comitant strabismus is a 'mechanical solution to a non-mechanical problem' (Dale, 1982). Strabismus between 10Δ and 20Δ may respond to non-surgical methods, and in angles less than 10Δ the accuracy of surgery may be inadequate. The question of whether to consider an operation is a matter of professional judgement and the parents and sometimes child also will have a view. Many prefer nonsurgical treatment to be tried first. In young patients, the sensory adaptations may disappear or be easier to treat once the motor deviation has been surgically corrected. If nonsurgical methods of treatment are proving unsuccessful, it is important to seek another opinion while the patient is still young enough for binocular vision to be restored.

Rutstein, Marsh-Tootle, Scheiman, and Eskridge (1991) studied 32 strabismic patients whose angle was altered surgically or spontaneously. Of the 20 patients with HARC, 13 continued to have HARC and 7 developed NRC. The cases who developed NRC had changes in angle that altered the direction of the strabismus. NRC is a prerequisite for fusion so the authors advocate overcorrection of deviations to normalise retinal correspondence, even in older patients, if presurgical testing demonstrates an ability to develop sensory and motor fusion (p. 291).

Smaller deviations may respond to nonsurgical treatment in the form of fusional reserve exercises and other methods. Where this approach is being followed, the first step is to break down the HARC. It is important to be sure that this has been done, before proceeding with the exercises to reduce the angle. The patient must, at the least, have NRC on an instrument with which the motor deviation can be treated (e.g., stereoscope).

It may help to treat any amblyopia first (Wright, 1994), particularly if the acuity of the strabismic eye is worse than 6/18. Occlusion is the best method, as it also weakens the HARC. Indeed, concurrent occlusion therapy for amblyopia is advisable because the treatment of HARC before the motor deviation is treated may result in diplopia during everyday vision.

TABLE 14.4 ■ **Visual Conditions that Influence Retinal Correspondence and Their Role in Treatment of HARC.**

Visual condition	Influence on retinal correspondence
Degree of dissociation	First try to achieve NRC under maximum dissociation, and then extend this to less and less dissociated conditions.
Retinal areas stimulated	Treatment must be bifoveal or stimulate other normally corresponding areas. Treatment should avoid conditions where the fovea of the dominant eye is presented with an image at the same time as the peripheral area in the other eye which coincides with the angle of strabismus.
Eye used for fixation	If possible, the patient should be taught to fixate with the strabismic eye as a preliminary to other treatment.
Constancy of deviation	Try to find conditions in which normal binocular fixation and correspondence is possible, and then extend them to a wider range of circumstances.
Relative illuminance of retinal images	Treatment should start from the least inequality of illuminance that will give NRC and move towards more equal illuminance.

HARC, Harmonious anomalous retinal correspondence; *NRC,* normal retinal correspondence.

Other types of treatment for HARC should have regard to the five factors which influence the type of correspondence (Table 14.3). The aim should be to begin treatment in the conditions which favour normal correspondence, and when this is achieved, move to the less favourable conditions. These factors are considered again in Table 14.4, with special reference to treatment.

The methods of treatment used for HARC also help in the treatment of the suppression area at the zero point in the strabismic eye. Hence, it may not be necessary to treat this suppression area. Any attempt to treat this suppression area has the danger of deepening the HARC, unless precautions are taken to ensure that there is always stimulation of innately corresponding points.

There are several approaches to the treatment of HARC. The choice of method will depend on the circumstances of the case. Prism therapy methods require less time in supervision and less effort from the patient; physiological diplopia methods can provide integrated binocular vision for one fixation distance, and quite early in treatment; haploscopic methods seem to be appropriate in more difficult cases. The following methods may be considered and are not necessarily mutually exclusive.

Prisms

It may be thought that to prescribe full prism relief would provide stimulation of corresponding points and NRC would be re-established. However, a relieving prism in most cases results in the angle of the deviation increasing, sometimes by as much as the original angle of the strabismus. This phenomenon of prism adaptation is sometimes referred to as 'eating up the prisms'. A prism adaptation test (Jampolsky, 1971) may help in deciding if the method will work. Experience shows that $8-10\Delta$ overcorrection is required, and even patients who show no prism adaptation at first may do so over a period of a few days. Hence, it has been stated that this method is unsuccessful for most patients (Dale, 1982).

Mallett (1979b) stated that prismatic techniques were the best method of treating HARC, and he advocated the use of adverse prism in breaking down anomalous correspondence: base-in for convergent strabismus. A prism of 16Δ base-in is recommended as it is generally too strong to be overcome by a divergent movement. This is said to produce a rapid breakdown in the HARC and has a good cosmetic appearance, as the convergent eye appears straighter when viewed through the prism.

Adverse or vertical prisms can produce diplopia. In cases where this is distressing, and in circumstances where it may be dangerous (e.g., driving or operating machinery) this type of therapy is inappropriate.

Synoptophore, Single Mirror Haploscope, and After-Image Methods

Most eyecare practitioners do not have access to a synoptophore, so synoptophore methods will not be described here in detail. A single mirror haploscope involves more natural viewing than the synoptophore (Earnshaw, 1962). This is more suitable for treatment in the clinic than at home.

Free-Space Methods

Because of the difficulties introduced when patients look through instruments at images rather that at real objects, 'free-space' methods of treatment have been developed by various workers in the field (Earnshaw, 1960; Calder Gillie, 1961; Jones, 1965; Gillie & Lindsay, 1969; Hugonnier & Clayette-Hugonnier, 1969; Pickwell, 1971). These methods have been suggested as a follow-up to other treatment at the final stages, but in cases where they are likely to be effective, it is better to use them as the primary form of treatment. Success has been demonstrated in many cases. These seem to be those cases with acuity of 6/24 or better in the amblyopic eye, and with an angle of strabismus between 5–15Δ. For most of these techniques, the starting point is being able to demonstrate a position in front of the eyes where bifoveal fixation can be achieved: the intersection of the visual axes in convergent strabismus.

After-Images in Free Space

After-images may be used in free-space methods as a starting procedure which ensures normal correspondence, or it can be used to supplement other procedures as a check on normal correspondence. Either a single after-image can be created in the strabismic eye or one can be created in each eye. The after-images (usually vertical lines centred on each macula) are best seen against a plain wall initially, to check the response is as expected. They are then superimposed on a fixation mark, such as a small letter. When this can be done, the patient is asked to touch the letter with the fingertip, and still see the after-images correctly localised. Where the angle of strabismus cannot be overcome, one eye is occluded.

Physiological Diplopia Method

This method (Pickwell & Sheridan, 1973) has been outlined in the previous chapter as a method for the treatment of amblyopia. Where there is HARC, the method needs very close supervision so that binocular fixation of the target is always maintained. The practitioner may be able to see by looking at the eyes if they are both fixating, and can carry out the cover test at any time that it appears to be in doubt. An intelligent patient can also usually tell when the appearance is correct, but younger children may not be sufficiently reliable in reporting their subjective responses.

As described in the previous chapter, the first step is to find a position where the patient can fixate a real object binocularly. This will be at the intersection of the visual axes in a convergent strabismus. This position is found by placing a small fixation object at what appears to be the correct distance and carrying out the cover test. The object is moved closer or further away from the eyes until no cover test movement is seen. The patient may have to be encouraged not to overconverge, by explaining that the eyes are looking too close and that one is turned inwards too much. In accommodative strabismus, a positive spherical addition in both eyes may be required to inhibit convergence. In those cases where a binocular fixation point can be found, the method may proceed.

A second object is introduced: where HARC is present, this second object is placed on the median line and a lot closer to the eyes. By having it closer to the eyes than the fixation object, its image will fall on the temporal retina in each eye. Accordingly, in HARC cases the nasal retina where sensory adaptations are deepest is avoided in the early stages until the physiological diplopia has been demonstrated to the patient. A card with differently coloured sides held edgewise against the nose is a useful second object for these early stages. This should be seen in crossed physiological diplopia: the patient should see the fixation object singly with the coloured patch from the right of the card in the left periphery of vision, and the coloured patch from the left of the card seen in the right periphery.

The fixation object and card are shown in Fig. 10.11, which also illustrates a length of string which can be introduced at a later stage. At this stage, rather than a continuous string it is better to use a third object further away from the fixation but of the same nature. Coloured pencils are suitable, or thin rods or needles mounted in blue-tack to stand vertically on a table. The third object should be about 15 cm beyond the first and also on the median line. The patient is encouraged to see this object in uncrossed physiological diplopia, but to maintain fixation on the first object. The patient is then taught to maintain physiological diplopia of the more distant object while it is moved slowly towards the fixation object. If physiological diplopia is lost or the practitioner sees that the eyes have converged, the more distant object is temporarily removed and fixation re-established.

If the patient sees both diplopic images on the same side (paradoxical diplopia) the fixation object is no longer at the intersection of the axes, and proper fixation needs to be re-established. A small vertical after-image on the fovea (or eccentrically fixating area) may assist as a subjective check on central fixation. The fixation object can also be changed for a small light, and this allows the use of Bagolini striated lenses as a check on retinal correspondence.

With practice and encouragement, the patient should be able to achieve steady fixation of the first object and physiological diplopia of the more distant one, while the latter is moved from its initial position to a position 4–5 cm from the fixation. The methods described in Chapter 10 can then proceed as an extension of this exercise. After some practice, patients who have become quite competent at appreciating physiological diplopia under a range of conditions can be given more interesting exercises.

It is very important not to move the fixation object from its best position until NRC is well established. In the very early stages of treatment, it is better to concentrate on establishing binocular fixation with physiological diplopia at one distance only (Calder Gillie, 1961), and develop this with some of the suppression exercises described in Chapter 10 or earlier in this chapter (e.g., wire reading, bar reading). This is to concentrate on the sensory aspects of the strabismus rather than the actual motor deviation. Indeed, in some cases, once the sensory problems are resolved, it is found that the deviation is present neither at near nor distance vision, but this spontaneous recovery for the deviation does not necessarily occur. It will then be necessary to give fusional reserve exercises.

Treatment of the Motor Deviation

When treating the motor deviation, the practitioner should always ensure that NRC is present during the therapy. It is possible that the patient has HARC and is exhibiting covariation, without changing the vergence. The cover test can be used to confirm NRC and the eyes should be observed to make sure appropriate vergence movements are occurring.

EYE EXERCISES

Some cases of intermittent strabismus can be treated in the same way as described for treating decompensated heterophoria in Chapters 6–10.

If the sensory adaptation to a constant strabismus is lightly ingrained, when the motor deviation is corrected (e.g., refractively or by exercises) NRC and fusion may occur. This can easily be tested by using prisms or spheres in the consulting room to temporarily correct the motor deviation and investigating the effect of this on the sensory status. If the sensory adaptation to the strabismus is still present when the motor deviation is temporarily (in the consulting room) corrected, the motor element should only be treated if it is certain that exercises to eliminate the sensory adaptation will be successful (see later).

Other cases, where deeper sensory adaptations to the strabismus are present, will require more sophisticated treatment regimens. When the sensory adaptations to the strabismus have been treated and a level of acuity of 6/12 or better has been established, attention should be given to the motor deviation by eye exercises. It is very important that this is not done too early or there will be a danger of HARC returning. Most of the fusional reserve and relative accommodation exercises described in Chapter 10 can be considered at this stage. It must be remembered, however, that treatment will begin at the angle of the strabismus and not the orthophoria position. In other words, the targets must be presented so the patient fuses them in NRC. The targets are then adjusted to train the fusional reserves or relative accommodation, whilst the patient maintains normal binocular single vision.

As mentioned earlier, it is very unlikely that angles of strabismus greater than 20Δ will respond to nonsurgical treatment alone, and in cases of $15-20\Delta$, all other factors need to be favourable before attempting eye exercises.

REFRACTIVE CORRECTION

In accommodative esotropia from hypermetropia, obviously the hypermetropia must be corrected. In cases of significant hypermetropia, wearing spectacles from the age of 6 months and within the first 18 months of life results in a better outcome in the amblyopic eye (Ingram, Lambert, & Gill, 2009). Contact lenses (Evans, 2006a) or refractive surgery are options, although owing to the more permanent nature of refractive surgery, detailed testing is required before intervention (Minnal & Rosenberg, 2011).

Many cases of strabismus can be controlled by modifying the refractive correction. The approach and types of deviation that can be treated are analogous to those described for treating heterophoria in Table 6.1 and p. 98. The success of this type of therapy depends on the angle of deviation, the AC/A ratio, and, in exotropia, the amount of accommodation which is comfortably available. For typical AC/A ratios, this method is unlikely to work if the deviation exceeds about 15Δ. Modification of the refractive error can be useful in cases where the patient is unable or unwilling to carry out orthoptic exercises. The aim is to gradually reduce the modification to the refractive correction over a period of months and, often, years, as patients gradually become better able to compensate for the deviation themselves, or until patients are able and willing to carry out eye exercises.

The most common use of refractive modification is for convergence excess eso-deviations (Case Study 14.5). The effect of a near addition of $+2.00$ DS on the deviation is investigated and the addition is varied until the deviation is corrected. If it cannot be corrected with $+3.00$ to $+4.00$ DS (depending on near working distance, which with young children can be quite close), this mode of treatment will be unsuccessful. Patients with abnormal binocular vision often do not show the usual adaptation to prisms or refractive corrections, but it is a sensible precaution with strabismic patients to leave the patient with the correction in place for about $2-3$ minutes to ensure its effectiveness is maintained (North & Henson, 1985).

When this type of correction is prescribed for children large segment bifocals should be used with the segment top placed at the centre of the pupil. Parents and teachers should be asked to ensure that the child does look through the near addition when reading. Some writers advocate the use of varifocals for the refractive management of binocular anomalies in children (Cho & Wild, 1990). A disadvantage of varifocals is that the child may not be looking through the correction part of the lens, so regular checks with a dispensing optician are required.

CASE STUDY 14.5

BACKGROUND
8-year-old girl whose recent cycloplegic refraction revealed R = L + 3.00DS. She was wearing glasses (most of the time) with this correction when she saw the author.

SYMPTOMS
Intermittent esotropia and diplopia when removes glasses. No symptoms as long as spectacles are worn.

RELEVANT CLINICAL FINDINGS
The following tests were normal: pupil reactions, ophthalmoscopic findings, ocular motility, amplitude of accommodation (with glasses).
  Vision with glasses: R = L = 6/6−.
  Cover test with glasses: D 8Δ SOP good recovery, N 10ΔRSOT
  Near cover test with add +2.00 over glasses 4Δ RSOT, with +2.50 orthophoria.

MANAGEMENT
Prescribed R = L = +3.00DS add +2.50, D − seg.

FOLLOW-UP 6 WEEKS LATER
Still 3Δ SOT at near, through bifocal segment. Add increased to +3.00.

FOLLOW-UP 6 WEEKS LATER
Constant wear of glasses, no strabismus seen, no diplopia. Cover test with glasses: D = N = 4Δ SOP, good recovery, no fixation disparity or foveal suppression on Mallett unit, 70″ stereo on Randot circles. Other results as before. Continue as now.

SUBSEQUENT FOLLOW-UPS
At each visit, patient was straight at D & N with glasses, and effect of reducing add was investigated. If cover test and Mallett fixation disparity test results were satisfactory with a lesser add, the add was reduced. Thus, the add reduced to +2.50 (age 9 years), +2.00 (age 9.5 years), +1.50 (age 10 years), +1.00 (age 10.25 years), +0.50 (age 10.5 years), and single vision distance (age 10.75 years: R +3.75/−0.50 × 90 = 6/6 L +3.75/−0.25 × 105 = 6/6). Seen regularly since then for >20 years, similar result: asymptomatic, ortho on cover test (now with single vision contact lenses), no aligning prism, Randot circles 20″ stereopsis.

D, Distance; *DS*, dioptre sphere; *L*, left; *N*, near; *R*, right; *RSOT*, right esotropia; *SOP*, esophoria.

Distance or near exotropia can be treated in a similar way by using a negative addition to the refractive error (i.e., over-minussing or under-plussing). The efficacy of this approach compares favourably with other modes of treatment and over-minus lenses do not induce clinically significant myopic changes (Rutstein, Marsh-Tootle, & London, 1989). These cases need to have adequate accommodation and the practitioner should be alert to the possibility of the negative addition causing asthenopic symptoms. It is rare for patients to be able to comfortably over-accommodate by more than 3.00D, less in older patients. Mallett (1988b) suggested that sometimes the benefit from negative additions is not immediately apparent but becomes apparent after a few months of wear.

The clinical technique for this approach is straightforward. If the patient experiences diplopia, the procedure is as illustrated in Fig. 14.3, with adjustments made to the spherical correction to bring the two targets together. If there is no diplopia, the cover test can be used to determine the prescription that eliminates the bulk of the deviation. Care should be taken with any approach involving repeated occlusion, as this can cause an increase in the angle. The Mallett fixation disparity test can be used to refine any correction once the axes are close to alignment, if NRC occurs. The required correction is the smallest that will eliminate a slip on the Mallett test and/or give good cover test recovery.

It is important to carefully explain to the patient/parent that the spectacles are not to correct a refractive error but are 'exercise glasses' to improve binocular coordination. Initially, the patient would be checked after a month, or sooner if there are any problems. In many cases, the refractive modification can be gradually reduced over time (e.g., every 3—6 months) when this is possible without inducing a slip on the Mallett test or poor cover test recovery.

A few cases of exotropia associated with high degrees of uncorrected hypermetropia have been described in whom the exotropia is eliminated when the hypermetropia is corrected (Iacobucci, Archer, & Giles, 1993). Patients were aged 2—4 years and it is possible that the patients failed to attempt to accommodate through their hypermetropia before correction.

RELIEVING PRISMS

The use of prisms to treat HARC is described earlier and, if prisms are to be prescribed to correct the motor deviation, the prism adaptation test already described should be carried out. Sometimes, prism adaptation takes a week rather than 5—10 minutes, so caution needs to be exercised before assuming a prism will be a long-term solution. If little or no prism adaptation occurs, bifoveal fixation is obtained and maintained and the case is not amenable to orthoptic or refractive therapy; prisms can provide an alternative management. Mallett (1979b) stressed that if HARC is present, this mode of treatment is very unlikely to be successful, although he felt that prisms could eliminate suppression. However, patients with suppression of the binocular field of their strabismic eye usually have a large angle of strabismus and there is a limit to the power of prism that can be prescribed, according to the size of spectacle frame and cosmetic considerations. Although Fresnel 'stick-on' prisms can be used, the optical degradation caused by these (Cheng & Woo, 2001) will reduce the stimulus to fusion and their main use is a temporary measure.

Cases that are more likely to respond to prism are those with a small angle deviation, NRC, and diplopia.

PHARMACOLOGICAL MANAGEMENT

Miotics are occasionally used therapeutically in the management of accommodative esotropia, particularly convergence excess (Chapter 15) and in the postoperative control of residual esotropia in patients with a good prognosis for binocular single vision (Ansons & Davis, 2001). The principle is that accommodation is brought about by the direct action on the ciliary muscle without synkinesis with convergence; and the small pupil increases depth of focus reducing the need for accommodation. The usual drug is pilocarpine, which is instilled every 6 hours (Ansons & Davis, 2001). Patients should be checked 2 weeks after treatment starts and regularly thereafter.

BOTULINUM TOXIN

Botulinum toxin can be used to treat comitant strabismus by injecting the medial rectus in esotropia and the lateral rectus in exotropia. The injected muscle is weakened and lengthened following the injection with a duration of action of about 3 months (Ansons & Spencer, 2001). The usual use is diagnostically, to see if surgery would be helpful. Occasional, long-term improvements in alignment occur following injection.

SURGERY

Large-angle strabismus or other cases which, for reasons discussed elsewhere in this chapter, are not amenable to nonsurgical management may need surgical management. These should be referred as soon as possible and there are psychosocial as well as physical benefits to surgery (Jackson, Harrad, Morris, & Rumsey, 2006). The main surgical techniques are summarised at the end of Chapter 17. Spiritus (1994) recommended a presurgical prism adaptation test (p. 291) lasting 1 day before surgery for comitant strabismus. The initial deviation increased (in 58% of esotropes and 37% of exotropes) even when NRC was present. Neikter (1994b) compared a prism adaptation test, lasting up to 14 days, with diagnostic occlusion (Chapter 5). She recommended carrying out both these investigative techniques to improve the accuracy of surgery for comitant intermittent exotropia. Other research indicates diagnostic occlusion can be useful in divergence-excess or convergence insufficiency types of exotropia with hypermetropia for determining the maximum angle before surgery (Han et al., 2014).

CLINICAL KEY POINTS

- Most cases of long-standing strabismus have good sensory adaptations and do not require treatment
- When treatment is sought, many cases of strabismus can be treated in community eyecare practices
- Attention needs to be paid to sensory and motor factors and neither of these should be treated unless both can be corrected
- Strabismic patients will either have diplopia, suppression, or HARC
- Patients with intractable diplopia can benefit from monovision, occlusion, or hypnosis
- If a patient is adapted to their sensory status, even if this is diplopia, they may be unhappy if their deviation is changed with new spectacles
- The best methods for assessing binocular sensory adaptations (HARC or suppression) are Bagolini lenses or the Mallett ARC and suppression in strabismus (MARCS) test. A neutral density filter bar can be used to assess the depth of adaptation
- Shallow HARC or suppression is often eliminated when the motor deviation is corrected
- The motor deviation can be treated by eye exercises, refractive modification, prisms, pharmacological management, botulinum toxin, or surgery

CHAPTER 15

An Overview of the Management of Strabismus

The previous chapters have described techniques that can be used to investigate and treat strabismus. This chapter provides a clinical guide on how these methods should be applied to different types of strabismus. Microtropia is a unique type of strabismus and the management of microtropia is discussed in Chapter 16.

Following the initial examination of a patient with strabismus, an evaluation of all the information available needs to be carried out to decide on the management of each patient. Many strabismic patients need referral for medical investigation and possible surgery, particularly where there is a recent onset. It is important to detect incomitancy, as a new or changing incomitant deviation has a high risk of a pathological aetiology and requires referral (Chapter 17). Table 15.1 helps identify those cases of comitant strabismus in which pathology may play a role. A useful approach, as suggested earlier in this book, is to look for both a positive sign of a likely aetiology that is correctable (e.g., refractive error) and a negative sign of pathology (eye examination normal and no suspicious general health problems). All cases of recently acquired strabismus need to be monitored closely in case the signs in Table 15.1 become apparent.

Most cases of comitant strabismus do not have a pathological aetiology and can be managed in community optometric practice. Patients may be adults of an age when it is not possible to restore binocular vision. Those with a recent onset and distressing symptoms obviously need medical investigation. Most of the other adult strabismics have come to terms with the anomaly and require spectacles for their refractive problems only, although strabismus can still effect quality of life (Hatt et al., 2007). Many children, however, respond to optometric treatment. The purpose of this chapter is to define the types of comitant strabismus likely to be found in optometric practice and understand the best form of approach to each. It is in nobody's interest to hold on to a patient who would be better referred. Indeed, to keep a patient on ineffective treatment too long can reduce the chance of success by other methods. Equally, if the treatment required is refractive, it should receive optometric attention.

Whereas this chapter is not a comprehensive list of all types of comitant strabismus, it is intended to cover those most frequently seen in primary eyecare practice. An indication of the type of approach in dealing with these is given in summary form. Detailed approaches to investigation and management are given in the preceding chapters.

Although this chapter concentrates on the binocular anomaly of strabismus, amblyopia may also require attention. Apart from the need to enhance monocular acuities in their own right, improving the acuity in amblyopia helps the binocular sensory and motor outcomes of strabismus treatment (Spiritus, 1994).

Most cases of strabismus that are seen in primary care are long-standing and have satisfactory sensory adaptation (Chapter 12). A dramatic change in the refractive status of these cases may interfere with the strabismus and cause symptoms. This may contraindicate monovision contact lenses (Evans, 2007a), refractive surgery (Kowal et al., 2005), or cataract surgery on the amblyopic eye before the nonamblyopic eye (Hale, Murjaneh, Frost, & Harrad, 2006).

TABLE 15.1 ■ Differential Diagnosis of Pathological Cause in Acquired Comitant Strabismus.

Sign associated with acquired comitant strabismus	Risk of pathology
Is there a refractive error that might account for the deviation?	Latent hypermetropia, if present, is very likely to be the cause of esotropia The onset of myopia can trigger a small exotropia
If new comitant strabismus, is there a history of previous large phoria or microtropia that may be decompensating?	If so, then a pathological cause is less likely
Is nystagmus present (may be only in abduction)?	If so, strongly suggests pathology in cases with onset after the age of 6 months
Are there pupil, field, disc, or fundus abnormalities?	Indicates pathology
Are there systemic neurological signs (seizures, headaches, mood changes, impaired coordination)?	Indicates pathology
Is the angle increasing?	Suggests pathology
Can motor and sensory fusion be demonstrated with prisms?	If not, pathology more likely
If comitant esotropia, is there an A pattern?	If so, may indicate hydrocephalus or Chiari type I
Is the strabismus responding to treatment?	If responding to treatment (e.g., refractive or exercises), pathology less likely

Modified after Hoyt, C.S., Fredrick, D.R. (1999). Serious neurologic disease presenting as comitant esotropia. In A.L. Rosenbaum & A.P. Santiago (Eds.), *Clinical Strabismus Management* (pp. 152–162). Philadelphia: W.B. Saunders Company.

Time of Onset

The first critical question is the time of onset of the strabismus. Parental recollections can be vague, but photographs taken in early life may help. The important thing to establish is whether the deviation was present during the first year of life.

Strabismus With an Onset in First Year

Retinoblastoma can cause strabismus and can present at any age from birth onwards, but is most commonly detected at about 18 months. Careful ophthalmoscopy, preferably with mydriatic, is required to search for this condition in infants with strabismus. Ophthalmoscopy should be repeated at follow-up and a cycloplegic refraction is required.

Early onset strabismus disrupts the emmetropisation process, often producing anisometropia (Smith et al., 2017).

INFANTILE ESOTROPIA SYNDROME

Brief **neonatal misalignments** of the visual axes commonly occur in the first month of life and should be becoming less frequent in the second month (Horwood, 2003a). It may be impossible to differentiate these episodes from emerging infantile esotropia syndrome, until the second month

(Horwood, 2004b). Even up to the age of 5 months, intermittent esotropia frequently resolves if the deviation is less than 40Δ and is intermittent or variable (PEDIG, 2002a). These cases should be monitored closely for amblyopia (PEDIG, 2002b), even if the deviation seems to be improving.

In contrast with intermittent esotropia, small-angle or variable-angle esotropia in the first year is much more likely to develop into constant large-angle esotropia (Fu, Stager, & Birch, 2007). Constant strabismus with an age of onset before 1 year is most commonly infantile esotropia syndrome, which requires referral (PEDIG, 2002a). This is also known as **early acquired esotropia** and used to be called congenital strabismus, although it is not usually present at birth. Infantile esotropia syndrome has a prevalence between 0.25% (Louwagie, Diehl, Greenberg, & Mohney, 2009) and 1% (Major, Maples, Toomey, DeRosier, & Gahn, 2007). Conventionally, infantile esotropia has been attributed to an innate defect of fusion (Spiritus, 1994), but it seems more likely to be a cortico-mesencephalic-cerebellar disorder where binocular cortical maldevelopment permits primitive subcortical visual pathways to remain operational (Brodsky, 2012). The incidence is influenced by several risk factors, including prematurity, family ocular history, maternal cardiovascular or systemic disease, pregnancy-associated hypertension, and low birth weight (Major et al., 2007). The clinical characteristics are listed in Table 15.2.

Infantile esotropia may be further subdivided into essential infantile esotropia, nystagmus blocking syndrome, or sixth nerve palsy (p. 52; Chapter 17; Chapter 18). None of these types of strabismus respond to optometric treatment regardless of the age at which the patient is seen. When these types of strabismus are found in young children, they should be referred promptly for a surgeon's opinion. The prognosis for sensory and motor fusion is poor (Kora et al., 1997), but is significantly improved by early surgical intervention, preferably at about 3 months of age (Leguire, Rogers, & Bremer, 1991) or before 10 months (Wong, 2008). There is no justification for waiting until the child is old enough for sensory testing (Ansons & Spencer, 2001). If the patient is over the age of 6 or 7 years, it is unlikely that anything other than a cosmetic improvement will result.

Children with infantile esotropia do not manifest the rapid decrease in hypermetropia (emmetropisation) that characterises normal development in the first 6 months of life (Birch, Stager, Wang, & O'Connor, 2010).

An early interruption to binocularity, typically from infantile esotropia syndrome, often results in four clinical signs which persist throughout life, even if the visual axes are surgically straightened. These conditions have been called dissociated eye movements and are latent nystagmus, dissociated vertical deviation (DVD), dissociated horizontal deviation, and inferior oblique overaction

TABLE 15.2 ■ Clinical Characteristics of Essential Infantile Esotropia.

Always present	Often present
Onset 0–6 months	Amblyopia
Large angle (30Δ or more)	Apparently defective abduction and excessive adduction
Stable angle	Dysfunction of oblique muscles
Initial alternation with crossed fixation	A- or V-pattern
Normal central nervous system	Dissociated vertical or horizontal deviation
Asymmetric optokinetic nystagmus	Manifest latent nystagmus
	Anomalous head posture
	Heredity

Modified after von Noorden, G.K. (1996) *Binocular Vision and Ocular Motility* (5th ed.). St. Louis: Mosby.

(Brodsky, 2012). Brodsky argued that these arise from subcortical visual reflexes and are triggered by cortical suppression of one eye. Latent nystagmus is discussed in Chapter 18 and DVD on p. 132. Dissociated horizontal deviations are asymmetric horizontal deviations which cannot be accounted for by incomitancy or anisometropia and occur in about 5% of patients who have had surgery for infantile esotropia syndrome (Enke, Stewart, Scott, & Wheeler, 1994).

After surgical treatment of infantile esotropia, children are still at risk of accommodative esotropia and, less commonly, nonrefractive accommodative esotropia (Uretmen, Civan, Kose, Yuce, & Egrilmez, 2007). The children at greatest risk are those with hypermetropia of 3D or more, and spectacle wear and close monitoring is recommended in these cases.

INFANTILE ACCOMMODATIVE ESOTROPIA

As many as 15% of patients with infantile esotropia may have infantile accommodative esotropia, nearly half of whom can be fully straightened with spectacles (Havertape, Whitfill, & Oscar, 1999), although another study found bifoveal fusion is rarely achieved (Black, 2006). The earlier correction begins, the better the chances of success, and if more than +2.25D is detected in an infant with esotropia, spectacles should be tried before surgery (Havertape et al., 1999). Surgery is only indicated on the portion of the deviation that spectacles do not control after a trial of 2—3 months, and spectacle wear should be continued after surgery (Koc, Ozal, & Firat, 2003).

INFANTILE EXOTROPIA

It has been said that it is very unusual to see congenital exotropia in an otherwise normal infant (Moore & Cohen, 1985), although others have argued that the onset of most exo-deviations is shortly after birth (von Noorden, 1996). Ethnicity is important, with infantile exotropia reported as more common than infantile esotropia in Asian populations (Gonzalez-Diaz Mdel & Wong, 2014). Intermittent exotropia (divergent drifts) are quite common up to the age of 6 months and should only be considered abnormal if it becomes more constant or persists beyond 6 months (Sondhi, Archer, & Helveston, 1990).

Strabismus With an Onset After First Year

REFRACTIVE (ACCOMMODATIVE ESOTROPIA)

In accommodative esotropia, the refractive error is part of the cause of the deviation and therefore the refractive correction is a part of the treatment. These cases are characterised by a significant degree of hypermetropia and/or a high AC/A ratio with a mean age of onset of 2.5 years, and over 90% can be treated successfully (Rutstein & Marsh-Tootle, 1998). The typical age of onset has been described as 3—5 years (Jennings, 1996) or 6 months to 6 years (Babinsky & Candy, 2013). Prompt treatment is therefore important because the critical period for susceptibility of human stereopsis continues to at least 4.5 years of age (Fawcett, Wang, & Birch, 2005). A retrospective study of 68 cases found that two-thirds achieve alignment with single vision spectacles, 22% with bifocals, and 12% require surgery (Reddy, Freeman, Paysse, & Coats, 2009). These authors found that a larger near deviation than distance at initial presentation is not a good indicator of whether the child requires bifocals, but they did not assess compensation (e.g., with a Mallett unit). Accommodative esotropia can decompensate (in about 20% of cases), so even those that are well-controlled by spectacles should be followed-up at least every 9—12 months (Raab, 2001).

Accommodative esotropia can be considered under four headings:

1. *Fully accommodative:* there is usually hypermetropia over +3.00 DS which causes excessive accommodation. Because of the relationship between accommodation and convergence,

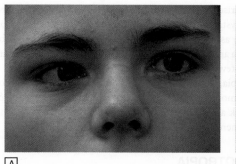
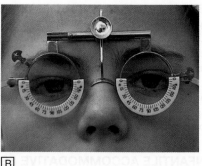

Fig. 15.1   A case of fully accommodative esotropia. The esotropia (A) is eliminated when the hyperme-tropia is corrected with spectacles (B). (Reproduced with permission.)

this stimulates excessive convergence which, in some young patients, is sufficient to cause strabismus (Fig. 15.1). The AC/A ratio in this type may be normal.

In some cases, the patient may overcome the hypermetropia without developing symptoms or esotropia until some episode, often a febrile illness, causes the patient to decompensate and develop esotropia. Often, the esotropia and hypermetropia is blamed on the febrile illness, although this was really a catalyst.

In fully accommodative strabismus, correction of the hypermetropia relieves the accommodation and eliminates the deviation. It is important that correction begins at as early an age as possible. The management of this type of strabismus therefore consists of prescribing the full cycloplegic refractive findings for constant wear. The success of full refractive correction has been given as the most likely explanation for the reduced need in recent years for strabismus surgery in children (MacEwen & Chakrabarti, 2004). Spectacles are the main treatment, but contact lenses (Evans, 2006a) and refractive surgery (Kirwan, O'Keefe, O'Mullane, & Sheehan, 2010; Magli, Forte, Gallo, & Carelli, 2014) are also effective.

It may be advisable to check the cover test with the proposed correction once the cycloplegic has worn off to ensure that an exo-deviation is not caused by the full prescription; if so, the prescription should be reduced. Patients with latent hypermetropia should be warned of the possibility of initial blur until their accommodation relaxes. If this is problematic, a cycloplegic can be instilled when the spectacles are collected to assist with adaptation. The effect on the binocular vision should be checked in 3—4 weeks.

In children, it is expected that binocular vision can be restored and that there will be an improvement in acuity of the amblyopic eye (Mulvihill, MacCann, Flitcroft, & O'Keefe, 2000). If vision does not improve then patching will be required (Chapter 13). Unfortunately, it is not uncommon for patients with refractive esotropia to become realigned with first refractive correction but deviate again at a later date (Babinsky & Candy, 2013).

Sometimes accommodative esotropes may stop wearing their refractive correction without any apparent problems. However, such cases can later present in adulthood with acute onset of comitant esotropia. In view of this, attempts to 'wean' children with accommodative esotropia out of wearing glasses (Hutcheson, Ellish, & Lambert, 2003) may be risky, although occasional success has been reported in cases with lower (e.g., +2.25 DS) hypermetropia (Hutcheson et al., 2003). A good amplitude of accommodation seems to be important for such attempts (Somer, Cinar, & Duman, 2006).

Although weaning may in some cases be possible (e.g., smaller angles), it is inappropriate to undercorrect every case of fully accommodative esotropia (MacEwen,

Lymburn, & Ho, 2008). Retrospective surveys show that accommodative esotropia needs to be monitored for many years and the condition nearly always requires continued optical correction (Mulvihill et al., 2000; Rutstein & Marsh-Tootle, 1998). One study found that hypermetropia can be gradually undercorrected in approximately two-thirds of patients, but undercorrection did not cause a greater rate of decrease of the hypermetropia and accommodative esotropia does not resolve in most patients (Black, 2006).

One approach is to reduce the full prescription in the consulting room in $-0.25D$ steps and prescribe the maximum undercorrection that does not result in an increase in the angle of deviation (Park, Kim, & Oh, 2011). For East Asian populations, the high incidence of myopia during school years may give the impression of successful weaning (Cho & Ryu, 2015).

If manifest refractive strabismus is left untreated, secondary sensory and motor sequelae may develop. As a result of these sequelae, the refractive correction may no longer be able to eliminate the strabismus in a case which once could have been fully corrected refractively. Therefore, all cases of hypermetropia associated with esophoria should be monitored routinely. This is also beneficial as an opportunity to encourage compliance with refractive correction. Poor compliance greatly increases the risk of poor sensory and motor outcomes (Hussein, Weakley, Wirazka, & Paysse, 2015).

It is, of course, inappropriate for people with fully accommodative esotropia to have surgery to correct their deviation. To do so may render the patient exotropic when they reach an age when the hypermetropia needs correction for clear vision.

2. *Partially accommodative:* in these cases, the deviation is reduced by hypermetropic or bifocal correction to a small residual angle. The management of this type of strabismus depends on size of the residual angle, depth of the sensory adaptations, age, and level of cooperation. It is a matter of clinical judgement whether to treat by nonsurgical methods or refer for a surgeon's opinion. Nonsurgical approaches are to correct the residual deviation with prisms (Choe, Yang, & Hwang, 2019) or eye exercises.

Where the residual angle is small, the patient is young, and the level of cooperation is good, these cases often will respond to eye exercises. A full cycloplegic refractive correction for constant wear is prescribed. A useful approach in suitable patients is to prescribe disposable contact lenses, starting with the noncycloplegic refractive findings and gradually increasing the prescription (every second week) until the visual acuity stabilises or symptoms cease (Abdi, Thunholm-Henriksson, & Pansell, 2016). The physiological diplopia methods can be successful in these cases (Chapter 14).

Some of these cases have a convergence excess element also. Physiological diplopia exercises may still be possible if binocular vision for near fixation can be established by an addition to the glasses for near vision as described at the end of Chapter 14. Other cases need referral.

If surgery is contemplated for partially accommodative strabismus, any occlusion therapy should be carried out first because the angle often reduces during occlusion and fewer patients will need surgery after occlusion therapy (Koc, Ozal, Yasar, & Firat, 2005).

3. *Convergence excess:* in some strabismus, there is a high AC/A ratio so an abnormally high degree of convergence is associated with accommodation for near vision. This results in a strabismus which is either present for near vision only or in which the angle is increased markedly for near fixation. These cases should be assessed with the distance correction in place to differentially diagnose convergence excess from fully accommodative strabismus. A different cause of convergence excess esotropia is a primary accommodative insufficiency (see later) causing excessive accommodative effort resulting in secondary overconvergence (Fresina, Schiavi, & Campos, 2010). These authors adopted the term 'hypo-accommodative esotropia', commenting these cases will require multifocal lenses indefinitely. Use of bifocals did not cause a decrease in accommodative ability.

Some cases of esotropia with a greater deviation at near than distance are not associated with convergence excess and have a normal AC/A ratio (Burke, 2015). These authors favour the term distance-near disparity esotropias to generically describe all esotropia where the deviation at near exceeds that at distance by 10Δ.

As noted on p. 97, in hypermetropes contact lenses should induce less accommodative convergence than spectacles, if the patient is suitable and willing to wear contact lenses.

Where the strabismus is only present for near fixation and there is binocular vision for distance vision, a binocular positive addition to the correction is likely to relieve the deviation for near vision, as described at the end of Chapter 14. Bifocals are not always successful and sometimes surgery is required (Vivian, Lyons, & Burke, 2002). A retrospective study found single vision spectacles result in better stereopsis than bifocals (Whitman et al., 2016). However, the authors prescribed bifocal adds of standard power and noted that the approach (advocated in this book) of tailoring the add to the minimum necessary to achieve full compensation at near might have produced different results. The authors advise against prescribing bifocals when the add does not eliminate the esotropia at near.

Surgery may be an alternative management to bifocals in some cases, but commonly more than one operation is required (Lueder & Norman, 2006). Antisuppression exercise for near vision, such as bar-reading, can be helpful.

Monovision contact lenses can be an effective alternative to bifocal spectacles in some cases (Eustis & Mungan, 1999). Less commonly, miotics (e.g., pilocarpine) may be used for convergence excess accommodative esotropia (Ansons & Davis, 2001). The treatment is thought to work in two ways: accommodation is brought about by direct action on the muscle and therefore without synkinesis with convergence; and increased depth of focus from the small pupil reduces the need for accommodation (Chapter 14).

4. *Accommodative insufficiency (hypo-accommodative esotropia):* this type of near esotropia is caused by a low amplitude of accommodation (Costenbader, 1958). The patient makes an excessive effort to accommodate to try and compensate for the low amplitude of accommodation, and this excessive effort induces accommodative convergence and, hence, a near esotropia. These cases may be treated by orthoptic exercises for the accommodative insufficiency (Chapter 10), or with bifocals. It is interesting to note that a similar, albeit milder (not resulting in strabismus), mechanism has been proposed to explain the finding that myopia onset is often proceeded by an increase in AC/A ratio, increased accommodative lag, and near esophoria (Mutti et al., 2017).

5. *Pseudo-accommodative insufficiency:* this is characterised by low divergent fusional reserves and a high AC/A ratio. It is believed that these patients habitually underaccommodate to prevent a manifest deviation and when they are forced to accommodate inside their near point of accommodation, they exceed the limit of their divergent fusional reserve and a near esotropia manifests.

NONREFRACTIVE

In many cases of strabismus, prescribing the refractive error does not markedly change the angle of deviation. Some of these patients will have a high refractive error and require refractive correction to relieve symptoms. Where there is anisometropia that blurs the vision of one eye more than the other, a prescription will be needed as part of the management of any sensory adaptations. However, care must be taken in older children that the correction does not produce intractable diplopia. Binocular sensory adaptations should only be treated if binocular single vision can be restored.

Rarely, cases are encountered in which a nonrefractive comitant strabismus is the result of pathology and these cases are likely to exhibit the characteristics highlighted in Table 15.1.

Esotropia

Acquired nonaccommodative esotropia is characterised by: sudden onset usually between 6–24 months of age, normal binocular vision before onset, constant comitant deviation of 30–70Δ, normal AC/A ratio, negligible effect of refractive correction on the angle, positive family history, and normal neurological health (Frane, Sholtz, Lin, & Mutti, 2000).

Some cases occur following a childhood febrile illness and these may be amenable to treatment by correcting significant refractive errors and strengthening the fusional reserves by the type of exercise described in Chapter 10. These patients have had binocular vision prior to the illness, and if they are seen soon after the recovery in general health, the binocular vision can often be restored. However, care must be taken to be sure that the strabismus was not present before the illness as parents are not always certain.

In some cases, the onset of strabismus may follow emotional trauma. These cases are much more difficult to treat as the traumatic scars do not have any optometric treatment and recovery from them may be very slow. Caution should be exercised before any treatment is given. A refractive correction and fusional reserve exercises may help, but the treatment can be very protracted. Patients in heroin detoxification become less exo/more eso at distance and this can trigger acute comitant esotropia (Firth et al., 2004).

Some esotropia may apparently occur spontaneously in children over the age of 1 year. A careful check for pathology must include searching for the white patches on the fundus indicative of retinoblastoma. This is rare but serious and, particularly where central areas of the fundus are involved, a strabismus may be the first sign. It usually occurs before the age of 4 years. Other neurological disorders usually produce incomitant deviations (e.g., sixth nerve palsy), so a motility test is essential (Chapter 17).

For acute acquired comitant esotropia in children, the main risk factors for intracranial disease are larger eso-deviation at distance, recurrence of the esotropia, neuro-ophthalmological signs (e.g., papilloedema), and age at onset over 6 years (Buch & Vinding, 2015).

Nonaccommodative esotropia with a spontaneous onset can occur without such pathology (Norbis & Malbran, 1956) and the aetiology may be an idiopathic increase in tonic convergence (Frane et al., 2000). It often occurs intermittently at first. If it can be detected at this stage, developing divergent fusional reserves can help to check it. If there is a significant anisometropia which may lead to amblyopia, this should be corrected. Although the strabismus is nonaccommodative, some cases benefit from bifocals which, even with a normal AC/A ratio, may correct the deviation at near. These are prescribed in the same way as for convergence excess deviations. Clearly, the bifocal will not help distance vision, but normal binocular vision at near is better than no binocular vision at all. This also makes eye exercises easier as they can build on the binocular vision at near.

One case has been described of sudden onset esotropia in a 4-year-old boy after watching a three-dimensional (3-D) movie (Tsukuda & Murai, 1988). It is unclear whether this is a chance finding or in fact the effect of the 3-D presentation (see p. 61).

Kothari (2007) described spontaneous late-onset comitant acute nonaccommodative esotropia (ANAET), with mean age of presentation of 7 years (range 2.5–13 years). The typical angle is 40Δ at distance and near, and early surgery is advocated to minimise the risk of amblyopia (Kothari, 2007).

Von Graefe and later Bielschowsky described acute onset esotropia that is associated with high myopia. It usually occurs in young adults at distance and then at near, and is associated with diplopia (von Noorden, 1996). Typically, this type of deviation is comitant (rarely, there is limited abduction), unlike another type of esotropia associated with very high myopia (−15D or more) characterised by a limitation of motility in all directions of gaze (von Noorden, 1996). This has been called 'heavy eye syndrome' and is described in Table 17.17. Acute onset esotropia in adults was reported to be associated with some degree of myopia in 9 out of 10 cases, and stereoacuity can be regained after surgery (Spierer, 2003).

Another type of nonaccommodative esotropia that can occur spontaneously is 'age-related distance esotropia' (Mittelman, 2006). Typically, an older patient reports a sudden onset of horizontal diplopia during distance vision. This has been termed divergence paralysis, although whether divergence is an active process is controversial (Lim, 1999) and it has been attributed instead to anatomical changes in the orbit or muscles (Mittelman, 2006). Prismatic correction is possible for many cases (Mittelman, 2006). The condition should be differentially diagnosed from a bilateral sixth nerve palsy (where an incomitancy will be detected on motility testing), but still requires referral to investigate possible neurological causes.

A retrospective study found a high correlation between adult onset distance esophoria or esotropia and cerebellar disease (Hufner et al., 2015). When nonaccommodative esotropia has become established for several years, nonsurgical treatment may not be successful; prism relief may assist (Chapter 14). Extraocular muscle surgery may be indicated when 20Δ or more of esotropia remains after full correction of the refractive error or if optical correction has no effect on the angle (Frane et al., 2000). The chances of achieving stereopsis after surgery for esotropia improve if the onset is after the second year, but coexisting hypertropia worsens the prognosis (Kora et al., 1997).

Exotropia

Exotropia (constant or intermittent) affects about 1% of children by the age of 11 years, with diagnosis most common at the ages of 3 years and 9 years (Govindan, Mohney, Diehl, & Burke, 2005). A more recent review estimated that 2% of children develop intermittent exotropia before the age of 3 years (Joyce, Beyer, Thomson, & Clarke, 2015). Indeed, intermittent exotropia is the most common form of exotropia (Mohney & Huffaker, 2003) to occur under the age of 19 years (50%); and other common types are exotropia associated with neurological abnormalities (21%; mostly cerebral palsy or developmental delay), convergence weakness (12%), and sensory exotropia (10%; mostly optic nerve hypoplasia or cataract). Intermittent exotropia is also discussed in Chapter 8 and this section should be read in conjunction with pp. 115—118. Intermittent exotropia is more likely to be associated with neurological disease (e.g., developmental delay, cerebral palsy, attention deficit disorder) if it is of the convergence weakness rather than the other types listed later (Phillips et al., 2005).

There is a lack of strong evidence concerning interventions for intermittent exotropia (Hatt & Gnanaraj, 2013; Joyce et al., 2015). The management options for intermittent exotropia were reviewed by Coffey, Wick, Cotter, Scharre, and Horner (1992) and negative lens therapy is said to often achieve long-term success (Caltrider & Jampolsky, 1983). For many patients with intermittent exotropia, the deviation reduces in angle and/or changes to an exophoria over time, and this seems to happen regardless of the management of the case (Rutstein & Corliss, 2003). In contrast, another study found that more than 50% of children with intermittent exotropia have an increase of 10Δ or more within 20 years of their diagnosis (Nusz et al., 2006). Surgery for intermittent exotropia may have a better prognosis than for constant exotropia (Wu, Sun, Xia, Xu, & Xu, 2006). In view of the weak evidence base, it is reassuring that most children with well-controlled intermittent exotropia receive no treatment within 12 months of the first hospital eye service appointment (Buck et al., 2009).

When a child is discovered to have both exotropia and significant hypermetropia there may be a concern that correction of the hypermetropia might cause the exotropia to worsen. This occasionally happens, but in more than half of such cases, the exotropia improves on full correction of the hypermetropia (Kassem, Rubin, & Kodsi, 2012).

Divergent strabismus can be classified under four headings, each with a different management and prognosis.

1. *Divergence excess:* presents typically as an intermittent divergent strabismus for distance vision only. It becomes most apparent during periods of inattention and day-dreaming,

and is worse during ill health. Patients are photophobic and bright light can cause the strabismus to occur (Eustace et al., 1973; Wiggins & von Noorden, 1990). Most patients are female, and there is little refractive error. Because of its intermittent nature, the acuities are generally good and nearly equal. There are usually no symptoms as there are sensory adaptations when the eye is deviated. Patients typically seek advice because some relative tells them that one eye sometimes deviates (see also Chapter 8). Where a V syndrome exists, optometric treatment may be more difficult.

In Chapter 8, the distinction is drawn between true and simulated divergence excess and it is noted that deterioration is rare and occlusion (e.g., 3 hours daily) may be an effective treatment for intermittent exotropia. The condition is usually improved by eye exercises designed to overcome sensory adaptations and to build up the convergent fusional reserves (Ma, Kang, Scheiman, & Chen, 2019). Also useful are exercises to teach an appreciation of physiological diplopia and the movement of the diplopic images during changes of fixation from near to distance and back.

If the patient has adequate accommodation and a moderate to high AC/A ratio, the deviation may be treated refractively by prescribing distance glasses that are over-minussed with a near addition (e.g., -2.00 DS at distance with a $+2.00$ add at near) to prevent the patient developing an eso-deviation at near (Mallett, 1988b). In a pilot randomised controlled trial, over-minus spectacles were found to improve distance control after 8 weeks in children aged 3–7 years (Chen et al., 2016). Parents should be warned that, regardless of any interventions they receive, over 90% of cases of intermittent exotropia become myopic by the age of 20 years (Ekdawi, Nusz, Diehl, & Mohney, 2010).

Surgical intervention is an option, but in a retrospective matched-group study, the cure rate was only slightly higher (30%) in the group receiving surgical intervention compared with 12% in the control group (Holmes, Hatt, & Leske, 2014). The authors concluded that active monitoring or nonsurgical treatment is reasonable unless clear deterioration occurs.

2. *Convergence weakness exotropia:* this is also called convergence insufficiency strabismus and is characterised by a near exotropia. The onset is usually in the mid-teens when binocular vision breaks down for near fixation. It seems that binocular vision has been maintained by the high convergence impulses which exist in children, but in these cases, it cannot be sustained for near when these impulses lessen. Binocular vision may also break down for distance vision, but the angle of the strabismus is greater for near. These patients complain of symptoms including diplopia. They are usually myopic and have equal acuities.

If the angle is over 20Δ, it is unlikely to be possible to restore binocular vision by optometric methods, and the patient should be referred for a surgeon's opinion. In other cases, one approach is to correct any significant refractive error and increase the convergent fusional reserves. With smaller angles, prism relief is also useful. Some patients with adequate amplitude of accommodation respond well to the prescribing of reading glasses which are 'over-minussed'. The minimum 'negative add' to transform the near exotropia into a compensated exophoria should be prescribed, and the effect of this on distance ocular motor balance should be investigated. Care must be taken to ensure that the glasses do not cause an eso-deviation for distance vision. If so, they should only be used for reading or executive bifocals glazed upside down can be prescribed (p. 122).

True convergence paralysis is rare and characterised by diplopia only at near from an inability to converge, but with normal adduction. The condition is commonly attributed to neurological lesions in the areas of the third nucleus, corpora quadrigemina, or pineal gland (Darko-Takyi et al., 2016).

3. *Basic exotropia:* in these cases, there is a constant divergent strabismus of approximately equal angle for distance and near vision. It is often alternating with nearly equal acuities. As the onset is likely to be early in life, there are no symptoms.

Any significant refractive error is corrected, following the general guide of maximum minus or minimum plus. In children young enough to have an adequate amplitude of accommodation, the effect of prescribing 'negative additions' to the prescription (over-minussing or under-plussing) can be tried, as described in Chapter 14. Exercises for simultaneous binocular vision may also be required. Divergent strabismus is sometimes accompanied by a vertical component which will make eye exercises more difficult. Surgical correction may be indicated for cosmetic reasons.

4. *Consecutive exotropia:* there are circumstances in which a convergent strabismus may become divergent. It is sometimes seen in patients who had accommodative esotropia on which an operation was performed in early childhood. No spectacles have been worn but, in adolescence or adulthood, these patients develop symptoms due to the hypermetropia. Correction of the refractive error relieves the facultative accommodation and a divergent strabismus with diplopia occurs. A partial correction and convergent fusional reserve exercises can sometimes help to maintain binocular vision. Other cases need further surgery.

Vertical Strabismus

About 1 in 400 people develop vertical strabismus by the age of 18 years (Tollefson, Mohney, Diehl, & Burke, 2006). When vertical strabismus presents in adulthood it is usually the result of an incomitant deviation (Chapter 17), typically fourth nerve palsy (Tollefson et al., 2006). This is a major reason why nearly 90% of cases of vertical strabismus are hypertropia, and hypotropia is very likely to be Brown syndrome (Tollefson et al., 2006) (Chapter 17). Hypertropia can, rarely, be exacerbated by convergence and accommodation (Thomas, Farooq, Proudlock, & Gottlob, 2005).

SPASM OF THE NEAR REFLEX (TRIAD)

Aetiology

The term **spasm of the near reflex** (Rutstein, 2000) is more accurate than its synonym, **convergent spasm** (Bishop, 2001), as all three components of the near triad (convergence, accommodation, miosis) are typically involved (Rutstein, 2000). It usually has a psychogenic origin, but can be organic (Bishop, 2001) when there may be other clinical findings such as nystagmus or papilloedema (Rutstein, 2000).

Investigation

Symptoms include headache, visual discomfort, dizziness, and print blurring, doubling, becoming smaller, or merging. A cycloplegic refraction is indicated to rule out latent hypermetropia (Table 2.11). The condition is characterised by intermittent and variable episodes of esotropia, pseudomyopia, and pupillary miosis. There may also be limited abduction and the condition has been observed in patients with previously well-controlled accommodative esotropia (Rutstein, 2000).

Management

The underlying cause should be treated, if it can be identified. The condition does not usually respond to exercises, but a near addition may help (Bishop, 2001) and cycloplegic agents (e.g., cyclopentolate 1%) are sometimes helpful (Rutstein, 2001).

CLINICAL KEY POINTS

- Look for active pathology: if present refer
- Infantile esotropia syndrome does not respond to optometric management. Exclude high hypermetropia and refer
- Only treat a motor deviation in strabismus if any sensory adaptation is very superficial or can be eliminated with treatment
- Microtropes are very often asymptomatic and best left alone (Chapter 16)
- Large (more than about 20Δ) deviations are difficult to treat and surgery is often the most appropriate management
- If you find an esotropia at near, suspect hypermetropia. If hypermetropia is not readily apparent, do a cycloplegic refraction. If you find significant hypermetropia in esotropia, prescribe
- If hypermetropia is causing accommodative esotropia, the hypermetropia will probably require correction for life
- 'Negative adds' can be an effective treatment for some exotropia

CHAPTER 16

Microtropia

Microtropia (Lang, 1966), or microsquint, may be found as an apparently primary condition, or may be present as a residual deviation after the treatment of a larger strabismus. It may have inherited characteristics (Burian & von Noorden, 1974). Anisometropia is often a major factor, and a foveal scotoma can result from the confusion of the blurred image with the sharp one in the other eye. The condition has also been called Parks monofixational syndrome (Parks, 1969; Parks & Eustis, 1961). Typically, microtropia develops before the age of 3 years, but it may break down into a larger-angle strabismus and give the impression that a strabismus has developed in later childhood. It is usually an eso-deviation, but microhypertropia (Lang, 1966) and microexotropia (Stidwill, 1998) have also been described.

Classification

Primary microtropia describes microtropia when there is no prior history of a larger deviation and **secondary microtropia**, when a primary comitant larger-angle deviation has been reduced as a result of treatment (Houston, Cleary, Dutton, & McFadzean, 1998). Another cause of secondary microtropia is a foveal lesion. It has been said that secondary microtropia is more common than primary microtropia (Griffin & Grisham, 1995).

Clinical Characteristics

The terminology surrounding small angle strabismus has been confused, but microtropia is now recognised as having certain characteristics in very many cases. These characteristics are listed below, and they are incorporated into a diagnostic algorithm at the end of the chapter. It is hoped that this will help to standardise the diagnosis of microtropia.

1. *Small angle.* The microtropia is less than 6Δ in angle. Some authors say less than 10Δ (Lang; cited by Mallett, 1988a) and others, less than 5Δ (Caloroso & Rouse, 1993). The deviation may not show on the cover test, not because it is too small, but because it is a fully adapted strabismus (see later). Microtropia is usually constant at all positions of gaze and fixation distances.
2. *Anisometropia.* There is usually a difference between the refractive errors in the two eyes (Hardman Lea et al., 1991) of more than 1.50D. Occasionally, microtropia will be found in patients without anisometropia.
3. *Amblyopia.* There is reduced acuity in one eye, and as the deviation may not be apparent on the cover test, amblyopia may be the first indication of the microtropia. Usually the acuity is only reduced to 6/9 or 6/12. Very rarely microtropia can be alternating, when there will be no amblyopia.
4. *Eccentric fixation.* Central fixation is lost in microtropia and there is likely to be a suppression scotoma in the foveal area of the amblyopic eye. The angle of the eccentric fixation is usually the same as the angle of the strabismus, and this is why the eye does not move on the cover test: the area of the retina on which the image falls in binocular vision is the same as the eccentrically fixating area (the area used for fixation when the

238

other eye is covered). Occasionally in microtropia, the degree of eccentric fixation is less than the angle of the strabismus, and in these cases a very small cover test movement may be seen. Some authors (e.g., Jennings, 1985) define microtropia as a strabismus in which no movement is seen on the cover test (Helveston & von Noorden, 1967), and hence would not classify this latter type as microtropia.

5. *Anomalous correspondence.* Harmonious anomalous retinal correspondence (HARC) is present in microtropia. Therefore, in most cases there will be identity of the retinal area on which the image falls in the patient's habitual vision with both the area used for fixation monocularly and the anomalously corresponding area. This has been referred to as **microtropia with identity**, and most microtropia is of this type. In these cases, the strabismus is said to be fully adapted.

6. *Peripheral fusion.* The eyes in microtropia seem to be held in the nearly straight position of the small angle by fusional impulses provided by peripheral vision. A form of 'pseudofusional reserves' can be measured. During the cover test it is therefore important to position the cover close to the eye to ensure complete dissociation, otherwise peripheral fusion may reduce the magnitude of any ocular movement and prevent accurate diagnosis.

7. *Pseudoheterophoria.* In many cases of microtropia, the angle of the deviation may increase on the alternating cover test or even if one eye is covered for a slightly longer time than normal for the cover test. When the cover is removed, the eye which was last covered will be seen to return to the microtropia position. It is as if a heterophoric movement is superimposed on the microtropia. This 'pseudoheterophoria' may be larger and more obvious than the microtropia, which may not show at all on the cover test. This cover test recovery movement can be described as an anomalous fusional movement.

Mallett (1988a) felt that these cases did not have a strabismus but in fact had a heterophoria with normal retinal correspondence (NRC) and a gross fixation disparity. This fixation disparity is much larger than that normally found in heterophoria, but does not cause diplopia because of a large foveal suppression area in the strabismic eye. Pickwell (1981) suggested a sequence of events which linked these features and could explain the development of some cases of microtropia. He argued that a decompensating heterophoria leads to an increasing fixation disparity which in time becomes associated with an enlargement of Panum's area and an increase in the deviation. This results in microtropia with identity. It is interesting that Pickwell suggested an enlargement of Panum's area, as had Goersch (1979), in contrast to the foveal suppression that Mallett proposed, and which is detected with the Mallett foveal suppression test (Jennings, 1996; see Fig. 4.8).

8. *Stereopsis.* A low grade of stereopsis has been reported in microtropia (Okuda, Apt, & Wanter, 1977), although it is not always detected with standard tests (Pickwell & Jenkins, 1978).

9. *Symptoms.* There are usually no symptoms and a good cosmesis.

Investigation and Diagnosis

The investigation and diagnosis of microtropia ensue from a full routine eye examination, but the following aspects are particularly useful in detecting the condition. These are summarised in Table 16.2.

AMBLYOPIA

The presence of amblyopia in one eye is usually the first clue that microtropia may be found. The amblyopic eye shows the crowding phenomenon referred to in Chapter 13, that is, single letter

TABLE 16.1 ■ Method of Use of the 4Δ Base-Out Test.

1. Select an appropriate target, which should be an isolated target on a large uniform field. A dot (resolvable by the amblyopic eye) on a white, otherwise featureless, wall in front of the patient is ideal. A dot in the centre of a blank sheet of A3 or A4 paper at 40 cm is acceptable.
2. Introduce the 4Δ base-out lens in front of one eye whilst the eyes fixate the target.
3. If the patient has no strabismus, then one of two normal responses, or a combination of both, will occur:
   a. Both eyes will make a saccadic version movement, followed by a vergence movement of the eye without the prism, or
   b. The eye with the prism will make a vergence movement, the other eye maintaining fixation.
4. If the patient has a microtropia and the prism is placed in front of the strabismic eye, the image will be displaced within the central suppression area and no movement of either eye will take place.
5. If the patient has a microtropia and the prism is placed in front of the nonstrabismic eye, then both eyes will make a saccadic version movement, but there will be no corrective vergence movement.
6. If an abnormal response is obtained, the better eye should be occluded and the test repeated with the prism just introduced in front of the strabismic eye. If this eye still fails to make a saccadic movement to the prism, this suggests pathology may be present, causing a central scotoma.

acuity is better than line acuity. The foveal scotoma may also result in the patient missing out letters when reading lines of Snellen letters, or they may read the line more easily backwards (Fig. 13.1).

The patient should be tested for eccentric fixation (Chapter 13 and Appendix 6). Eccentric fixation in microtropia is usually parafoveal and slightly nasal and superior to the fovea in microesotropia. The other diagnostic features of strabismic amblyopia are summarised in Table 13.1. The depth of amblyopia seems to be the main factor influencing binocularity (Tomac & Birdal, 2001).

COVER TEST

For microtropia without identity, the diagnosis is usually made from a strabismic result on the unilateral cover test of between 1Δ and 10Δ. As explained earlier, microtropia with identity is unlikely to be detected as a strabismic movement with the cover test. There may be an apparent heterophoria movement when the cover is removed, and this could result in the microtropia being missed.

FOUR-PRISM DIOPTRE TEST (IRVINE PRISM TEST)

In this test (Irvine, 1948; Jampolsky, 1964), a 4Δ base-out prism is placed before one eye and the eye movements are observed. The typical response in normal eyes (Ciuffreda & Tannen, 1995) is a small initial vergence movement (which may not be seen), followed by a conjugate saccade (version movement) and then a symmetric vergence movement. The theory behind the test (Frantz, Cotter, & Wick, 1992) is that, in microtropia, if the prism is placed before the strabismic eye the image will move within the suppression area, and there will be no movement of either eye. If the prism is placed before the nonmicrotropic eye, both eyes will make the initial version movement, but the microtropic eye will fail to make the subsequent vergence movement. When the patient has HARC, the test can still reveal a small suppression area at the fovea which can coexist with HARC (Chapter 12).

Surprisingly, in most descriptions of the test the fixation target is not mentioned. The test should only work if the patient is fixating an angular, isolated, target on a large featureless background. If this is not the case (e.g., if the patient fixates a letter chart), other detail in the field of view will also appear to move, not just the fixation target. The importance of fixation target (Irvine, 1948) was highlighted by Irvine shortly after the initial description of the test (Irvine, 1944), but has since then been omitted from descriptions of the test. This factor probably explains some confusing results from publications that do not specify whether a featureless background was used (Tomac, Sener, & Sanac, 2002). As the strength/depth of suppression is likely to vary with target conditions, it is best to avoid an unusually high contrast target (e.g., spotlight). One study evaluated the effect of target parameters, but only included eight cases of microtropia, all of whom had HARC without central suppression and who exhibited normal responses on the 4Δ base-out test (Savino, Di Nicola, Bolzani, & Dickmann, 1998).

In some cases where there is amblyopia in one eye and no movement on the cover test, it is important to differentiate microtropia from organic amblyopia. It is possible that a central scotoma in organic amblyopia could cause a 4Δ test result similar to that in microtropia. In these cases, it may be useful to occlude the good eye and repeat the 4Δ base-out test monocularly. If there is a large pathological scotoma, as in many cases of organic amblyopia, there will be no monocular response to the prism. Because any monocular suppression area in a microtropic eye is likely to be lighter than the larger suppression area that occurs under binocular viewing, a microtropic eye should make a version movement to a 4Δ lens that is introduced monocularly. The test method is summarised in Table 16.1.

Although the 4Δ base-out test has been proposed as a diagnostic test for microtropia, the test can give atypical responses, particularly in esophoric patients where the 4Δ base-out may correct the eso-deviation (Romano & von Noorden, 1969). Frantz et al. (1992) also advised caution in using this test. They found test-retest repeatability to be low and that normal and microtropic children and adults exhibit many atypical responses. The present author speculates that this may be because too little attention has been paid to the test target. Concurrent testing for suppression with Bagolini lenses during the 4Δ base-out test indicates that in some cases there is a positive response to the test in the absence of suppression, so a positive test implies only that there is no normal motor fusion (Bagolini, Campos, & Chiesi, 1985). A polarised letter chart can also be used to detect central suppression (Epstein & Tredici, 1973) and may be a preferable approach (p. 83).

HARC

The Bagolini lens test or MARCS test will show the response typical of HARC (Chapter 14). The HARC is usually deeply ingrained and will require a neutral-density filter value of 1.0 log units or more to suppress the Bagolini streak.

AMSLER CHARTS

The scotoma may show on the Amsler charts or as a disturbance of a page of print (Table 13.1 and Appendix 6).

STEREOPSIS

This will depend on the type of test used. The TNO test measures random dot stereopsis and microtropic patients are unlikely to do better than 2000 seconds of arc, whereas the result from the Randot or Titmus stereotest circles, which measure contoured stereopsis, may be as high as 100 seconds of arc (Stidwill, 1998).

SUMMARY OF THE DIAGNOSIS OF MICROTROPIA

In summary, there is a consensus about some characteristics which are invariably present for a diagnosis of microtropia. There are several other characteristics which some authors argue are necessary for such a diagnosis, and others consider are only sometimes present in microtropia. The algorithm

TABLE 16.2 ■ **Algorithm to Assist in the Diagnosis of Microtropia.**

All the following characteristics must be present for a diagnosis of microtropia:
Angle less than 10Δ
Amblyopic eye with morphoscopic acuity at least one line worse than dominant eye, unless alternating microtropia (rare)
Eccentric fixation (Chapter 13), unless rare alternating microtropia
HARC detected by Bagolini striated lens test, or by modified Mallett Unit (Chapter 14)
And at least three of the following characteristics should also be present:
Angle less than 6Δ
Anisometropia over 1.50D
Microtropia with identity: angle of anomaly = angle of eccentric fixation, so no movement when dominant eye is covered
Monofixational syndrome: apparent phoria movement on cover test
Motor fusion: 'pseudofusional reserves' can be measured
Stereopsis of 100″ or more on contoured tests such as Titmus circles, or Randot contoured circles
Four-prism dioptre test shows positive response (with appropriate target)
Lang's one-sided scotoma demonstrated with Amsler charts

in Table 16.2 summarises these factors and it is hoped this helps to standardise the definition and diagnosis of this condition.

Management

Microtropia is a fully adapted strabismus and does not give rise to symptoms unless other conditions are present. Management consists, initially, of correcting the refractive error. This is particularly important if the patient is under 5 years of age and has anisometropia. Amblyopia and eccentric fixation should be treated in the usual way (Chapter 13).

Houston et al. (1998) recommended aggressive treatment with patching of patients with microtropia under the age of 10 years, which they found to be effective without inducing intractable diplopia. Cleary, Houston, McFadzean, and Dutton (1998) noted that for one-third of their sample, aggressive occlusion therapy not only restored monocular acuities of 6/5 but also eliminated the microtropia.

Adults with microtropia are usually not likely to benefit from any treatment (Harwerth & Fredenburg, 2003). Special caution is needed in treating any case of adapted strabismus because, if the adaptation is broken down, this could result in intractable diplopia.

THE MANAGEMENT OF DECOMPENSATED MICROTROPIA

In a study, 14 adults whose microtropia had decompensated (causing diplopia) were compared to 16 controls with stable microtropia (Siatkowski, 2011). The decompensated cases were more likely to have a vertical strabismus and had lower convergent and divergent fusional reserves.

If microtropia breaks down into a larger deviation, or if monofixational heterophoria is decompensated and giving rise to symptoms, treatment for these conditions may restore the microtropia to its compensated and fully adapted state. The situation here is rather analogous to a heterophoria decompensating and the factors described in Chapter 4 as causing decompensation may be responsible. The sensory and motor adaptations to microtropia described earlier seem to be less well-established and less stable in microexotropia and microhypertropia than in the more common microesotropia (Arnoldi, 2001). Practitioners should be particularly alert to the possibility of decompensation in nonesotropic microtropia.

The treatment in cases that are decompensating will consist of that described in the earlier chapters for heterophoria and strabismus and a change to the refractive correction (Siatkowski, 2011) or eye exercises can be successful (Griffin & Grisham, 1995).

When a microtropia decompensates, symptoms are often alleviated by treatment (exercises, refractive correction, prisms, or surgery) to reestablish the original asymptomatic angle (Siatkowski, 2011). Case Study 16.1 is an example of such a case.

CASE STUDY 16.1 | **First Appointment (Aged 42 Years: Occupation, Surgeon)**

SYMPTOMS & HISTORY
At age 4 years, surgery for convergent strabismus; age 13 years recurred requiring further surgery. For as long as can remember, has had intermittent diplopia but more frequent in last 3 months. Distance vision is clear but has to strain to keep single; easier with glasses than without, but still problematic. Frontal headaches, especially after concentrated vision (e.g., viewing x-ray scans). Family history: father glaucoma.

RELEVANT CLINICAL FINDINGS
Normal ocular health, pupil reactions, fields, IOP, OCT.
   Ocular motility: full, smooth, diplopia only in extreme L gaze

Current glasses:	R +1.50/−0.50 × 75 6/7.5−	L −1.00DS 6/5−
Subjective:	R +2.25/−0.50 × 75 6/7.5−	L −0.75/−0.25 × 20 6/5−
	N.B., RE VA test misses central letters (Fig. 13.1)	
	[all tests below with spectacles]	
Amp. Acc. (with Rx):	R 5D	L 7D
Stereoacuity:	Randot 2 shapes nil, circles nil	
Cover test (with Rx):	D 6Δ R SOT, nil vertical	
	N 10Δ R SOT, nil vertical	
MARC (large OXO) test:	when single vision, HARC	
Mallett aligning prism:	D crossed dip, 2Δ in R	0.5Δ up R
	N consistent suppression RE for horizontal & vertical tests	
Dissociation tests:	D initially 2Δ exo, then small variable eso, 0.75Δ up R	
	N 2Δ in L	2Δ L hyper
Fusional reserves:	D convergent −/9/6	divergent −/4/2
	N convergent 10/6/12	divergent 6/supp/−
Subjective prism:	With subjective in trial frame, viewing isolated target:	
	0.5Δ up R reduces diplopia. With this left in trial frame:	
	additional 1Δ in RE lessens diplopia, this removed and	
	2Δ in RE eliminates diplopia at D & N	

COMMENT
The patient has a microesotropia and superimposed on this is a decompensating pseudoexophoria. Although this was not seen on cover test, it is inferred from the other results. The base-in prism (and small vertical prism) aids compensation of the pseudoexophoria, evidenced by the fixation disparity test and subjective response to prism. The prism restores the patient to the compensated microtropia with which he is comfortable.

MANAGEMENT
Prescribe Rx below, check at spectacle collection and patient to return if diplopia no better or recurs
R +2.00/−0.50 × 75 0.5Δ up 2Δ in
L −0.75/−0.25 × 20

NEXT EXAMINATION (4 YEARS)
Patient reports prisms helped a lot, resolved headaches and diplopia, only very rare diplopia now if exceptionally tired; never when driving. D and N clear with spectacles (still managing without presbyopic correction). Findings, similar to above.

Amp. Acc, Accommodative amplitude; *D*, distance/dioptre; *DS*, dioptre sphere; *HARC*, harmonious anomalous retinal correspondence; *IOP*, intraocular pressure; *L*, left; *N*, near; *OCT*, optical coherence tomography; *R*, right; *RE*, right eye; *Rx*, prescription; *SOT*, esotropia; *VA*, visual acuity.

CLINICAL KEY POINTS

- Microtropia can be primary or secondary, when it is the residual deviation after correction of a larger deviation
- Literally, microtropia is a small-angle strabismus (less than 6−10Δ)
- Microtropia is usually associated with amblyopia, eccentric fixation, HARC, anisometropia, 'pseudofusional reserves', 'pseudostereopsis', and an abnormal response on the 4Δ base-out test
- In microtropia the angle of the deviation is often equal to the angle of eccentric fixation so no strabismic movement is seen on the cover test. A 'pseudoheterophoric movement' may be seen
- Microtropia is a fully adapted strabismus and patients are usually asymptomatic

PART 4

Incomitant Deviations and Nystagmus

CHAPTER 17

Incomitant Deviations

Nature of Incomitant Deviations

In some deviations, strabismus or heterophoria, the angle of the deviation varies as the patient moves the eyes to look in different parts of the field. Such deviations are incomitant. For most causes of incomitancy, there is a consistency in the way the angle changes: it increases in one particular direction of gaze each time the eyes are turned in that direction. Also, the angle will differ according to which eye is fixating (p. 250). Incomitant deviations are usually caused by abnormalities in the anatomy of the ocular motor apparatus or by one or more muscles being unable to function normally. These deviations can either be congenital, or may be acquired at any age:

1. *Congenital* incomitancy is due to some developmental anomaly of the motor system, either in the anatomy or in the functioning of the muscles or the parts of the nervous system that serve them. This type of deviation gradually becomes more comitant over time but is very much less likely to respond to eye exercises than comitant (concomitant) deviations.
2. *Acquired* incomitant deviations are caused by injury or disease of the ocular motor system. For example, they may be the result of a fracture of the skull, or of pathology affecting the muscles, nerves, or brain centres. Such conditions may be long-standing, static, and requiring no further medical attention, or can be due to recently acquired injury or active disease process. In the latter case, the patient needs referral for medical attention to the ocular condition or to the disease causing the anomaly.

The complete loss of action of a muscle is called a muscle **paralysis**. A partial loss is referred to as **paresis**. The term **palsy** is used generically to include both paralysis and paresis. In incomitant deviations of all kinds, treatment with spectacles or exercises is very limited in remedying the patient's deviation. The first priority is to recognise those cases which require urgent medical attention.

A refractive correction may be required by the patient but is likely to have minimal effect on the deviation. Incomitancy is present in about 13% of cases of strabismus, but is rarer in heterophoria (Flom, 1990). Prolonged occlusion in normal subjects may reveal small incomitancies (Neikter, 1994a). It may be that there is a continuum between the extremes of perfect comitancy and frank incomitancy, with most people having a slight anatomical incomitancy which is only revealed by prolonged periods of dissociation.

Before detailing the investigation and management of incomitancies, the normal actions of the extraocular muscles will be reviewed.

ACTIONS OF THE EXTRAOCULAR MUSCLES

The basis of muscle actions arises from their anatomy (Evans, 2004a). Fig. 17.1 is a scale plan view of the orbit. The eye is in the primary position, so the visual axis is parallel to the medial wall of the orbit. The centre of rotation of the eye is marked (C). Fig. 17.1A shows the centre of the attachment of the superior rectus muscle is medial to the plane containing the visual axis. This muscle's attachment is neither symmetrical nor quite central, and its general line of pull is slightly nasal to the plane containing the centre of rotation. This means that it does not act vertically over the centre of rotation and this influences the secondary actions of this muscle. By

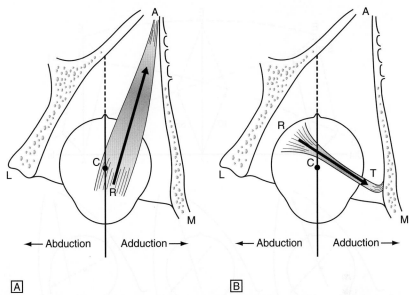

Fig. 17.1 Plan view of right orbit. (A) The plane and direction of pull of the superior and inferior recti muscles, *RA*, which passes medial *(M)* to the plane of the centre of rotation of the eye *(C)*. (B) The plane containing the superior and inferior oblique muscles: their direction of pull is almost the same. It passes behind and medial to the centre of rotation. See text for further explanation. *L*, Lateral.

reference to Fig. 17.1A, when the eye is looking straight ahead the primary action must be to elevate the eye, and the secondary actions are adduction and intorsion. The secondary actions will increase on adduction.

On abduction of the eye, the attachment of the muscle will move outwards, and the line of pull will be carried directly over the centre of rotation when the eye is abducted by about 25 degrees. In this position, two factors are obvious: the secondary actions can no longer occur, and the primary action will be at its greatest mechanical advantage. When the eye is abducted by 25 degrees, the superior rectus muscle will be a pure elevator and at its maximum power as an elevator (Fig. 17.2).

A similar state of affairs applies to the depressor action of the inferior rectus muscle, as this lies very nearly in the same vertical plane as the superior rectus. When the eye is turned out by about 25 degrees, the inferior rectus has its strongest action as a depressor and has no secondary actions. The primary action of the superior rectus muscle opposes that of the inferior rectus: the muscles are antagonists.

The oblique muscles are illustrated in Fig. 17.1B. From its attachment to the eye, the superior oblique pulls towards the trochlea (T). The line of pull is also medial to the centre of rotation, and its actions in the primary position, intorsion, depression, and abduction follow from this one anatomical detail. Also, as the eye turns inwards its vertical action (depression) is increased and the other actions are very much reduced. If the eye were to be adducted by about 50 degrees, the line of pull would lie in the same plane as the centre of rotation. In this position, its power as a depressor would be maximum, and it would have no other actions.

From the point of view of clinical diagnosis, we can regard the inferior oblique muscle as lying in the same vertical plane as the superior oblique. Its actions can therefore be deduced in a similar way and the primary actions of the two muscles are opposite, so they are antagonists.

The single anatomical detail from which the muscle actions arise is that the two vertical planes containing the lines of pull of the vertically acting pairs of muscles cross medially to the centre of

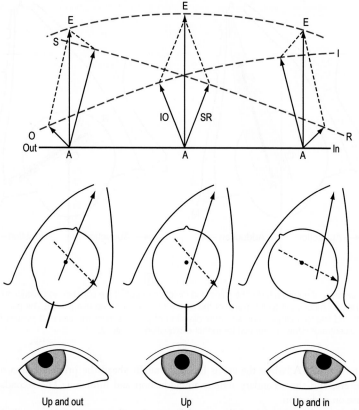

Fig. 17.2 Relative actions of the elevator muscles: the superior rectus *(SR)* and inferior oblique *(IO)*. The centre diagrams show the plan views of elevated right eye abducted, central, and adducted. The upper diagrams show a simple vector analysis of the relative actions of the elevator muscles as the eye moves across the upper motor field. In abduction, the superior rectus muscle is responsible for maintaining elevation. As the eye moves across the top of the field to the central position, the power of the superior rectus declines, while that of the inferior oblique increases. In the adducted position, the inferior oblique maintains the elevation and the elevating power of the superior rectus is at a minimum. For further description, see text.

rotation of the eye. Once this is understood, not only can the primary and secondary actions of these muscles be deduced, but also incomitant deviation can be analysed.

Fig. 17.2 shows the interaction of the two elevator muscles: the superior rectus and the inferior oblique. The central diagram shows the eye turned upwards from the primary position. Its elevation is maintained by the combined actions of both these muscles. Their individual contributions to the maintenance of elevation (E) is shown in the vector construction above the central diagram. The diagrams on the left of the figure show the way these two muscles contribute to elevation when the eye is turned outwards (abducted), and those on the right show the contribution of each when the eye is turned inwards (adducted). In the vector construction (Fig. 17.2), the sloping line SR shows how the power of the superior rectus to elevate the eye is at its maximum when the eye is abducted, and declines as the eye moves across the top of the motor field to the adducted position. The other sloping line IO indicates that the reverse is true of the oblique muscle: its elevating power is at a minimum when the eye is abducted and increases as the eye adducts. One muscle gradually takes over from the other as the eye moves across the top of the field. Fig. 17.3 shows a similar

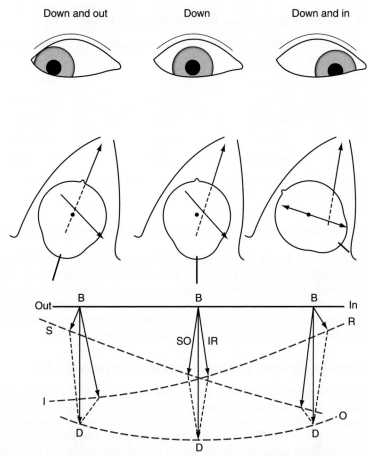

Fig. 17.3 The relative actions of the depressor muscles: the inferior rectus *(IR)* and superior oblique *(SO)*. The centre diagrams show the right orbit in plan view and the lower diagrams a simple vector analysis indicating the relative strengths of the depressor muscles as the eye moves in the lower motor field. For further explanation, see text.

treatment of the depressor muscles (the inferior rectus and the superior oblique) as the eye moves across the lower motor field in the depressed (D) positions.

The actions of the extraocular muscles in the primary position can be deduced from Figs. 17.1 and 17.2 and are given in Table 17.1. It is stressed that the actions of each muscle will change as the eye moves away from the primary position. The cardinal diagnostic positions of gaze are important in interpretation of the ocular motility test (see later), but knowledge of the actions of the muscles in the primary position is required to interpret the results of the cover test carried out in the primary position. An easy way to remember the secondary and tertiary actions of the cyclovertical muscles is RadSin: recti adduct, superiors intort (Hosking, 2001).

It has been suggested that fibroelastic sleeves, **muscle pulleys**, act as mechanical origins of the muscles and modify their actions (Kono, Poukens, & Demer, 2002; Demer, 2006), although this has been disputed (Jampel and Shi, 2006). In any event, a palsy or malfunction of one muscle will show as a failure of the eye to turn fully in the direction for which the muscle has the greatest mechanical advantage. For example, a palsy of the superior rectus muscle usually will be detected by

TABLE 17.1 ■ Actions of the Extraocular Muscles in the Primary Position.

Muscle	Primary action	Secondary action	Tertiary action
Medial rectus	adduction	none	none
Lateral rectus	abduction	none	none
Superior rectus	elevation	intorsion	adduction
Inferior rectus	depression	extorsion	adduction
Superior oblique	intorsion	depression	abduction
Inferior oblique	extorsion	elevation	abduction

From Ciuffreda, K.J., & Tannen, B. (1995). *Eye movement basics for the clinician*. St. Louis: Mosby.

the restricted movement when an attempt is made to elevate the eye when it is turned outwards (Fig. 17.2).

It can also be noted that as the primary functions of the vertically acting muscles decrease, their secondary functions increase slightly. Thus, when the eye is turned down and inwards, the inferior rectus is pulling nearly at right-angles to the visual axis and plays little part in depression. However, its ability to adduct the eye is increased as is its ability to cyclorotate the eye (extorsion) (Fig. 17.3).

The medial rectus muscle in each orbit is an adductor with little secondary function, and the lateral rectus is an abductor with little other function. These muscles are antagonists.

MUSCLE PAIRS, HERING'S LAW, AND SHERRINGTON'S LAW

Within one eye, **synergistic muscles** move the eye in the same direction. For example, the superior rectus and inferior oblique are ipsilateral synergists for elevation (but they are not synergists for horizontal or torsional movements). Conversely, the pair of extraocular muscles that move the eye in opposite directions can be thought of as **agonist/antagonist pairs**. For example, the superior and inferior rectus muscles are antagonistic for vertical and torsional movements (but not for horizontal movements). **Sherrington's law** of reciprocal innervation states that the contraction of a muscle is accompanied by simultaneous and proportional relaxation of its ipsilateral antagonist.

Sherrington's law applies to the muscles of one eye. The movements of two eyes as a team are described by Hering's law. Yoke muscles are pairs of muscles, consisting of one muscle from each eye, that produce simultaneous rotations of the eyes in either the same direction (conjugate movement) or opposite direction (disjugate movement). Hering's law relates the innervation of a muscle in one eye (the agonist) to its yoked muscle in the other eye, the contralateral synergist. Normally, the agonist in one eye and its contralateral synergist move the eyes in the same direction (e.g., the right superior oblique is the contralateral synergist of the left inferior rectus). **Hering's law of equal innervation** states that nerve impulses stimulating an agonist are equal to those stimulating its contralateral synergist.

PRIMARY AND SECONDARY DEVIATIONS

It was noted at the beginning of this chapter that if an incomitancy is present, the angle of deviation will differ according to which eye is fixating. This occurs because of Hering's law of equal innervation and will be explained by the example in Fig. 17.4. The top panel shows normal binocular fixation. ' + ' signifies innervation to the lateral and medial recti muscles. In the second and third panels, the left lateral rectus has suffered a paresis. In the second panel the nonparetic (right) eye

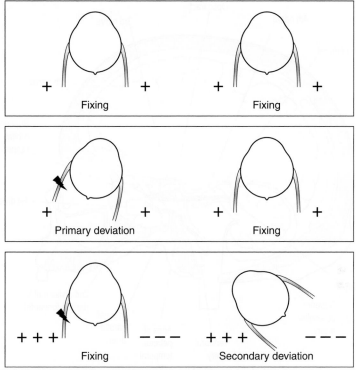

Fig. 17.4   Illustration of primary and secondary deviations. See text for explanation.

fixates, as is most commonly the case. There will be approximately equal innervation to the right lateral and medial recti, and therefore equal innervation to the left lateral and medial recti. Since the left lateral rectus is paretic, the left eye will be deviated inwards: the **primary deviation**.

In the bottom panel of Fig. 17.4, the same left lateral rectus muscle is paretic but now the less common situation pertains, when the patient fixates with the paretic eye. Excessive innervation (+++) is required to the paretic left lateral rectus to maintain fixation in the primary position, and inhibition to the left medial rectus (−−−). Hering's law means that the nonparetic right eye will also receive much greater innervation to the right medial rectus causing a very large **secondary deviation**, which is greater than the primary deviation that resulted when the nonparetic eye was fixating.

The difference between primary and secondary deviations has several clinical manifestations. During the cover test in the primary position, the size of the deviation when each eye is covered can be compared and if the deviation differs, this indicates the patient may have an incomitant deviation and can also indicate which eye has the under-acting muscle. Later in this chapter the use of the Maddox rod for comparing primary and secondary deviations will be discussed. The difference between primary and secondary deviations also explains why Hess and Lees screen plots are carried out twice, once with each eye fixating.

CLASSIFICATION OF INCOMITANT DEVIATIONS

Incomitant deviations can be classified as neurogenic (a problem with the nervous supply), myogenic (a problem with the muscle), or mechanical (where a muscle is mechanically restricted).

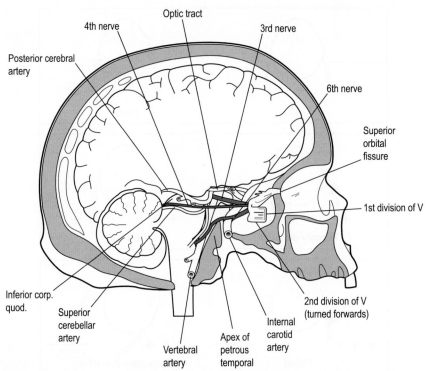

Fig. 17.5 Diagram illustrating part of the course of the nerves innervating the extraocular muscles. (Modified after Lindsay, R. (1941). *Neuro-ophthalmology* (p. 49). London: Heinemann.)

Three cranial nerves control the movements of the extraocular muscles: the fourth nerve (IV; trochlear) controlling the superior oblique muscle, the sixth nerve (VI; abducens) controlling the lateral rectus, and the third nerve (III; oculomotor) controlling the other extraocular muscles. These nerves have nuclei, and neurogenic deviations can be supranuclear, nuclear, or infranuclear depending on whether the lesion occurs above, at, or below the level of the relevant nucleus. Nuclear palsies are rarely isolated due to the extensive size of the causative lesion in most cases, so the clinical findings are complicated by involvement of adjacent supranuclear eye movement control centres (Ansons & Davis, 2001).

Fig. 17.5 illustrates the ocular cranial nerve pathways. The long pathway of the fourth and sixth nerves makes them prone to damage. The fourth nerve is particularly slender. Where the sixth nerve bends at the petrous temporal bone it is particularly prone to damage from compressive lesions from above following raised intracranial pressure, or from below such as following otitis media infection.

In myogenic palsies the primary problem affects the muscle itself rather than influencing its nerve supply or mechanically constricting the muscle. The most common example is myasthenia gravis.

Incomitancies that result from mechanical restriction are caused by elements within the orbit which either interfere with muscle contraction or otherwise prevent free movement of the globe. The restriction may be direct (e.g., tight or shortened muscle or tendon) or indirect (e.g., large retinal explant following retinal detachment surgery).

Incomitant deviations can also be classified as congenital or acquired. The main causes of acquired incomitant deviations are summarised in Table 17.2. Myasthenia gravis is not strictly neurological in origin: it results from an anomaly at the neuromuscular junction.

TABLE 17.2 ■ Main Causes of Acquired Incomitant Deviations.

Vascular	Neurological	Other
Diabetes	Tumour	Trauma
Vascular hypertension	Multiple sclerosis	Thyroid eye disease
Stroke	Migraine	Toxic
Aneurysm	(Myasthenia gravis)	Iatrogenic
Giant cell arteritis		Idiopathic

Acquired neurogenic palsies can be a sign of life-threatening pathology or of trauma. Nearly all myogenic palsies are acquired. Mechanical incomitancies can be congenital (e.g., Duane syndrome) or acquired (e.g., blow-out fracture). Depending on the cause, acquired incomitancies may undergo spontaneous partial or complete recovery. So, surgical intervention is often postponed until consecutive Hess plots have been stable for at least 6 months.

INCOMITANT DEVIATIONS AS A CAUSE OF DIPLOPIA

Moorfields Eye Hospital carried out a retrospective review of 171 patients presenting with diplopia (Comer, Dawson, Plant, Acheson, & Lee, 2006). One in five patients originated from optometrists. Monocular diplopia accounted for 11.5%, caused by factors relating to refractive error, bifocal segment, ectropion, entropion, corneal lesions, cataract, retinal lesions, and migraine (rarely, monocular diplopia or polyopia can result from central nervous system disease; Miller, 2011). Of the 146 patients with binocular diplopia, cranial nerve palsies accounted for 67% and the results are summarised in Table 17.3. Overall, 78.5% of cases had resolved after 12 months, with the best prognosis for incomitancies of a vascular origin.

A similar study from Scotland found 54% had an isolated nerve palsy (III, IV, or VI), 11% a mechanical cause, 10% dysfunction of higher control, 8% decompensation of existing phoria, 7% idiopathic, 5% monocular diplopia, and 5% another diagnosis. Fewer than 5% had serious underlying pathology that required immediate management.

A retrospective review of 300 hospital cases of vertical diplopia revealed the most common causes were congenital fourth nerve palsy (23%), thyroid eye disease (21%), and acquired fourth nerve palsy (9%) (Tamhankar, Kim, Ying, & Volpe, 2011). Other causes included ocular surgery, orbital fracture, neurosurgery, childhood strabismus, skew deviation, third nerve palsy, myasthenia gravis, and decompensated hyperphoria. The authors concluded that in most cases of hypertropia, the aetiology can be ascertained by history and eye examination alone. Two-thirds of patients did not have an observable limitation of eye movements.

Several systemic medications, particularly for epilepsy, can cause diplopia (Table 17.4), often from neurogenic palsies (Alves, Miranda, Narciso, Mieiro, & Fonseca, 2015). When a patient reports recent onset diplopia, it is advisable to ask about any new medication that was started around the time of the onset of the diplopia.

Investigation

Most of the remainder of this chapter is concerned with the detection of incomitant deviations and the interpretation of their significance. Most patients in need of urgent medical attention have symptoms that lead them to consult medical practitioners in the first instance. It is, however, important to be able to detect incomitancy, as it does not respond well to eye exercises and occasionally cases of

TABLE 17.3 ■ **Causes of Binocular Diplopia. The % column indicates the proportion of the cases who presented with binocular diplopia.**

Condition	%	Aetiology
Isolated VI nerve palsy	31	Commonly: hypertension or diabetes Occasionally: unknown Rarely: trauma, herpes zoster, myasthenia gravis, migraine, demyelination, Miller Fisher, neurosarcoidosis, malignancy, blocked ventriculoperitoneal shunt
Isolated IV nerve palsy	25	Commonly: hypertension or diabetes Occasionally: trauma, congenital, unknown Rarely: herpes zoster, migraine
Trauma	11	Occasionally: soft tissue trauma, orbital floor fracture
Myogenic	11	Occasionally: thyroid, myasthenia gravis Rarely: myositis, superior oblique myokymia, previous surgery
Isolated III nerve palsy	8	Commonly: vascular hypertension or diabetes Rarely: herpes zoster, myasthenia gravis, sinusitis, unknown
Decompensating heterophoria	3	Rarely: esophoria, exophoria, hyperphoria
Orbital	2	Rarely: metastases, cellulitis, dacryoadenitis
Combined IV & VI nerve palsy	1	Rarely: herpes zoster, migraine
Bilateral VI nerve palsy	1	Rarely: raised intracranial pressure

From Comer R.M., Dawson E., Plant G., Acheson J.F., Lee J.P. (2006). Causes and outcomes for patients presenting with diplopia to an eye casualty department. *Eye* 21(3), 413–418.

active pathology present themselves to community optometrists. The first indication of incomitancy may emerge during a routine eye examination, and additional tests may be required to confirm the diagnosis. The sections of the routine and appropriate additional tests are reviewed later.

HISTORY AND SYMPTOMS

Incomitant deviations due to recent injury or to active pathology nearly always have a sudden and dramatic onset of symptoms, sudden diplopia being the most usual. In long-standing deviations, the symptoms are seldom so disturbing to the patient, and of course they are usually reported as having been present for as long as the deviation. The following symptoms may be present:

1. *Diplopia* is often present in incomitancy but may not be present in heterophoric incomitancy nor in long-standing strabismic incomitancy. The patient may be able to recognise the variation in the degree of doubling in different direction of gaze. There is usually a vertical element in the diplopia. In long-standing cases, it may be intermittent due to sensory adaptations. Two-thirds of patients who acquire strabismus following brain damage (usually stroke or trauma) do not experience diplopia (Fowler et al., 1996).
2. *Asthenopia* may be present (Smith, 1979).
3. *Blurred vision* may be present if the condition involves the third cranial nerve which also serves the ciliary muscle. For the same reason, the pupil reflexes may be abnormal. Some patients describe small degrees of diplopia as blur.
4. *Dizziness or vertigo* may accompany incomitant heterophoria (Rabbetts, 2007). Normally, a change in the pattern of innervation to the extraocular muscles is associated with a particular movement of the retinal image. Incomitancy results in an imbalance between innervation

TABLE 17.4 ■ Drugs Associated with Diplopia.

Likelihood of diplopia	Drug	Main uses of drug
Very common (≥1 in 10)	Lacosamide	Epilepsy, diabetic neuropathic pain
	Zonisamide	Epilepsy, Parkinson disease
Common (between 1 in 10 and 1 in 100)	Eslicarbazepine	Epilepsy
	Botulinum toxin	Hemifacial spasm, cosmesis, EOM palsy
	Rufinamide	Epilepsy
	Pregabalin	Epilepsy, neuropathic pain
	Perampanel	Epilepsy
	Temozolomide	Cancer
	Sildenafil (Viagra)	Erectile dysfunction, pulmonary artery hypertension
	Gabapentin	Epilepsy, neuropathic pain
	Topiramate	Epilepsy, migraine
Uncommon (between 1 in 100 and 1 in 1000)	Zaleplon	Insomnia
	Levetiracetam	Epilepsy
	Bortezomib	Cancer
	Amlodipine	High blood pressure, coronary artery disease
	Adalimumab	Arthritis, spondylitis, Crohn disease
	Pravastatin	Hypercholesterolemia
	Lamotrigine	Epilepsy
	Capecitabine	Cancer
Rare (between 1 in 1000 and 1 in 10,000)	Telithromycin	Bacterial pneumonia
	Voriconazole	Fungal infections
	Dextromethorphan/Quinidine	PBA (an emotional disturbance)
	Sertraline	Depression, anxiety
	Ciprofloxacin	Bacterial infections

Modified after Alves M., Miranda A., Narciso M.R., Mieiro L., Fonseca T. (2015). Diplopia: a diagnostic challenge with common and rare etiologies. *American Journal of Case Reports* 16, 220–223.

and retinal image movement and this can make the patient's surroundings appear to move. If the paresis is mild, there may be an incomitant heterophoria rather than strabismus with diplopia. Hence, the symptoms of vertigo and dizziness may be reported.

5. *Other symptoms* due to the disease causing the incomitant deviation may be present; for example, headache in intracranial conditions, neoplasms, vascular disturbances, etc. The diseases most likely to be associated with incomitant deviations are dealt with in a later section of this chapter, where their symptoms are also summarised.

6. *General health deterioration* may also occur in accompanying metabolic disorders: loss of weight, changed appetite, general fatigue, loss of muscular ability, muscular tremor, breathlessness, etc.

7. *Injury* to the head or orbital regions may be reported, and this could cause damage to the muscular apparatus, intracranial bruising, and damage or pressure from haemorrhage. This can be recent or be the explanation of a long-standing incomitant deviation. In some cases, the patient may not have thought the injury serious enough to seek medical advice at the time. Injury during birth sometimes causes lateral rectus palsy or superior oblique palsy. An operation for a previous strabismus can sometimes cause a degree of incomitancy.

8. *Previous comitant strabismus* can result in an acquired incomitancy (see later).

ANOMALOUS HEAD POSTURES AND FACIAL ASYMMETRY

Acquired ocular torticollis is a type of anomalous head posture (AHP) that occurs in some patients with incomitant deviations, most commonly superior oblique paresis (Nucci, Kushner, Serafino, & Orzalesi, 2005). In nearly every case, the purpose of the AHP is to reduce the effect of the incomitancy, so the AHP turns the head towards the field of action of the affected muscle. Generally speaking, if the underacting muscle is horizontally acting, then there will be a head turn; if it is a torsional muscle (obliques), then there will be a head tilt; and if it is a vertically acting muscle, there will be an elevation or depression of the head. The most commonly encountered AHPs are for lateral rectus palsies (right lateral rectus palsy: head turn to right), superior oblique pareses (right superior oblique paresis: top of head tilted to patient's left), Duane syndrome (head turn), pattern deviations (elevation or depression), and Brown syndrome (may be turn, elevation, and tilt). Sometimes, a head tilt is adopted in a vertical incomitancy to level the diplopic images and so aid fusion. Common AHPs are detailed in Appendix 8. Normal amounts of head tilt (up to 30 degrees) do not affect reading speed (Firth, Machin, & Watkins, 2007).

The typical AHPs outlined earlier apply to the usual situation, when the purpose of the AHP is to reduce the effect of the incomitancy. Very rarely, an AHP may be adopted for the opposite reason: to exaggerate the effect of an incomitancy (von Noorden, 1996). For these rare cases, this can have two advantages: it can cause the deviation to break down and hence eliminate a symptomatic heterophoria, or it can cause diplopic images to move further apart making them easier to ignore. These cases are easy to detect because the patient will be strabismic when they view a straight-ahead object using their normal AHP. Another complication is that a compensatory head posture may be provoked not so much by the primary paralysis as by the modifications of other muscles induced by the paralysis (secondary sequelae).

An AHP that has been present for many years is frequently associated with facial asymmetry and this is found in more than 75% of patients with congenital palsy, typically from a congenital superior oblique palsy. The shallower side of the face is always on the side of the head tilt (Plager, 1999). The presence of a facial asymmetry is such a strong sign of an early onset that it may preclude the need for neurological investigation (Plager, 1999).

Because the usual purpose of an AHP is to preserve or enhance binocularity, the presence of an AHP suggests the patient has had binocularity at least at some time in the past. This improves the prognosis for treating sensory factors.

Other visual causes of AHPs are a visual field loss and to move the visual axes into the null zone in congenital nystagmus (Chapter 18). However, most (60%) cases of torticollis in children are nonvisual, mainly orthopaedic (Nucci et al., 2005), but also sometimes from unilateral deafness, shyness, or just habit.

EXTERNAL EXAMINATION OF THE EYES

General inspection may show an obvious strabismus. Scars or asymmetry of the orbital region may indicate previous injury. Some eye-signs of systemic disease may be seen in conditions which are sometimes accompanied by strabismus: exophthalmos, ciliary hyperaemia, ptosis, etc.

EYELID SIGNS

Eyelid abnormalities may sometimes be useful in indicating the presence of an incomitant deviation. The width of the palpebral fissure should be noted:
1. In the primary position when the right and left lid openings are compared. The width may be judged by the amount of the limbus visible through the lid openings. An abnormally wide fissure (Dalrymple's sign of thyrotoxicosis) may be accompanied by

hypophoria or hypotropia which increases on elevation of the eyes. Ptosis and diplopia which are both worse at the end of the day can be an early sign of myasthenia gravis. Ptosis can also be a sign of third nerve palsy. A hypotropic position of one eye may show a 'pseudoptosis'; the lid is slightly lower as the eye is turned down.

2. During the motility test, a lag of the lids on downward gaze (von Graefe's sign) may be present in thyrotoxicosis. A change in lid fissure, when looking left or right, usually accompanies Duane retraction syndrome (p. 279).

OPHTHALMOSCOPY AND FUNDUS PHOTOGRAPHY

The internal examination of the eyes may also provide further evidence of pathology such as those present in vascular conditions or metabolic disease. Indirect ophthalmoscopy and fundus photography can be used to provide an objective measure of ocular torsion in which the relative positions of the fovea and optic disc are noted. Normally, the fovea is 0.3 disc diameters below a horizontal line extending through the geometric centre of the optic disc. A variation of more than 0.25 disc diameters between the two eyes indicates cyclodeviation (von Noorden, 1996). Visual field analysis can also be used in a similar way. A problem with these approaches is their sensitivity to improper head position (Phillips and Hunter, 1999).

OCULAR MOTILITY TEST

The examination of ocular motility is an essential part of the detection of incomitancy. The ocular motility test allows a subjective, and an objective, check that:

1. both eyes move smoothly and follow the target;
2. there is a corresponding lid movement accompanying the vertical eye movements; and
3. there is no underaction or overaction of the movement of one eye in any direction of gaze.

The details of procedure for investigating the motility in routine examination are given in Chapter 2. This chapter is mainly concerned with determining the significance of any anomaly and with any additional tests which may give further information. The site of a muscle palsy can be determined from an understanding of the actions of the extraocular muscles, as described at the beginning of this chapter.

In the motility test, the patient is asked to keep the head still and to follow, with the eyes, a pen torch as it is moved into the different parts of the visual motor field. The patient is asked to report any diplopia, although patients with an incomitancy may not report any diplopia, owing to sensory adaptations. Often, the most useful information that the motility test gives relates to the practitioner's observation of the eye movements.

The fixation light is moved up and down in the median plane, so that lid movements and vertical eye movements (e.g., detecting gaze palsies) can be observed. In the method recommended by Boylan and Clement (1987), the light is then moved across the field at three levels: at the top, at eye level, and in the lower part of the motor field. This is done with the patient following the light with both eyes, so one eye's position can be judged relative to the other. A failure of one eye to follow the light in the top of the field indicates an anomaly of one of the elevators. To the patient's right and top, the affected muscle is likely to be either the right superior rectus or the left inferior oblique. Failure of one eye to turn to the right or to the left at eye level is likely to show an anomaly of either medial recti muscles or either lateral recti, and failure in the lower field shows a problem with one of the depressor muscles (Fig. 17.6). In these directions of gaze, each muscle has little or no secondary actions. Alternatively, some authors recommend that a 'star' technique is used where the pen torch is moved in the vertical, horizontal (at eye level), and four oblique positions (Mallett, 1988a).

It should be noted that Fig. 17.6 does not show muscle actions but shows the approximate directions in which the muscles have their greatest ability to move the eyes, excluding torsional

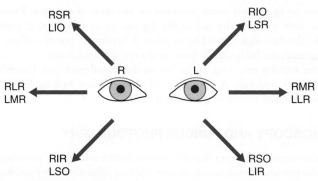

Fig. 17.6 The six cardinal diagnostic positions of gaze, indicating the muscles which should have maximum power to maintain the eyes in these directions. The paired synergists (muscles, one from each eye, which act together) are shown. *IO,* Inferior oblique; *IR,* inferior rectus; *L,* left; *LR,* lateral recti; *MR,* medial recti; *R,* right; *SO,* superior oblique; *SR,* superior rectus.

movements. These diagnostic positions of gaze are very different from the actions of the extraocular muscles in the primary position (Table 17.1). This is because the actions of each muscle will change as the eye moves. The cardinal diagnostic positions of gaze are important in interpretation of ocular motility results, but knowledge of the actions of the muscles in the primary position is required to interpret the results of the cover test carried out in the primary position.

The motility test is the only objective method available for standard clinical investigation of muscle paresis. Small deviations of one eye when it is in a tertiary position are not easy to detect. Observation of the corneal reflection of the fixation light will help, as will the symmetry of the lid and eye positions comparing dextroversion with laevoversion. Fortunately, from the detection point of view, underaction of a muscle is usually accompanied by an overaction in the paired synergic muscle which exaggerates the deviation.

Patients with active pathology usually have diplopia and this helps detection. Very small degrees of diplopia may be detected subjectively, which makes diagnosis more certain. During the motility test, therefore, the patient is asked to report any doubling and how this varies in different parts of the field. A diplopic image due to a paretic muscle is displaced in the same direction as the rotation which contraction of that muscle normally produces. The eye which sees the outermost diplopic image when the eyes look in the direction of maximum separation of the images is therefore the eye with the paretic muscle, and this eye can be identified by covering one eye. Subjective analysis of ocular motility can be assisted by using red and green diplopia goggles. A red goggle is worn before the right eye and a green one before the left. However, goggles prevent the eyes being observed.

It is useful to quantify the degree to which a deviation is incomitant, so any change can be monitored to assess if the condition is getting better or worse. This can be done by several methods and Appendix 8 is a worksheet for recording these results. This includes three variations of the motility test, including cover testing in peripheral gaze as described next. Incomitant deviations can be difficult to diagnose, and in incomitant cases, three versions of the motility test are often easiest to interpret if they are carried out separately (Chapter 2).

COVER TEST

In the primary position, the cover test can be used to compare the size of the deviation when the patient is fixating with either eye. The deviation is larger (secondary deviation) when the patient is fixating with their paretic eye than when they are fixating with the nonparetic eye (p. 250).

The cover test also can be used to measure the deviation in different positions of gaze during the motility test. The cover/uncover test, alternating cover test, or prism cover test can be used in peripheral gaze to provide further objective information on the motility test results. The alternating cover test is often easiest to interpret, but with just two to three alternate covers in each position of gaze to avoid causing greater dissociation than is necessary.

THE MADDOX ROD OR HAND FRAME

Primary and Secondary Deviations

The difference between primary and secondary deviations was explained earlier in this chapter. This phenomenon can be investigated (Appendix 8) with a Maddox rod test in the primary position, with the rod first in front of the strabismic eye (measuring the primary deviation) and then in front of the nonstrabismic eye (measuring the secondary deviation). If the two readings are different, this suggests an incomitancy (Borish, 1975). Unfortunately, the author has been unable to find any norms for determining what represents a significant difference between the two eyes with this test.

Deviation in Different Positions of Gaze

The Maddox rod can be used to measure the horizontal and vertical deviations in different directions of gaze (Appendix 8). Using a pen torch for fixation, the patient's head is kept still whilst measurements are taken in different parts of the field. It is important that the light is at a fixed distance and is moved to definite peripheral positions, so the test is repeatable. It is suggested that it is held at 50 cm from the eyes, and at the corners of a square formation in front of the patient, of 50 cm dimension.

Double Maddox Rod Test and Similar Approaches

In the double Maddox rod test, two Maddox rod lenses are placed, one in front of each eye, to measure cyclodeviation (Phillips & Hunter, 1999). The method is described on p. 133 and illustrated in Fig. 9.1. A significant cyclodeviation suggests the involvement of an oblique muscle.

The tilt of the retinal image is opposite to the tilt of the line as seen by the observer. So, if the patient reports that the line seen by their right eye is tilted with the outer end up, they have right ex-cyclodeviation, suggesting underaction of the right superior oblique. In summary, **the line is perceived to be tilted in the direction in which the underacting muscle would rotate the eye**.

Paresis of the superior oblique muscle can be very difficult to detect on motility testing (Brazis, 1993) and Simons, Arnoldi, and Brown (1994) stated that the double Maddox rod test is the standard test for investigating a superior oblique paresis. Theoretically, the test can demonstrate which eye(s) manifest the paresis. However, von Noorden (1996) cautioned that an ex-cyclodeviation in superior oblique paresis may occur in the nonparetic eye in patients who habitually fixate with the paretic eye owing to a monocular sensorial adaptation to the cyclodeviation. Sensory adaptations (harmonious anomalous retinal correspondence (HARC) or sensory cyclofusion) and motor cyclofusion (Phillips & Hunter, 1999) may explain why some patients with congenital superior oblique palsies have minimal subjective torsion with the double Maddox rod test (Plager, 1999).

Simons et al. (1994) stressed that both eyes should view through the same colour Maddox rod, in which case the paretic eye is correctly diagnosed in 94% of cases. A comparison of five methods of measuring ocular torsional movements found that the double Maddox rod was reliable when used in the primary position (Capdepon, Klainguti, Strickler, & van Melle, 1994), although Kraft, O'Reilly, Quigley, Allan, and Eustis (1993) found that the test was best at discriminating superior oblique palsies (normal/single/double pareses) in down-gaze.

A pair of Bagolini lenses can be used, with axes parallel, in an analogous way to the double Maddox rod test (von Noorden, 1996). When Bagolini lenses are used, the eyes are not dissociated, so the test is unlikely to work in strabismic cases where there is suppression and will be confounded in HARC. The result with this test may be similar to an assessment of the cyclodeviation with the Mallett fixation disparity test, which might be expected to have the same shortcomings with strabismic patients.

The Maddox wing test can be used to measure cyclodeviations and is straightforward to interpret. Very large cyclodeviations cannot be measured in this way. It is important to keep the patient's head and the instrument level.

Rabbetts (1972) described a prototype instrument, the cyclophorometer, that used polarised filters to dissociate the eyes. A similar principle is used in the commercially available torsionometer, in which the patient views a red and a green line on card through red/green goggles (Georgievski & Kowal, 1996). One of the lines is rotated until they are parallel, and the degree of torsion is recorded from the required rotation of the line. The test is less dissociating than the double Maddox rod test, but probably more dissociating than the Bagolini lens test. Even for patients with diplopia, where the eyes are effectively already dissociated, there is some variation (more than 5 degrees in 10% of patients) between different methods of measuring cyclodeviations (double Maddox rod, Maddox wing, synoptophore, torsionometer), although no particular test was responsible for the variation (Georgievski & Kowal, 1996).

SCREEN TESTS

Alternatives to the Hess screen, the Foster and Lancaster screens, employ similar principles to those described for the Hess screen. These methods provide the most thorough way of recording the degree of incomitancy and other information which will help assess progress of the condition. During all these tests, it is essential that the patient's head does not move.

Screen tests are essentially dissociation tests that are carried out in different positions of gaze. The deviation is plotted in space, and chart plots can give a precise measure of the deviation in different positions of gaze. Another important feature of the test is that it is carried out first with one eye fixating and then the plot is repeated, but with the other eye fixating. This is to differentiate between the primary and secondary deviation (p. 250).

Hess Screen

Modern Hess screens are grey in colour, so that the light from two projector torches can be seen on the screen. The patient sits at a distance of 50 cm. The screen is divided into 'squares' representing 5-degree rotations of the eyes. As the screen is flat, tangential to the line of sight, the squares are distorted into a pincushion pattern. The practitioner holds the red torch and the patient wears red/green diplopia goggles. On the screen, a red bar image from this torch can be seen only by the eye with the red goggle before it. Thus, when the patient is asked to look at the red bar image on the screen, the eye will be positioned so the red image falls on the fovea of that eye. The patient holds a green torch and is asked to shine its bar image on the screen so that it appears to cross the red bar. This subjective cross will be formed when the green bar of light is in such a position that its image falls on the fovea, as the fovea in each eye are corresponding points and have the same visual direction. Therefore, the positions of the bar images on the screen mark the points of intersection of the visual axes with the screen. The degree of any deviation can be estimated from the 5-degree marking. The relative positions are plotted in nine positions of gaze. Then, the goggles are changed round so that the red goggle is in front of the other eye, and the plot is repeated with this eye fixating and the first one deviated. A copy of the plot is made on a paper chart with each eye fixating in turn.

Some versions are internally illuminated, so that an LED is illuminated in the appropriate position (Fig. 17.7).

A computerised version of the Hess screen is available (Fig. 17.7 and Appendix 12) which allows plots (Fig. 17.10) to be obtained on standard desktop or laptop computers. Head position

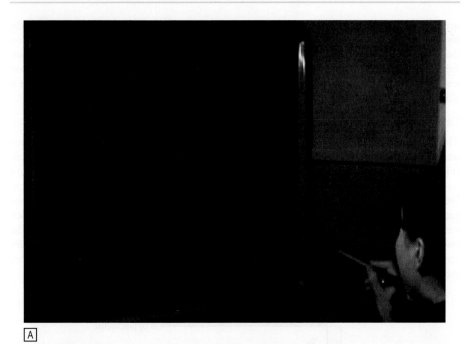

A

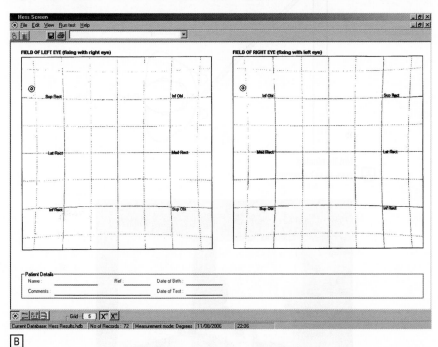

B

Fig. 17.7 The Hess screen test. The top panel (A) shows the conventional test and the low panel (B) shows the PC Hess screen.

needs to be carefully monitored, and too close a working distance might reduce the ability of the test to detect subtle lateral rectus palsies. The absence of the peripheral points that are present on the standard Hess chart might be a disadvantage with rare cases of subtle mechanical limitations, although in the author's experience this has not been a significant problem. A prototype of the test was described by Thomson, Desai, and Russell-Eggitt (1990) and a result recorded with the test is illustrated in Fig. 17.9.

Lees Screen

The Lees screen is a pair of Hess screens mounted at right angles, the markings showing only when internally illuminated. A pair of mirrors mounted back to back bisects the angle between the screens (Fig. 17.8). The patient initially faces the unilluminated screen and views the illuminated right screen with his or her right eye by reflection in the mirror. The patient is thus fixating with the right eye. The examiner uses a pointer to indicate a test position on the illuminated right screen and the patient uses a pointer to indicate the position to which the right pointer is projected on the left screen. The practitioner then presses a foot switch to briefly illuminate the left screen and plots the result relative to the correct position on a record chart (Fig. 17.8). This procedure is repeated for various test positions, as with the Hess screen. The standard pointers have circular targets, but they can be modified to bar targets to aid the investigation of torsional palsies.

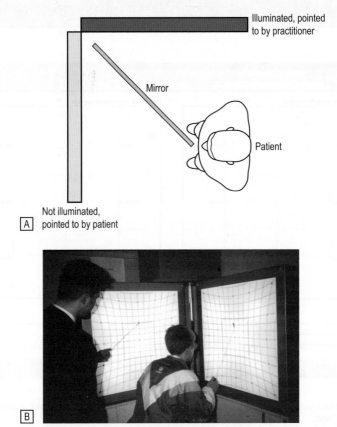

Fig. 17.8 The Lees screen test. The top panel (A) illustrates the principle of the test and the lower panel (B) shows the test in use (both panels are illuminated, as they are when the practitioner records the result).

Interpretation of Hess or Lees Screen Plots

It is important with these techniques that the results are plotted correctly, with the fixating eye recorded as such. With the Hess screen, the fixating eye sees the image projected by the examiner. With the Lees screen, the fixating eye sees the image which is constantly illuminated.

General Points (Worksheet in Appendix 8)

1. All counting of squares must be from the centre of the plot (result recorded), not from the centre of the chart (Fig. 17.9).
2. The test is, fundamentally, a dissociation test in different positions of gaze. When the central point is plotted, this is equivalent to a dissociation test in the primary position and the deviation should be revealed. If the deviation varies when different eyes are fixating, this suggests incomitancy.
3. The test is based on foveal projection, so the position of the plots indicates the position of the eyes. For example, if the left eye's plot is higher than the right, then there is left hypertropia.
4. It follows from (3) that the smallest plot will be from the eye with the underacting muscle(s) (Fig. 17.9). If it is difficult to tell which is the smaller plot, concentrate on a comparison of the height of the plot in vertical incomitancies and on the width in horizontal incomitancies.
5. The paretic muscle(s) can be found by looking for the smallest distance from the centre of the plot.
6. There should be an overaction of the contralateral synergist to the palsied muscle(s), and this will be very marked in a recent onset incomitancy. This overaction occurs because of Hering's law of equal innervation.
7. In a long-standing incomitancy, secondary sequelae usually will be apparent, as described later.
8. Sloping fields are indicative of an A- or V-pattern, not a cyclodeviation (although this may be present as well).
9. In mechanical incomitancies, secondary sequelae (see later) are not likely to be present and the deviation in the primary position does not reflect the extent of the defect.

LOCALISATION DISTURBANCES

The localisation of objects in space is determined visually by a combination of two mechanisms: retinal localisation, and the motor system's directional mechanism. The position of the image on the retina determines the direction in which it is perceived: its visual localisation. Because the eyes and head move, the brain must also take these movements into account in localising an object with respect to the egocentre. Eccentric fixation can cause a disturbance of the retinal system when the fixation point moves away from the centre of localisation at the fovea: past pointing occurs (Chapter 13).

The motor localisation system uses two types of information to register eye position. One of these is feedback from the extraocular muscles themselves (inflow), which is called muscle proprioception. The other is information which is copied within the brain from the centres that control movement to those that monitor eye position (**efferent copy**: outflow). Proprioception is a back-up to efferent copy (Bridgeman & Stark, 1991). If the eyes do not move correctly in response to the nerve impulses sent to the muscles, as in paretic strabismus, then the motor localisation system will be disturbed.

The past pointing test may be used to demonstrate these motor disturbances. The test is applied monocularly to each eye in turn, as described in Chapter 13. Past pointing will be demonstrated in the eye having the affected muscle and in the field of action of this muscle. The degree of past pointing will increase as the eye turns further into the direction of its action and will not occur in the opposite direction of gaze. This test can be made more effective by holding a card horizontally

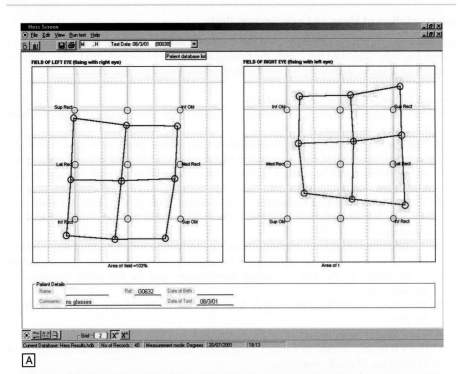

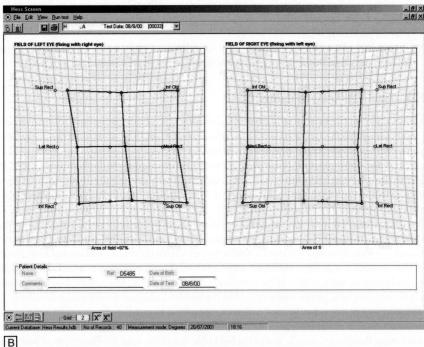

Fig. 17.9 Example plots from the PC Hess screen test. (A) right superior oblique muscle paresis; (B) mild left lateral rectus underaction; (C) recent paresis of left lateral rectus (caused by vascular hypertension); (D) same as (C) but partially resolved 1 month later (see also Appendix 13 and Digital Resource).

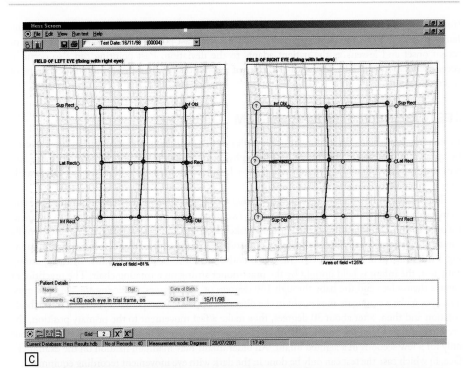

C

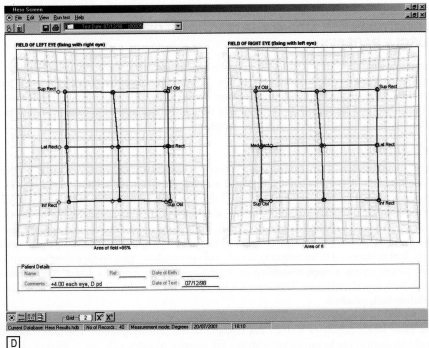

D

Fig. 17.9 (Continued).

(for horizontal deviations) at the level of the patient's chin, so that it occludes the patient's pointing hand from view while the target appears above the card. Past pointing only occurs with paresis of recent onset and lessens as the patient adapts to the deviation. Past pointing can also occur in eccentric fixation (p. 184), where it is typically of a lesser degree than in incomitant deviations of recent onset.

TESTING THE VESTIBULAR SYSTEM

In supranuclear lesions the vestibular ocular reflex (VOR) will be maintained, but in those caused by infranuclear lesions it will not. The VOR is phylogenetically the oldest slow eye movement system and, because it does not require visual feedback, it has a short latency. Horizontal VOR is well-developed at birth; the vertical VOR develops a little later.

The VOR can be tested to investigate whether a gaze palsy is supranuclear or infranuclear, and to investigate poor abduction in an infant. The two most common ways of testing the VOR are as follows. In the Doll's head test, the patient is asked to fixate an object while the examiner rapidly rotates the patient's head, first in the horizontal and then in the vertical plane. A normally functioning VOR will result in eye movements equal and opposite to head movements. In the spinning baby test, the infant is held upright by the practitioner sitting on a rotating chair. The practitioner rotates themselves and the baby through 180 degrees or 360 degrees, observing the patient's eyes. The eyes make a conjugate movement in the direction opposite (compensatory) to that of the body rotation and then, after about 30 degrees, they make a fast movement to the primary position, the cycle repeating. Once the rotation is stopped there may be some post-rotational nystagmus, but only for a few seconds in a sighted infant. An older infant may maintain fixation on the examiner's face, in which case the test can only be done in the dark with eye movement recording equipment.

ALGORITHMS FOR AIDING THE DIAGNOSIS OF VERTICAL MUSCLE PARESES

The diagnosis of the paretic muscle(s) is fairly straightforward in horizontal deviations, but is more complicated in cyclovertical deviations (Spector, 1993). Three algorithms (e.g., three-steps tests) have been developed to help practitioners detect the paretic muscle(s) in cyclovertical deviations, and these will now be described. The principles behind the various tests in these methods can be understood from the earlier sections of this chapter.

The Lindblom 70-cm Rod Method

A very simple method of qualitatively investigating cyclovertical incomitancies is to use a 70-cm rod held horizontally, 1 m in front of the patient (Lindblom, Westheimer, & Hoyt, 1997). If a 70-cm rod cannot be found, a 50-cm ruler will suffice (Table 17.5). The patient is asked to describe whether the rod is single or double and, if double, whether tilted (indicating faulty oblique muscle(s)) or parallel (indicating faulty vertical recti muscle(s)). If tilted, the patient's perception typically resembles an arrow (e.g., ∠) which points towards the side of the eye with the paretic muscle. The muscle can be further identified by investigating the effect of up- and down-gaze on the patient's perception. If the patient reports a shape resembling an ✕, it suggests there may be a double oblique paresis, usually both superior obliques. This approach is summarised in Table 17.5, and is included in the worksheet in Appendix 8.

This test is delightfully straightforward, and a modified version can be used in patients who have more subtle deviations and are not diplopic in the primary position. For these cases, the Lindblom method can be carried out with two full aperture Maddox rods, one in front of each eye, placed so that the patient sees two horizontal lines when viewing a spotlight, if necessary with a vertical prism as in the double Maddox rod test.

TABLE 17.5 ■ **Procedure for Lindblom's Method of Differentially Diagnosing Cyclovertical Incomitancies.**

THE PATIENT VIEWS A 70-CM WOODEN ROD, OR USE MADDOX RODS (SEE TEXT).

Test instructions	Indicative paretic muscles
1. Move the wooden rod (or spotlight) up and down. Where is the vertical diplopia (or separation of the red lines) greatest, in upgaze or downgaze?	Upgaze: RSR, RIO, LSR, LIO Downgaze: RIR, RSO, LIR, LSO
2. In the position of maximum diplopia, are the two images parallel or tilted (torsional)?	Parallel: RSR, RIR, LSR, LIR Torsional: RSO, RIO, LSO, LIO
3. If parallel, does the separation increase on right or left gaze?	Right gaze: RSR, RIR Left gaze: LSR, LIR
4. If tilted, does the illusion of tilt increase in upgaze or downgaze?	Upgaze: RIO, LIO Downgaze: RSO, LSO
5. If tilted, the two rods will resemble an arrow (< or >) or an X. If they resemble an arrow, which way does the arrow point?	Arrow to R: RSO, RIO Arrow to L: LSO, LIO
6. If crossed, does the tilt angle increase in upgaze or downgaze?	Upgaze: bilateral IO paresis[a] Downgaze: bilateral SO paresis

[a]Very unlikely. *IO*, Inferior oblique; *IR*, inferior rectus; *L*, left; *R*, right; *SO*, superior oblique; *SR*, superior rectus.

TABLE 17.6 ■ **Parks' Method.**

Test instructions	Indicative paretic muscles
1. Which eye is hyper (relatively, elevated)?	R/L: RSO, RIR, LIO, LSR L/R: RIO, RSR, LSO, LIR
2. Is the vertical deviation greater in right or left gaze?	R gaze: RSR, RIR, LIO, LSO L gaze: LSR, LIR, RIO, RSO
3. Is the vertical deviation greater with head tilt to R or L?	R tilt: RSO, RSR, LIO, LIR L tilt: RIO, RIR, LSO, LSR

IO, Inferior oblique; *IR*, inferior rectus; *L*, left; *R*, right; *SO*, superior oblique; *SR*, superior rectus.

Parks' Method

There are three questions that are considered in Parks' method, each of which narrows down the paretic extraocular muscle. These questions are summarised in Table 17.6: each question is followed by a list of the muscles which are suggested as possibly paretic by the answer to the question. A right hypotropia is treated as a left hypertropia, and a left hypotropia as a right hypertropia. A clinical worksheet is included in Appendix 8. Vazquez described a simple graphical method of recording and analysing the results (Vazquez, 1984).

When the results of the three questions are combined, the paretic muscle should be identified. The last question utilises the Bielschowsky head tilt test, which should be carried out with the patient seated upright fixating at 3 m (Finlay, 2000). When the head is tilted to the right, normally the right eye intorts from actions of the right superior oblique and right superior rectus. With weakness of the right superior oblique, the right superior rectus acts alone to accomplish intorsion and this causes a marked elevation of the right eye. The elevation occurs because the superior rectus

TABLE 17.7 ■ Scobee's Method.

Test instructions	Indicative paretic muscles
1. Which eye is hyper (relatively, elevated)?	R/L: RSO, RIR, LIO, LSR L/R: RIO, RSR, LSO, LIR
2. Is the vertical deviation greater at distance (primary position) or at near (adducted)?	D: RSR, RIR, LSR, LIR N: RSO, RIO, LSO, LIO
3. Which eye is fixating when there is the greatest vertical deviation?	R: RSR, RIR, RSO, RIO L: LSR, LIR, LSO, LIO

IO, Inferior oblique; *IR*, inferior rectus; *L*, left; *R*, right; *SO*, superior oblique; *SR*, superior rectus.

receives a larger signal than usual, has a primary action of elevation, and receives less opposition than usual from the superior oblique.

Parks' method is not infallible, and the result is confounded by several factors (Spector, 1993): contracture of vertical recti muscles, paresis of more than one muscle, where there is a restrictive (mechanical) aetiology, skew deviation, previous strabismus surgery, myasthenia gravis, dissociated vertical divergence, and small nonparetic vertical deviations with horizontal strabismus. Many, if not all, of these factors will also affect the result of Scobee's method described next.

Research indicates the test is particularly poor at detecting cases where there is superior oblique atrophy, which is found in the three-quarters of cases where there is denervation (Manchandia & Demer, 2014). The sensitivity of the test can be improved in these cases from 70% to 84% if step two is omitted, although there will be an as yet unknown loss of specificity. These authors cautioned 'the cumulative evidence argues that it may not be possible to reliably diagnose superior oblique palsy on clinical grounds'.

Scobee's Method

Another three-step method was described by Scobee (1952), particularly for hyperphoria, and is given in Table 17.7. Again, each question is followed by a list of the muscles which are suggested as possibly paretic by the answer to the question. The second question in Scobee's method relies on the greater action of the vertical recti when the eyes are abducted, as during distance vision, and the maximal vertical actions of the oblique muscles when the eyes are adducted, as during near vision. The third question relies on the secondary deviation being greater than the primary deviation (p. 250). The clinical worksheet in Appendix 8 includes Scobee's method.

Evaluation

MUSCLE SEQUELAE OF PALSIES

Clearly, a muscle palsy will result in an underaction of the affected muscle (the primary deviation). When the patient is fixating with the affected eye (or binocularly), there will also be an overaction of the contralateral synergist (the secondary deviation; see Fig. 17.4), as predicted by Hering's law. This is the largest overaction in the sequelae, and occurs at onset, increasing over the first week (Stidwill, 1998).

Over time, other muscles become affected: motor secondary sequelae occur. It is important to accurately recognise secondary sequelae, because they help the practitioner to decide whether an incomitancy is new or old. In a long-standing incomitancy, one of the following two secondary sequelae may also occur (Mallett, 1988a).

1. If the nonparetic eye is used for everyday fixation, the ipsilateral antagonist to the palsied muscle will be in a permanently contracted state. Consequently, some of the elastic tissue in this muscle may be replaced by fibrous tissue. This results in contracture, which occurs within days to weeks (Finlay, 2000) or about 4 weeks (Stidwill, 1998) after the original palsy. This exaggerates the original deviation and manifests as an enlargement of the Hess plot in the field of action of the ipsilateral antagonist (Fig. 17.9). If possible, this contracture should be avoided, for example by prescribing alternate occlusion.

2. If the patient fixates with the paretic eye in everyday vision, Hering's law may result in a constant overaction of the contralateral synergist to the palsied muscle (the secondary deviation; Fig. 17.4). There may also be an inhibitional palsy of the contralateral antagonist (Mallett, 1969). To give a common example, if a patient has a right superior oblique palsy and fixates with the right eye, there will be an overaction of the contralateral synergist (left inferior rectus) and underaction (inhibition) of the contralateral antagonist (left superior rectus). This inhibitional palsy can be greater than the original palsy (Stidwill, 1998) and the effect of this may be to make the patient's ocular motility less incomitant with time. This is sometimes referred to as a 'spreading of the comitance' and occurs between 2 and 9 months after the original palsy (Stidwill, 1998).

If the patient sometimes fixates with either eye, secondary sequelae are less frequently found (Mallett, 1969). The literature is not clear about the situation when the patient has a palsy but is most of the time heterophoric, as often happens with superior oblique palsies. It seems likely these cases are unlikely to exhibit secondary sequelae, at least if they are binocular most of the time.

DIFFERENTIATING INCOMITANCIES THAT ARE LONG-STANDING FROM THOSE OF RECENT ONSET

The first priority with incomitant deviations is to decide if there is an active pathological cause requiring immediate medical attention, or if it is a long-standing deviation. Table 17.8 summarises the factors that help in this evaluation.

The Aetiology of the Incomitancy

One of the differences between deviations of recent pathological cause and more long-standing deviations is that there may be other symptoms of the general pathological condition. It is therefore useful to be aware of the primary conditions which can give rise to incomitant deviations and of the other signs and symptoms that may accompany them. There is a very large number of these conditions and general categories are summarised in Table 17.2, with more specific examples in Table 17.3. In Table 17.2, the conditions are divided into three categories to make them easier to remember rather than as a strict taxonomy. Some of these aetiologies may have incomitant diplopia as an early sign. In other conditions, the deviation may occur as part of the possible progress of the disease for which the patient is already under treatment. The patient's medical adviser needs to be made aware of this development. An awareness of relevant anatomy is helpful (Evans, 2004a, 2004b).

Some of the most common of the conditions which may be associated with ocular muscle palsy are described here. The other general symptoms that can accompany the diplopia are also given as a means of helping to confirm the diagnosis of the deviation as of recent pathological cause.

1. *Diabetes:* Ocular palsy from diabetes usually affects the third cranial nerve and may sometimes involve the pupil reflex and reduce the amplitude of accommodation. The palsy is usually unilateral and of sudden onset, often with pain. Most cases recover within 2–3 months, but can recur (Baker, 2000). The symptoms of diabetes may include, in addition to the diplopia, generalised headache, increased thirst and urination, increased appetite with loss of weight, constipation, boils, or other skin conditions. Older patients are mostly overweight.

2. *Thyroid Eye Disease:* This can occur with muscle palsy and is described on p. 281.

TABLE 17.8 ■ Summary of Main Factors to be Considered in Assessing Incomitant Deviations for Active Pathology.

Factor	Congenital or long-standing	Recent onset
Diplopia	Unusual	Usually present in at least one direction of gaze
Onset	Patient does not know when the deviation began	Usually sudden and distressing
Amblyopia	Often present	Absent (almost always)
Comitance	More comitant with time	Always incomitant
Secondary sequelae	Usually present	Absent, except for overaction of contralateral synergist
Fusion range	May be large in vertical incomitancies	Usually normal
Facial asymmetry	May be present	Absent, unless from trauma
Abnormal head posture (AHP) (if present)	Slight, but persists on covering paretic eye; patient often unaware of reason for AHP	More marked; the patient is aware of it (to avoid diplopia); disappears on covering paretic eye
Past pointing in field of paretic muscle	Absent	Present
Old photographs	May show strabismus or anomalous head posture	Normal
Other symptoms	Unlikely	May be present due to the primary cause

3. *Vascular hypertension:* the chances of hypertension being accompanied by ocular palsy increases with age as the blood supply to the cranial nerves becomes involved. In addition to the vascular changes seen on the fundus, symptoms may include headache, dizziness, breathlessness, and ringing in the ears.

4. *Aneurysms:* The ocular palsy may be accompanied by frontal pain on the same side. The symptoms of hypertension may also be present.

5. *Temporal (giant cell) arteritis:* Marked temporal pain and tenderness is present with intermittent diplopia, loss of appetite and general lassitude. The pain may be noticed on brushing the hair or chewing and there may also be a sudden loss of vision. The ocular palsy occurs in a minority of patients and before the loss of vision begins.

6. *Multiple sclerosis:* Ocular palsy is an early sign in about half the patients, who are usually under 40 years. Other symptoms include paresthesias, and weakness or clumsiness of a leg or hand. This condition can begin with optic neuritis and be associated with reduced visual acuity, scotomata, pain in one eye, as well as diplopia.

7. *Myasthenia gravis:* This is an uncommon myogenic incomitancy which can occur at any age and is described on p. 277.

8. *Tumours:* For example, sixth nerve palsies can be associated with acoustic neuroma, when there is a loss of hearing, corneal sensitivity, and sometimes an impaired blink reflex, and acquired nystagmus (Douglas, 2002).

While it is useful, in diagnosis of a pathological cause, to note some of the symptoms mentioned here, it must be remembered that many other conditions can cause incomitant deviations. Additionally, a long-standing palsy can **decompensate** at any time. Sometimes this decompensation can be explained by other factors such as poor general health, pregnancy (Jacobson, 1991), trauma, stress, or interruption to sensory fusion (Schuler, Silverberg, Beade, & Moadel, 1999). In other cases, the decompensation can be spontaneous.

DIFFERENTIATING NEUROGENIC FROM MYOGENIC AND MECHANICAL INCOMITANCIES

Several methods can be used to differentially diagnose a neurogenic from a myogenic or mechanical incomitancy. These are summarised in Table 17.9 (Spector, 1993). In 62% of ocular motor cranial nerve palsies from microvascular ischaemia, there is pain, typically in the ipsilateral brow or eye (Wilker, Rucker, Newman, Biousse, & Tomsak, 2009). There was no significant difference in the prevalence of pain in participants who were diabetic or not.

NEUROGENIC PALSIES

Another aspect which can help in the diagnosis of incomitant deviations is the recognition of particular cranial nerve palsies which are given here. Reviews have detailed the pathway of the cranial nerves (Evans, 2004a) and vasculature of these and the extraocular muscles (Evans, 2004b). A summary of the relative likelihood of a cranial nerve palsy affecting a given nerve is included in Table 17.3 and on p. 253.

Migraine is a rare cause of incomitancy (ophthalmoplegic migraine) in children and adults with migraines of worsening severity and with diplopia occurring nearly always during (rarely within 24 hours of) a migraine attack (Lal, Sahota, Singh, Gupta, & Prabhakar, 2009). It can involve VI (57%), III (34%), or IV (8%) nerves and complete recovery is expected with migraine medication, accelerated by steroids (Lal et al., 2009).

TABLE 17.9 ■ Summary of the Differential Diagnosis of Neurogenic, Myogenic, and Mechanical Incomitancies.

Test	Neurogenic	Myogenic	Mechanical
Comparison of results of binocular and monocular motility testing	Apparent on binocular testing but most cases are not apparent on monocular testing	Likely to be apparent on monocular motility test as well as binocular. The muscle may be unable to contract or relax	
Appearance of underaction on motility testing	Underaction becomes gradually apparent as target moves into field of action of the affected muscle	Difficult to interpret because several muscles may be involved	Underaction becomes abruptly apparent as move into field of action of affected muscle. Sometimes, crossing of diplopia – the eye that sees the outermost image changes in opposite directions of gaze
Secondary sequelae	Usually present	Not usually present	Not present. Only over-action of the contralateral synergist will occur
Intraocular pressures in different positions of gaze	Will not vary	Will not vary	Will vary
Forced duction test	No resistance to passive movement	No resistance to passive movement	Resistance to passive movement
Saccadic velocities	Abnormally slow	Abnormally slow	Close to normal limits

Fourth Nerve (Superior Oblique) Palsy

A fourth nerve palsy is the most frequently diagnosed form of vertical strabismus (Tollefson et al., 2006). In 92 patients presenting with superior oblique palsy under the age of 8 years, there were no cases where it was associated with the development of new intracranial pathology (Tarczy-Hornoch & Repka, 2004). Sometimes, a superior oblique palsy can decompensate following refractive surgery, particularly if monovision is induced (Godts et al., 2004; Schuler et al., 1999). Contact lens monovision can also induce decompensation (Evans, 2007a).

Congenital Fourth Nerve Palsy

About three-quarters of superior oblique pareses are congenital, but many cases do not present until adulthood when they decompensate (Plager, 1999), sometimes during pregnancy (Jacobson, 1991), and sometimes secondary to a different extraocular muscle palsy (Metz, 1986). A review of high-resolution MRI scan research concluded that approximately three-quarters of congenital cases (the ones most likely to have a head tilt from the first year of life) have an absence of the trochlear nerve and significantly smaller superior oblique muscle and the other quarter had a normal nerve and muscle (Engel, 2015).

Superior oblique palsies may be characterised by a head tilt away from the affected side and, in long-standing cases, there may be a corresponding facial asymmetry (Plager, 1999). Surgical intervention in the first year of life may prevent the facial asymmetry, but this advantage needs to be balanced against the risks of surgery at this age (Engel, 2015).

Acquired Fourth Nerve Palsy

The trochlear nerve is the thinnest of the cranial nerves and is the only motor nerve that arises from the dorsal aspect of the central nervous system (Warwick, 1976). Its long pathway means that it is particularly prone to damage in closed head injuries (Table 17.3). According to Plager (1999), more than half of acquired superior oblique palsies result from trauma, one-third are iatrogenic, and other causes include tumour and, very rarely, aneurysm. Another study agreed that most cases result from indirect injury to the skull, with most spontaneous cases having a vascular aetiology (Neetens & Janssens, 1979). These authors report vascular cases usually recover spontaneously but traumatic cases do not.

Plager (1999) stated that to cause a superior oblique paresis, trauma had to be substantial, whereas von Noorden (1996) argued that it often followed only a mild concussion. Trauma can cause bilateral superior oblique palsies (discussed later), which can be asymmetric and thus easy to misdiagnose as unilateral (Lee & Flynn, 1985).

Investigation

Superior oblique palsies can be difficult to detect on motility testing (Brazis, 1993) and patient descriptions of the position of gaze in which there is maximum vertical diplopia are often unhelpful (Fig. 17.10 and Appendix 13 with the cases on **Digital Resource**). The double Maddox rod test is a useful tool for investigating superior oblique palsies, but it has only limited usefulness for diagnosing bilateral superior oblique involvement. This test is discussed on p. 133. The cyclodeviation may be manifest in the eye that is contralateral to the one with the original palsy.

If the patient is asked to tilt the head to the other side, the affected eye elevates (the Bielschowsky head tilting test; p. 267). The head tilt can disappear in early adolescence, and there may be binocular vision in the primary position.

Congenital palsies may be hard to detect, even with the double Maddox rod or torsionometer tests (p. 260) because of sensory adaptations (HARC or sensory cyclofusion) and motor cyclofusion (Phillips & Hunter, 1999). Objective cyclotorsion can be assessed from fundus photography, but objective (and subjective) torsion can switch to the nonpalsied eye over a 6-month period (Kushner & Hariharan, 2009). Therefore, the eye in which the objective torsion is present is not necessarily the eye with the palsy. Indeed, in acquired unilateral superior oblique palsy, the eye manifesting

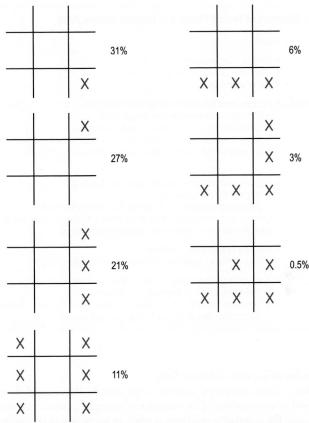

Fig. 17.10 Position of gaze for maximum hypertropia in right superior oblique palsies (illustrated from practitioner's perspective). The diagrams show, for a right superior oblique palsy, the position of gaze in which the hyperdeviation is greatest. For example, the first panel shows that 31% of cases have a maximum hyperdeviation when looking down and in, the next panel down shows 27% of cases have maximum hyperdeviation when looking up and in, and so on. Most cases do not exhibit the predicted pattern of maximum hypertropia in the field of action of the superior oblique muscle. (Modified after von Noorden, G.K. (1996). *Binocular vision and ocular motility* (5th ed.). St. Louis: Mosby).

the excyclotorsion is not necessarily the same eye that manifests hypertropia (Lee, Chun, Baek, & Kim, 2013).

A useful sign in congenital superior oblique palsies is the patient may have vertical fusional reserves in excess of 10Δ (Finlay, 2000). Reports of image tilting are said to be diagnostic for acquired superior oblique palsy (von Noorden, Murray, & Wong, 1986). Patients with superior oblique pareses who can achieve binocular single vision and who have astigmatism over 1.00DC should have their astigmatic axes determined under binocular viewing conditions (Rutstein & Eskridge, 1990).

Management
The superior oblique muscle has been described as the 'reading muscle' and patients often adapt to the palsy by holding text higher than usual. Bifocals and varifocals may therefore be contraindicated or may require a vertical prism in the near vision portion of the lens (Erickson & Caloroso, 1992). Prisms may be of benefit to patients with a small relatively comitant deviation from a unilateral (Plager, 1999) or bilateral (Lee & Flynn, 1985) superior oblique palsy.

The key typical features of a superior oblique palsy are summarised in Table 17.10.

TABLE 17.10 ■ Summary of Typical Features of Superior Oblique Palsy.

Feature	Detail
Aetiology	• Can be congenital or acquired • Trauma (quite commonly road traffic accident) • Other aetiologies

Symptoms (if recent onset)	• Diplopia that is predominantly vertical and is
	  • Possibly described as one image tilted
	  • More marked at near (downgaze) than distance
	  • More marked when looking down and inward (for the affected eye)
	• Also, may be symptoms related to the aetiology of the palsy

Clinical signs	• Head tilt and/or chin tucked down
	• Hyperdeviation in the affected eye, which is larger:
	  • At near than at distance
	  • When looking down and inward (for the affected eye)
	• Underaction of superior oblique on motility testing. In long-standing cases, there can be a variety of secondary sequelae (see below)

Management	• If recent onset: urgent referral • If long-standing: varifocals or bifocals are contraindicated

Additional comments	• A superior oblique palsy can be difficult to detect on motility because:
	  • The main action of the muscle is torsional
	  • The nose and lids can obstruct the view of the eye when looking down and in
	  • Secondary sequelae may be present (see below)

Secondary Sequelae of Superior Oblique Palsy

In superior oblique palsies, secondary sequelae often obscure the original deviation (p. 268). Typically, there will be an overaction of the contralateral synergist (contralateral inferior rectus). In cases that fixate with the nonparetic eye, there is often an overaction of the ipsilateral antagonist (inferior oblique). This can cause the hypertropia to be greatest when the eye with the original paresis looks up and in (von Noorden, 1996).

Patients who habitually fixate with their paretic eye may develop an inhibitional palsy of the contralateral antagonist (contralateral superior rectus). This can cause the hyperdeviation to be greatest in upgaze (Fig. 17.10). Von Noorden (1996) argued that this occurs even when patients do not fixate with their paretic eye and is attributable to an overaction of the ipsilateral inferior oblique when the patient is looking up and in. His data from 200 patients explain why reports of vertical diplopia during the motility test so often lead to confusion in diagnosing a superior oblique paresis (Fig. 17.10). The key to uncovering whether a superior rectus palsy results from a contralateral superior oblique paresis is to test for a cyclodeviation, and to carry out Bielschowsky's head tilt test.

Some patients who fixate with their paretic eye also manifest a pseudo-overaction of the contralateral superior oblique, which has been attributed to a contracture of the ipsilateral superior rectus (von Noorden, 1996), which prevents the paretic eye from looking downwards when abducting (Plager, 1999). Surgical overcorrection of a unilateral superior oblique paresis can masquerade as an apparent contralateral superior oblique muscle paresis (masked bilateral superior oblique muscle paresis) (Ellis, Stein, & Guyton, 1998).

Bilateral Superior Oblique Palsy

Bilateral superior oblique palsy is nearly always acquired, typically following closed head trauma (e.g., in a road accident) or, uncommonly, from a tumour in the dorsal midbrain (Barr et al., 1997).

Although it is rare, it should be suspected in all severe head injuries (Lee & Flynn, 1985). The condition can be asymmetric and may appear to be unilateral on motility testing, so bilateral cases are often misdiagnosed as unilateral (Lee & Flynn, 1985). It is unusual for a single superior oblique muscle palsy to cause an excyclotropia over 8 degrees (Spector, 1993); a bilateral superior oblique palsy causes an excyclotropia that is nearly always over 5 degrees (Lee & Flynn, 1985) and often over 10 degrees (Plager, 1999). However, Plager (1999) cautioned that this type of measurement does not allow an infallible diagnosis and von Noorden (1996) found little difference between the magnitude of the excyclotropia for unilateral and bilateral cases. Von Noorden (1996) listed two signs which are never present in unilateral cases and which may be present in bilateral cases: right hypertropia in left gaze and left hypertropia in right gaze and a positive Bielschowsky test with the head tilted to either side. Additionally, bilateral superior oblique palsies often cause subjective complaints of torsion, a chin-down head posture, and a V-syndrome.

Sixth Nerve (Lateral Rectus) Palsy

According to some authors, this is the most common ocular cranial nerve palsy (King, Stacey, Stephenson, & Trimble, 1995; Santiago & Rosenbaum, 1999).

Congenital Sixth Nerve Palsy

Congenital bilateral lateral rectus palsy produces an alternating convergent strabismus with equal acuities. In unilateral cases, the face is turned towards the affected side.

Acquired Sixth Nerve Palsy

The long intracranial path of the sixth nerve makes it particularly susceptible to lesions associated with skull fractures and raised intracranial pressure. Raised intracranial pressure is most likely to involve the nerve where it passes over the apex of the petrous temporal bone (Fig. 17.5). Rare cases of benign intracranial hypertension, which can result from endocrine disorders including obesity, can result in sixth nerve palsy, headache, and transient visual loss (Ramadan, 1996). Because of the close association of the sixth and seventh cranial nerves in the mid-brain, the facial muscles also may be involved in some sixth nerve palsies. Children may have a transient sixth nerve paresis following a viral illness that should improve in about 6 weeks. However, prompt referral is still appropriate. Vascular hypertension is a cause in adults.

Bacterial infection of the middle ear can spread to the petrous temporal bone affecting both the sixth and fifth (causing head pain) nerves. This condition (Gradenigo syndrome) was common before antibiotics became widely used. The sixth nerve may be involved in acoustic neuroma, and these cases will exhibit diminished hearing and corneal sensitivity (Swann, 2001).

Arnold-Chiari or Chiari malformations are congenital structural defects in the cerebellum. The indented bony space at the lower rear of the skull is smaller than normal, causing the cerebellum and brainstem to be pushed downward. Symptoms including dizziness, muscle weakness, numbness, vision problems, headache, and problems with balance and coordination. There are three primary types of Arnold-Chiari malformations. The most common is type I, which sometimes only produces symptoms in late childhood or early adulthood. Acute esotropia can be an early sign, as can downbeat nystagmus (Russell, Wick, & Tang, 1992). The esotropia may be comitant, divergence palsy (Lewis, Kline, & Sharpe, 1996), or lateral rectus palsy (Miki, Ito, Kawai, & Nakanishi, 1999). Patients need to be referred for early decompression surgery (Russell et al., 1992).

A report of over 200 patients with sixth nerve palsy of unknown aetiology found that 36% recovered in 8 weeks, and 84% recovered in 4 months (King et al., 1995). About half of those who failed to recover had serious underlying pathology, emphasising the need for optometrists to refer any recent sixth nerve palsy. Another sign of underlying pathology is an A-pattern; a small V-pattern (Fig. 17.9B) should be expected in normal sixth nerve pareses (Hoyt & Fredrick, 1999).

Investigation

Lateral rectus palsy can be confused with Duane syndrome (p. 279), and the patient should be watched from the side during horizontal eye movements to detect the retraction which is usually characteristic of Duane syndrome. The degree of separation of the diplopic images may be greater in the inferior than in the superior field on the affected side (Percival, 1928).

Surprisingly, a lateral rectus palsy can produce a hyperdeviation as well as a horizontal deviation, and there may be a vertical element to the diplopia (Slavin, 1989). The hyperdeviation is maximal when the patient looks to the side of the affected lateral rectus muscle (during upgaze, downgaze, or straight lateral gaze) and may also be present in the primary position and, to a much lesser extent, for near vision. There can even be a cyclodeviation and, very rarely, a positive Bielschowsky head tilt test (Slavin, 1989). If the vertical deviation is more than 5Δ, then it may indicate a skew deviation (p. 284) or that another nerve or muscle is involved (Wong et al., 2002).

A video clip of the motility test result for a lateral rectus palsy can be found on the **Digital Resource** (Appendix 13). Once a case of recently acquired sixth nerve palsy has been referred and medically investigated, there is often a need for prismatic correction and the required prism will need to reduce if the condition improves. When investigating these cases, great care needs to be taken to control the head position. For example, when attempting to measure the dissociated deviation in the primary position, a slight change in head position can cause a large change in the measurement. A Hess screen plot can be useful in these cases and Fig. 17.9 shows consecutive Hess screen plots for a patient with a resolving lateral rectus palsy which was caused by vascular hypertension.

Management

The patient described earlier and illustrated in Fig. 17.9, benefited from base-out prisms in her distance vision spectacles, which reduced as the palsy improved. Fresnel prisms were not tolerated due to blurring.

The key typical features of lateral rectus palsy are summarised in Table 17.11.

Third Nerve Palsy

If only the extrinsic muscles supplied by this nerve are affected, this is **external ophthalmoplegia**. A paresis of the ciliary muscle and the iris sphincter is known as **internal ophthalmoplegia**, and when both the extrinsic and intrinsic muscles are affected, there is **total ophthalmoplegia**. Some

TABLE 17.11 ■ Typical Features of Lateral Rectus (Sixth Nerve) Palsy.

Feature	Detail
Aetiology	• Can be congenital or acquired

Symptoms (if recent onset)	• Head turn
	• Diplopia that is predominantly horizontal and is
	  • More marked at distance than near
	  • More marked when looking to the side of the affected muscle
	• Also, may be symptoms related to the aetiology of the palsy

Clinical signs	• Eso-deviation, which is larger:
	  • At distance than near
	  • When looking to the side of the affected muscle
	• Underaction of lateral rectus on motility testing, with overaction of contralateral synergist (medial rectus in the other eye)

Management	• If recent onset: urgent referral • If long-standing: base-out prism in distance glasses may help
Additional comments	• It can be difficult to differentially diagnose lateral rectus palsy from one type of Duane syndrome

authors make the distinction that if the lid muscles are involved then it is ocular myopathy. Total ophthalmoplegia is also known as **complete oculomotor palsy**: there will be a divergent strabismus with slightly depressed eyes, ptosis, and a loss of pupil action and accommodation. Ophthalmoplegia can result from a blow on the frontal region of the head, vascular disease (e.g., diabetes, hypertension), neoplasia, aneurysm, and ophthalmoplegic migraine (Swann, 2001). Other accompanying symptoms therefore may include headache, a tremor of the contralateral limbs (due to the involvement of the red nucleus where the third nerve fibres pass), and other symptoms of diabetes (earlier).

Classically, it was said if the pupil is dilated, it is likely to be an aneurysm, and if the pupil is spared, the cause is probably ischaemia as in diabetes and hypertension. However, this 'rule' is not absolute, and the optometrist should refer all new cases as an emergency (Swann, 2001). In particular, this 'rule' does not apply to children (Ng & Lyons, 2005).

In cases of third nerve palsy it is important to test fourth nerve function, as pathology may involve this as well. The patient is asked to look down and outwards and, if the superior oblique is normal, intorsion should be seen.

During the recovery of acquired third nerve paralysis, **aberrant regeneration** of nerve fibres may occur. This can result in failure of the upper lid to follow the eye as it moves downward or retraction of the upper lid in downward gaze or adduction, sometimes accompanied by contraction of the pupil (von Noorden, 1996). Typically, aberrant regeneration occurs over weeks to months following trauma or aneurysm (Rowe, 2004).

A superior rectus palsy sometimes occurs as a congenital isolated muscle palsy, usually accompanied by ptosis. As discussed earlier, a superior rectus palsy also occurs as a secondary sequel to a superior oblique palsy in the other eye. So, in apparent cases of superior rectus palsy it is important to carefully check the function of the contralateral superior oblique.

The medial and inferior recti and inferior oblique muscles are seldom affected as congenital isolated anomalies but may be involved with other muscles. An acquired inferior oblique palsy with diplopia can result from injections of botulinum toxin around the eyes for facial rejuvenation (Aristodemou, Watt, Baldwin, & Hugkulstone, 2006).

A Brown superior oblique tendon sheath syndrome can resemble an inferior oblique palsy and the differential diagnosis of inferior oblique palsies from Brown syndrome is discussed on p. 280. As noted later, unilateral or bilateral underaction of the inferior rectus can be a sign of myasthenia gravis.

The key features of third nerve palsy are summarised in Table 17.12.

Multiple Neurogenic Paresis

There are some rare syndromes affecting several extraocular muscles. Double elevator pareses involve the superior rectus and inferior oblique muscles, and double depressor pareses affect the inferior rectus and superior oblique muscles. Moebius syndrome is congenital and affects the sixth, seventh, and sometimes the ninth and twelfth cranial nerve nuclei. It can cause esotropia, Bell's phenomenon, facial paralysis, and tongue and hand abnormalities. Typically, infants will present with a bilateral lateral rectus palsy and expressionless face.

MYOGENIC DISORDERS

Myasthenia Gravis

This is a chronic disorder characterised by weakness and fatigability of striated muscles caused by impaired transmission across the neuromuscular junction. About 50% of patients with this condition present with purely ocular signs and symptoms, half of whom progress to develop the generalised disease (Benatar & Kaminski, 2012). Estimates of prevalence range from 1 in 50,000 to 1 in 10,000 and it is three times more common in people of Chinese origin than in those of Caucasian origin (Lee, 1999). The condition can occur at any age and diplopia and ocular palsy is an early sign in about half the cases. Symptoms are often transitory, and variability and fatigability are key

TABLE 17.12 ■ **Typical Features of Third Nerve Palsy.**

Feature	Detail
Aetiology	• Various aetiologies • The presentation of a third nerve palsy varies greatly: some or all of the muscles served by the third nerve may be affected
Symptoms (if recent onset)	• Diplopia, which in a full third nerve palsy will be constant (although sometimes ameliorated by ptosis) • Also, likely to be symptoms related to the aetiology of the palsy
Clinical signs	• In full third nerve palsy, the eye will be down and out with a fixed dilated pupil and ptosis
Management	• If recent onset painful third nerve palsy: emergency referral
Additional comments	• This condition is rarely seen in primary eyecare practice

features (Lee, 1999). The ocular muscle most often involved is the levator, so ptosis is the most common ocular sign, although this is not always present. If the patient is asked to look downwards for 15 seconds and then quickly back to the primary position, an upward twitch of the upper lid is seen before it resumes the ptosis position (Cogan's sign). Myasthenia gravis is an autoimmune disorder and can be associated with thyroid eye disease, or with a family history of thyroid dysfunction.

Although any extraocular muscle can be affected, Lee (1999) cautioned that isolated underaction of one or both inferior rectus muscles should be assumed to be due to myasthenia until proved otherwise. Bilateral and multiple extraocular muscle involvement is typical, with weakness of both elevator muscles (superior rectus and inferior oblique) common (Cleary, Williams, & Metcalfe, 2008). Even if visual symptoms are not severe, referral is important because if muscles involved in breathing become affected, the disease can be life threatening.

Giant Cell (Temporal) Arteritis

Diplopia can occur in giant cell arteritis reflecting extraocular muscle ischaemia (Gurwood & Malloy, 2001). The resulting ocular motility dysfunctions do not take on the stereotypical pattern of common cranial nerve palsies. Restriction of upgaze appears to be the most common manifestation (Gurwood & Malloy, 2001).

Incomitant Deviation from Long-Standing Comitancy

Even where the extraocular muscles are anatomically and physiologically normal before the onset of comitant strabismus, months or years of deviation may eventually produce secondary changes in the muscles. For example, in an uncorrected large accommodative esotropia, the lateral rectus muscle may be permanently elongated while the medial rectus remains in contracture. Eventually, the ability of the eye to abduct may become restricted causing an incomitancy. A strabismus which was initially comitant and easily correctable refractively may become very difficult to treat after only a few years (Rabbetts, 2007).

Other Myogenic Disorders

As described later, the 'wet stage' of thyroid eye disease is a form of myogenic disorder. **Myotonic dystrophy** can cause a symmetrical external ophthalmoplegia. **Ocular myositis** (orbital pseudotumour) can cause extraocular muscle inflammation with resultant impairment of function. **Kearns-Sayre ophthalmoplegia** is a mitochondrial abnormality of extraocular muscles causing progressive external ophthalmoplegia and may be associated with cardiac defects.

Chronic progressive external ophthalmoplegia (ocular myopathy of von Graefe) is a rare progressive disorder characterised by progressive bilateral ptosis and restriction of the extraocular muscles in all directions of gaze (Noorden & Campos, 2002). It results from mitochondrial myopathy (Schoser & Pongratz, 2006).

MECHANICAL DISORDERS

Duane Retraction Syndrome

The characteristic feature of Duane syndrome is **retraction** of the globe on attempted adduction caused by co-contraction of the medial and lateral recti. There may also be an elevation or depression of the affected eye. DeRespinis, Caputo, Wagner, and Guo (1993) felt that convergence insufficiency was also an invariable feature. Duane retraction syndrome occurs in approximately 1 in 50 patients with strabismus (Jampolsky, 1999), is four times more common in females, and both eyes are affected in about 20% of cases.

Conventionally, the condition was classified into type A, restricted abduction and slightly defective adduction; type B, restricted abduction and normal adduction; and type C, restricted adduction and slightly defective abduction. However, the alternative **Huber's classification** (Appendix 13 and **Digital Resource**) appears now to be more common:

1. *Type 1:* marked limitation or absence of abduction with normal or slightly limited adduction. This is the most common type (78%; von Noorden, 1996) and is invariably associated with an absence of the abducens nerve on the affected side (Kim & Hwang, 2005).
2. *Type 2:* limited or absent adduction with normal or mildly limited abduction. This is the least common (7%) and the abducens nerve on the affected side is present (Kim & Hwang, 2005).
3. *Type 3:* limitation or absence of both abduction and adduction (Appendix 13 and **Digital Resource**). This type affects 15% of cases (von Noorden, 1996) and is sometimes associated with an absence of the abducens nerve on the affected side (Kim & Hwang, 2005).

More complicated classifications have been proposed (Romero-Apis & Herrera-Gonzalez, 1995), but the most straightforward approach is to simply describe the clinical characteristics. For example, 'Duane syndrome of right eye with no abduction, normal adduction, retraction on adduction'. If this descriptive terminology is used in reports, the reader does not have to be familiar with whatever classification the writer uses.

Although Duane retraction syndrome is considered a mechanical restriction, Jampolsky (1999) states that the condition results from a maldevelopment or injury of the abducens nucleus and nerve(s) in the fourth to eighth weeks of gestation. He argues there is no credible evidence that the sixth nerve branches are redirected to innervate any of the third nerve muscles. However, the medial rectus is said to rarely manifest subnormal innervation, presumably owing to some of its nerve fibres being redirected to the lateral rectus. Von Noorden (1996) believed more aetiologic factors are involved.

Occasionally, Duane syndrome is associated with other abnormalities (von Noorden, 1996) which can be ocular (iris dysplasia, pupillary anomalies, cataracts, heterochromia, persistent hyaloid arteries, choroidal colobomas, distichiasis, crocodile tears, microphthalmos, and others) or systemic (e.g., Goldenhar syndrome, facial hemiatrophy, dystrophic defects, arthrogryposis multiplex congenital, cervical spina bifida, cleft palate, facial anomalies, sensorimotor hearing deficits, Chiari I malformation, deformities of the external ear, and anomalies of the limbs, feet, and hands). Previously uninvestigated cases in children should therefore be referred for medical investigation, which may also be advisable for siblings as the condition and the associated factors can be inherited (Marshman, Dawson, Neveu, Morgan, & Sloper, 2001).

Many cases are orthotropic in the primary position and do not require treatment. Approximately 75% of cases have fusion and measurable stereoacuity, but only 25% demonstrate normal binocularity (Tomac, Mutlu, & Altinsoy, 2007). These authors found type 1 cases tend to have the best clinical features.

Patients often adopt a head position which allows comfortable binocular vision during normal viewing, although stereoacuity is subnormal (Sloper, Garnham, Gous, Dyason, & Plunkett, 2001). The orthoptic status of these patients should be investigated with their own glasses (if used) or with a trial frame, but not with a refractor head which can force an uncharacteristic head position. Testing these patients in different positions of gaze often reveals a full gamut of binocular anomalies including compensated heterophoria in their preferred position of gaze, decompensated heterophoria, and strabismus in positions of gaze that are progressively more affected by the incomitancy. Typical features are summarised in Table 17.13.

Brown (Superior Oblique Tendon Sheath) Syndrome

In this condition, the sheath of the superior oblique muscle tendon between the trochlea and the insertion into the globe is too short, or mechanically restricted (Kushner, 2013), or there is paradoxical innervation of a noninnervated superior oblique muscle (Kaeser, Kress, Rohde, & Kolling, 2012). This prevents elevation when the eye is turned inwards, giving the appearance of paresis of the inferior oblique (Appendix 13 and **Digital Resource**). A suspected paresis of the inferior oblique is much more likely to be a Brown syndrome and the differential diagnosis of these conditions is considered in Table 17.14. Brown syndrome has a prevalence of approximately 1 in 20,000 (Weakley, Stager, & Stager, 1999). It is usually congenital, when it occasionally spontaneously resolves; or it can be acquired (Kushner, 2013).

Most cases of Brown syndrome are congenital, with both eyes affected in about 10% of cases. The rare acquired cases can be unilateral or bilateral and result from trauma, neoplasm, systemic inflammatory conditions, or sinusitis (Sturm, Landau, Grossglauser, & Sturmer, 2008). Acquired cases may be intermittent and sometimes resolve spontaneously or with medical treatment.

TABLE 17.13 ■ **Typical Features of Duane Syndrome.**

Feature	Detail
Aetiology	• Congenital restrictive anomaly affecting abduction and/or adduction of one or both eye(s)
Symptoms	• Usually, there are no symptoms as the patient compensates with a head turn and/or there is suppression when the person looks in the field of action of the affected muscle
Clinical signs	• Head turn • On motility testing, it is as if one eye is 'tethered' 　• The eye does not move (or barely moves) beyond the horizontal in abduction and/or adduction 　• There may be up-shoots: an eye aberrantly moves upwards when trying to look to one side 　• Usually, globe retraction is present causing the palpebral aperture to narrow on adduction • There are three types depending on whether abduction, adduction, or both are affected. Two different classifications, so best to describe the features rather than the label • Even when the adduction is normal, the near point of convergence is often remote
Management	• If long-standing: no management is usually necessary • If detected in a child and has not been previously investigated, referral is advisable as there can (rarely) be other associated abnormalities
Additional comments	• This is one of the most common incomitancies seen in primary eyecare • In cases where only abduction is affected, it can be difficult to differentially diagnose from a lateral rectus palsy. The presence of palpebral aperture narrowing aids diagnosis, as does a convergence abnormality

TABLE 17.14 ■ Differential Diagnosis of Brown Syndrome and Inferior Oblique Palsy.

Factor	Brown syndrome	Inferior oblique palsy
Prevalence	Relatively common	Relatively rare
Incyclotropia	Usually absent	Present from unopposed ipsilateral superior oblique
Anomalous head posture	May not be present. If present, main feature is chin lifted, but also head tilted towards involved side	Almost always present in congenital cases. Head tilted towards palsied side and turned towards the uninvolved side
Pattern strabismus	V-syndrome present (Kushner, 2013)	A-pattern esotropia common, particularly in bilateral cases
Overaction of ipsilateral superior oblique muscle	Absent	Usually present
Overaction of contralateral superior rectus	Usually absent	Usually present
Bielschowsky head tilt test	Usually negative	Usually positive
Discomfort elevating affected eye when adducted	Often present, may be actually painful	Absent
Improvement of elevation in adduction on repeated testing	May be present, sometimes with click	Usually absent
Forced duction test (definitive test)	Marked mechanical restriction	No mechanical restriction

Rarely, acquired Brown syndrome can occur in pregnancy, when it may be a sign of an underlying inflammatory process (Eneh, Johnson, Schweitzer, & Strube, 2018). Occasionally, a click can be heard or felt, with a finger placed over the trochlea. Congenital cases do not require treatment, unless there is a deviation in the primary position or a marked abnormal head posture. The condition can spontaneously improve as the child ages (Swann, 2001).

Brown syndrome is sometimes associated with **trochleodynia (trochleitis, trochlear headache)**, which is a term used to describe a spectrum of disorders characterised by pain arising from the trochlear region (Tran et al., 2019). It may result from several structures in the trochlear region and can be misdiagnosed as migraine or tension-type headache. This requires referral for medical investigation and treatment (Tran et al., 2019).

Thyroid Eye Disease

Thyroid dysfunction is an autoimmune disease typically with onset in women aged 30—50 years (Weiler, 2017). During the active (inflammatory, wet) stage the extraocular muscle bellies are the primary site of the disease. During this stage it is technically a myogenic disorder, but optometrists are more likely to see the disease during the inactive, fibrotic, phase which is characterised by a mechanical incomitancy. The condition is bilateral but can be asymmetric, typically with gradual onset of diplopia. The systemic and ocular signs are listed in Table 17.15. Rarely, the condition is associated with myasthenia gravis. Smoking is the most important risk factor for thyroid eye disease.

The severity of visual loss in thyroid eye disease can be graded according to the mnemonic in Table 17.16. These patients require medical attention (Cawood, Moriarty, & O'Shea, 2004), and should be monitored for compressive optic nerve damage and exposure keratitis. If visual function is compromised (visual acuity or field loss), the medical team should be notified as medical, surgical,

TABLE 17.15 ■ Systemic and Ocular Signs of Thyroid Eye Disease.

Sign	Details
Systemic	
Weight loss	Despite good appetite
Enlarged thyroid gland	
Raised body temperature	Causes sweating and heat intolerance. Sometimes, clammy hands and tremor of outstretched arm
Raised blood pressure	Can lead to tachycardia, nervous agitation, tremors
Mood changes	Irritability, emotional lability
Ocular	
Upper lid retraction	Dalrymple's sign: raised upper lid due to overaction of Muller's muscle
Lid lag	Von Graefe's sign: upper lid does not follow the eye fully when changing fixation from up- to down-gaze
Reduced blink rate and dry eye disease	(Gupta, Sadeghi, & Akpek, 2009)
Poor convergence	Moebius' sign: in cases where the medial rectus is involved
Inability to hold gaze	Typically, in peripheral gaze
Staring appearance	Kocher's sign: manifestation of lid retraction and proptosis
Resistance to retrodisplacement of the eye	
Conjunctival hyperaemia and oedema	Patients may report gritty sensation
Tremor on gentle lid closure	
Extraocular muscle restriction	Most commonly affected muscles: inferior rectus, medial rectus, superior rectus, lateral rectus Limited elevation is most common, which may have the appearance of superior rectus palsy. May also be limited abduction, depression, and adduction
Raised intraocular pressure on attempted elevation	
Abnormal head posture	Often allows binocular single vision in primary position
Corneal exposure	
Optic nerve involvement	Causing reduced visual acuity and possibly visual field
Hypermetropia	Occasionally, from raised intraocular pressure
Abnormal to forced duction test	Restriction of ocular movements

or radio treatment for decompression of the orbit is indicated. These patients often respond well to relieving prisms (Ansons & Davis, 2001). Regular monitoring is required as the prism strength may need to be changed frequently. Steroids are the mainstay of treatment (Weiler, 2017).

Blow-Out Fracture

This is an acquired anomaly resulting from a blow on the front of the face, for example, from a cricket ball or from falling on the face. The diplopia usually results from direct muscle injury

TABLE 17.16 ■ NOSPECS Mnemonic for Grading Severity of Thyroid Eye Disease.

Grade	Mnemonic	Description
0	N	No signs or symptoms
1	O	Only symptoms
2	S	Soft tissue involvement
3	P	Proptosis
4	E	Extraocular muscle involvement
5	C	Corneal exposure
6	S	Sight loss due to optic nerve involvements

From Cawood, T., Moriarty, P., O'Shea, D. (2004). Recent developments in thyroid eye disease. *British Medical Journal* **329**, 385–390.

(Pitts, 1996), but can be associated with a fracture of the thin orbital wall. Orbital fascial tissue can become trapped in the maxillary sinus preventing the eye from elevating above the horizontal. The motility defect varies depending on the site of the lesion, but restriction of elevation is most common (Spector, 1993). There may be retraction of the eye in attempted elevation, which can be seen from the side. The condition can resolve spontaneously, or may require surgery (Pitts, 1996). Symptoms can improve and then recur (Turnbull, Vingrys, & Kalloniatis, 2007). There may also be hypaesthesia of the area of the face under the eye due to entrapment of the V2 branch of the trigeminal nerve.

Iatrogenic Incomitancies

Iatrogenic incomitancies can occur as a rare complication of surgery, including neurosurgical procedures, dental procedures, endoscopic paranasal sinus surgery, and several ophthalmic procedures (Gonzalez-Martin-Moro et al., 2014). A restrictive incomitancy can result from filtering devices used to treat glaucoma (Wright, 1994). The device typically causes a restrictive hypertropia (Sun, Leske, Holmes, & Khanna, 2016), sometimes with the appearance of an acquired Brown syndrome (Gonzalez-Martin-Moro et al., 2014). The patient may report confusion rather than diplopia, possibly because of a field defect (Wright, 1994). Incomitancies can also result from a scleral buckle in retinal detachment surgery.

Other Mechanical Incomitancies

Strabismus fixus is an extremely rare condition in which one or both eyes are anchored, typically in a position of extreme adduction. This is believed to result from a fibrous tightening of the medial rectus muscle (von Noorden, 1996). Strabismus fixus of the lateral rectus can also occur (Caloroso & Rouse, 1993). **Fibrosis of the extraocular muscles** is an extremely rare condition, which can be inherited, involving fibrosis of one or all of the extraocular muscles (von Noorden, 1996). Typically, there is downward deviation of one or both eyes with marked ptosis and chin elevation.

SUPRANUCLEAR AND INTERNUCLEAR DISORDERS

Internuclear Ophthalmoplegia

Internuclear ophthalmoplegia (INO) results from a lesion in the medial longitudinal fasciculus between the third and fourth nerve nuclei. It results in poor adduction of the eye on the affected side and abducting nystagmus in the contralateral eye. Convergence is often, but not always, intact. Subtle cases can be detected by having the patient make rapid horizontal eye movements to show the slowness of adduction. Unilateral cases are usually due to a vascular or ischaemic lesion, and bilateral mostly due to multiple sclerosis (Wu, Cafiero-Chin, & Marques, 2015). Bilateral INO in the young is almost always associated with multiple sclerosis.

Wall-eyed bilateral INO (WEBINO) is an uncommon variant of INO characterised by primary gaze exotropia, adduction impairment, and nystagmus of the abducting eye (Wu et al., 2015). Spontaneous resolution is common, typically within a few months. The management involves eliminating diplopia and treating any underlying systemic condition.

Gaze Palsies

Gaze palsies, arising from supranuclear disorders, do not necessarily manifest a deviation between the two visual axes so may not meet the definition of an incomitancy, but are nonetheless included in this chapter. These can occur due to lesions in the frontal motor centre, gaze centres in the pons, or in the interconnecting pathways. There is seldom diplopia, and the eyes move together in most directions of gaze. In one direction, the eyes cannot move reflexly to take up fixation or, more rarely, cannot follow a moving target (pursuit palsy). In lateral gaze palsy, the two eyes will not move beyond the mid-line. In vertical gaze palsy, movements above and/or below the horizontal are restricted. Parkinson disease can be associated with restrictions of upgaze and convergence (Naylor, 2005). New or changing gaze palsies should be referred because possible aetiologies include neoplasms and emboli.

Parinaud Syndrome

Parinaud syndrome is also known as **dorsal midbrain syndrome**. It is characterised by: gaze palsy for elevation and/or depression for saccades and later pursuit, convergence retraction nystagmus, upper eyelid retraction, large pupils with light-near dissociation, and papilloedema. Causes include tumours of the pineal gland and vascular accidents or trauma.

Skew Deviation

Skew deviation is a hypertropia of supranuclear origin resulting from a disturbance of the vestibular input to ocular motor nuclei (Hernowo & Eggenberger, 2014). The deviation may be comitant or may vary in different positions of gaze. Skew deviation is differentiated from fourth nerve palsy by two signs: in skew deviation, the hypertropic eye is incyclotorted and the vertical deviation decreases from upright to supine head position (Hernowo & Eggenberger, 2014). Skew deviation can be intermittent but usually occurs in association with brain stem, cerebellar, or vestibular disease (Lee, 1999). A common cause is ischaemia of the brainstem or cerebellum (Hernowo & Eggenberger, 2014). Skew deviation is usually accompanied by binocular torsion, torticollis, and a tilt in the subjective visual vertical: this constellation of findings has been termed the ocular tilt reaction (Brodsky, Donahue, Vaphiades, & Brandt, 2006). If there is minimal ocular torsion, the deviation can be managed with prisms (Hernowo & Eggenberger, 2014).

OTHER DISORDERS

Pattern Deviations (Alphabet Patterns; Pattern Strabismus; A- and V-Syndromes)

Quite commonly, cases are encountered in which the patient appears to be fairly comitant on motility testing in the six cardinal positions of gaze, but the horizontal deviation is seen to increase or decrease with the eyes elevated or depressed. The simplest examples of these cases are A-syndrome, in which the eyes are relatively convergent in upgaze, and V-syndrome, where the eyes are relatively convergent in downgaze. V-syndrome is about twice as common as A-syndrome (von Noorden, 1996). An estimated one in five patients with strabismus have an A- or V-pattern (von Noorden, 1996; Biglan, 1999), and subtle variants of the conditions are very common in 'normal' heterophoria. Von Noorden (1996) discussed the aetiology of the condition, concluding that several factors play a role, including dysfunction of the oblique muscles and various anatomical factors, including the configuration and rotation of the orbit (Biglan, 1999).

Both A- and V-syndromes can be present in patients with exo- or eso-deviations. For example, in A-esotropia, the esotropia increases in upgaze and decreases in downgaze. In V-exotropia the deviation increases in upgaze and reduces in downgaze. Other variants also exist, although they are less common. For example, in X-syndrome, the eyes may be straight in the primary position, and exotropic in upgaze and downgaze. Other forms include Y-pattern and λ-pattern. It is not surprising that the generic terms 'pattern strabismus' or 'alphabetic pattern' have been coined.

These patterns may be present as congenital anomalies, or may accompany an acquired strabismus, particularly where the oblique muscles are affected. Anomalous head postures are common. The presence of A- or V-patterns can improve the prognosis because binocular single vision may be developed or maintained in up- or downgaze. However, most pattern deviations do not require treatment (Ansons & Davis, 2001). When treatment is required, some authors have found success with oblique prisms, but others do not advocate this approach (von Noorden, 1996). Surgical approaches are also available (Biglan, 1999).

Pattern deviations can be diagnosed with cover testing in upgaze and downgaze and, more accurately, with a Hess or Lees screen. Von Noorden (1996) suggested criteria for diagnosis: V-pattern with a difference of 15Δ or more from up- to downgaze and an A-pattern with a difference of 10Δ. Several disorders are commonly associated with pattern deviations: infantile esotropia syndrome, Duane retraction syndrome, Brown syndrome, acquired fourth nerve palsy, thyroid eye disease (Ansons & Davis, 2001).

Superior Oblique Myokymia

Benign superior oblique myokymia is an episodic small amplitude nystagmoid intorsion and depression of one eye, accompanied by visual shimmer and oscillopsia (Case Study 17.1). The condition was originally called **unilateral rotary nystagmus** (Plager, 1999). The onset is in adulthood, the symptoms troublesome, whilst the 'diagnosis is often missed' (von Noorden, 1996). Episodes usually last from 20 seconds to several minutes and can be triggered by physical activity (von Noorden, 1996), fatigue, and stress (Plager, 1999). The prevalence of this condition does not appear to be quoted in the literature.

Superior oblique myokymia is usually benign, but there have been at least two cases of association with a posterior fossa tumour (von Noorden, 1996). Plager (1999) felt that neuro-imaging was unnecessary, unless there are other neurological complaints.

Although the precise aetiology is unclear (von Noorden, 1996), superior oblique myokymia may be the result of regeneration (Plager, 1999) after prior clinical or subclinical injury to the trochlear nerve (Mehta & Demer, 1994) or compression of the trochlear nerve (Strupp, Dieterich, Brandt, & Feil, 2016). Medical treatments may have improved since Case Study 17.1 (Tomsak, Kosmorsky, & Leigh, 2002; Strupp et al., 2016). Surgical approaches are sometimes successful, although second operations may be required (von Noorden, 1996). Optical correction with prisms may be helpful if there is a habitual vertical imbalance (Case Study 17.1).

CASE STUDY 17.1

BACKGROUND
47-year-old businessman referred by neurologist to optometrist to investigate vertical diplopia and photosensitivity. Possible history of binocular anomaly at age 9 years.

SYMPTOMS
For the last 18 months, patient experiences momentary vertical diplopia at some time most days; people who are with him do not notice any abnormalities. Headaches, particularly with office work. Reading is

blurred, unstable, and tiring; patient has given up reading for pleasure. Two ophthalmologists diagnosed superior oblique myokymia, one discharged patient, the other tried medical treatment, to no avail.

RELEVANT CLINICAL FINDINGS
Minimal myopia and early presbyopia. At distance and near, dissociation testing revealed 2Δ R hyperphoria with same aligning prism on Mallett unit. Motility appeared normal, but Lees screen revealed mild underaction of right superior oblique muscle, confirmed by Scobee's three-step test (Parks' inconclusive) and double Maddox rod test.

MANAGEMENT
Prescribed distance spectacles and near spectacles, both with vertical prism.

FOLLOW-UP 5 WEEKS LATER
Virtually no vertical diplopia or headaches, reading much easier.

COMMENT
It seems likely that the patient had a long-standing superior oblique paresis, with secondary superior oblique myokymia. The comitancy had spread, so it was now possible to correct the vertical deviation with a prism which alleviated the symptoms.

R, Right.

Inferior Oblique Overaction

Inferior oblique overaction is a common sequel to an early onset interruption to binocularity, typically infantile esotropia syndrome (Brodsky, 2005; Koc et al., 2003). It is often accompanied by latent nystagmus and/or dissociated vertical deviation (Chapter 18).

Rare Causes of Incomitant Deviations

There are several rare syndromes and pathologies that can cause incomitancies. These are summarised in Table 17.17.

Management

Considerable attention has been given in this chapter to the diagnosis of conditions requiring medical attention, which is obviously the first priority. The speed of onset of symptoms is a good guide to the urgency required for referral. If a patient awoke today with sudden onset diplopia, they need emergency referral. If they have been experiencing intermittent diplopia when reading for many months that is not changing markedly, routine referral may be appropriate if there are no other suspicious symptoms or signs.

The number of patients who have incomitant deviations as an early sign of disease requiring urgent medical attention is not large, and many of them will take medical advice in the first place. Therefore, most incomitant deviations seen in primary eyecare practice will be long-standing, and most of these will already have received medical attention. The question which arises is whether there is anything further that can be done in these long-standing cases. Incomitant deviations do not respond at all well to eye exercises. Very occasionally, congenital conditions in children may be helped by exercises to extend the area of the binocular field over which there is binocular vision, or to re-establish it when it has broken down due to general ill-health. In the latter case, the patient may suddenly experience diplopia, which may be remedied by orthoptic exercises if it is established that the general condition has cleared.

Patients with childhood onset strabismus will have suppression or HARC which prevents diplopia over most of the visual field. There may be some diplopia in one peripheral part of the motor field. If there are no significant symptoms, it is better not to disturb this adapted or partially

TABLE 17.17 ■ Rare Causes of Incomitant Deviations.

Condition	Classification	General signs	Nature of incomitancy
Dental surgery (Gonzalez-Martin-Moro et al., 2014)	Iatrogenic		Usually transitory, resolving after a few hours Secondary to diffusion of local anaesthesia
Extraocular muscle cysticercosis (Sundaram, Jayakumar, & Noronha, 2004)	Myogenic	Adult-onset seizures. Cysticercosis is endemic in many regions of Central & South America, sub-Saharan Africa, India, Asia	Diplopia, pain, redness, all EOM involved, predominantly lateral rectus, medial rectus, superior oblique
Inferior oblique muscle adherence syndrome (Kushner, 2007)	Mechanical	Complication of previous surgery on the inferior rectus or scleral buckle surgery	Restrictive hypotropia and excyclotropia
'Heavy eye syndrome' or 'strabismus fixus' (Ranka & Steele, 2015)	Restrictive	Gradual onset diplopia in an adult with high myopia	From nasal displacement of SR & inferior displacement of LR. Esotropia and hypotropia, limitation of abduction and elevation
Lumbar puncture (Gonzalez-Martin-Moro et al., 2014)	Iatrogenic neurogenic (VI palsy)	Sixth nerve palsy is an uncommon complication of lumbar puncture	Diplopia from lateral rectus underaction
Miller-Fisher syndrome		Variant of Guillain-Barré syndrome. Abnormal muscle coordination causing poor balance and coordination, absence of tendon reflexes	Complete or partial ophthalmoplegia, with inferior oblique muscle most commonly affected
'Sagging eye syndrome' (Goseki et al., 2020)	Connective tissue degeneration	Diplopia in an older patient. May also have changes to levator causing ptosis	Often cyclovertical strabismus, sometimes with esotropia
Silent sinus syndrome (Numa, Desai, Gold, Heher, & Annino, 2005)	Mechanical	Progressive enophthalmos and hypoglobus due to gradual collapse of the orbital floor with opacification of the maxillary sinus, from subclinical chronic maxillary sinusitis	Vertical diplopia and pseudo-retraction of the superior lid are sometimes reported

(Continued)

TABLE 17.17 ■ Rare Causes of Incomitant Deviations.—cont'd

Condition	Classification	General signs	Nature of incomitancy
Systemic lupus erythematosus (Arevalo, Lowder, & Muci-Mendoza, 2002)	Neurogenic Myogenic	Chronic immunologic disorder affecting multiple organs. Can cause keratoconjunctivitis sicca, retinal, and neuro-ophthalmic manifestations	Cranial nerve palsies Enlargement of extraocular muscles
Vitamin B12 deficiency (Akdal, Yener, Ada, & Halmagyi, 2007)	Brain stem		Bilateral internuclear ophthalmoplegia or downbeat nystagmus
Wegener's granulomatosis with polyangiitis (Salam, Meligonis, & Malhotra, 2008)	Myogenic (myositis)	Inflammation of various tissues, including blood vessels, respiratory tract, kidneys	Usually, horizontal recti, rarely superior oblique
Wernicke-Korsakoff syndrome (Isenberg-Grzeda, Rahane, DeRosa, Ellis, & Nicolson, 2016)	Neurogenic	Neuropsychiatric deficiency caused by Vitamin B1 deficiency, can occur in alcoholics or cancer patients	Palsy of VI nerve and III nerve Gaze palsy Nystagmus

EOM, Extraocular muscles; *LR,* lateral rectus; *SR,* superior rectus.

adapted state. If one eye has been neglected or has had a blurred image for many years, correcting the refractive error can produce troublesome diplopia. It may be better to give a balancing lens or a blurring lens to maintain the status quo. In some cases, correction may be appropriate, particularly in children, if it is likely that some binocular vision can be restored, perhaps with relieving prisms. However, this is a difficult procedure, and should only be attempted with great caution. Once diplopia is created, it is difficult for the patient to revert to suppression. Very occasionally, the sensory adaptation in these incomitant deviations seems to break down spontaneously, and a patient presents complaining of diplopia and a long-standing deviation not due to recently acquired pathology. The management of intractable diplopia is discussed on p. 206.

It has been suggested that some patients with acquired incomitant deviations benefit from monovision, where each eye is given its own 'domain' (London, 1987; Phillips, 2007; Migneco, 2008). Case study 17.2 describes such a case. However, care should be taken not to force patients to fixate with an eye which has had long-standing strabismus (p. 208), as this may cause **fixation switch diplopia** (Kushner, 1995).

CASE STUDY 17.2

BACKGROUND
46-year-old male healthcare professional, hobby sailing.

SYMPTOMS
For the last 6 months, notices vertical diplopia of isolated small objects (navigational buoys) and road signs. Consulted a neuro-ophthalmologist who diagnosed ocular myasthenia gravis and suggested no treatment.

RELEVANT CLINICAL FINDINGS
Refraction −0.75 DS each eye, near add +1.50. At distance and near, dissociation testing revealed 1Δ R hyperphoria with 5–10 degrees extorsion, worse in elevation. Motility suggestive of mild right superior oblique underaction. Repeat Hess plots variable, sometimes showing superior oblique and other times inferior rectus mild underaction. Prisms in consulting room unable to consistently eliminate diplopia.

MANAGEMENT
Trial with distance vision contact lens right eye only (monovision). Good distance and near acuity with no diplopia.

FOLLOW-UP 2 MONTHS LATER
Monovision has eliminated diplopia; but recurs in consulting room with bilateral distance vision correction. Clinical tests of ocular motor status unchanged.

COMMENT
Successful monovision requires foveal suppression of the blurred image from one eye, with the suppressed eye varying with fixation distance (Evans, 2007a). This suppression may be effective at eliminating a small degree of diplopia, in this case cyclovertical.

DS, Dioptre sphere; *R*, right.

PRISMS

In some cases of diplopia from incomitant deviations, prisms may be prescribed to extend the area of comfortable single vision. These need to be a compromise, as the deviation varies with gaze position. The aim is to give prism relief for the central part of the motor field. This is usually adequate because the head is generally moved rather than making very large eye movements. A good starting point is prism of the power of the deviation shown by a Mallett fixation disparity test or with the Maddox rod with the eyes in the primary position. It should be checked this gives good cover test recovery, first with the eyes in the primary position, and then with the fixation looking further into the affected motor field. A judgement needs to be made in each case as to how strong a prism is reasonable in terms of weight and edge thickness, and how much binocularity in peripheral gaze can be restored. Patients who have lacked binocular vision for many months may not exhibit fusion with the appropriate prism in the consulting room but may develop binocular vision with the prism over time (Ansons & Davis, 2001).

In large angles, Fresnel stick-on prisms can be used. With incomitancies, several Fresnel lenses can be cut and placed adjacent to one another on the lens, so that the power increases in the direction of action of the affected muscle. However, these are cosmetically unattractive, cause blurred vision, and are best thought of as a temporary measure.

BOTULINUM TOXIN AND OTHER MEDICAL INTERVENTIONS

Botulinum toxin can be used to treat incomitant strabismus by injecting the ipsilateral antagonist of the affected muscle (Ansons & Spencer, 2001). The duration of action is usually about 3 months. Typically, in a lateral rectus paresis, the palsy will have improved during this time, so fusion is maintained. Its main uses are to determine the state of recovery of the lateral rectus following a sixth nerve palsy; the risk of developing postoperative diplopia; the potential for binocular single vision; and as an adjunct to strabismus surgery (Ansons & Spencer, 2001). Cochrane reviews find the evidence concerning botulinum toxin for strabismus (Rowe & Noonan, 2017) and sixth nerve palsy (Rowe et al., 2018) is uncertain. Botulinum toxin injections are also used for other conditions, including blepharospasm (Elston, 1994), hemifacial spasm, and spasmodic torticollis (Jamieson, 1994).

Medical treatments are available for myasthenia gravis, but a Cochrane review was unable to draw firm conclusions about their efficacy (Benatar & Kaminski, 2012).

SURGERY

Surgery is the principal management option for incomitant and large angle (over about 20Δ) comitant strabismus, and for other cases of comitant strabismus that do not respond to nonsurgical management (Case Study 17.3). Surgery is indicated in these cases when there is poor cosmesis, symptoms (principally diplopia), a recent onset within the sensitive period, or marked ocular torticollis which could cause permanent neck problems. The aims of surgery are to straighten the visual axes and, if possible, to restore binocular vision. Eye exercises, occlusion (p. 207), prisms, and refractive correction may be required in addition to surgery (Chapter 14).

CASE STUDY 17.3	First Appointment (Aged 81 Years, Retired GP)

SYMPTOMS & HISTORY

First examination at this practice (not local), referred by his optometrist. Patient reports diplopia since 2002, of gradual onset, which his optometrist has been controlling by increasing prisms (now 3Δ down R, 3Δ up L). At the recent appointment, local optometrist said the prism can be increased no further in spectacles and referred to the author. Spectacles (with the prism) are worn constantly, but diplopia returns when he is tired causing him to close RE to resolve diplopia. The diplopia is worse in left gaze and is vertical and torsional, for D & N. Has not been referred previously for investigation of aetiology of the diplopia. Takes aspirin, statin, diuretic. No other relevant PH or FH.

RELEVANT CLINICAL FINDINGS

Normal: ocular health, pupil reactions, 25-degree fields, IOP.

Subjective:	R +4.00/−2.00 × 100	L +3.25/−1.75 × 60	Add +2.00
	6/6	6/6	
Cover test*:	D orthophoria	N 5Δ R hyperphoria,	
		Grade 3 recovery	
Dissociation tests*:	D 7Δ eso 10Δ R/L	N 5Δ exo 13Δ R/L 10 degrees excyclo-deviation	

*cover test & dissociation test through spectacles, including total 6Δ down R, split

Motility: moderate underaction R superior oblique

MANAGEMENT

Explained – likely progressive right superior oblique palsy. Needs referral to investigate aetiology and consider surgery as reaching limit of prism, which cannot correct cyclotorsional deviation. Detailed referral letter sent via GP with copy given to patient to present to ophthalmologist. Copy sent to local optometrist.

FOLLOW-UP

No reply received to referral letter, but patient wrote to thank for referral as received surgery which eliminated diplopia.

COMMENT

The patient should have been referred by the previous practitioner when the incomitancy first manifested. The lack of a reply to the author's referral is unhelpful as it would be useful to know the presumed cause of the incomitancy in case it recurs.

D, Distance; *FH*, family history; *IOP*, intraocular pressure; *L*, left; *PH*, personal history; *R*, right; *RE*, right eye.

Before surgery, the surgeon should carry out the forced duction test (Table 17.9) to investigate the influence of the extraocular muscles, Tenon's capsule, and other nonmuscular tissues on globe rotation in different positions of gaze (Bruenech, 2001).

Two randomised controlled trials of strabismus surgery for adults were positive (Mills, Coats, Donahue, & Wheeler, 2004) and surgical correction of acquired strabismus can result in recovery of stereoacuity, particularly if surgery occurs within 12 months of the onset of strabismus (Fawcett, Stager, & Felius, 2004). However, Cochrane reviews have identified a lack of high-quality evidence on several questions relating to strabismus surgery (Korah, Philip, Jasper, Antonio-Santos, & Braganza, 2014; Hatt et al., 2015; Chang, Coleman, Tseng, & Demer, 2017; Hassan, Haridas, & Sundaram, 2018).

Complications from strabismus surgery are rare, estimated to be 1 in 400 operations, with the most common perforation of the globe (0.08%), suspected slipped muscle (0.07%), severe infection (0.06%), scleritis (0.02%), and lost muscle (0.02%) (Bradbury & Taylor, 2013). A poor or very poor clinical outcome was only recorded as one operation in 2400.

Presurgical Prism Adaptation Test

The presurgical prism adaptation test is different to the short-term prism adaptation test that is rarely required when prescribing prisms in heterophoria (p. 104). The presurgical prism adaptation test is useful for determining the presence of binocular vision and for planning surgery (Rutstein et al., 1991), commonly in esotropia (Moore & Drack, 2000). It is still useful for adults who are considering surgery for esotropia of childhood onset (Kutschke & Scott, 2004). The patient should have equal or nearly equal visual acuities and an angle of deviation not exceeding 40Δ (Ansons & Spencer, 2001).

The deviation is completely corrected or slightly overcorrected with prisms, which are usually split between the eyes. These are prescribed, typically as Fresnel prisms, and the patient is re-assessed one week later. If the patient has adapted to the prisms so there is a manifest deviation greater than 8Δ, the prism strength is increased. The process is repeated until the deviation is 8Δ or less or the magnitude of the prism exceeds 50Δ.

There are three possible responses to the test (Ansons & Spencer, 2001):

1. The visual axes become straight and binocular single vision is confirmed.
2. There is a residual microtropia with a good sensory adaptation (Chapter 16).
3. The visual axes keep re-converging ('eating up the prisms').

If options 1 or 2 occur, the patient is described as a 'prism responder' and surgery is performed to correct the maximum angle measured (Ansons & Spencer, 2001). If the test results in 3, the patient is classed as a nonresponder and any surgery performed is based on the angle of deviation first measured.

Prism Testing for Diplopia

Sometimes, adults or children over the age of 5 years with no potential for binocular single vision request strabismus surgery for cosmetic reasons. In these cases, the possibility of postoperative diplopia must be considered (Ansons & Spencer, 2001) and Kushner (2002) advocated testing for diplopia with prisms in all adults before strabismus surgery. Diplopia can occur even in the presence of very poor acuity (Case Study 14.3).

The patient views a fixation target at distance and near. The prism is introduced (base-out for esotropia), and the strength is slowly increased until the patient notices diplopia (Ansons & Davis, 2001). The range of prismatic strength which elicits diplopia should be recorded and will help the surgeon in planning the surgery. If diplopia is likely to occur, the patient should be informed and the diplopia demonstrated with prisms so they can decide whether to have the operation (Ansons & Spencer, 2001). The surgeon may use Botulinum toxin to temporarily correct the strabismus and provide additional information about postoperative diplopia risk and its likely tolerance.

Overview of Surgical Techniques

The decision to surgically undercorrect, fully correct, or overcorrect strabismus is influenced by whether there is potential binocular single vision and the duration of the strabismus (Ansons & Spencer, 2001). Adjustable sutures can be used in some cases. A detailed description of surgical procedures is beyond the scope of this book, but the main procedures (Bruenech, 2001; Kanski, 1994) are summarised below:

1. *Weakening procedures*, which decrease the pull of a muscle.
   (a) **Recession**, where the insertion of a muscle is moved posteriorly. It can be used on any extraocular muscle.
   (b) **Marginal myotomy**, which lengthens a muscle without moving its insertion. It is used to weaken a previously fully recessed rectus muscle.
   (c) **Myectomy**, which involves severing a muscle from its insertion without reattachment. It is most often used in weakening an overactive inferior oblique muscle.
   (d) **Posterior fixation suture (Faden procedure)**, which is used mainly to treat dissociated vertical deviation.
2. *Strengthening procedures*, which enhance the pull of a muscle.
   (a) **Resection**, which shortens the length of a muscle to enhance its effective pull. It is suitable only for a rectus muscle.
   (b) **Tucking** of a muscle or its tendon is usually reserved to enhance the action of the superior oblique muscle.
   (c) **Advancement**, which moves the insertion of a muscle nearer to the limbus to enhance the action of a previously recessed rectus muscle.
3. *Transposition procedures*, which change the direction of action of a muscle.
   (a) **Vertical transposition of the horizontal recti**, to correct A- and V-patterns in cases which do not show significant oblique muscle overaction.
   (b) **Hummelsheim's procedure**, to improve abduction in sixth nerve palsy.
   (c) **Jensen's procedure**, also to improve abduction in sixth nerve palsy, in conjunction with recession of the medial rectus or injection of botulinum toxin.

CLINICAL KEY POINTS

- In incomitant deviations, the angle varies in different positions of gaze and according to which eye is fixating
- An understanding of the actions of the extraocular muscles is essential to the diagnosis of incomitant deviations
- The actions of the muscles change as the eyes move into different positions of gaze
- Incomitant deviations can be classified as neurogenic, myogenic, or mechanical
- Primary care practitioners need to refer all new or changing incomitancies
- Symptoms and signs usually make it clear whether an incomitancy is long-standing or recent (Table 17.8)
- Superior oblique muscle pareses are difficult to diagnose from motility testing and testing the cyclodeviation is helpful
- Ideally, incomitancies should be quantified with a Hess screen (e.g., computerised Hess screen)
- Algorithm methods (Lindblom, Parks' or Scobee's) are useful but require practice

CHAPTER 18

Nystagmus

Introduction

Nystagmus is an eye movement disorder characterised by abnormal, involuntary rhythmic oscillations of one or both eyes, initiated by a slow phase (Self et al., 2020). Jerk nystagmus is nystagmus with a slow phase and a fast phase; pendular nystagmus is nystagmus with only slow phases (Eggers et al., 2019). Nystagmus affects 0.24% of the UK population (Self et al., 2020). Physiological nystagmus can occur with certain types of visual (optokinetic nystagmus) or vestibular stimulation (e.g., by rotating the subject or by introducing warm or cold water into the ear). End point nystagmus can also occur during motility testing, particularly if the child is tired (Grisham, 1990) and if the target is held at the end point position for 15–30 seconds. This chapter will concentrate on nonphysiological nystagmus.

There are several factors, listed here, which cause the investigation of nystagmus to be complicated. The aim of this chapter is to provide an overview of the subject for clinicians who may only encounter nystagmus occasionally, and who need to know when to refer and what optometric management, if any, is appropriate.

PROBLEMS IN THE EVALUATION OF NYSTAGMUS

1. Nystagmus is not a condition, but a sign. Many different ocular anomalies can cause nystagmus, or nystagmus can be idiopathic, with no apparent cause.
2. Attempts to classify the type of nystagmoid eye movement by simply watching the patient's eye movements often do not agree with the results of objective eye movement analysis (Dell'Osso & Daroff, 1975).
3. The pattern of nystagmoid eye movements cannot be used with certainty to predict the aetiology of the nystagmus (Dell'Osso & Daroff, 1975). Some general rules exist; for example, infantile nystagmus (INS) is usually horizontal. However, there are exceptions, when INS is not purely horizontal, and there are many cases of horizontal nystagmus which do not have an infantile onset.
4. The same patient may exhibit different types of nystagmoid eye movements on different occasions (Abadi & Dickinson, 1986). In INS, the eye movements worsen under stressful conditions (Cham, Anderson, & Abel, 2008b; Jones et al., 2013). In the absence of stress, the eye movements in nystagmus may improve a little with demanding visual tasks (Wiggins, Woodhouse, Margrain, Harris, & Erichsen, 2007). INS is not exacerbated by visual demand per se, rather the need to do something visually demanding of importance to the individual (Tkalcevic & Abel, 2005).
5. Visual loss in nystagmus is only loosely correlated with the type of nystagmoid eye movements (Bedell & Loshin, 1991). There may be an underlying pathology causing poor vision resulting in nystagmus; a pathology causing, independently, the nystagmus and the poor vision; or a pathology (hypothesised in infantile idiopathic nystagmus) causing the nystagmus which then causes poor vision. Amblyopia may develop secondary to early onset nystagmus (Abadi & King-Smith, 1979; Spierer, 1991; Currie, Bedell, & Song, 1993).

CLASSIFICATION

There are two fundamentally different approaches to classifying nystagmus, based on the aetiology and the eye movement characteristics. This chapter concentrates on the two types of nystagmus that eyecare practitioners will encounter most frequently (infantile nystagmus and latent nystagmus). Eggers et al. (2019) provide a more comprehensive classification of nystagmus from a neurological/vestibular perspective.

Classification Based on Aetiology

1. *Infantile nystagmus (infantile nystagmus syndrome; INS)*, occurring in infancy (Committee for the Classification of Eye Movement Abnormalities and Strabismus, 2001), usually the first 6 months of life (Self et al., 2020). The condition was previously called **congenital nystagmus** or **early onset nystagmus**.

   (a) *Infantile nystagmus with a sensory defect*, associated with an ocular anomaly causing poor vision, e.g., congenital cataract, optic atrophy, aniridia. A relatively common form of sensory defect nystagmus is **albinism**, both oculocutaneous (lack of skin and eye pigmentation) and ocular (only lacking eye pigmentation). Many albinos have INS and latent nystagmus (see later), which should be labelled as 'INS with a latent component' (Harris, 2013).

   (b) *Infantile nystagmus without a sensory defect*, also known as infantile idiopathic **nystagmus**. Previous terminology (sensory nystagmus and motor nystagmus) is deprecated because the waveform of the two types is indistinguishable and both result from the same deficit in the smooth pursuit motor subsystem (Dell'Osso, Hertle, & Daroff, 2007).

   (c) *Nystagmus blockage syndrome* is probably a rare subdivision of INS in which a reduction of the nystagmus during convergence appears to have resulted in an esotropia. The fixating eye is adducted during binocular or monocular vision giving the appearance of a lateral rectus palsy and resulting in an anomalous head posture (Grisham, 1990).

2. *Latent nystagmus (fusion maldevelopment nystagmus syndrome)* is a common sequel to infantile esotropia syndrome and is characteristically only present, or greatly increased, on monocular occlusion. However, it is very occasionally found in monocular individuals. The fast phase of the eye movement always beats towards the uncovered eye. Therefore, the direction of the nystagmus reverses when the cover is moved from one eye to the other and this is pathognomonic of latent nystagmus (Repka, 1999). Dell'Osso (1994) stated that both types of latent nystagmus (see below) are always accompanied by strabismus and a cyclotorsional element is usually present, together with dissociated vertical deviation (Guyton, 2000).

   (a) *Latent latent nystagmus*, or true latent nystagmus, which only becomes apparent on monocular occlusion.

   (b) *Manifest latent nystagmus*, which is present without occlusion.

3. *Acquired (neurological) nystagmus*, occurring usually after the first few months of life, owing to some pathological lesion or trauma affecting the motor pathways (e.g., multiple sclerosis, closed head trauma). All uninvestigated cases, except voluntary nystagmus, should be referred.

   (a) *Gaze paretic (evoked) nystagmus*, a jerk nystagmus that appears on eccentric gaze and beats in the direction of the gaze. It is associated with cerebellar disorders (Harris, 1997) or some substances (e.g., sedatives, anticonvulsants, alcohol).

   (b) *Acquired pendular nystagmus*, which is associated with brain stem or cerebellar disease, or demyelinating diseases (Averbuch-Heller and Leigh, 1996).

(c) *Acquired jerk nystagmus* is usually associated with cerebellar or brainstem disease. Down-beating nystagmus is strongly suggestive of Arnold-Chiari malformation when vertical pursuit and the vestibulo-ocular reflex also may be abnormal.

(d) *Convergence-retraction nystagmus (induced convergence-retraction)* is caused by co-contraction of the extraocular muscles, particularly the medial recti. There is a jerk nystagmus (with discomfort) stimulated by attempted upgaze in which the fast phase brings the two eyes together in a convergence movement with retraction of the globe.

(e) *Vestibular nystagmus* is usually acquired and sometimes has a 'saw tooth' waveform where a slow constant velocity drift takes the eyes off target, followed by a quick corrective saccade (Grisham, 1990).

(f) *See-saw nystagmus*, one eye elevates and usually intorts as the other depresses and extorts. It is rare, usually associated with parasellar or chiasmal lesions; there may be bitemporal hemianopia.

(g) *Dissociated nystagmus*, with eye movements that are dissimilar in direction, amplitude, or speed. May occur in internuclear ophthalmoplegia.

4. Other eye movement phenomena.

(a) *Square wave jerks* occur in up to 60% of normal subjects and are small horizontal saccades which are quickly corrected by a second saccade (Worfolk, 1993). Square wave jerks and saccadic intrusions are common in Parkinson's disease.

(b) *Ocular flutter* is a burst of horizontal back to back saccades with no resting interval between them and can be unidirectional or multidirectional (**opsoclonus**). It can occur transiently in healthy infants, as a side effect of some drugs, or from pathology. About 5% of the population can simulate ocular flutter as **voluntary nystagmus**.

(c) *Spasmus nutans* is characterised by the triad of nystagmus, head nodding, and abnormal head posture and usually presents in the first year of life. The nystagmus is a pendular oscillation of variable conjugacy (Dell'Osso, 1994). It is generally benign and only lasts a year or two, but can be associated with pathology (Grisham, 1990).

(d) *Microsaccadic opsoclonus* are high frequency, small amplitude, back-to-back multivectorial saccadic movements which are visible with slit lamp biomicroscopy and direct ophthalmoscopy (Foroozan and Brodsky, 2004). The condition can cause intermittent blurred vision and oscillopsia. Differential diagnosis includes superior oblique myokymia (p. 285).

5. Other saccadic disturbances. These include unilateral oculomotor apraxia, Huntington's chorea, and saccadic dysfunction in dementia and multiple sclerosis.

Rare Causes of Nystagmus

There are a number of rare syndromes and pathologies that can cause nystagmus which are uncommonly encountered by community optometrists. These are summarised in Table 18.1.

Classification Based on Eye Movement Characteristics

The classification of nystagmus by eye movement characteristics requires apparatus for objectively recording eye movements. Nystagmoid eye movements may be pendular (Fig. 18.1A), or jerky, consisting of a fast (saccadic eye movement) phase and a slow (slow eye movement) phase. The direction of jerk nystagmus is defined by the direction of the fast component. In jerk nystagmus, it is important to know whether the slow phase is accelerating (Fig. 18.1B), or decelerating (Fig. 18.1C) and this requires an eye movement recording of the type shown in Fig. 18.1. Ideally, a trace of velocity versus time should also be obtained.

The waveform in infantile and many forms of acquired nystagmus can be pendular or jerk. The jerk movement in INS characteristically has an accelerating slow phase (Dell'Osso & Daroff, 1975),

TABLE 18.1 ■ Rare Causes of Nystagmus.

Condition	Classification	Systemic signs	Nature of nystagmus
Heimann-Bielschowsky phenomenon (dissociated vertical nystagmus) (Jeong, Oh, Hwang, & Kim, 2008)	Vertical oscillation of an eye with impaired vision	Cases reported following cataract surgery with complications resulting in impaired vision in one eye. Several years later, patient reports vertical diplopia or oscillopsia	Only affects the eye with impaired vision Vertical oscillation of equal velocity in both vertical directions. Can resolve spontaneously or respond to gabapentin
Vestibular migraine (Polensek & Tusa, 2009)	Vestibular	Nystagmus associated with vertigo, nausea, headache. The nystagmus resolves when the headache abates	Positional nystagmus, commonly sustained, low velocity, can be horizontal, vertical, or torsional
Vitamin B12 deficiency (Akdal et al., 2007)	Brain stem		Bilateral internuclear ophthalmoplegia or downbeat nystagmus
Wernicke-Korsakoff syndrome (Isenberg-Grzeda et al., 2016)	Neurogenic	Neuropsychiatric deficiency caused by Vitamin B1 deficiency, can occur in alcoholics or cancer patients	Horizontal or vertical nystagmus Palsy of 6th nerve & 3rd nerve Gaze palsy

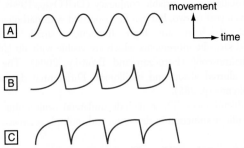

Fig. 18.1 Schematic eye movement traces to illustrate (A) pendular nystagmus and (B) jerk nystagmus with an accelerating slow phase and (C) with a decelerating slow phase. Faster eye movements are represented by lines which are more vertical: the eyes are stationary when the trace is horizontal.

suggesting a deficit in the slow eye movement subsystem. Latent nystagmus, on the other hand, has a decelerating slow phase and always beats towards the viewing eye. However, there are occasional patients who have INS with a decelerating slow phase (Abadi & Dickinson, 1986) and Bourron-Madignier (1995) believed that intermediary and mixed forms exist. Dell'Osso (1994) noted that since INS persists in the dark, it is not likely to be a primary deficit of the fixation mechanism. The waveform in INS usually has a torsional component (Maybodi, 2003).

Dell'Osso and Daroff (1975) presented a classification of INS waveforms into 12 different types. The situation is complicated because most people with INS exhibit more than one type of waveform and the waveform cannot be used to determine the type of nystagmus, as classified in the previous section (Abadi & Dickinson, 1986). Indeed, the waveform in a person with INS may evolve with time to develop adaptations which increase the foveation period, described below (Abadi & Dickinson, 1986).

The **foveation period** is the proportion of time that the object of regard is imaged at or very close to the fovea and during which the image is moving slowly enough for useful information to be assimilated. The precision of foveation is a better of predictor of acuity than the intensity of the nystagmus (Abadi & Dickinson, 1986). Dell'Osso (1994) argued that the ability to use a foveation period explains why patients with infantile and manifest latent nystagmus do not often report oscillopsia. However, Waugh and Bedell (1992) found that people with nystagmus sample visual information continuously, not just during one phase of the nystagmus. Extraretinal signals are likely to play a role in alleviating the perception of motion smear from the eye movements in INS, in the same way as they do during eye movements in normal observers (Bedell, 2000). It is not just the duration of the foveation period that is important in INS, but also the period of temporal integration of the visual system (Chung & Bedell, 1997).

Investigation

SYMPTOMS AND HISTORY

Children with a low birth weight (<2000 g) or birth complications are seven times more likely to have nystagmus than other children (Stayte, Johnson, & Wortham, 1990). Approximately 1 in 10 children with cerebral palsy or visual impairment have nystagmus (Grisham, 1990), and it is also more common in children with spina bifida (Caines, Dahl, & Holmstrom, 2007) and vitamin B12 deficiency (Akdal et al., 2007).

Idiopathic INS is diagnosed by exclusion, and the lengths to which ophthalmologists go to exclude sensory defects varies. As noted later, electrophysiological testing is required.

Many patients with nystagmus adopt an anomalous head position so they are looking in their null position (see later). A patient who reports recent onset oscillopsia (usually accompanied by dizziness) and poor vision is very likely to have acquired nystagmus, requiring referral. Acquired nystagmus may also be associated with diplopia and, in recent cases, past pointing. Most patients with INS do not spontaneously report oscillopsia, but on careful questioning might report this under certain viewing conditions (Cham, Anderson, & Abel, 2008a).

Nystagmus is a sign with many different causes and some of these causes are genetically determined, so nystagmus often runs in families. However, in INS many aspects of the waveform are not genetically determined (Abadi, Dickinson, Lomas, & Ackerley, 1983).

OCULAR HEALTH

Ocular pathology must be excluded in all cases of nystagmus. Particular attention should be paid to the optic discs and visual fields. The degree of ocular pigmentation should be noted: ocular albinos do not have hypopigmentation of the hair and skin but do have reduced iris and fundus pigment, and foveal hypoplasia. Optical coherence topography is useful in differential diagnosis of foveal hypoplasia (Self et al., 2020). An iris transillumination test should be carried out in all cases, as even brown irides can demonstrate the transillumination characteristic of ocular albinism (Day & Narita, 1997). A slit lamp biomicroscope is used with the illumination directed through the centre of the pupil, to create retroillumination. The iris is observed under low magnification and if the red retinal reflex can be seen through the iris, this suggests that there is either iris atrophy or ocular albinism. Ocular albinism usually causes transillumination throughout the iris, but the hypopigmentation can be sectoral on the iris or fundus (Shiono, Mutoh, Chida, & Tamai, 1994). Some normal, nonalbinotic, patients also demonstrate iris transillumination, and this can be seen where there is history of iritis.

REFRACTION

Chung and Bedell (1995) found that, in INS, contour interaction (crowding) is greater when stimuli are presented against a black background than against white. This effect can reduce the visual acuity (VA) by two Snellen lines.

Many patients with INS have a high refractive error and early onset nystagmus appears to interfere with normal refractive development (Sampath & Bedell, 2002). With-the-rule astigmatism is especially common (Jethani, Prakash, Vijayalakshmi, & Parija, 2006). This was initially attributed to lid pressure (Spielmann, 1994), but may in fact be due to meridional emmetropisation (Wang et al., 2010). A very careful refraction is required; often the patient will notice a significant improvement with updated spectacles. Some cases of INS have a latent component to the nystagmus (the nystagmus increases when one eye is covered) and monocular refraction is best carried out with a high-power fogging lens over the other eye, rather than an occluder. Similarly, binocular acuities are much more useful in predicting vision in everyday life than monocular acuities (Norn, 1964). The contrast sensitivity function is a useful measure of visual function in nystagmus (Abadi, 1979; Dickinson & Abadi, 1985). Accommodative function is often below normal limits in people with INS (Ong, Ciuffreda, & Tannen, 1993).

BINOCULAR VISION

Latent nystagmus is usually (Grisham, 1990), or always (Dell'Osso, 1994), associated with strabismus and INS is often associated with strabismus. Normal criteria should be applied in deciding whether to treat binocular anomalies. Anecdotal reports suggest that improving sensory and motor fusion can help to stabilise nystagmus in some cases (Leung, Wick, & Bedell, 1996; Scheiman & Wick, 1994). Many, if not all, patients with ocular or cutaneous albinism have abnormal visual pathways in the chiasma and no potential for true binocular vision.

CLINICAL INVESTIGATION OF NYSTAGMUS

The eye movements should be observed for a couple of minutes (Worfolk, 1993) and the nystagmus described (Table 18.2). In INS, there is often a **gaze null position** (a position of gaze in which the nystagmus is reduced), and the null position may change over time (Abadi & Dickinson, 1986). In about 8% of infantile-onset cases, the nystagmus is reduced markedly upon near fixation (Abadi & Dickinson, 1986): a convergent null position.

Foveation precision is an important index of VA and can be appraised ophthalmoscopically using a small projected fixation target and a red-free filter to enhance foveal contrast (Abadi & Dickinson, 1986).

There are many methods for objectively recording eye movements (Terao, Fukuda, & Hikosaka, 2017). They are not usually available in primary care practice and will not be described here. Methods that are claimed to assess eye movements using a simulated reading task (e.g, reading digits) were discussed on p. 29.

Evaluation

An important clinical judgement for the optometrist is whether the nystagmus is infantile, latent, or acquired. The characteristic features of these conditions are summarised in Table 18.3.

Management

Patients with nystagmus that has not been previously investigated in a hospital clinic should be referred because of the risk of an underlying pathology (Holmstrom, Bondeson, Eriksson,

TABLE 18.2 ■ Clinical Observations of Nystagmus.

Characteristic	Observations
General observations	General posture, facial asymmetries, head posture
Type of nystagmus	Pendular, jerk, or mixed (N.B., this is the apparent type, possibly different to the actual type by eye movement recording)
Direction	Horizontal, vertical, torsional, or combination
Amplitude	Small (<2 degrees), moderate (2–10 degrees), large (>10 degrees; cornea moves by more than 3 mm)
Frequency	Slow (<0.5 cycles per second; Hz), moderate (0.5–2 Hz), fast (>2 Hz)
Constancy	Constant, intermittent, periodic
Conjugacy	Conjugate (both eyes' movements approximately parallel), disjunctive (eyes move independently), or monocular
Latent component	Does nystagmus increase or change with occlusion of one eye? If so, does it always beat towards the uncovered eye?
Field of gaze changes	Null point: does nystagmus increase or decrease in any field of gaze or with convergence?

Modified after Grisham, D. (1990). Management of nystagmus in young children. *Problems in Optometry*, **2**(3), 496–527.

Akerblom, & Larsson, 2013). Electrodiagnostic testing (electroretinography and pattern visual evoked potentials) are required, without which some sensory defects (e.g., congenital stationary night blindness, cone dysfunction) can be missed (Self et al., 2020). Optometrists' referrals should therefore recommend that the patient should be seen in a tertiary centre with the appropriate facilities.

There is no cure for nystagmus and an apparent improvement following vision therapy for any condition could be attributable to a placebo effect. Patients with INS are likely to become more relaxed with each subsequent measurement of their visual acuities, causing an improvement simply because they are less stressed. It is therefore important that any treatment for nystagmus should be evaluated with double-masked randomised placebo-controlled trials, and yet there have been few such studies (Evans, 2006b). Even when an improvement is shown during or immediately after treatment, the patient has only really been helped if this improvement transfers into everyday life.

In the UK, for Group 1 (car and motorcycle) and Group 2 (bus and lorry) drivers, the Driver and Vehicle Licensing Agency (DVLA) need not be notified of nystagmus providing the vision standards for driving are achieved and any associated medical condition is declared (DVLA, 2020).

GOALS OF THE TREATMENT OF NYSTAGMUS

The four goals of nystagmus treatment are to improve: VA, cosmesis from the ocular oscillation, cosmesis from any abnormal head position, and (in acquired nystagmus) oscillopsia. An informal survey by the author at an open day of the Nystagmus Network demonstrated that the first of these, an improvement in VA, was by far the highest priority of most people with nystagmus.

Whatever the underlying aetiology of the nystagmus, some of the reduced VA is likely to be attributable to the constant oscillation of the eyes, causing reduced foveation time (Bedell, White, & Abplanalp, 1989). Treatment of this motor element should not just be aimed at reducing the nystagmus, but also at changing the waveform to one (pseudocycloid) with a longer percentage foveation

TABLE 18.3 ■ Characteristic Features of Infantile, Latent, and Acquired Nystagmus to Aid Differential Diagnosis.

INS	Latent nystagmus	Acquired nystagmus
Nearly always presents in first 6 months of life	Usually presents in first 6 months of life, and almost always in first 12 months	Onset at any age and usually associated with other symptoms (e.g., nausea, vertigo, movement or balance disorders)
Family history often present (X-linked or, less commonly, autosomal modes of inheritance)	May be family history of underlying cause (e.g., infantile esotropia)	History may include head trauma or neurological disease such as cerebellar degeneration or multiple sclerosis
Oscillopsia absent or rare under normal viewing conditions	Oscillopsia absent or rare under normal viewing conditions	Oscillopsia common; may also have diplopia
Usually horizontal, although small vertical and torsional movements may be present. Pure vertical or torsional presentations are rare	Always horizontal, and, on monocular occlusion, saccadic, beating away from the covered eye	Oscillations may be horizontal, vertical, or torsional depending on the site of the lesion. Vertical or torsional nystagmus has been described as a 'red flag' for pathology (Self et al., 2020)
The eye movements are bilateral and conjugate to the naked eye	Oscillations are always conjugate	Oscillations may be disconjugate and in different planes
Eye movement recordings show accelerating slow phase	Decelerating slow phase	Jerk, pendular, or saw-toothed waveform
May be present with other ocular conditions: albinism, achromatopsia, aniridia, optic atrophy	Usually occurs secondary to an early-onset interruption of binocular vision, particularly infantile esotropia; may be associated with DVD (p. 132)	Results from pathological lesion or trauma affecting motor areas of brain or motor pathways
A head turn may be present to utilise a null zone, although nystagmus is present in all directions of gaze	May be a head turn in the direction of the fixating eye	There may be a gaze direction in which nystagmus is absent, and a corresponding head turn
Intensity may lessen on convergence, but is worse when fatigued or under stress	More intense when the fixating eye abducts, less on adduction	
Pursuit and optokinetic reflexes may be 'inverted'		Peripheral vestibular disease (e.g., Ménière's) usually has linear slow phases and worsens if fixation target is removed

DVD, Dissociated vertical deviation; INS, infantile nystagmus syndrome.

time per cycle (Dickinson & Abadi, 1985). Because INS occurs during the sensitive period, this reduced acuity can cause meridional amblyopia (Abadi & King-Smith, 1979). As the child ages, the amplitude of nystagmus usually reduces (Harris, 1997), so the residual reduced vision may be attributable in part to the ocular oscillation and in part to amblyopia that occurred secondary to the oscillation (Chung & Bedell, 1995, 1996; Spierer, 1991).

One interesting feature of INS is that most patients do not experience oscillopsia; they are unaware that their eyes are 'wobbling' (Bedell, 1992). This is in most respects advantageous, but the lack of feedback about the nystagmus might be one reason why they are unable to control their ocular oscillations (Abplanalp & Bedell, 1983). Some interventions have aimed to provide this feedback.

REFRACTIVE MANAGEMENT: SPECTACLES AND CONTACT LENSES

Patients with INS often prefer contact lenses to spectacles (Biousse et al., 2004), possibly owing to optical factors and the contact lenses providing a form of bio-feedback (Abadi, 1979). The lenses seem to provide tactile feedback from the inner eyelids that dampens INS and results in better acuity (Dell'Osso, Traccis, Abel, & Erzurum, 1988).

A small study of patients with INS suggested the reported improvement in visual function with contact lenses is from better optical correction of the refractive error rather than a dampening of the nystagmus (Biousse et al., 2004). A small crossover trial found no significant differences between soft contact lenses and rigid contact lenses and spectacles for any nystagmus characteristics and similar VA in all conditions (Jayaramachandran, Proudlock, Odedra, Gottlob, & McLean, 2014). However, 40% of participants reported that rigid contact lenses gave better vision than spectacles (55% said about the same). It was not reported whether the 40% had any particular characteristics. A pilot randomised controlled trial (RCT) found a slight improvement in VA with contact lenses and a larger UK RCT is planned (Theodorou et al., 2018).

Dell'Osso (1994) recommended that patients with a convergent null position could benefit from prisms with −1.00 overcorrection to create accommodative-convergence. A case study of a pre-presbyopic patient with INS and convergence excess found a near addition helpful (Evans, 2001e). The important point is to evaluate whether patients are capable of binocular single vision and, if so, to carefully investigate the effect of refractive correction on their binocular status.

RELIEVING PRISMS

It was noted earlier that the intensity of INS is sometimes reduced in near vision. This effect is not mediated by convergence or accommodation and is determined solely by the angle between the visual axes: binocular viewing is not necessary (Abadi & Dickinson, 1986). Prescribing base-out prisms might be helpful in these cases. This is not a universal treatment: most cases of INS do not show reduced nystagmus at near (Abadi & Dickinson, 1986), and there may even be an increase in intensity at near in some cases (Ukwade & Bedell, 1992).

Some cases of INS benefit from the correction of small vertical deviations (Evans, 2001e). Yoked prisms can also be used in nystagmus to cause a version movement, so the eyes look through the null gaze position without an anomalous head position, or with a reduced, anomalous head position.

EYE EXERCISES/VISION THERAPY

Latent nystagmus can be a barrier to conventional occlusion therapy for strabismic amblyopia. Stegall (1973) reported the latent nystagmus can be overcome by using a narrow band transmission red filter over the unoccluded eye. He also described two studies which found a reduction in latent nystagmus in the unoccluded eye when a cycloplegic was instilled. In addition to penalisation methods, Scheiman and Wick (1994) recommended using anaglyph techniques to treat amblyopia in latent nystagmus and suggested vision therapy can be effective at reducing latent nystagmus, supporting Healy (1962). Leung et al. (1996) reported improvements in a few case studies of INS following vision therapy; but there have been no RCTs (Evans, 2006a). Similarly, vision therapy for 'oculomotor rehabilitation' following mild traumatic brain injury has been criticised for providing very low-certainty evidence (Rowe et al., 2018).

Auditory Bio-Feedback

Apparatus was developed that measures eye movements and translates these into auditory signals (Abadi, Carden, & Simpson, 1980; Abadi, Carden, & Simpson, 1981). Eye movements to the right or left can be converted to sounds in the appropriate earphone and the pitch of the sound made proportional to the magnitude of the eye movement (Abplanalp & Bedell, 1983). Case studies and open trials produced encouraging results in several types of nystagmus (Abplanalp & Bedell, 1987; Ciuffreda, Goldrich, & Neary, 1982; Kirschen, 1983). However, there have been no RCTs of auditory feedback (Evans, 2006b).

Visual (After-Image) Bio-Feedback

Visual bio-feedback can be achieved using an after-image (Stegall, 1973; Stohler, 1973), and this may be more effective at translating into everyday life than treatment solely based on auditory bio-feedback (Abplanalp & Bedell, 1983). People with nystagmus usually spontaneously comment that they perceive an after-image to be 'wobbling'. This movement is related (but not equal in magnitude; Kommerell, Horn, & Bach, 1986) to their eye movements and it has been suggested that patients can improve their nystagmus by trying to reduce the movement of the after-image (Mallett, personal communication).

An alternative after-image technique (Stegall, 1973) is to allow the patient to adopt a head position to reduce the 'wobble' and then slowly straighten their head. Goldrich (1981) described a perceptual effect, **emergent textual contours**, which he claimed allowed nystagmus patients to monitor their nystagmus as an alternative to an after-image.

Active Amblyopia Therapy: Intermittent Photic Stimulation

People with INS may have some level of amblyopia associated with their nystagmus (Abadi & King-Smith, 1979; Currie et al., 1993). Mallett (1983) described the use of intermittent photic stimulation (IPS) for the treatment of infantile idiopathic nystagmus. Scheiman and Wick (1994) described a case study where IPS had been used to treat nystagmus successfully. An RCT of this treatment is described next.

Combining Treatment Approaches

The greatest chance of success will probably be obtained by combining two or more of the aforementioned methods. Ciuffreda et al. (1982) described a combination of auditory and visual biofeedback. Mallett and Radnam (1992) advocated a combination of after-image feedback and IPS treatment for infantile (including albinotic) nystagmus.

Evans et al. (1998) carried out an RCT of the combined treatment described by Mallett and Radnam (1992). They studied 38 subjects which, according to a statistical sample size calculation, should have been enough for a clinically significant treatment effect to reach statistical significance. The VA and contrast sensitivity (CS) were assessed three times before undergoing treatment for 6 weeks, and then once more after treatment.

Evans et al.'s RCT clearly demonstrates that the improvement in high contrast VA of the group receiving the experimental treatment is not significantly different to the improvement in those receiving a placebo treatment (Fig. 18.2). If we just look at the data for the experimental group, we can investigate what the outcome of the study would have been if it had been a noncontrolled trial, like most other studies of treatments for nystagmus. Fig. 18.3 illustrates the improvement in VA of the experimental group from the first VA measurement to the final, posttreatment, assessment. A matched pairs t-test on the pre- and posttreatment data in Fig. 18.3 shows that the apparent improvement in VA is statistically significant ($P = .031$). Yet Fig. 18.2 shows that this improvement

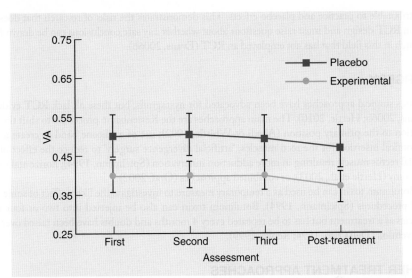

Fig. 18.2 Graph of high contrast Bailey-Lovie visual acuity *(VA)* at each research visual assessment (error bars represent 1 standard error of the mean). VA is in LogMAR units, so smaller values represent better VA (0.4 represents 6/15 and 0.5 represents 6/18). VA was measured three times before treatment, to investigate the practice effect, and once after treatment. (Reproduced with permission from Evans B.J., Evans B.V., Jordahl-Moroz J., Nabee M. (1998). Randomised double-masked placebo-controlled trial of a treatment for congenital nystagmus. *Vision Research*, 38(14), 2193–2202.)

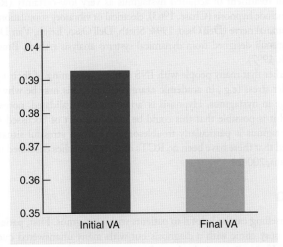

Fig. 18.3 Bar chart representing the improvement in LogMAR VA of the experimental group of Evans et al. (1998). VA is in LogMAR units, so that smaller figures represent better VA. Note: This figure deliberately misrepresents the overall results of the study to illustrate the dangers of researching therapies for INS without using an RCT design (text). *INS*, Infantile nystagmus; *RCT*, randomised controlled trial; *VA*, visual acuity. (From Evans B.J., Evans B.V., Jordahl-Moroz J., Nabee M. (1998). Randomised double-masked placebo-controlled trial of a treatment for congenital nystagmus. *Vision Research*, 38(14), 2193–2202.)

is attributable to practice and placebo effects. This demonstrates the risks of research that does not use an RCT design and must raise questions about whether any safe conclusions can be drawn from research in this field that has not employed an RCT (Evans, 2006b).

SURGERY

Various surgical approaches have been advocated for nystagmus, but these all lack RCT evidence (Evans, 2006b; Hertle, 2010). The main approaches are the Kestenbaum procedure to shift the null position to the primary position (Abadi & Whittle, 1992); use of a silicone band to create a new anatomical insertion for the recti muscles; 'artificial divergence surgery' to reduce the effect of the medial rectus muscle resulting in more adduction innervation (Spielmann, 1994); horizontal rectus tenotomy (Hertle et al., 2003); or combined approaches (Graf, 2002).

Botulinum toxin can be used as a temporary measure to investigate the likely effect of some surgical procedures (Spielmann, 1994). Botulinum toxin can also be injected into two or four recti muscles as a treatment but has to be repeated every 4 months and doubts have been raised over this intervention (Dell'Osso, 1994; Repka, 1999).

OTHER TREATMENT APPROACHES

Leigh, Rushton, Thurston, Hertle, and Yaniglos (1988) used an electronic device to stabilise the retinal image and reduce oscillopsia in patients with acquired nystagmus due to neurological disease. This can be used to calculate the power required for a telescopic contact lens system (high minus contact lens with high plus spectacle lens) which provides partial optical stabilisation of the retinal image (Yaniglos & Leigh, 1992).

Pharmacological agents have been used to treat nystagmus, most commonly acquired nystagmus (Grisham, 1990; Richman, Garzia, & Cron, 1992) and may also have a role in INS (Shery, Proudlock, Sarvananthan, McLean, & Gottlob, 2006). A Cochrane review described the evidence for pharmacological treatment of acquired nystagmus as very low-certainty (Rowe et al., 2018). Other approaches include hypnosis (Chase, 1963), electrical or vibratory stimulation of the ophthalmic division of the trigeminal nerve (Dell'Osso, 1994; Sheth, Dell'Osso, Leigh, Van Doren, & Peckham, 1995), and visual stimuli designed from dynamical systems analysis (Abadi, Broomhead, Clement, Whittle, & Worfolk, 1997).

It was noted earlier that many people with INS suffer a worsening of their nystagmus and VA when they are under stress (e.g., in academic examinations). This may be why the placebo effect seems to be so large in nystagmus. Hypnosis is 'an empirically-validated, non-deceptive placebo' (Kirsch, 1996) and it is possible that this could be used as a sort of 'focussed relaxation' to help patients whose nystagmus is particularly troublesome in certain stressful situations. Once again though, it is stressed that there have been no RCTs of the approaches described in this 'other treatments' section (Evans, 2006b).

COUNSELLING

Three sorts of counselling can be helpful to patients with nystagmus. First, patients are sometimes discharged from a busy clinic with a diagnosis but with many unanswered questions (Budge & Derbyshire, 2005). If the diagnosis is clear, the community optometrist can explain what this means. The hospital should provide a report with clear discharge information, including a diagnosis to the patient and community optometrist (Self et al., 2020). Optometrists can advise, for example, a diagnosis of idiopathic INS does not mean the infant is, or will go, blind. Although the nystagmus will always be present, it usually reduces a little as the child ages (Harris, 1997) and the level of vision usually permits most everyday activities, although driving will probably not be possible.

The second type of counselling is genetic counselling to discuss whether an underlying pathology or idiopathic nystagmus is likely to be passed to future generations. This should be provided by appropriate experts, genetic counsellors, who are usually found in major hospitals.

The third type of counselling is to give patients or their parents advice that will help them deal with the nystagmus on a day-to-day basis. For example, if there is a null zone in a certain direction of gaze, a child should be allowed to sit at a position in class that takes advantage of this. Maximum reading speeds can be near normal in INS when optimal font sizes are provided, even in individuals with poor VA or intense nystagmus (Barot, McLean, Gottlob, & Proudlock, 2013). These researchers showed that reading performance in INS is acutely sensitive to font size, which may need to be as much as 6 LogMAR lines larger than the near VA.

People with nystagmus or their families can often receive considerable support from talking to other people with the condition. The Nystagmus Network provides this type of support and has excellent literature (www.nystagmusnetwork.org).

CLINICAL KEY POINTS

- The main types of nystagmus are infantile nystagmus syndrome (INS), latent nystagmus (usually from early onset strabismus) and (more rarely) acquired (neurological) nystagmus
- INS can occur secondary to a sensory defect, including albinism, or idiopathic where there is assumed to be a motor defect
- The apparent pattern of nystagmoid eye movements cannot be used to determine the aetiology of the nystagmus nor the level of vision
- All new cases in adults need referral to a neuro-ophthalmologist; new cases in children to a paediatric hospital eye clinic
- Nystagmus often varies over time and at different gaze positions and fixation distances
- There may be an anomalous head position, so the gaze is in a 'null position'
- High refractive errors are common
- Orthoptic problems should be treated if causing symptoms, but patients with albinism are probably unable to exhibit true binocular vision
- There is no cure for nystagmus and claims about treatments should be viewed cautiously in the absence of randomised controlled trials

REFERENCES

Abadi, R. V. (1979). Visual performance with contact lenses and congenital idiopathic nystagmus. *British Journal of Physiological Optics, 33*(3), 32–37.

Abadi, R. V., Broomhead, D. S., Clement, R. A., Whittle, J. P., & Worfolk, R. (1997). Dynamical systems analysis: a new method of analysing congenital nystagmus waveforms. *Experimental Brain Research, 117*, 355–361.

Abadi, R. V., Carden, D., & Simpson, J. (1980). A new treatment for congenital nystagmus. *British Journal of Ophthalmology, 64*, 2–6.

Abadi, R. V., Carden, D., & Simpson, J. (1981). Listening for eye movements. *Ophthalmic and Physiological Optics, 1*, 19–27.

Abadi, R. V., & Dickinson, C. M. (1986). Waveform characteristics in congenital nystagmus. *Documenta Ophthalmologica, 64*, 153–167.

Abadi, R. V., Dickinson, C. M., Lomas, M. S., & Ackerley, R. (1983). Congenital idiopathic nystagmus in identical twins. *British Journal of Ophthalmology, 67*, 693–695.

Abadi, R. V., & King-Smith, P. E. (1979). Congenital nystagmus modifies orientation detection. *Vision Research, 19*, 1409–1411.

Abadi, R. V., & Whittle, J. (1992). Surgery and compensatory head postures in congenital nystagmus. *Archives of Ophthalmology, 110*, 632–635.

Abbott, M. L., Schmid, K. L., & Strang, N. C. (1998). Differences in the accommodation stimulus response curves of adult myopes and emmetropes. *Ophthalmic & Physiological Optics, 18*(1), 13–20.

Abd Manan, F., Jenkins, T. C. A., & Collinge, A. J. (2001). The effect of clinical visual stress on stereoacuity measured with the TNO test. *Malaysian Journal Medical Sciences, 8*(2), 25–31.

Abdi, S., Lennerstrand, G., Pansell, T., & Rydberg, A. (2008). Orthoptic findings and asthenopia in a population of Swedish schoolchildren aged 6 to 16 years. *Strabismus, 16*(2), 47–55.

Abdi, S., Thunholm-Henriksson, I.-L., & Pansell, T. (2016). Stepwise increase of hypermetropic correction using contact lenses in intermittent partially accommodative esotropia. *Clinical and Experimental Optometry, 99*(3), 258–263.

Abplanalp, P., & Bedell, H. (1987). Visual improvement in an albinotic patient with an alteration of congenital nystagmus (case report). *American Journal of Optometry and Physiological Optics, 64*(12), 944–951.

Abplanalp, P. L., & Bedell, H. (1983). Biofeedback therapy in rehabilitative optometry. *Rehabilitative Optometry Journal, 1*, 11–14.

Abrahamsson, M., & Sjostrand, J. (2003). Astigmatic axis and amblyopia in childhood. *Acta Ophthalmologica Scandinavica, 81*, 33–37.

Abramson, D. H., Beaverson, K., Sangani, P., Vora, R. A., Lee, T. C., Hochberg, H. M., ... Ranjithan, M. (2003). Screening for retinoblastoma: presenting signs as prognosticators of patient and ocular survival. *Pediatrics, 112*(6 Pt 1), 1248–1255.

Adams, G. G. W., & Karas, M. P. (1999). Effect of amblyopia on employment prospects. *British Journal of Ophthalmology, 83*, 378.

Adams, W. E., Leske, D. A., Hatt, S. R., & Holmes, J. M. (2009). Defining real change in measures of stereoacuity. *Ophthalmology, 116*(2), 281–285.

Adler, P. (2001). Optometric evaluation of binocular vision anomalies. In B. Evans, & S. Doshi (Eds.), *Binocular Vision and Orthoptics* (pp. 1–12). Oxford: Butterworth-Heinemann.

Adler, P., Scally, A. J., & Barrett, B. T. (2012). Test-retest variability of Randot stereoacuity measures gathered in an unselected sample of UK primary school children. *The British Journal of Ophthalmology, 96*(5), 656–661.

Adler, P., Scally, A. J., & Barrett, B. T. (2013). Test-retest reproducibility of accommodation measurements gathered in an unselected sample of UK primary school children. *British Journal of Ophthalmology, 97*, 592–597.

Adler, P. M., Cregg, M., Viollier, A. J., & Woodhouse, J. M. (2007). Influence of target type and RAF rule on the measurement of near point of convergence. *Ophthalmic and Physiological Optics, 27*(1), 22–30.

Adoh, T. O., & Woodhouse, J. M. (1994). The Cardiff Acuity Test used for measuring visual acuity development in toddlers. *Vision Research, 34*(4), 555–560.

Ahn, S. J., Yang, H. K., & Hwang, J. M. (2012). Binocular visual acuity in intermittent exotropia: role of accommodative convergence. *American Journal of Ophthalmology, 154*(6), 981–986.

Ainsworth, J. R. (1999). Clinical decision making in paediatric ophthalmology. *Optometry Today,* 26–33, May 7.

Aitchison, D. A., Capper, E. J., & McCabe, K. L. (1994). Critical subjective measurement of amplitude of accommodation. *Optometry and Vision Science, 71,* 699–706.

Akdal, G., Yener, G. G., Ada, E., & Halmagyi, G. M. (2007). Eye movement disorders in vitamin B12 deficiency: two new cases and a review of the literature. *European Journal of Neurology, 14*(10), 1170–1172.

Akinci, A., Guven, A., Degerliyurt, A., Kibar, E., Mutlu, M., & Citirik, M. (2008). The correlation between headache and refractive errors. *Journal of AAPOS, 12*(3), 290–293.

Al-Bagdady, M., Stewart, R. E., Watts, P., Murphy, P. J., & Woodhouse, J. M. (2009). Bifocals and Down's syndrome: correction or treatment? *Ophthalmic & Physiological Optics, 29*(4), 416–421.

Aletaha, M., Daneshvar, F., Mosallaei, M., Bagheri, A., & Khalili, M. R. (2018). Comparison of three vision therapy approaches for convergence insufficiency. *Journal of Ophthalmic and Vision Research, 13*(3), 307–314.

Al-Haddad, C. E., Mollayess, G. M., Cherfan, C. G., Jaafar, D. F., & Bashshur, Z. F. (2011). Retinal nerve fibre layer and macular thickness in amblyopia as measured by spectral-domain optical coherence tomography. *The British Journal of Ophthalmology, 95*(12), 1696–1699.

Alhassan, M., Hovis, J. K., & Chou, R. B. (2015). Repeatability of associated phoria tests. *Optometry and Vision Science, 92,* 900–907.

Alhassan, M., Hovis, J. K., & Chou, B. R. (2016). Comparison of MKH-Haase associated phoria charts with other common clinical tests. *Optometry & Visual Performance, 4*(5), 254–264.

Allen, P. M., & O'Leary, D. J. (2006). Accommodation functions: co-dependency and relationship to refractive error. *Vision Research, 46*(4), 491–505.

Aller, T. A., Laure, A., & Wildsoet, C. (2006). Results of a one-year prospective clinical trial (CONTROL) of the use of bifocal soft contact lenses to control myopia progression. *Ophthalmic and Physiological Optics, 26*(Suppl. 1), 8–9.

Almer, Z., Klein, K. S., Marsh, L., Gerstenhaber, M., & Repka, M. X. (2011). Ocular motor and sensory function in Parkinson's disease. *Ophthalmology, 119*(1), 178–182.

Almog, Y. (2008). A benign syndrome of transient loss of accommodation in young patients. *Archives of Ophthalmology, 126*(12), 1643–1646.

Alves, M., Miranda, A., Narciso, M. R., Mieiro, L., & Fonseca, T. (2015). Diplopia: a diagnostic challenge with common and rare etiologies. *The American Journal Of Case Reports, 16,* 220–223.

Amrhein, V., Greenland, S., & McShane, B. (2019). Scientists rise up against statistical significance. *Nature, 567*(7748), 305–307.

Anderson, H. A., & Stuebing, K. K. (2014). Subjective versus objective accommodative amplitude: preschool to presbyopia. *Optometry & Vision Science, 91*(11).

Anderson, J. E., Brown, S. M., Mathews, T. A., & Mathews, S. M. (2006). Opaque contact lens treatment for older children with amblyopia. *Eye & Contact Lens, 32*(2), 84–87.

Anker, S., Atkinson, J., Braddick, O., Nardini, M., & Ehrlich, D. (2004). Non-cycloplegic refractive screening can identify infants whose visual outcome at 4 years is improved by spectacle correction. *Strabismus, 12,* 227–245.

Ansons, A., & Spencer, A. (2001). The medical management of strabismus. In B. Evans, & S. Doshi (Eds.), *Binocular vision and orthoptics* (pp. 101–109). Oxford: Butterworth-Heinemann.

Ansons, A. M., & Davis, H. (2001). *Diagnosis and management of ocular motility disorders.* Oxford: Blackwell Science.

Anstice, N. S., Jacobs, R. J., Simkin, S. K., Thomson, M., Thompson, B., & Collins, A. V. (2017). Do picture-based charts overestimate visual acuity? Comparison of Kay Pictures, Lea Symbols, HOTV and Keeler logMAR charts with Sloan letters in adults and children. *PLoS One, 12*(2), e0170839.

Anstice, N. S., & Thompson, B. (2014). The measurement of visual acuity in children: an evidence-based update. *Clinical and Experimental Optometry, 97*(1), 3–11.

Antona, B., Barra, F., Barrio, A., Gonzalez, E., & Sanchez, I. (2007). Validity and repeatability of a new test for aniseikonia. *Investigative Ophthalmology Visual Science, 48*(1), 58–62.

Antona, B., Barrio, A., Barra, F., Gonzalez, E., & Sanchez, I. (2008). Repeatability and agreement in the measurement of horizontal fusional vergences. *Ophthalmic & Physiological Optics, 28*(5), 475–491.

Antonio-Santos, A., Vedula, S. S., Hatt, S. R., & Powell, C. (2020). Occlusion for stimulus deprivation amblyopia. *Cochrane Database of Systematic Reviews, 3*CD005136.

Arevalo, J. F., Lowder, C. Y., & Muci-Mendoza, R. (2002). Ocular manifestations of systemic lupus erythematosus. *Current Opinion in Ophthalmology, 13*(6), 404–410.

Aristodemou, P., Watt, L., Baldwin, C., & Hugkulstone, C. (2006). Diplopia associated with the cosmetic use of botulinum toxin a for facial rejuvenation. *Ophthalmic Plastic and Reconstructive Surgery, 22*, 134–136.

Arnoldi, K. (2001). Monofixation with eso-, exo-, or hypertropia: is there a difference? *American Orthoptic Journal, 51*, 55.

Aslin, R. N. (1993). Infant accommodation and convergence. In K. Simons (Ed.), *Early visual development: normal and abnormal* (pp. 30–38). New York: Oxford University Press.

Asper, L., Watt, K., & Khuu, S. (2018). Optical treatment of amblyopia: a systematic review and meta-analysis. *Clinical & Experimental Optometry, 101*(4), 431–442.

Assaf, A. A. (1982). The sensitive period: transfer of fixation after occlusion for strabismic amblyopia. *British Journal of Ophthalmology, 66*, 64–70.

Astin, C. L. K. (1998). The use of occluding tinted contact lenses. *Contact Lens Association of Ophthalmologists Journal, 24*, 125–127.

Atkinson, J., Anker, S., Evans, C., et al. (1988). Visual acuity testing of young children with the Cambridge crowding cards at 3 and 6 m. *Acta Ophthalmologica, 66*, 505–508.

Atkinson, J., Braddick, O., Nardini, M., & Anker, S. (2007). Infant hyperopia: detection, distribution, changes and correlates-outcomes from the Cambridge infant screening programs. *Optometry and Vision Science, 84*(2), 84–96.

Attebo, K., Mitchell, P., Cumming, R., Smith, W., Jolly, N., & Sparkes, R. (1998). Prevalence and causes of amblyopia in an adult population. *Ophthalmol, 105*, 154–159.

Averbuch-Heller, L., & Leigh, R. J. (1996). Eye movements. *Current Opinion in Neurology, 9*, 26–31.

Ayton, L. N., Abel, L. A., Fricke, T. R., & McBrien, N. A. (2009). Developmental eye movement test: what is it really measuring? *Optometry and Vision Science, 86*(6), 722–730.

Babinsky, E., & Candy, T. R. (2013). Why do only some hyperopes become strabismic? *Investigative Ophthalmology & Visual Science, 54*(7), 4941–4955.

Backus, B. T., Dornbos, B. D., Tran, T. A., Blaha, J. B., & Gupta, M. Z. (2018). Use of virtual reality to assess and treat weakness in human stereoscopic vision. *Electronic Imaging, Stereoscopic Displays and Applications XXIX, 6*, 109-1–109-6.

Bade, A., Boas, M., Gallaway, M., Mitchell, G. L., Scheiman, M., Kulp, M. T., ... Rouse, M. (2013). Relationship between clinical signs and symptoms of convergence insufficiency. *Optometry and Vision Science, 90*(9), 988–995.

Bagolini, B. (1967). Anomalous correspondence: definition and diagnostic methods. *Documenta Ophthalmologica, 23*, 346–386.

Bagolini, B. (1999). Bagolini's striated glasses: a reappraisal. *Binocular Vision & Strabismus Quarterly, 14*, 266–271.

Bagolini, B., Campos, E. C., & Chiesi, C. (1985). The Irvine 4 diopter prism test for the diagnosis of suppression: a reappraisal. *Binocular vision, 1*(2), 77–84.

Bagolini, B., Falsini, B., Cermola, S., & Porciatti, V. (1994). Binocular interactions and steady-stated VEPs. *Graefe's Archive for Clinical and Experimental Ophthalmology, 232*, 737–744.

Bailey, I. L., & Lovie, J. E. (1976). New design principles for visual acuity letter charts. *American Journal of Optometry and Physiological Optics, 53*, 740–745.

Baker, L. (2000). Ocular motor nerve palsies in diabetes. *CE Optometry, 3*(2), 72–76.

Bandyopadhyay, S. K., Chatterjee, A., & Banerjee, R. (2012). Peripapillary nerve fibre layer thickness and macular thickness in children with anisometropic amblyopia attending a referral centre in Eastern India. *Journal of the Indian Medical Association, 110*(8), 542–545.

Banks, R. V., Campbell, F. W., Hess, R., & Watson, P. G. (1978). A new treatment for amblyopia. *British Orthoptic Journal, 35*, 1–12.

Barbur, J. L., Hess, R. F., & Pinney, H. D. (1994). Pupillary function in human amblyopia. *Ophthalmic and Physiological Optics, 14*, 139–149.

Barnard, N. A. S., & Edgar, D. F. (1996). Examination techniques and routines. *Pediatric Eye Care* (pp. 105–136). Oxford: Blackwell.

Barnard, N. A. S., & Thomson, W. D. (1995). A quantitative analysis of eye movements during the cover test - a preliminary report. *Ophthalmic and Physiological Optics, 15*, 413–419.

Barnard, S. (1995). Ocular signs of child abuse. In S. Barnard, & D. Edgar (Eds.), *Pediatric eye care* (pp. 273–279). Oxford: Blackwell Science.

Barnett, A. G., van der Pols, J. C., & Dobson, A. J. (2005). Regression to the mean: what it is and how to deal with it. *International Journal of Epidemiology, 34*(1), 215–220.

Barot, N., McLean, R. J., Gottlob, I., & Proudlock, F. A. (2013). Reading performance in infantile nystagmus. *Ophthalmology, 120*(6), 1232–1238.

Barr, D. B., McFadzean, R. M., Hadley, D., Ramsay, A., Houston, C. A., & Russell, D. (1997). Acquired bilateral superior oblique palsy: a localising sign in the dorsal midbrain. *European Journal of Ophthalmology, 7*, 271–276.

Barrett, B. T., Candy, R. T., McGraw, P. V., & Bradley, A. (2005). Probing the causes of visual acuity loss in patients diagnosed with functional amblyopia. *Ophthalmic and Physiological Optics, 25*, 175–178.

Barrett, B. T., Pacey, I. E., Bradley, A., Thibos, L. N., & Morrill, P. (2003). Nonveridical visual perception in human amblyopia. *Investigative Ophthalmology and Visual Science, 44*, 1555–1567.

Barrett, B. T. (2008). A critical evaluation of the evidence supporting the practice of behavioural vision therapy. *Ophthalmic and Physiological Optics, 29*, 4–25.

Barrett, B. T., Bradley, A., & Candy, T. R. (2013). The relationship between anisometropia and amblyopia. *Progress in Retinal and Eye Research, 36*, 120–158.

Barrett, C. D. (1945). Sources of error and working methods in retinoscopy. *British Journal of Physiological Optics, 5*, 35–40.

Barry, S. R., & Bridgeman, B. (2017). An assessment of stereovision acquired in adulthood. *Optometry and Vision Science, 94*(10), 993–999.

Bates, D., Blau, J. N., Campbell, M. J., et al. (1993). *Migraine management guidelines*. Richmond: Synergy Medical Education.

Bauer, A., Dietz, K., Kolling, G., Hart, W., & Schiefer, U. (2001). The relevance of stereopsis for motorists: a pilot study. *Graefe's Archive for Clinical and Experimental Ophthalmology, 239*(6), 400–406.

Bauer, A., Kolling, G., Dietz, K., Zrenner, E., & Schiefer, U. (2000). Are cross-eyed persons worse drivers? The effect of stereoscopic disparity on driving skills. *Klinische Monatsblatter fur Augenheilkunde, 217*, 183–189.

Bayramlar, H., Gurturk, A. Y., Sari, U., & Karadag, R. (2016). Overcorrecting minus lens therapy in patients with intermittent exotropia: should it be the first therapeutic choice? *International Ophthalmology*, 1–6.

Beardsell, R., Clarke, S., & Hill, M. (1999). Outcome of occlusion treatment for amblyopia. *Journal of Pediatric Ophthalmology and Strabismus, 36*, 19–24.

Becker, R., Hubsch, S., Graf, M. H., & Kaufmann, H. (2002). Examination of young children with Lea symbols. *The British Journal of Ophthalmology, 86*, 513–516.

Bedell, H. E. (1992). Sensitivity to oscillatory target motion in congenital nystagmus. *Investigative Ophthalmology and Visual Science, 33*, 1811–1821.

Bedell, H. E. (2000). Perception of a clear and stable visual world with congenital nystagmus. *Optometry and Vision Science, 77*, 573–581.

Bedell, H. E., Lee Yap, Y., & Flom, M. C. (1990). Fixational drift and nasal-temporal pursuit asymmetries in strabismic amblyopes. *Investigative Ophthalmology and Visual Science, 31*, 968–976.

Bedell, H. E., & Loshin, D. S. (1991). Interrelations between measures of visual acuity and parameters of eye movement in congenital nystagmus. *Investigative Ophthalmology and Visual Science, 32*(2), 416–421.

Bedell, H. E., White, J. M., & Abplanalp, P. L. (1989). Variability of foveations in congenital nystagmus. *Clinical Vision Sciences, 4*, 247–252.

Benatar, M., & Kaminski, H. (2012). Medical and surgical treatment for ocular myasthenia. *Cochrane Database of Systematic Reviews* (12).

Beneish, R. G., Polomeno, R. C., Flanders, M. E., & Koenekoop, R. K. (2009). Optimal compliance for amblyopia therapy: occlusion with a translucent tape on the lens. *Canadian Journal of Ophthalmology*, *44*(5), 523−528.

Benzoni, J. A., Collier, J. D., McHugh, K., Rosenfield, M., & Portello, J. K. (2009). Does the dynamic cross cylinder test measure the accommodative response accurately? *Optometry*, *80*(11), 630−634.

Bhoola, H., Bruce, A. S., & Atchison, D. A. (1995). Validity of clinical measures of the AC/A ratio. *Clinical and Experimental Optometry*, *78*(1), 3−10.

Biglan, A. W. (1999). Pattern strabismus. In A. L. Rosenbaum, & A. P. Santiago (Eds.), *Clinical Strabismus Management* (pp. 202−216). Philadelphia: Saunders.

Biousse, V., Tusa, R. J., Russell, B., Azran, M. S., Das, V., Schubert, M. S., ... Newman, N. J. (2004). The use of contact lenses to treat visually symptomatic congenital nystagmus. *Journal of Neurology, Neurosurgery, and Psychiatry*, *75*(2), 314−316.

Birch, E. E., Fawcett, S. L., Morale, S. E., Weakley, D. R., Jr., & Wheaton, D. H. (2005). Risk factors for accommodative esotropia among hypermetropic children. *Investigative Ophthalmology & Visual Science*, *46*, 526−529.

Birch, E. E., Jost, R. M., Wang, Y.-Z., Kelly, K. R., & Giaschi, D. E. (2019). Impaired fellow eye motion perception and abnormal binocular function. *Investigative Ophthalmology & Visual Science*, *60*(10), 3374−3380.

Birch, E. E., Shimojo, S., & Held, R. (1985). Preferential-looking assessment of fusion and stereopsis in infants aged 1-6 months. *Investigative Ophthalmology & Visual Science*, *26*, 366−370.

Birch, E. E., & Stager, D. R. (1995). *The critical period for surgical treatment of dense congenital unilateral cataract, . Technical digest: vision science and its applications* (1, pp. 224−227). Optical Society of America.

Birch, E. E., Stager, D. R., Sr., Wang, J., & O'Connor, A. (2010). Longitudinal changes in refractive error of children with infantile esotropia. *Eye (Lond)*, *24*(12), 1814−1821.

Birch, E. E., & Swanson, W. H. (2000). Hyperacuity deficits in anisometropic and strabismic amblyopes with known ages of onset. *Vision Research*, *40*, 1035−1040.

Birnbaum, M. H. (1993). *Optometric management of nearpoint disorders*. Boston: Butterworth-Heinemann.

Birnbaum, M. H. (1994). Behavioral optometry: a historical perspective. *Journal of the American Optometric Association*, *65*(4), 255−264.

Bishop, A. (1991). *Vision in childhood: young children at visual risk*. British College of Optometrists, London.

Bishop, A. (2001). Convergence and convergent fusional reserves - investigation and treatment. In B. Evans, & S. Doshi (Eds.), *In Binocular vision and orthoptics* (pp. 28−33). Oxford: Butterworth-Heinemann.

Black, B. C. (2006). The influence of refractive error management on the natural history and treatment outcome of accommodative esotropia (an American Ophthalmological Society thesis). *Transactions of the American Ophthalmological Society*, *104*, 303−321.

Bobier, W. R., & McRae, M. (1996). Gain changes in the accommodative convergence cross-link. *Ophthalmic and Physiological Optics*, *16*, 318−325.

Borish, I. M. (1975). *Clinical refraction*. Chicago: The Professional Press Inc..

Borsting, E., Chase, C. H., & Ridder, W. H., III (2007). Measuring visual discomfort in college students. *Optometry and Vision Science*, *84*(8), 745−751.

Borsting, E., Rouse, M. W., & De Land, P. N. (1999). Prospective comparison of convergence insufficiency and normal binocular children on CIRS symptom survey. *Optometry and Vision Science*, *76*, 221−228.

Bourron-Madignier, M. (1995). Nystagmus. *Current Opinion in Ophthalmology*, *6*, 32−36.

Boylan, C., & Clement, R. A. (1987). Excursion tests of ocular motility. *Ophthalmic and Physiological Optics*, *7*, 31−35.

Bradbury, J. A., & Taylor, R. H. (2013). Severe complications of strabismus surgery. *Journal of AAPOS*, *17*(1), 59−63.

Bradford, G. M., Kutschke, P. J., & Scott, W. E. (1992). Results of amblyopia therapy in eyes with unilateral structural abnormalities. *Ophthalmology*, *99*, 1616−1621.

Brautaset, R., Wahlberg, M., Abdi, S., & Pansell, T. (2008). Accommodation insufficiency in children: are exercises better than reading glasses? *Strabismus*, *16*(2), 65−69.

Brautaset, R. L., & Jennings, J. A. (2006a). Measurements of objective and subjective fixation disparity with and without a central fusion stimulus. *Medical Science Monitor*, *12*, MT1−MT4.

Brautaset, R. L., & Jennings, J. A. M. (2001). Associated heterophoria and the measuring and correcting methodology after H.J. Haase (MKH). *Strabismus*, *9*, 165−176.

Brautaset, R. L., & Jennings, J. A. M. (2005a). Distance vergence adaptation is abnormal in subjects with convergence insufficiency. *Ophthalmic and Physiological Optics, 25*, 211–214.

Brautaset, R. L., & Jennings, J. A. M. (2005b). Horizontal and vertical prism adaptation are different mechanisms. *Ophthalmic and Physiological Optics, 25*, 215–218.

Brautaset, R. L., & Jennings, J. A. M. (2006b). Effects of orthoptic treatment on the CA/C and AC/A ratios in convergence insufficiency. *Investigative Ophthalmology Visual Science, 47*, 2876–2880.

Brautaset, R. L., & Jennings, J. A. (1999). The influence of heterophoria measurements on subsequent associated phoria measurement in a refractive routine. *Ophthalmic & Physiological Optics, 19*(4), 347–350.

Brazis, P. W. (1993). Palsies of the trochlear nerve: diagnosis and localization--recent concepts. *Mayo Clinic Proceedings. Mayo Clinic, 68*, 501–509.

Breinin, G. N. (1957). The nature of vergence revealed by electromyography, Part III. *Archives of Ophthalmology, 58*, 623–635.

Bremner, F. D. (2000). Pupil abnormalities. *Optometry Today, April 7*, 32–39.

Bridgeman, B., & Stark, L. (1991). Ocular proprioception and efference copy in registering visual direction. *Vision Research, 31*, 1903–1913.

Brodsky, M. C. (2005). Visuo-vestibular eye movements: infantile strabismus in 3 dimensions. *Archives of Ophthalmology, 123*, 837–842.

Brodsky, M. C. (2012). An expanded view of infantile esotropia: Bottoms up! *Archives of Ophthalmology, 130*(9), 1199–1202.

Brodsky, M. C., Donahue, S. P., Vaphiades, M., & Brandt, T. (2006). Skew deviation revisited. *Survey of Ophthalmology, 51*, 105–128.

Brownlee, G. A., & Goss, D. A. (1988). Comparisons of commercially available devices for the measurement of fixation disparity and associated phorias. *Journal of the American Optometric Association, 59*, 451–460.

Bruce, A., Pacey, I. E., Bradbury, J. A., Scally, A. J., & Barrett, B. T. (2013). Bilateral changes in foveal structure in individuals with amblyopia. *Ophthalmology, 120*(2), 395–403.

Bruenech, D. (2001). Surgical management of binocular vision anomalies. In B. Evans, & S. Doshi (Eds.), *Binocular vision and orthoptics* (pp. 110–115). Oxford: Butterworth-Heinemann.

Bucci, M. P., Kapoula, Z., Bernotas, M., & Zamfirescu, F. (1999). Role of attention and eye preference in the binocular coordination of saccades in strabismus. *Neuro-ophthalmology, 22*, 115–126.

Buch, H., & Vinding, T. (2015). Acute acquired comitant esotropia of childhood: a classification based on 48 children. *Acta Ophthalmologica, 93*(6), 568–574.

Buck, D., Hatt, S. R., Haggerty, H., Hrisos, S., Strong, N. P., Steen, N. I., & Clarke, M. P. (2007). The use of the Newcastle Control Score in the management of intermittent exotropia. *British Journal of Ophthalmology, 91*(2), 215–218.

Buck, D., Powell, C., Cumberland, P., Taylor, R., Sloper, J., Tiffin, P., ... Clarke, M. P. (2009). Presenting features and early management of childhood intermittent exotropia in the UK: inception cohort study. *The British Journal of Ophthalmology, 93*(12), 1620–1624.

Budge, F., & Derbyshire, N. (2005). *Social impact study results*. Focus 69. 2005. Nystagmus Network.

Burian, H. M. (1939). Fusional movements: role of peripheral retinal stimuli. *Archives of Ophthalmology, 21*, 486–491.

Burian, H. M., & von Noorden, G. K. (1974). *Binocular vision and ocular motility* (p. 295) St. Louis: Mosby.

Burke, J. P. (2015). Distance-near disparity esotropia: can we shrink the gap? *Eye (Lond), 29*(2), 208–213.

Burns, D. H., Allen, P. M., Edgar, D. F., & Evans, B. J. W. (2020). Sources of error in clinical measurement of the amplitude of accommodation. *Journal of Optometry, 13*(1), 3–14.

Burns, D. H., Evans, B. J. W., & Allen, P. M. (2014). Clinical measurement of amplitude of accommodation: a review. *Optometry in Practice, 15*(3), 75–86.

Cacho, P., Garcia-Munoz, A., Garcia-Bernabeu, G., & Lopez, A. (1999). Comparison between MEM and Nott dynamic retinoscopy. *Optometry and Vision Science, 76*, 650–655.

Cacho-Martinez, P., Garcia-Munoz, A., & Ruiz-Cantero, M. T. (2010). Do we really know the prevalence of accomodative and nonstrabismic binocular dysfunctions? *Journal of Optometry, 3*(4), 185–197.

Cackett, P., Weir, C., & Houston, C. A. (2003). Transient monocular diplopia resulting from the treatment of amblyopia. *Journal of Pediatric Ophthalmology and Strabismus, 40*(4), 245–246.

Cagnolati, W. (1991). Qualification and quantification of binocular disorders with Zeiss Polatest. *European Society of Optometry Communications, 134*, 9–12.

Caines, E., Dahl, M., & Holmstrom, G. (2007). Longterm oculomotor and visual function in spina bifida cystica: a population-based study. *Acta Ophthalmologica Scandinavica, 85*(6), 662–666.

Calder Gillie, J. (1961). *Aberrant vergence movements in heterophoria and heterotropia. Transactions of the international ophthalmic optical congress* (pp. 596–605). Crosby Lockwood.

Calloway, S. L., Lloyd, I. C., & Henson, D. B. (2001). A clinical evaluation of random dot stereoacuity cards in infants. *Eye, 15*, 629–634.

Caloroso, E. (1972). After-image transfer: a therapeutic procedure for amblyopia. *American Journal of Optometry, 49*, 65–69.

Caloroso, E. E., & Rouse, M. W. (1993). *Clinical management of strabismus.* Boston: Butterworth-Heinemann.

Caltrider, N., & Jampolsky, A. (1983). Overcorrecting minus lens therapy for treatment of intermittent exotropia. *Ophthalmology, 90*, 1160–1165.

Campbell, H., Doughty, M. J., Heron, G., & Ackerley, R. G. (2001). Influence of chronic alcohol abuse and ensuing forced abstinence on static subjective accommodation function in humans. *Ophthalmic and Physiological Optics, 21*, 197–205.

Cantonnet, A., & Filliozat, J. (1938). *Strabismus, its re-education: physiology and pathology of binocular vision* (2nd ed.). London: Wiseman.

Capdepon, E., Klainguti, G., Strickler, J., & van Melle, G. (1994). Superior oblique muscle paralysis and ocular torsion. What is the effect of measuring method on the results? *Klinische Monatsblatter fur Augenheilkunde, 204*(5), 370–377.

Carter, D. B. (1963). Effects of prolonged wearing of prism. *American Journal of Optometry and Archives of American Academy of Optometry, 40*, 265–273.

Carter, D. B. (1965). Fixation disparity and heterophoria following prolonged wearing of prisms. *American Journal of Optometry, 42*(3), 141–153.

Casillas, C. E., & Rosenfield, M. (2006). Comparison of subjective heterophoria testing with a phoropter and trial frame. *Optometry and Vision Science, 83*, 237–241.

Castagno, V. D., Vilela, M. A., Meucci, R. D., Resende, D. P., Schneid, F. H., Getelina, R., ... Fassa, A. G. (2016). Amplitude of accommodation in schoolchildren. *Current Eye Research*, 1–7.

Cawood, T., Moriarty, P., & O'Shea, D. (2004). Recent developments in thyroid eye disease. *BMJ, 329*, 385–390.

Cham, K. M., Anderson, A. J., & Abel, L. A. (2008a). Factors influencing the experience of oscillopsia in infantile nystagmus syndrome. *Investigative Ophthalmology Visual Science, 49*(8), 3424–3431.

Cham, K. M., Anderson, A. J., & Abel, L. A. (2008b). Task-induced stress and motivation decrease foveation-period durations in infantile nystagmus syndrome. *Investigative Ophthalmology & Visual Science, 49*(7), 2977–2984.

Chang, J. W. (2017). Refractive error change and vision improvement in moderate to severe hyperopic amblyopia after spectacle correction: restarting the emmetropization process? *PLoS One, 12*(4), e0175780.

Chang, M. Y., Coleman, A. L., Tseng, V. L., & Demer, J. L. (2017). Surgical interventions for vertical strabismus in superior oblique palsy. *Cochrane Database of Systematic Reviews*, 11CD012447.

Charman, W. N., & Jennings, J. A. M. (1995). Letter: recognition of TNO stereotest figures in the absence of true stereopsis. *Optometry and Vision Science, 72*, 535–536.

Charnwood, Lord (1950). *An essay on binocular vision.* London: Hatton Press.

Chase, W. W. (1963). An experiment in controlled nystagmus using hypnosis. *American Journal of Optometry and Archives of the American Academy of Optometry, 40*, 463–468.

Chen, A. H., O'Leary, D. J., & Howell, E. R. (2000). Near visual function in young children. Part 1: near point of convergence. Part 2: amplitude of accommodation. Part 3: near heterophoria. *Ophthalmic and Physiological Optics, 20*, 185–198.

Chen, A. M., Holmes, J. M., Chandler, D. L., Patel, R. A., Gray, M. E., Erzurum, S. A., ... Jensen, A. A. (2016). A randomized trial evaluating short-term effectiveness of overminus lenses in children 3 to 6 years of age with intermittent exotropia. *Ophthalmology, 123*(10), 2127–2136.

Cheng, D., & Woo, G. C. (2001). The effect of conventional CR39 and Fresnel prisms on high and low contrast acuity. *Ophthalmic and Physiological Optics, 21*, 312–316.

Cheng, D., Woo, G. C., Irving, E. L., Charman, W. N., & Murray, I. J. (1998). Clinical research note: scattering properties of Bagolini lenses and their effects on spatial vision. *Ophthalmic and Physiological Optics, 18*, 438–445.

Cho, M. H., & Wild, B. W. (1990). Spectacles for children. In A. A. Rosenbloom, & M. W. Morgan (Eds.), *Pediatric optometry* (pp. 198–199). Philadelphia: Lippincott.

Cho, Y. A., & Ryu, W. Y. (2015). Changes in refractive error in patients with accommodative esotropia after being weaned from hyperopic correction. *The British Journal of Ophthalmology, 99*(5), 680–684.

Choe, H. R., Yang, H. K., & Hwang, J.-M. (2019). Long-term outcomes of prismatic correction in partially accommodative esotropia. *PLoS One, 14*(12), e0225654.

Choong, Y. F., Lukman, H., Martin, S., & Laws, D. E. (2004). Childhood amblyopia treatment: psychosocial implications for patients and primary carers. *Eye, 18*, 369–375.

Chopin, A., Bavelier, D., & Levi, D. M. (2019). The prevalence and diagnosis of 'stereoblindness' in adults less than 60 years of age: a best evidence synthesis. *Ophthalmic and Physiological Optics, 39*(2), 66–85.

Christian, L. W., Nandakumar, K., Hrynchak, P. K., & Irving, E. L. (2018). Visual and binocular status in elementary school children with a reading problem. *Journal of Optometry, 11*(3), 160–166.

Chua, B., & Mitchell, P. (2004). Consequences of amblyopia on education, occupation, and long term vision loss. *British Journal of Ophthalmology, 88*, 1119–1121.

Chung, S. T. L., & Bedell, H. E. (1996). Velocity criteria for 'foveation periods' determined from image motions simulating congenital nystagmus. *Optometry and Vision Science, 73*, 92–103.

Chung, S. T. L., & Bedell, H. E. (1997). Congenital nystagmus image motion: influence on visual acuity at different luminances. *Optometry and Vision Science, 74*, 266–272.

Chung, T. L., & Bedell, H. E. (1995). Effect of retinal image motion on visual acuity and contour interaction in congenital nystagmus. *Vision Research, 35*, 3071.

Ciner, E. B., Schanel-Klitsch, E., & Herzberg, C. (1996). Stereoacuity development: 6 months to 5 years. A new tool for testing and screening. *Optometry and Vision Science, 73*, 43–48.

Ciner, E. B., Schanel-Klitsch, E., & Scheiman, M. (1991). Stereoacuity development in young children. *Optometry and Vision Science, 68*(7), 533–536.

CITT. (2008). Randomized clinical trial of treatments for symptomatic convergence insufficiency in children. *Archives of Ophthalmology, 126*(10), 1336–1349.

CITT-ART Investigator Group. (2019). Treatment of symptomatic convergence insufficiency in children enrolled in the Convergence Insufficiency Treatment Trial-Attention & Reading Trial: a randomized clinical trial. *Optometry and Vision Science, 96*(11), 825–835.

Ciuffreda, K. J., Goldrich, S. G., & Neary, C. (1982). Use of eye movement auditory feedback in the control of nystagmus. *American Journal of Optometry and Physiological Optics, 59*, 396–409.

Ciuffreda, K. J., Hokoda, S. C., Hung, G. K., Semmlow, J. L., & Selenow, A. (1983). Static aspects of accommodation in human amblyopia. *American Journal of Optometry and Physiological Optics, 60*, 436–449.

Ciuffreda, K. J., Rosenfield, M., & Chen, H. W. (1997). The AC/A ratio, age and presbyopia. *Ophthalmic and Physiological Optics, 17*(4), 307–315.

Ciuffreda, K. J., & Tannen, B. (1995). *Eye movement basics for the clinician.* St. Louis: Mosby.

Clark, T. Y., & Clark, R. A. (2015). Convergence insufficiency symptom survey scores for reading versus other near visual activities in school-age children. *American Journal of Ophthalmology, 160*(5), 905–912.e902.

Clarke, M. P., Wright, C. M., Hrisos, S., Anderson, J. D., Henderson, J., & Richardson, S. R. (2003). Randomised controlled trial of treatment of unilateral visual impairment detected at preschool vision screening. *BMJ, 327*, 1251–1254.

Cleary, M., & Thompson, C. M. (2001). Diagnosis of eccentric fixation using a calibrated ophthalmoscope: defining clinically significant limits. *Ophthalmic and Physiological Optics, 21*, 461–469.

Cleary, M., Houston, C. A., McFadzean, R. M., & Dutton, G. N. (1998). Recovery in microtropia: implications for aetiology and neurophysiology. *The British Journal of Ophthalmology, 82*, 225–231.

Cleary, M., Williams, G. J., & Metcalfe, R. A. (2008). The pattern of extra-ocular muscle involvement in ocular myasthenia. *Strabismus, 16*(1), 11–18.

Coats, D. K., Paysse, E. A., & Kim, D. (2001). Excessive blinking in childhood: a prospective evaluation of 99 children. *Ophthalmology, 108*, 1556–1561.

Coffey, B., Wick, B., Cotter, S., Scharre, J., & Horner, D. (1992). Treatment options in intermittent exotropia: a critical appraisal. *Optometry and Vision Science, 69*, 386–404.

Cole, R. G., & Boisvert, R. P. (1974). Effect of fixation disparity on stereo-acuity. *American journal of optometry and physiological optics, 51*, 206–213.

College of Optometrists. (2012). *F02: Guidance for the issuing of small prescriptions and making small changes to existing prescriptions. www.college-optometrists.org.* College of Optometrists.

College of Optometrists. (2017). *Guidance for professional practice. Professional excellence in eye health.* London: College of Optometrists.

Collewijn, H., Steinman, R. M., Erkelens, C. J., & Regan, D. (1991). Binocular fusion, stereopsis and stereoacuity with a moving head. In J. Cronly-Dillon (Ed.), *Vision and visual dysfunction* (pp. 121–136). London: Macmillan.

Comer, R. M., Dawson, E., Plant, G., Acheson, J. F., & Lee, J. P. (2006). Causes and outcomes for patients presenting with diplopia to an eye casualty department. *Eye, 21*(3), 413–418.

Committee for the Classification of Eye Movement Abnormalities and Strabismus. (2001). A classification of eye movement abnormalities and strabismus (CEMAS). http://www.nei.nih.gov/news/statements/cemas.pdf. 2001. Last accessed May 2020.

Constantinescu, C. S., & Gottlob, I. (2001). Possible role of corticosteroids in nervous system plasticity: improvement in amblyopia after optic neuritis in the fellow eye treated with steroids. *Neurorehabilitation and Neural Repair, 15*, 223–227.

Conway, M. L., Thomas, J., & Subramanian, A. (2012). Is the aligning prism measured with the Mallett unit correlated with fusional vergence reserves? *PLoS One, 7*(8), e42832.

Cook, R. C., & Glasscock, R. E. (1951). Refractive and ocular findings in the newborn. *American Journal of Optometry, 34*, 1407–1413.

Cooper, J. (1977). Intermittent exotropia of the divergence excess type. *Journal of the American Optometric Association, 48*, 1261–1273.

Cooper, J. (1979). Clinical stereopsis testing: contour and random dot stereograms. *Journal of the American Optometric Association, 50*, 41–46.

Cooper, J. (1987). Accommodative dysfunction. In J. F. Amos (Ed.), *Diagnosis and management in vision care* (pp. 431–459). Boston: Butterworths.

Cooper, J. (1988a). Orthoptic treatment of vertical deviations. *Journal of the American Optometric Association, 59*(6), 463–468.

Cooper, J. (1988b). Review of computerized orthoptics with specific regard to convergence insufficiency. *Optometry and Vision Science, 65*(6), 455–463.

Cooper, J., & Feldman, J. (1978). Random-dot-stereogram performance by strabismic, amblyopic, and ocular-pathology patients in an operant-discrimination task. *American Journal of Optometry and Physiological Optics, 55*(9), 599–609.

Cooper, J., & Feldman, J. (1979). Assessing the Frisby Stereo Test under monocular viewing conditions. *Journal of the American Optometric Association, 50*, 807–809.

Cooper, J., Feldman, J., Horn, D., & Dibble, C. (1981). Short report: Reliability of fixation disparity curves. *American Journal of Optometry and Physiological Optics, 11*, 960–964.

Cooper, J., Selenow, A., Ciuffreda, K. J., Feldman, J., Faverty, J., Hokoda, S., & Silver, J. (1983). Reduction of asthenopia in patients with convergence insufficiency after fusional vergence training. *American Journal of Optometry and Physiological Optics, 60*, 982–989.

Cooper, J., & Warshowsky, J. (1977). Lateral displacement as a response cue in the Titmus stereotest. *American Journal of Optometry and Physiological Optics, 54*, 537–541.

Cordonnier, M., & de Maertelaer, V. (2005). Screening for amblyogenic factors in preschool children with the retinomax hand-held refractor: do positive children have amblyopia and is treatment efficacious? *Strabismus, 13*, 27–32.

Cornell, E. D., MacDougall, H. G., Predebon, J., & Curthoys, I. S. (2003). Errors in binocular fixation are common in normal subjects during natural conditions. *Optometry and Vision Science, 80*, 764–771.

Costenbader, F. D. (1958). Clinical cause and management of esotropia. In J. H. Allen (Ed.), *Strabismus: ophthalmic symposium II.* Kimpton.

Costenbader, F. D., & Mousel, D. K. (1964). Cyclic esotropia. *Archives of Ophthalmology, 71*, 180–183.

Cotter, S. A. (2007). Management of childhood hyperopia: a pediatric optometrist's perspective. *Optometry and Vision Science, 84*(2), 103–109.

Coulter, R. A., Bade, A., Tea, Y., Fecho, G., Amster, D., Jenewein, E., . . . Quint, N., et al. (2014). Eye examination testability in children with autism and in typical peers. *Optometry and Vision Science, 92*(1), 31–43.

Coulter, R. A., & Shallo-Hoffmann, J. (2000). The presumed influence of attention on accuracy in the developmental eye movement (DEM) test. *Optometry and Vision Science*, 77, 428–432.

Coutant, B. E., & Westheimer, G. (1993). Population distribution of stereoscopic ability. *Ophthalmic and Physiological Optics*, 13, 3–7.

Cregg, M., Woodhouse, J. M., Stewart, R. E., Pakeman, V. H., Bromham, N. R., Gunter, H. L., ... Fraser, W. I. (2003). Development of refractive error and strabismus in children with Down syndrome. *Investigative Ophthalmology and Visual Science*, 44, 1023–1030.

Cullen, A. P., & Jacques, R. A. (1960). Bates' method of ocular treatment. *The British Journal of Physiological Optics*, 17, 240–247.

Cumberland, P. M., Czanner, G., Bunce, C., Dore, C. J., Freemantle, N., & Garcia-Finana, M. (2014). Ophthalmic statistics note: the perils of dichotomising continuous variables. *The British Journal of Ophthalmology*, 98(6), 841–843.

Currie, D. C., Bedell, H. E., & Song, S. (1993). Visual acuity for optotypes with image motions simulating congenital nystagmus. *Clinical Vision Sciences*, 8(1), 73–84.

Dale, R. T. (1982). *Fundamentals of ocular motility and strabismus*. New York: Grune & Stratton.

Dalziel, C. C. (1981). Effect of vision training on patients who fail Sheard's criterion. *American Journal of Optometry and Physiological Optics*, 58(1), 21–23.

Daniel, F., & Kapoula, Z. (2019). Induced vergence-accommodation conflict reduces cognitive performance in the Stroop test. *Scientific Reports*, 9(1), 1247.

Darko-Takyi, C., NIrghin, U., & Khan, N. E. (2016). A review of the classification of nonstrabismic binocular vision anomalies. *Optometry Reports*, 6(5626), 1–7.

Daum, K. (1984). Divergence excess: characteristics and results of treatment with orthoptics. *Ophthalmic and Physiological Optics*, 4, 15–24.

Daum, K. M., Rutstein, R. P., & Eskridge, J. B. (1978). Efficacy of computerized vergence therapy. *American Journal of Optometry and Physiological Optics*, 64, 83–89.

Davis, A. R., Sloper, J. J., Neveu, M. M., Hogg, C. R., Morgan, M. J., & Holder, G. E. (2006). Differential changes of magnocellular and parvocellular visual function in early- and late-onset strabismic amblyopia. *Investigative Ophthalmology Visual Science*, 47(11), 4836–4841.

Davis, A. R., Sloper, J. J., Neveu, M. M., Hogg, C. R., Morgan, M. J., & Holder, G. E. (2003). Electrophysiological and psychophysical differences between early- and late-onset strabismic amblyopia. *Investigative Ophthalmology and Visual Science*, 44, 610–617.

Daw, N. W. (1997). Critical periods and strabismus: what questions remain? *Optometry and Vision Science (Editorial)*, 74, 690–694.

Day, S. (1997). Normal and abnormal visual development. In D. Taylor (Ed.), *Paediatric ophthalmology* (2nd ed., pp. 13–28). Oxford: Blackwell Science Ltd.

Day, S., & Narita, A. (1997). The uveal tract. In D. Taylor (Ed.), *Paediatric ophthalmology* (2nd ed., pp. 410–444). Oxford: Blackwell Science.

de Jongh, E., Leach, C., Tjon-Fo-Sang, M. J., & Bjerre, A. (2014). Inter-examiner variability and agreement of the alternate prism cover test (APCT) measurements of strabismus performed by 4 examiners. *Strabismus*, 22(4), 158–166.

de Pool, M. E., Campbell, J. P., Broome, S. O., & Guyton, D. L. (2005). The dragged-fovea diplopia syndrome: clinical characteristics, diagnosis, and treatment. *Ophthalmology*, 112, 1455–1462.

de Weger, C., Boonstra, N., & Goossens, J. (2019). Bifocals reduce strabismus in children with Down syndrome: evidence from a randomized controlled trial. *Acta Ophthalmologica*, 97(4), 378–393.

de Wit, G. C. (2003). Evaluation of a new direct-comparison aniseikonia test. *Binocular Vision & Strabismus Quarterly*, 18(2), 87–94.

DeAngelis, G. C. (2000). Seeing in three dimensions: the neurophysiology of stereopsis. *Trends in Cognitive Sciences*, 4(3), 80–90.

DeCarlo, D. K., Bowman, E., Monroe, C., Kline, R., McGwin, G., Jr., & Owsley, C. (2014). Prevalence of attention-deficit/hyperactivity disorder among children with vision impairment. *Journal of AAPOS*, 18(1), 10–14.

Dell'Osso, L. F. (1994). Congenital and latent/manifest latent nystagmus: diagnosis, treatment, foveation, oscillopsia, and visual acuity. *Japanese Journal of Ophthalmology*, 38, 329–336.

Dell'Osso, L. F., & Daroff, R. B. (1975). Congenital nystagmus waveforms and foveation strategy. *Documenta Ophthalmologica*, 39, 155–182.

Dell'Osso, L. F., Hertle, R. W., & Daroff, R. B. (2007). "Sensory" and "motor" nystagmus: erroneous and misleading terminology based on misinterpretation of David Cogan's observations. *Archives of Ophthalmology*, *125*(11), 1559–1561.

Dell'Osso, L. F., Traccis, S., Abel, L., & Erzurum, S. I. (1988). Contact lenses and congenital nystagmus (Research Report). *Clinical Vision Sciences*, *3*, 229–232.

Demer, J. L. (2006). Evidence supporting extraocular muscle pulleys: refuting the platygean view of extraocular muscle mechanics. *Journal of Pediatric Ophthalmology and Strabismus*, *43*(5), 296–305.

Dengler, B., & Kommerell, G. (1993). Stereoscopic cooperation between the fovea of one eye and the periphery of the other eye at large disparities. Implications for anomalous retinal correspondence in strabismus. *Graefe's Archive for Clinical and Experimental Ophthalmology*, *231*, 199–206.

DeRespinis, P. A., Caputo, A. R., Wagner, R. S., & Guo, S. (1993). Duane's retraction syndrome. *Survey of Ophthalmology*, *38*, 257–288.

Dickinson, C. M., & Abadi, R. V. (1985). The influence of nystagmoid oscillation on contrast sensitivity in normal observers. *Vision Research*, *8*, 1089–1096.

Ding, J., & Levi, D. M. (2014). Rebalancing binocular vision in amblyopia. *Ophthalmic and Physiological Optics*, *34*(2), 199–213.

Doble, J. E., Feinberg, D. L., Rosner, M. S., & Rosner, A. J. (2010). Identification of binocular vision dysfunction (vertical heterophoria) in traumatic brain injury patients and effects of individualized prismatic spectacle lenses in the treatment of postconcussive symptoms: a retrospective analysis. *PM R*, *2*(4), 244–253.

Doherty, S. E., Doyle, L. A., McCullough, S. J., & Saunders, K. J. (2019). Comparison of retinoscopy results with and without 1% cyclopentolate in school-aged children. *Ophthalmic and Physiological Optics*, *39*(4), 272–281.

Donahue, S. P. (2006). Relationship between anisometropia, patient age, and the development of amblyopia. *American Journal of Ophthalmology*, *142*(1), 132-132.

Douglas, R. (2002). Acoustic neuroma and its ocular implications: a personal view. *Optometry Today*, *January 25*, 29–33.

Douthwaite, W. A., Jenkins, T. C. A., Pickwell, L. D., & Sheridan, M. (1981). The treatment of amblyopia by the rotating grating method. *Ophthalmic and Physiological Optics*, *1*, 97–106.

Dowley, D. (1987). The orthophorization of heterophoria. *Ophthalmic and Physiological Optics*, *7*(2), 169–175.

Dowley, D. (1990). Heterophoria. *Optometry and Vision Science*, *67*, 456–460.

Doyle, L. A., McCullough, S. J., & Saunders, K. J. (2019). Cycloplegia and spectacle prescribing in children: attitudes of UK optometrists. *Ophthalmic & Physiological Optics*, *39*(3), 148–161.

Drew, S. A., Borsting, E., Stark, L. R., & Chase, C. (2012). Chromatic aberration, accommodation, and color preference in asthenopia. *Optometry & Vision Science*, *89*(7).

Driver and Vehicle Licensing Authority (DVLA). (2020). *Guidance. Visual disorders: assessing fitness to drive*. DVLA.

Drover, J. R., Morale, S. E., Wang, Y. Z., Stager, D. R., Sr., & Birch, E. E. (2010). Vernier acuity cards: examination of development and screening validity. *Optometry and Vision Science*, *87*(11), E806–E812.

Duane, A. (1896). A new classification of the motor anomalies of the eyes based upon physiological principles. *Annals of Ophthalmology*, *5*, 969.

Duane, A. (1897). A new classification of the motor anomalies of the eye. *Annals of Ophthalmology*, *6*, 250.

Duke-Elder, S., & Abrams, D. (1970). *Eye-strain. System of ophthalmology, vol. V. Ophthalmic optics and refraction* (pp. 559–578). London: Henry Kimpton.

Duke-Elder, S. (1970). *System of ophthalmology, vol. V. Ophthalmic optics and refraction* (p. 459) London: Kimpton.

Duke-Elder, S. (1973). *System of Ophthalmology, vol. VI. Ocular motility and strabismus* (p. 326) London: Kimpton.

Dusek, W., Pierscionek, B. K., & McClelland, J. F. (2010). A survey of visual function in an Austrian population of school-age children with reading and writing difficulties. *BMC Ophthalmology*, *10*, 16.

Dusek, W. A., Pierscionek, B. K., & McClelland, J. F. (2011). An evaluation of clinical treatment of convergence insufficiency for children with reading difficulties. *BMC Ophthalmology*, *11*, 21.

Duwaer, A. L. (1983). New measures of fixation disparity in the diagnosis of binocular oculomotor deficiencies. *American Journal of Optometry and Physiological Optics*, *60*, 586–597.

Dwyer, P., & Wick, B. (1995). The influence of refractive correction upon disorders of vergence and accommodation. *Optometry and Vision Science, 72*(4), 224−232.

Eames, T. H. (1934). Low fusion convergence as a factor in reading disability. *American Journal of Ophthalmology, 17,* 709−710.

Earnshaw, J. R. (1960). The use of knitting needles in the treatment of strabismus. *The Optician, 139,* 465−466.

Earnshaw, J.R. (1962). The single mirror haploscope. *Transactions of the international congress of the British optical association* (pp. 673-674).

Eastgate, R. M., Griffiths, G. D., Waddingham, P. E., Moody, A. D., Butler, T. K., Cobb, S. V., ... Brown, S. M. (2006). Modified virtual reality technology for treatment of amblyopia. *Eye, 20,* 370−374.

Edgar, D., & Barnard, S. (1996). Refraction. In S. Barnard, & D. Edgar (Eds.), *Pediatric eye care* (pp. 151−167). Oxford: Blackwell.

Edwards, M. H., Law, L. F., Lee, C. M., Leung, K. M., & Lui, W. O. (1993). Clinical norms for amplitude of accommodation in Chinese. *Ophthalmic & Physiological Optics, 13*(2), 199−204.

Eggers, S. D. Z., Bisdorff, A., von Brevern, M., Zee, D. S., Kim, J. S., Perez-Fernandez, N., ... Newman-Toker, D. E. (2019). Classification of vestibular signs and examination techniques: nystagmus and nystagmus-like movements. *Journal of Vestibular Research, 29*(2-3), 57−87.

Ehrenstein, W. H., Arnold-Schulz-Gahmen, B. E., & Jaschinski, W. (2005). Eye preference within the context of binocular functions. *Graefe's Archive for Clinical and Experimental Ophthalmology, 243*(9), 926−932.

Ekdawi, N. S., Nusz, K. J., Diehl, N. N., & Mohney, B. G. (2010). The development of myopia among children with intermittent exotropia. *American Journal of Ophthalmology, 149*(3), 503−507.

El Ghrably, I. A., Longville, D., & Gnanaraj, L. (2007). Does compliance with amblyopia management improve following supervised occlusion treatment? *European Journal of Ophthalmology, 17*(5), 823−827.

El Mallah, M. K., Chakravarthy, U., & Hart, P. M. (2000). Amblyopia: is visual loss permanent? *The British Journal of Ophthalmology, 84,* 952−956.

Elliott, D. B. (2013). The Bates method, elixirs, potions and other cures for myopia: how do they work? *Ophthalmic & Physiological Optics, 33*(2), 75−77.

Elliott, D. B. (2014). Refraction and prescribing. In D. B. Elliott (Ed.), *Clinical procedures in primary eye care* (4th ed., pp. 68−111). Oxford: Elsevier.

Ellis, F. J., Stein, L. A., & Guyton, D. L. (1998). Masked bilateral superior oblique muscle paresis. A simple overcorrection phenomenon? *Ophthalmology, 105*(3), 544−551.

Elston, J. (1994). Idiopathic blepharospasm. *Eye News, 1,* 5.

Eneh, A., Johnson, D., Schweitzer, K., & Strube, Y. N. J. (2018). Brown's syndrome during pregnancy: a case report and review of literature. *Canadian Journal of Ophthalmology, 53*(6), e256−e258.

Engel, J. M. (2015). Treatment and diagnosis of congenital fourth nerve palsies: an update. *Current Opinion in Ophthalmology, 26*(5), 353−356.

Enke, E. S., Stewart, S. A., Scott, W. E., & Wheeler, D. T. (1994). The prevalence of dissociated horizontal deviations in congenital esotropia. *American Orthoptic Journal, 44,* 109−111.

Eperjesi, F. (2000). Optometric assessment and management in dyslexia. *Optometry Today, Dec 15,* 20−25.

Epstein, D. L., & Tredici, T. J. (1973). Microtropia (monofixation syndrome) in flying personnel. *American Journal of Ophthalmology, 76*(5), 832−841.

Erickson, G. B., & Caloroso, E. E. (1992). Vertical diplopia onset with first-time bifocal. *Optometry and Vision Science, 69,* 645−651.

Erkelens, C. J., & Collewijn, H. (1985). Eye movements and stereopsis during dichoptic viewing of moving random dot stereograms. *Vision Research, 25,* 1689−1700.

Escalante, J. B., & Rosenfield, M. (2006). Effect of heterophoria measurement technique on the clinical accommodative convergence to accommodation ratio. *Optometry, 77*(5), 229−234.

Espana-Gregori, E., Montes-Mico, R., Bueno-Gimeno, I., Diaz-Llopi, M., & Menezo-Rozalen, J. L. (2001). Latent ocular deviations in patients with advanced AIDS. *Documenta Ophthalmologica, 103,* 195−200.

Eustace, P., Weston, E., & Druby, D. J. (1973). The effect of illumination on intermittent divergent squint of the divergence excess type. *Transactions of the Ophthalmological Society of Great Britain, 93,* 559−590.

Eustis, H. S., & Mungan, N. K. (1999). Monovision for treatment of accommodative esotropia with a high AC/A ratio. *Journal of AAPOS, 3,* 87−90.

Evans, B. J. W. (1991). *Ophthalmic factors in dyslexia.* Vision Sciences, Aston University.

Evans, B. (2000a). Binocular vision problems in children: their investigation and management. *Ophthalmic and Physiological Optics, 20*(2), S11–S13.

Evans, B. (2000b). Efficacy of hypnosis in treating double vision and nystagmus. *Contemporary Hypnosis, 17*, 218.

Evans, B. (2004a). The diploma in orthoptics. Part 1: A "how to" guide. *The Optician, 226*, 26–27.

Evans, B. (2004b). The diploma in orthoptics. Part 3: Certificate A clinical portfolio. *The Optician, 227*, 32–34.

Evans, B. J., Evans, B. V., Jordahl-Moroz, J., & Nabee, M. (1998). Randomised double-masked placebo-controlled trial of a treatment for congenital nystagmus. *Vision Research, 38*(14), 2193–2202.

Evans, B. J. W. (1994). American Academy of Optometry Conference Report: papers relating to binocular vision and orthoptics. *Optometry Today, April 11*, 26–29.

Evans, B. J. W. (1997a). The evidence-based approach in optometry: Part 1. *Optometry Today, 37*, 32–35.

Evans, B. J. W. (1997b). The evidence-based approach in optometry: Part 3, Interventions. *Optometry Today, 38*, 35–38.

Evans, B. J. W. (2000). An open trial of the Institute Free-space Stereogram (IFS) exercises. *British Journal of Optometry & Dispensing, 8*, 5–14.

Evans, B. J. W. (2001a). *Dyslexia and vision.* London: Whurr.

Evans, B. J. W. (2001b). Decompensated exophoria at near, convergence insufficiency and binocular instability: diagnosis and the development of a new treatment regimen. In B. Evans, & S. Doshi (Eds.), *Binocular vision and orthoptics* (pp. 39–49). Oxford: Butterworth-Heinemann.

Evans, B. J. W. (2001c). Diplopia: when can intractable be treatable? In B. Evans, & S. Doshi (Eds.), *Binocular vision and orthoptics* (pp. 50–57). Oxford: Butterworth-Heinemann.

Evans, B. J. W. (2001d). Anomalous retinal correspondence. In B. Evans, & S. Doshi (Eds.), *Binocular vision and orthoptics* (pp. 65–72). Oxford: Butterworth-Heinemann.

Evans, B. J. W. (2001e). Case studies. In B. Evans, & S. Doshi (Eds.), *Binocular vision and orthoptics* (pp. 116–126). Oxford: Butterworth-Heinemann.

Evans, B. J. W. (2005a). *Eye essentials: binocular vision.* Oxford: Elsevier.

Evans, B. J. W. (2005b). Case reports: The need for optometric investigation in suspected Meares-Irlen syndrome or visual stress. *Ophthalmic and Physiological Optics, 25*, 363–370.

Evans, B. J. W. (2006a). Orthoptic indications for contact lens wear. *Contact Lens & Anterior Eye, 29*, 175–181.

Evans, B. J. W. (2006b). Interventions for infantile nystagmus syndrome: towards a randomized controlled trial? *Survey of Ophthalmology, Semin Ophthalmol, 21*(2), 111–116.

Evans, B. J. W. (2007a). Monovision: a systematic review. *Ophthalmic and Physiological Optics, 27*, 417–439.

Evans, B. J. W. (2007b). *Pickwell's binocular vision anomalies.* Oxford: Elsevier.

Evans, B. J. W. (2010). The investigation and management of heterophoria. *Optometry Today*, 40–47.

Evans, B. J. W. (2018a). The role of the optometrist with underachieving children (case studies). *Optometry Today, 58*(6), 73–78.

Evans, B. J. W. (2018b). The role of the optometrist with underachieving children (further case studies). *Optometry Today.* (August 2018).

Evans, B. J. W., & Allen, P. M. (2016). A systematic review of controlled trials on visual stress using intuitive overlays or the intuitive colorimeter. *Journal of Optometry, 9*(4), 205–218.

Evans, B. J. W., Allen, P. M., & Wilkins, A. J. (2017). A Delphi study to develop practical diagnostic guidelines for visual stress (pattern-related visual stress). *Journal of Optometry, 10*(3), 161–168.

Evans, B. J. W., Barnard, N. A. S., & Arkush, C. (1996). Optometric uses of hypnosis. *Contemporary Hypnosis, 13*(2), 69–73.

Evans, B. J. W., Busby, A., Jeanes, R., & Wilkins, A. J. (1995). Optometric correlates of Meares-Irlen Syndrome: a matched group study. *Ophthalmic and Physiological Optics, 15*(5), 481–487.

Evans, B. J. W., Drasdo, N., & Richards, I. L. (1994). Investigation of accommodative and binocular function in dyslexia. *Ophthalmic and Physiological Optics, 1*, 5–19.

Evans, B. J. W., Evans, B. V., Jordahl-Moroz, J., & Nabee, M. (1998). Double-masked randomised placebo-controlled trial of a treatment for congenital nystagmus. *Vision Research, 38*, 2193–2202.

Evans, B. J. W., Patel, R., & Wilkins, A. J. (2002). Optometric function in visually sensitive migraine before and after treatment with tinted spectacles. *Ophthalmic and Physiological Optics, 22*, 130–142.

Evans, B. J. W., & Rowlands, G. (2004). Review article. Correctable visual impairment in older people: a major unmet need. *Ophthalmic and Physiological Optics, 24.*

Evans, B. J. W., & Stevenson, S. J. (2008). The Pattern Glare Test: a review and determination of normative values. *Ophthalmic and Physiological Optics, 28,* 295–309.

Evans, B. J. W., Wilkins, A. J., Brown, J., Busby, A., Wingfield, A. E., Jeanes, R., & Bald, J. (1996). A preliminary investigation into the aetiology of Meares-Irlen Syndrome. *Ophthalmic and Physiological Optics, 16*(4), 286–296.

Evans, B. J. W., Yu, C. S., Massa, E., & Mathews, J. E. (2011). Randomised controlled trial of intermittent photic stimulation for treating amblyopia in older children and adults. *Ophthalmic & Physiological Optics, 31*(1), 56–68.

Fahle, M. (1987). Naso-temporal asymmetry of binocular inhibition. *Investigative Ophthalmology & Visual Science, 28,* 1016–1017.

Fahle, M., & Bachmann, G. (1996). Better performance through amblyopic than through normal eyes. *Vision Research, 36,* 1939–1944.

Fawcett, S. L., Stager, D. R., & Felius, J. (2004). Factors influencing stereoacuity outcomes in adults with acquired strabismus. *American Journal of Ophthalmology, 138,* 931–935.

Fawcett, S. L., Wang, Y. Z., & Birch, E. E. (2005). The critical period for susceptibility of human stereopsis. *Investigative Ophthalmology & Visual Science, 46,* 521–525.

Feldman, J. M., Cooper, J., & Eichler, R. (1993).). The effect of stimulus parameters (size, complexity, depth and line thickness) on horizontal fusional amplitudes in normal humans. *Binocular Vision and Eye Muscle Surgery Quarterly, 8*(1), 23–30.

Fellows, B. (1995). Critical issues arising from the APA description of hypnosis. *Contemporary Hypnosis, 12*(2), 74–80.

Fells, P., & Lee, J. P. (1984). In D. J. Spalton, R. A. Hitchings, & R. A. Hunter (Eds.), Strabismus. *Atlas of clinical ophthalmology* (p. 188). Edinburgh: Churchill-Livingstone.

Fender, D. H., & Julesz, B. (1967). Extension of Panum's fusional area in binocularly stabilized vision. *Journal of the Optical Society of America, 57,* 819–830.

Fern, K. D., Manny, R. E., & Garza, R. (1998). Screening for anisometropia in preschool children. *Optometry and Vision Science, 75,* 407–423.

Field, A. (2002). Vision therapy over the internet. *The Optician, March 22,* 21.

Finlay, A. (2000). The differential diagnosis of diplopia. *Optometry Today, October 6,* 31–40.

Finlay, A. L. (2007). Binocular vision and refractive surgery. *Contact Lens & Anterior Eye, 30*(2), 76–83.

Firth, A. Y., Machin, J., & Watkins, C. L. (2007). Tilt and reading speed. *Journal of AAPOS, 11*(1), 52–54.

Firth, A. Y., Pulling, S., Carr, M. P., & Beaini, A. Y. (2004). Orthoptic status before and immediately after heroin detoxification. *British Journal of Ophthalmology, 88,* 1186–1190.

Firth, A. Y., & Whittle, J. P. (1994). Clarification of the correct and incorrect use of ophthalmic prisms in the measurement of strabismus. *British Orthoptic Journal, 51,* 15–18.

Firth, A. Y., & Whittle, J. P. (1995). Further clarification on the use of ophthalmic prisms in the measurement of strabismus. *British Orthoptic Journal, 52,* 48–49.

Fisher, S. K., Ciuffreda, K. J., Levine, S., & Wolf-Kelly, K. S. (1987). Tonic adaptation in symptomatic and asymptomatic subjects. *American Journal of Optometry and Physiological Optics, 64,* 333–343.

Flitcroft, D. I. (2012). The complex interactions of retinal, optical and environmental factors in myopia aetiology. *Progress in Retinal and Eye Research, 31*(6), 622–660.

Flodin, S., Pansell, T., Rydberg, A., & Andersson Grönlund, M. (2019). Clinical measurements of normative subjective cyclotorsion and cyclofusion in a healthy adult population. *Acta Ophthalmologica, 98*(2), 177–181.

Flom, M. C. (1990). Issues in the clinical management of binocular anomalies. In A. A. Rosenbloom, & M. W. Morgan (Eds.), *Pediatric optometry* (pp. 219–244). Philadelphia: Lippincott.

Flynn, J. T. (1991). Amblyopia revisited. *The Journal of Pediatric Ophthalmology & Strabismus, 28,* 183–201.

Fogt, N., & Jones, R. (1998). Comparison of fixation disparities obtained by objective and subjective methods. *Vision Research, 38,* 411–421.

Fogt, N., Baughman, B., & Good, G. (2000). The effect of experience on the detection of small eye movements. *Optometry and Vision Science, 77,* 670–674.

Foroozan, R., & Arnold, A. C. (2005). Diplopia after cataract surgery. *Survey of Ophthalmology, 50,* 81–84.

Foroozan, R., & Brodsky, M. C. (2004). Microsaccadic opsoclonus: an idiopathic cause of oscillopsia and episodic blurred vision. *American Journal of Ophthalmology, 138,* 1053–1054.

Fortenbacher, D. L., Bartolini, A., Dornbos, B., & Tran, T. (2018). Vision therapy and virtual reality applications. *Advances in Ophthalmology and Optometry, 3*(1), 39–59.

Fortuin, M. F., Lambooij, M. T., Ijsselsteijn, W. A., Heynderickx, I., Edgar, D. F., & Evans, B. J. (2011). An exploration of the initial effects of stereoscopic displays on optometric parameters. *Ophthalmic & Physiological Optics, 31*(1), 33–44.

Fowler, M. S., Riddell, P. M., & Stein, J. F. (1988). The effect of varying vergence speed and target size on the amplitude of vergence eye movements. *British Orthoptic Journal, 45,* 49–55.

Fowler, M. S., Wade, D. T., Richardson, A. J., & Stein, J. F. (1996). Squints and diplopia seen after brain damage. *Journal of Neurology, 243,* 86–90.

Franceschetti, A. T., & Burian, H. M. (1970). Gradient accommodative convergence/accommodative ratio in families with and without esotropia. *American Journal of Ophthalmology, 70*(4), 558–562.

Francis, J. L., Rabbetts, R. B., & Stone, J. (1979). Depressed accommodation in young people. *Ophthalmic Optician, 19,* 803–811.

Francois, J., & James, M. (1955). Comparative study of amblyopic treatment. *American Orthoptic Journal, 5,* 61-44.

Frane, S. L., Sholtz, R. I., Lin, W. K. I., & Mutti, D. O. (2000). Ocular components before and after acquired, nonaccommodative esotropia. *Optometry and Vision Science, 77,* 633–636.

Frantz, K. A., Cotter, S. A., & Wick, B. (1992). Re-evaluation of the four prism diopter base-out test. *Optometry and Vision Science, 69*(10), 777–786.

Frantz, K. A., & Scharre, J. E. (1990). Comparison of disparometer fixation disparity curves as measured with and without the phoropter. *Optometry and Vision Science, 67,* 117–122.

Freeman, A. W., & Jolly, N. (1994). Visual loss during interocular suppression in normal and strabismic subjects. *Vision Research, 34*(15), 2043–2050.

Freeman, C., & Evans, B. J. W. (2010). Investigation of the causes of non-tolerance to optometric prescriptions for spectacles. *Ophthalmic and Physiological Optics, 30*(1), 1–11.

Freeman, R. S., & Isenberg, S. J. (1989). The use of part-time occlusion for early onset unilateral exotropia. *Journal of Pediatric Ophthalmology and Strabismus, 26,* 94–96.

Freidburg, D., & Kloppel, K. P. (1996). Early correction of hyperopia and astigmatism in children leads to better development of visual acuity. *Klinische Monatsblatter fur Augenheilkunde, 209,* 21–24.

Freier, B. E., & Pickwell, L. D. (1983). Physiological exophoria. *Ophthalmic and Physiological Optics, 3,* 267–272.

Fresina, M., Schiavi, C., & Campos, E. C. (2010). Do bifocals reduce accommodative amplitude in convergence excess esotropia? *Graefe's Archive for Clinical and Experimental Ophthalmology, 248*(10), 1501–1505.

Fricke, T., & Siderov, J. (1997). Non-stereoscopic cues in the Random-Dot E stereotest: results for adult observers. *Ophthalmic and Physiological Optics, 17,* 122–127.

Friedman, D. S., Katz, J., Repka, M. X., Giordano, L., Ibironke, J., Hawse, P., & Tielsch, J. M. (2008). Lack of concordance between fixation preference and HOTV optotype visual acuity in preschool children: the Baltimore Pediatric Eye Disease Study. *Ophthalmology, 115*(10), 1796–1799.

Fronius, M., & Sireteanu, R. (1994). Pointing errors in strabismics: complex patterns of distorted visuomotor coordination. *Vision Research, 34*(5), 689–707.

Fu, V. L. N., Stager, D. R., & Birch, E. E. (2007). Progression of intermittent, small-angle, and variable esotropia in infancy. *Investigative Ophthalmology Visual Science, 48*(2), 661–664.

Fulk, G. W., Cyert, L. A., & Parker, D. E. (2000). Authors response to Press. *Optometry and Vision Science, 77,* 631–632.

Fullard, R. J., Rutstein, R. P., & Corliss, D. A. (2007). The evaluation of two new computer-based tests for measurement of Aniseikonia. *Optometry and Vision Science, 84*(12), 1093–1100.

Fulton, A. B., Hansen, R. M., Moskowitz, A., & Mayer, D. L. (2013). Normal and abnormal visual development. In C. S. Hoyt, & D. Taylor (Eds.), *Pediatric ophthalmology and strabismus* (pp. 23–35). Elsevier Saunders.

Fulton, A. B., & Mayer, D. L. (1988). Esotropic children with amblyopia: effects of patching on acuity. *Graefe's Archive for Clinical and Experimental Ophthalmology, 226*(4), 309–312.

Gall, R., & Wick, B. (2003). The symptomatic patient with normal phorias at distance and near: what tests detect a binocular vision problem? *Optometry, 74*(5), 309−322.

Gall, R., Wick, B., & Bedell, H. (1998a). Vergence facility: establishing clinical utility. *Optometry and Vision Science, 75,* 731−742.

Gall, R., Wick, B., & Bedell, H. (1998b). Vergence facility and target type. *Optometry and Vision Science, 75,* 727−730.

Garcia, A., Cacho, P., Lara, F., & Megias, R. (2000). The relation between accommodative facility and general binocular dysfunction. *Ophthalmic and Physiological Optics, 20,* 98−104.

Garcia-Garcia, M. A., Belda, J. I., Schargel, K., Santos, M. J., Ruiz-Colecha, J., Rey, C., … Mompean, B. (2018). Optical coherence tomography in children with microtropia. *Journal of Pediatric Ophthalmology and Strabismus, 55*(3), 171−177.

Garnham, L., & Sloper, J. J. (2006). Effect of age on adult stereoacuity as measured by different types of stereotest. *British Journal of Ophthalmology, 90,* 91−95.

Gasson, A., & Morris, J. (1998). *Contact lens manual* (pp. 280−282). Oxford: Butterworth-Heinemann.

Geer, I., & Westall, C. A. (1996). A comparison of tests to determine acuity deficits in children with amblyopia. *Ophthalmic and Physiological Optics, 16,* 367−374.

Georgievski, Z., & Kowal, L. (1996). Evaluating torsion with the torsionometer, synoptophore, double Maddox rod test and Maddox wing test: a reliability study. *Australian Orthoptic Journal, 32,* 9−12.

Gerling, J., Ball, M., Bomer, T., Bach, M., & Kommerell, G. (1998). Fixationsdisparation am Pola-Zeigertest: nicht reprasentativ fur die Augenstellung unter naturlichen Sehbedingungen. *Klinische Monatsblatter fur Augenheilkunde, 212,* 226−233.

Gersztenkorn, D., & Lee, A. G. (2015). Palinopsia revamped: a systematic review of the literature. *Survey of Ophthalmology, 60*(1), 1−35.

Giannaccare, G., Primavera, L., & Fresina, M. (2018). Photorefractive keratectomy influences the angle of ocular deviation in strabismus patients with hyperopia. *International Ophthalmology, 39,* 737−744.

Giaschi, D. E., Regan, D., Kraft, S. P., & Kothe, A. C. (1993). Crowding and contrast in amblyopia. *Optometry and Vision Science, 70*(3), 192−197.

Gibson, H. W. (1947). *Clinical orthoptics.* London: Hatton Press.

Gibson, H. W. (1955). *Textbook of orthoptics.* London: Hatton Press.

Gifford, K. L., Gifford, P., Hendicott, P. L., & Schmid, K. L. (2020). Zone of clear single binocular vision in myopic orthokeratology. *Eye & Contact Lens, 46*(2), 82−90.

Gifford, K. L., Richdale, K., Kang, P., Aller, T. A., Lam, C. S., Liu, Y. M., … Rose, K. A., et al. (2019). IMI - Clinical Management Guidelines Report. *Investigative Ophthalmology & Visual Science, 60*(3), M184−M203.

Giles, G. H. (1960). *The principles and practice of refraction.* London: Hammond & Hammond.

Gillie, C., & Lindsay, L. (1969). *Orthoptics: a discussion of binocular anomalies.* London: Hatton Press.

Godts, D., Tassignon, M. J., & Gobin, L. (2004). Binocular vision impairment after refractive surgery. *Journal of Cataract and Refractive Surgery, 30,* 101−109.

Goersch, H. (1979). Decompensated heterophoria and its effects on vision. *The Optician, 177*(13-16), 29.

Goldrich, S. G. (1981). Emergent textural contours: a new technique for visual monitoring in nystagmus, oculomotor dysfunction, and accommodative disorders. *American Journal of Optometry and Physiological Optics, 58,* 451−459.

Golnik, K. C., Lee, A. G., & Eggenberger, E. R. (2004). The monocular vertical prism dissociation test. *American Journal of Ophthalmology, 137*(1), 135−137.

Gonzalez-Diaz Mdel, P., & Wong, A. M. (2014). Low positive predictive value of referrals for infantile esotropia among children of Chinese descent. *Journal of AAPOS, 18*(5), 502−504.

Gonzalez-Martin-Moro, J., Sales-Sanz, A., Gonzalez-Martin-Moro, J., Gomez-Sanz, F., Gonzalez-Manrique, M., Pilo-de-la-Fuente, B., & Garcia-Leal, R. (2014). Iatrogenic diplopia. *International Ophthalmology, 34*(4), 1007−1024.

Goseki, T., Suh, S. Y., Robbins, L., Pineles, S. L., Velez, F. G., & Demer, J. L. (2020). Prevalence of sagging eye syndrome in adults with binocular diplopia. *American Journal of Ophthalmology, 209,* 55−61.

Goss, D. A. (1995). *Ocular accommodation, convergence, and fixation disparity: a manual of clinical analysis.* Boston: Butterworth-Heinemann.

Goss, D. A., Groppel, P., & Dominguez, L. (2005). Comparison of MEM retinoscopy and Nott retinoscopy: their interexaminer repeatability. *Journal of Behavioral Optometry, 16*(6), 149−155.

Goss, D. A., & Grosvenor, T. (1990). Rates of childhood myopia progression with bifocals as a function of nearpoint phoria: consistency of three studies. *Optometry and Vision Science*, *67*(8), 637−640.

Goss, D. A., & Patel, J. (1995). Comparison of fixation disparity curve variables measured with the Sheedy Disparometer and the Wesson Fixation Disparity Card. *Optometry and Vision Science*, *72*, 580−588.

Goss, D. A., & Rosenfield, M. (1998). Vergence and myopia. In B. Gilmartin (Ed.), *Myopia and nearwork* (pp. 147−161). Oxford: Butterworth-Heinemann.

Gould, A., Fishkoff, D., & Galin, M. A. (1970). Active visual stimulation: a method of treatment of amblyopia in the older patient. *The American Orthoptic Journal*, *20*, 39−45.

Govindan, M., Mohney, B. G., Diehl, N. N., & Burke, J. P. (2005). Incidence and types of childhood exotropia: a population-based study. *Ophthalmology*, *112*, 104−108.

Gowen, E., Porter, C., Baimbridge, P., Hanratty, K., Pelham, J., & Dickinson, C. (2017). Optometric and orthoptic findings in autism: a review and guidelines for working effectively with autistic adult patients during an optometric examination. *Optometry in Practice*, *18*(3), 145−154.

Gowrisankaran, S., & Sheedy, J. E. (2015). Computer vision syndrome: a review. *Work*, *52*(2), 303−314.

Graefe, A.von. (1862). Cited by Burian and von Noorden (see above), p. 395.

Graf, M. (2002). Kestenbaum and artificial divergence surgery for abnormal head turn secondary to nystagmus. Specific and nonspecific effects of artificial divergence. *Strabismus*, *10*, 69−74.

Grant, S., Melmoth, D. R., Morgan, M. J., & Finlay, A. L. (2007). Prehension deficits in amblyopia. *Investigative Ophthalmology Visual Science*, *48*(3), 1139−1148.

Gresset, J. A., & Meyer, F. M. (1994). Risk of accidents among elderly car drivers with visual acuity equal to 6/12 or 6/15 and lack of binocular vision. *Ophthalmic and Physiological Optics*, *14*, 33−37.

Griffin, J. R., & Grisham, J. D. (1995). *Binocular anomalies: procedures for vision therapy* (3rd ed.). Boston: Butterworth-Heinemann.

Grisham, D. (1990). Management of nystagmus in young children. *Problems in Optometry*, *2*(3), 496−527.

Grosvenor, T., Perrigin, D. M., Perrigin, J., & Maslivitz, B. (1987). Houston myopia control study: a randomized clinical trial. Part II. Final report by the patient care team. *American Journal of Optometry and Physiological Optics*, *64*(7), 482−498.

Grzybowski, A., & Brona, P. (2017). Nutritional optic neuropathy instead of tobacco-alcohol amblyopia. *Canadian Journal of Ophthalmology*, *52*(5), 533.

Guggenheim, J. A., & Farbrother, J. E. (2005). A deficit in visits to the optometrist by preschool age children: implications for vision screening. *The British Journal of Ophthalmology*, *89*, 246−247.

Gunton, K. B., & Armstrong, B. (2010). Diplopia in adult patients following cataract extraction and refractive surgery. *Current Opinion in Ophthalmology*, *21*(5), 341−344.

Gupta, A., Sadeghi, P. B., & Akpek, E. K. (2009). Occult thyroid eye disease in patients presenting with dry eye symptoms. *American Journal of Ophthalmology*, *147*(5), 919−923.

Gur, S., Ron, S., & Heicklenklein, A. (1994). Objective evaluation of visual fatigue in VDU workers. *Occupational Medicine*, *44*, 201−204.

Gurwood, A. S., & Malloy, K. A. (2001). Review: giant cell arteritis. *Clinical & Experimental Optometry*, *85*, 19−26.

Guyton, D. L. (2000). Dissociated vertical deviation: etiology, mechanism, and associated phenomena. Costenbader Lecture. *Journal of American Association for Pediatric Ophthalmology and Strabismus*, *4*, 131−144.

Gwiazda, J., Bauer, J., Thorn, F., & Held, R. (1997). Development of spatial contrast sensitivity from infancy to adulthood: psychophysical data. *Optometry and Vision Science*, *74*(10), 785−789.

Gwiazda, J., Grice, K., & Thorn, F. (1999). Response AC/A ratios are elevated in myopic children. *Ophthalmic and Physiological Optics*, *19*, 173−179.

Gwiazda, J. E., Hyman, L., Norton, T. T., Hussein, M. E., Marsh-Tootle, W., Manny, R., ... Everett, D. (2004). Accommodation and related risk factors associated with myopia progression and their interaction with treatment in COMET children. *Investigative Ophthalmology & Visual Science*, *45*(7), 2143−2151.

Haase, H. J. (1962). Binocular testing and distance correction with the Berlin Polatest (transl. W. Baldwin). *Journal of the American Optometric Association*, *34*, 115−124.

Habeeb, S. Y., Arthur, B. W., & ten Hove, M. W. (2012). The effect of neutral density filters on testing in patients with strabismic amblyopia. *Canadian Journal of Ophthalmology*, *47*(4), 348−350.

Hadid, O. H., Wride, N. K., Griffiths, P. G., Strong, N. P., & Clarke, M. P. (2008). Opaque intraocular lens for intractable diplopia: experience and patients' expectations and satisfaction. *The British Journal of Ophthalmology*, *92*(7), 912–915.

Haggerty, H., Richardson, S., Hrisos, S., Strong, N. P., & Clarke, M. P. (2004). The Newcastle Control Score: a new method of grading the severity of intermittent distance exotropia. *British Journal of Ophthalmology*, *88*, 233–235.

Hainline, L. (2000). Development of accommodation and vergence in infancy. In O. Fransen, H. Richter, & L. Stark (Eds.), *Accommodation and vergence mechanisms in the visual system* (pp. 161–181). Basel, Switzerland: Birkhauser.

Halass, S. (1959). Aniseikonic lenses of improved design and their application. *Australian Journal of Optometry*, *42*, 387–393.

Hale, J. E., Murjaneh, S., Frost, N. A., & Harrad, R. A. (2006). How should we manage an amblyopic patient with cataract? *The British Journal of Ophthalmology*, *90*, 132–133.

Hall, C. (1982). Relation between clinical stereotests. *Ophthalmic and Physiological Optics*, *2*, 135–143.

Hall, D. M. B. (1996). *Chapter 11. Screening for vision defects. Health for All Children*. Oxford.

Hammond, R. S., & Schmidt, P. P. (1986). A random dot E stereogram for the vision screening of children. *Archives of Ophthalmology*, *104*, 54–60.

Han, J., Hong, S., Lee, S., Kim, J. K., Lee, H. K., & Han, S. H. (2014). Changes in fusional vergence amplitudes after laser refractive surgery for moderate myopia. *Journal of Cataract and Refractive Surgery*, *40*(10), 1670–1675.

Han, J. M., Yang, H. K., & Hwang, J. M. (2014). Efficacy of diagnostic monocular occlusion in revealing the maximum angle of exodeviation. *British Journal of Ophthalmology*, *98*(11), 1570–1574.

Hardman Lea, S. J., Loades, J., & Rubinstein, M. P. (1991). Microtropia versus bifoveal fixation in anisometropic amblyopia. *Eye*, *5*, 576–584.

Harle, D. E. (2007). The optometric correlates of migraine. *PhD thesis*. City University, London.

Harle, D. E., & Evans, B. J. (2004). The optometric correlates of migraine. *Ophthalmic & Physiological Optics*, *24*, 369–383.

Harle, D. E., & Evans, B. J. (2006). Subtle binocular vision anomalies in migraine. *Ophthalmic & Physiological Optics*, *26*(6), 587–596.

Harrad, R. (1996). Psychophysics of suppression. *Eye*, *10*(Pt 2), 270–273.

Harris, C. (1997). Nystagmus & eye movement disorders. In D. Taylor (Ed.), *Paediatric ophthalmology* (2nd ed., pp. 869–896). Oxford: Blackwell Science.

Harris, C. (2013). Latent nystagmus. *Optometry Today*, *53*(10), 49–53.

Harris, C. M., Jacobs, M., Shawkat, F., & Taylor, D. (1993). The development of saccadic accuracy in the first seven months. *Clinical Vision Sciences*, 85–96.

Harwerth, R. S., & Fredenburg, P. M. (2003). Binocular vision with primary microstrabismus. *Investigative Ophthalmology and Visual Science*, *44*, 4293–4306.

Harwerth, R. S., Moeller, M. C., & Wensveen, J. M. (1998). Effect of cue context on the perception of depth from combined disparity and perspective cues. *Optometry and Vision Science*, *75*, 433–444.

Harwerth, R. S., Smith, E. L., Duncan, G. C., Crawford, M. L. J., & Von Noorden, G. K. (1986). Multiple sensitive periods in the development of the primate visual system. *Science*, *232*, 235–238.

Hasebe, S., Nonaka, F., & Ohtsuki, H. (2005). Accuracy of accommodation in heterophoric patients: testing an interaction model in a large clinical sample. *Ophthalmic and Physiological Optics*, *25*(6), 582–591.

Hashemi, H., Pakzad, R., Heydarian, S., Yekta, A., Aghamirsalim, M., Shokrollahzadeh, F., … Khabazkhoob, M. (2019). Global and regional prevalence of strabismus: a comprehensive systematic review and meta-analysis. *Strabismus*, 1–12.

Hassan, S., Haridas, A., & Sundaram, V. (2018). Adjustable versus non-adjustable sutures for strabismus. *Cochrane Database of Systematic Reviews*, *3*CD004240.

Hatch, S. W., & Laudon, R. (1993). Sensitive period in stereopsis: random dot stereopsis after long-standing strabismus. *Optometry and Vision Science*, *70*, 1061–1064.

Hatt, S. R., & Gnanaraj, L. (2013). Interventions for intermittent exotropia. *Cochrane Database of Systematic Reviews* (5).

Hatt, S. R., Leske, D. A., Kirgis, P. A., Bradley, E. A., & Holmes, J. M. (2007). The effects of strabismus on quality of life in adults. *American Journal of Ophthalmology*, *144*(5), 643–647.

Hatt, S. R., Leske, D. A., Klaehn, L. D., Kramer, A. M., Iezzi, R., Jr., & Holmes, J. M. (2019). Treatment for central-peripheral rivalry-type diplopia and dragged-fovea diplopia syndrome. *American Journal of Ophthalmology, 208*, 41–46.

Hatt, S. R., Leske, D. A., Liebermann, L., Mohney, B. G., & Holmes, J. M. (2012). Variability of angle of deviation measurements in children with intermittent exotropia. *Journal of AAPOS, 16*(2), 120–124.

Hatt, S. R., Mohney, B. G., Leske, D. A., & Holmes, J. M. (2007). Variability of control in intermittent exotropia. *Ophthalmology, 115*(2), 371–376.e2.

Hatt, S. R., Wang, X., & Holmes, J. M. (2015). Interventions for dissociated vertical deviation. *Cochrane Database of Systematic Reviews* (11), CD010868.

Havertape, S., Whitfill, C., & Oscar, C. (1999). Early-onset accommodative esotropia. *Journal of Pediatric Ophthalmology and Strabismus, 36*, 69–73.

Hayes, G. J., Cohen, B. E., Rouse, M. W., & DeLand, P. N. (1998). Normative values for the nearpoint of convergence of elementary schoolchildren. *Optometry and Vision Science, 75*, 506–512.

Hazel, C. A. (1996). The efficacy of sports vision practice and its role in clinical optometry. *Optometry Today*, 29–34, **November 18**.

Healy, E. (1962). Nystagmus treated by orthoptics: a second report. *The American Orthoptic Journal, 12*, 89–91.

Helveston, E. M., & von Noorden, G. K. (1967). Microtropia. A newly defined entity. *Archives of Ophthalmology, 78*(3), 272–281.

Hendricks, T. J., De Brabander, J., van Der Horst, F. G., Hendrikse, F., & Knottnerus, J. A. (2007). Relationship between habitual refractive errors and headache complaints in schoolchildren. *Optometry and Vision Science, 84*(2), 137–143.

Henson, D. B., & North, R. (1980). Adaptation to prism-induced heterophoria. *American Journal of Optometry and Physiological Optics, 57*, 129–137.

Henson, D. B., & Williams, D. E. (1980). Depth perception in strabismus. *British Journal of Ophthalmology, 64*, 349–353.

Hernowo, A., & Eggenberger, E. (2014). Skew deviation: clinical updates for ophthalmologists. *Current Opinion in Ophthalmology, 25*(6), 485–487.

Heron, G., Dholakia, S., Collins, D. E., & McLaughlan, H. (1985). Stereoscopic threshold in children and adults. *American Journal of Optometry and Physiological Optics, 62*, 505–515.

Hertle, R. W. (2010). Nystagmus in infancy and childhood: characteristics and evidence for treatment. *The American Orthoptic Journal, 60*, 48–58.

Hertle, R. W., Dell'Osso, L. F., Fitzgibbon, E. J., Thompson, D., Yang, D., & Mellow, S. D. (2003). Horizontal rectus tenotomy in patients with congenital nystagmus: results in 10 adults. *Ophthalmology, 110*, 2097–2105.

Hess, R. F. (1977). On the relationship between strabismic amblyopia and eccentric fixation. *British Journal of Ophthalmology, 61*, 767–773.

Hess, R. F. (2002). Sensory processing in human amblyopes: snakes and ladders. In M. Moseley, & A. Fielder (Eds.), *Amblyopia: a multidisciplinary approach* (pp. 19–42). Butterworth Heinemann: Oxford.

Hess, R. F., & Pointer, J. S. (1985). Differences in the neural basis of human amblyopia: the distribution of the anomaly across the visual field. *Vision Research, 25*, 1577–1594.

Hess, R. F., Thompson, B., & Baker, D. H. (2014). Binocular vision in amblyopia: structure, suppression and plasticity. *Ophthalmic and Physiological Optics, 34*(2), 146–162.

Hill, A. B. (1966). Reflections on controlled trial. *Annals of the Rheumatic Diseases, 25*(2), 107–113.

Hillis, J. M., & Banks, M. S. (2001). Are corresponding points fixed? *Vision Research, 41*, 2457–2473.

Hodd, F. A. B. (1951). The measurement of spherical refraction by retinoscopy. *Transactions of the International Congress of the British Optical Association*, 191–291.

Hoeg, T. B., Moldow, B., Ellervik, C., Klemp, K., Erngaard, D., la Cour, M., & Buch, H. (2014). Danish Rural Eye Study: the association of preschool vision screening with the prevalence of amblyopia. *Acta Ophthalmologica, 93*(4), 322–329.

Hokoda, S. C., & Ciuffreda, K. J. (1983). Theoretical and clinical importance of proximal vergence and accommodation. In C. M. Schor, & K. J. Ciuffreda (Eds.), *Vergence eye movements: basic and clinical aspects* (pp. 75–97). Boston: Butterworths.

Holmes, J. M., Hatt, S. R., & Leske, D. A. (2014). Is intermittent exotropia a curable condition? *Eye (Lond), 29*, 171–176.

Holmes, J. M., & Kaz, K. M. (1994). Recovery of phorias following monocular occlusion. *Journal of Pediatric Ophthalmology and Strabismus, 31*, 110−113.

Holmes, J. M., Leske, D. A., & Hohberger, G. G. (2008). Defining real change in prism-cover test measurements. *American Journal of Ophthalmology, 145*(2), 381−385.

Holmes, J. M., Liebermann, L., Hatt, S. R., Smith, S. J., & Leske, D. A. (2013). Quantifying diplopia with a questionnaire. *Ophthalmology, 120*(7), 1492−1496.

Holmes, J. M., Manh, V. M., Lazar, E. L., Beck, R. W., Birch, E. E., Kraker, R. T., ... Pediatric Eye Disease Investigator G. (2016). Effect of a binocular iPad game vs part-time patching in children aged 5 to 12 years with amblyopia: a randomized clinical trial. *JAMA Ophthalmology, 134*(12), 1391−1400.

Holmes, J. M., Melia, M., Bradfield, Y. S., Cruz, O. A., & Forbes, B. (2007). Factors associated with recurrence of amblyopia on cessation of patching. *Ophthalmology, 114*(8), 1427−1432.

Holmstrom, G., Bondeson, M. L., Eriksson, U., Akerblom, H., & Larsson, E. (2013). 'Congenital' nystagmus may hide various ophthalmic diagnoses. *Acta Ophthalmologica, 95*(5), 412−416.

Hopkins, S., Black, A. A., White, S. L. J., & Wood, J. M. (2019). Visual information processing skills are associated with academic performance in Grade 2 school children. *Acta Ophthalmologica, 97*(8), 1141−1148.

Horan, L. A., Ticho, B. H., Khammar, A. J., Allen, M. S., & Shah, B. A. (2015). Is the convergence insufficiency symptom survey specific for convergence insufficiency? A prospective, randomized study. *The American Orthoptic Journal, 65*, 99−103.

Horwood, A. (2003a). Neonatal ocular misalignments reflect vergence development but rarely become esotropia. *British Journal of Ophthalmology, 87*, 1146−1150.

Horwood, A. (2003b). Too much or too little: neonatal ocular misalignment frequency can predict later abnormality. *British Journal of Ophthalmology, 87*, 1142−1145.

Horwood, A., & Toor, S. (2014). Clinical test responses to different orthoptic exercise regimes in typical young adults. *Ophthalmic & Physiological Optics, 34*(2), 250−262.

Horwood, A. M., & Riddell, P. M. (2012). Evidence that convergence rather than accommodation controls intermittent distance exotropia. *Acta Ophthalmologica, 90*(2), e109−117.

Horwood, A. M., Toor, S., & Riddell, P. M. (2014). Screening for convergence insufficiency using the CISS is not indicated in young adults. *The British Journal of Ophthalmology, 98*(5), 679−683.

Hosking, S. (2001). Incomitant strabismus. In B. Evans, & S. Doshi (Eds.), *Binocular vision and orthoptics* (pp. 83−91). Oxford: Butterworth-Heinemann..

Houston, C. A., Cleary, M., Dutton, G. N., & McFadzean, R. M. (1998). Clinical characteristics of microtropia: is microtropia a fixed phenomenon? *The British Journal of Ophthalmology, 82*, 219−224.

Houston, C. A., Jones, D., & Weir, C. R. (2000). An unusual cause of asthenopia: "pseudo-accommodative insufficiency" associated with a high AC:A ratio. *The British Journal of Ophthalmology, 84*(12), 1438.

Howard, C., & Firth, A. Y. (2006). Is the Cardiff Acuity Test effective in detecting refractive errors in children? *Optometry and Vision Science, 83*(8), 577−581.

Howard, I. P., Fang, X., Allison, R. S., & Zacher, J. E. (2000). Effects of stimulus size and eccentricity on horizontal and vertical vergence. *Experimental Brain Research, 130*, 124−132.

Howarth, P. A. (2011). Potential hazards of viewing 3-D stereoscopic television, cinema and computer games: a review. *Ophthalmic & Physiological Optics, 31*(2), 111−122.

Howell-Duffy, C., Umar, G., Ruparelia, N., & Elliott, D. B. (2010). What adjustments, if any, do UK optometrists make to the subjective refraction result prior to prescribing? *Ophthalmic & Physiological Optics, 30*(3), 225−239.

Hoyt, C. S., & Fredrick, D. R. (1999). Serious neurologic disease presenting as comitant esotropia. In A. L. Rosenbaum, & A. P. Santiago (Eds.), *Clinical strabismus management* (pp. 152−162). Philadelphia: W. B. Saunders Company.

Hrisos, S., Clarke, M. P., Kelly, T., Henderson, J., & Wright, C. M. (2006). Unilateral visual impairment and neurodevelopmental performance in preschool children. *British Journal of Ophthalmology, 90*(7), 836−838.

Hrisos, S., Clarke, M. P., & Wright, C. M. (2004). The emotional impact of amblyopia treatment in preschool children: randomized controlled trial. *Ophthalmology, 111*, 1550−1556.

Hudak, D. T., & Magoon, E. H. (1997). Poverty predicts amblyopia treatment failure. *Journal of American Association for Pediatric Ophthalmology and Strabismus, 1*, 214−215.

Hufner, K., Frenzel, C., Kremmyda, O., Adrion, C., Bardins, S., Glasauer, S., ... Strupp, M. (2015). Esophoria or esotropia in adulthood: a sign of cerebellar dysfunction? *Journal of Neurology, 262*(3), 585−592.

Hugonnier, R., & Clayette-Hugonnier, S. (translated by S. Veronneau-Troutman) (1969). *Strabismus, Heterophoria, Ocular Motor Paralysis*, 158.

Hulme, C., & Snowling, M. J. (2016). Reading disorders and dyslexia. *Current Opinion in Pediatrics, 28*(6), 731−735.

Humphriss, D., & Woodruff, E. W. (1962). Refraction by immediate contrast. *British Journal of Physiological Optics, 19*, 15−23.

Hung, G. K. (1998). Saccade-vergence trajectories under free- and instrument-space environments. *Current Eye Research, 17*(2), 159−164.

Hung, G. K., Ciuffreda, K. J., & Semmlow, J. L. (1986). Static vergence and accommodation: population norms and orthoptic effects. *Documenta Ophthalmologica, 62*, 165−179.

Hung, L.-F., Crawford, M. L. J., & Smith, E. L. (1995). Spectacle lenses alter eye growth and the refractive status of young monkeys. *Nature Medicine, 1*, 761−765.

Hunt, O. A., Wolffsohn, J. S., & Garcia-Resua, C. (2006). Ocular motor triad with single vision contact lenses compared to spectacle lenses. *Contact Lens & Anterior Eye, 29*(5), 239−245.

Hussaindeen, J. R., Rakshit, A., Singh, N. K., Swaminathan, M., George, R., Kapur, S., ... Ramani, K. K. (2018). The minimum test battery to screen for binocular vision anomalies: report 3 of the BAND study. *Clinical and Experimental Optometry, 101*(2), 281−287.

Hussein, M. A., Weakley, D., Wirazka, T., & Paysse, E. E. (2015). The long-term outcomes in children who are not compliant with spectacle treatment for accommodative esotropia. *Journal of American Association for Pediatric Ophthalmology and Strabismus {JAAPOS}, 19*(2), 169−171.

Hutcheson, K. A., Ellish, N. J., & Lambert, S. R. (2003). Weaning children with accommodative esotropia out of spectacles: a pilot study. *British Journal of Ophthalmology, 87*, 4−7.

Hyson, M. T., Julesz, B., & Fender, D. H. (1983). Eye movements and neural remapping during fusion of misaligned random dot stereograms. *Journal of the Optical Society of America, 73*, 1665−1673.

Hyvarinen, L., Nasanen, R., & Laurinen, P. (1980). New visual acuity test for pre-school children. *Acta Ophthalmol (Copenh), 58*(4), 507−511.

Iacobucci, I., Archer, S., & Giles, C. (1993). Children with exotropia responsive to spectacle correction of hypermetropia. *American Journal of Ophthalmology, 116*, 79−83.

Iacobucci, I. L., Archer, S. M., Furr, B. A., Beyst Martonyi, J., & Del Monte, M. A. (2001). Bangerter foils in the management of moderate amblyopia. *American Orthoptic Journal, 51*, 84−91.

Ingram, R. M. (1977). Refraction as a basis for screening children for squint and amblyopia. *The British Journal of Ophthalmology, 61*, 8−15.

Ingram, R. M., Gill, L. E., & Lambert, T. W. (2000). Effect of spectacles on changes of spherical hypermetropia in infants who did, and did not, have strabismus. *The British Journal of Ophthalmology, 84*, 324−326.

Ingram, R. M., Lambert, T. W., & Gill, L. E. (2009). Visual outcome in 879 children treated for strabismus: insufficient accommodation and vision deprivation, deficient emmetropisation and anisometropia. *Strabismus, 17*(4), 148−157.

Ip, J. M., Robaei, D., Rochtchina, E., & Mitchell, P. (2006). Prevalence of eye disorders in young children with eyestrain complaints. *American Journal of Ophthalmology, 142*(3), 495−497.

Irvine, S. R. (1944). A simple test for binocular fixation: clinical application useful in the appraisal of ocular dominance, amblyopia ex anopsia, minimal strabismus, and malingering. *American Journal of Ophthalmology, 27*, 740−746.

Irvine, S. R. (1948). Amblyopia ex anopsia. *Transactions of the American Ophthalmological Society, 46*, 527.

Irving, E. L., & Robertson, K. M. (1996). Influences of monocular image degradation on the monocular components of fixation disparity. *Ophthalmic and Physiological Optics, 16*, 326−335.

Isenberg-Grzeda, E., Rahane, S., DeRosa, A. P., Ellis, J., & Nicolson, S. E. (2016). Wernicke-Korsakoff syndrome in patients with cancer: a systematic review. *The Lancet Oncology, 17*(4), e142−e148.

Jackson, S., Harrad, R. A., Morris, M., & Rumsey, N. (2006). The psychosocial benefits of corrective surgery for adults with strabismus. *British Journal of Ophthalmology, 90*(7), 883−888.

Jacobson, D. M. (1991). Superior oblique palsy manifested during pregnancy. *Ophthalmology, 98*, 1874−1876.

Jainta, S., Bucci, M. P., Wiener-Vacher, S., & Kapoula, Z. (2011). Changes in vergence dynamics due to repetition. *Vision Research, 51*(16), 1845−1852.

Jainta, S., & Jaschinski, W. (2009). "Trait" and "state" aspects of fixation disparity during reading. *Journal of Eye Movement Research, 3*(3), 1–13.

Jamieson, D. R. S. (1994). Conference report: focus on botulinum toxin. *Hospital Update, October,* 509–510.

Jampel, R. S., & Shi, D. X. (2006). Evidence against mobile pulleys on the rectus muscles and inferior oblique muscle: central nervous system controls ocular kinematics. *Journal of Pediatric Ophthalmology and Strabismus, 43*(5), 289–295.

Jampolsky, A. (1964). The prism test for strabismus screening. *Journal Pediatric Ophthalmology, 1,* 30–34.

Jampolsky, A. (1971). *A simplified approach to strabismus diagnosis. Symposium of Strabismus* (pp. 3–4). St. Louis: Mosby.

Jampolsky, A. (1999). Duane syndrome. In A. L. Rosenbaum, & A. P. Santiago (Eds.), *Clinical Strabismus Management* (pp. 325–346). Philadelphia: W.B. Saunders Company.

Jaschinski, W. (2001). Methods for measuring the proximity fixation disparity curve. *Ophthalmic and Physiological Optics, 21,* 368–375.

Jaschinski, W. (2018). Individual objective versus subjective fixation disparity as a function of forced vergence. *PLoS One, 13*(7), e0199958.

Jaschinski, W., Brode, P., & Griefahn, B. (1999). Fixation disparity and nonius bias. *Vision Research, 39,* 669–677.

Jaschinski, W., Jainta, S., & Kloke, W. B. (2010). Objective vs subjective measures of fixation disparity for short and long fixation periods. *Ophthalmic & Physiological Optics, 30*(4), 379–390.

Jaschinski-Kruza, W., & Schubert-Alshuth, E. (1992). Variability of fixation disparity and accommodation when viewing a CRT visual display unit. *Ophthalmic and Physiological Optics, 12,* 411–419.

Jayaramachandran, P., Proudlock, F. A., Odedra, N., Gottlob, I., & McLean, R. J. (2014). A randomized controlled trial comparing soft contact lens and rigid gas-permeable lens wearing in infantile nystagmus. *Ophthalmology, 121,* 1827–1836.

Jenkins, T. C. A., Abd-Manan, F., Pardhan, S., & Murgatroyd, R. N. (1994). Effect of fixation disparity on distance binocular visual acuity. *Ophthalmic and Physiological Optics, 14,* 129–131.

Jenkins, T. C. A., Abd-Manan., & Pardhan, S. (1995). Clinical research note: fixation disparity and near visual acuity. *Ophthalmic and Physiological Optics, 15*(1), 53–58.

Jenkins, T. C. A., Pickwell, L. D., & Sheridan, M. (1979). After-image transfer – evaluation of short-term treatment. *British Journal of Physiological Optics, 33*(3), 33–37.

Jenkins, T. C. A., Pickwell, L. D., & Yekta, A. A. (1989). Criteria for decompensation in binocular vision. *Ophthalmic and Physiological Optics, 9,* 121–125.

Jennings, A. (1996). Investigation of binocular vision. In S. Barnard, & D. Edgar (Eds.), *Pediatric eye care* (pp. 168–190). Oxford: Blackwell Science.

Jennings, A. (2000). Behavioural optometry: a critical review. *Optometry in Practice, 1,* 67–78.

Jennings, A. (2001a). Anomalies of convergence. In B. Evans, & S. Doshi (Eds.), *Binocular vision and orthoptics* (pp. 34–38). Oxford: Butterworth-Heinemann.

Jennings, A. (2001b). Amblyopia and eccentric fixation. In B. Evans, & S. Doshi (Eds.), *Binocular vision and orthoptics* (pp. 73–78). Oxford: Butterworth-Heinemann.

Jennings, J. A. M. (1985). Anomalous retinal correspondence - a review. *Ophthalmic and Physiological Optics, 5*(4), 357–368.

Jeong, S. H., Oh, Y. M., Hwang, J. M., & Kim, J. S. (2008). Emergence of diplopia and oscillopsia due to Heimann-Bielschowsky phenomenon after cataract surgery. *The British Journal of Ophthalmology, 92*(10), 1402.

Jethani, J., Prakash, K., Vijayalakshmi, P., & Parija, S. (2006). Changes in astigmatism in children with congenital nystagmus. *Graefe's Archive for Clinical and Experimental Ophthalmology, 244*(8), 938–943.

Jimenez, J. R., Ponce, A., & Anera, R. G. (2004). Induced aniseikonia diminishes binocular contrast sensitivity and binocular summation. *Optometry and Vision Science, 81,* 559–562.

Jimenez, J. R., Ponce, A., Jimenez-del Barco, L., Diaz, J. A., & Perez-Ocon, F. (2002). Impact of induced aniseikonia on stereopsis with random-dot stereogram. *Optometry and Vision Science, 79,* 121–125.

Jimenez, R., Martinez-Almeida, L., Salas, C., & Ortiz, C. (2011). Contact lenses vs spectacles in myopes: is there any difference in accommodative and binocular function? *Graefe's Archive for Clinical and Experimental Ophthalmology, 249*(6), 925–935.

Jimenez, R., Perez, M. A., Garcia, J. A., & Gonzalez, M. D. (2004). Statistical normal values of visual parameters that characterize binocular function in children. *Ophthalmic & Physiological Optics, 24,* 528–542.

Jimenez, J. R., Rubino, M., Diaz, J. A., Hita, E., & del Barco, L. J. (2000). Changes in stereoscopic depth perception caused by decentration of spectacle lenses. *Optom Vis Sci., 77*(8), 421–427.

Jin, Y. H., & Son, J. H. (1991). The effect of occlusion in intermittent exotropia. *Journal of the Korean Ophthalmological Society, 32,* 307–311.

Jones, H. A. (1965). Orthoptic handling of fusion vergences. *American Orthoptic Journal, 15,* 21–29.

Jones, P. H., Harris, C. M., Woodhouse, J. M., Margrain, T. H., Ennis, F. A., & Erichsen, J. T. (2013). Stress and visual function in infantile nystagmus syndrome. *Investigative Ophthalmology & Visual Science, 54*(13), 7943–7951.

Joosse, M. V., Esme, D. L., Schimsheimer, R. J., Verspeek, S. A. M., Vermeulen, M. H. L., & van Minderhout, E. M. (2005). Visual evoked potentials during suppression in exotropic and esotropic strabismics: strabismic suppression objectified. *Graefe's Archive for Clinical and Experimental Ophthalmology, 243,* 142–150.

Joslin, C. E., McMahon, T. T., & Kaurman, L. M. (2002). The effectiveness of occluder contact lenses in improving occlusion compliance in patients that have failed traditional occlusion therapy. *Optometry and Vision Science, 79,* 376–380.

Joubert, C., & Bedell, H. E. (1990). Proximal vergence and perceived distance. *Optometry and Vision Science, 67*(1), 29–35.

Joyce, K. E., Beyer, F., Thomson, R. G., & Clarke, M. P. (2015). A systematic review of the effectiveness of treatments in altering the natural history of intermittent exotropia. *British Journal of Ophthalmology, 99*(4), 440–450.

Julesz, B. (1971). *Foundations of cyclopean perception.* Chicago: University of Chicago Press.

Justo, M. S., Bermudez, M. A., Perez, R., & Gonzalez, F. (2004). Binocular interaction and performance of visual tasks. *Ophthalmic & Physiological Optics, 24,* 82–90.

Kaban, T., Smith, K., Beldavs, R., Cadera, W., & Orton, R. B. (1995). The 20-prism-dioptre base-out test: an indicator of peripheral binocularity. *Canadian Journal of Ophthalmology, 30,* 247–250.

Kaeser, P. F., Kress, B., Rohde, S., & Kolling, G. (2012). Absence of the fourth cranial nerve in congenital Brown syndrome. *Acta Ophthalmologica, 90*(4), e310–e313.

Kang, P., Watt, K., Chau, T., Zhu, J., Evans, B. J. W., & Swarbrick, H. (2018). The impact of orthokeratology lens wear on binocular vision and accommodation: a short-term prospective study. *Contact Lens & Anterior Eye, 41*(6), 501–506.

Kanonidou, E., Proudlock, F. A., & Gottlob, I. (2010). Reading strategies in mild to moderate strabismic amblyopia: an eye movement investigation. *Investigative Ophthalmology & Visual Science, 51*(7), 3502–3508.

Kanski, J. J. (1994). *Clinical ophthalmology.* Oxford: Butterworth-Heinemann.

Kaplan, R. (1983). Changes in form visual fields in reading disability children produced by syntonic (coloured-light) stimulation. *International Journal of Biosocial Research, 5,* 20–33.

Karania, R., & Evans, B. J. (2006a). Authors' reply. *Ophthalmic & Physiological Optics, 26*(5), 524.

Karania, R., & Evans, B. J. (2006b). The Mallett Fixation Disparity Test: influence of test instructions & relationship with symptoms. *Ophthalmic and Physiological Optics, 26,* 507–522.

Karlén, E., Milestad, L., & Pansell, T. (2019). Accommodation and near visual function in children with albinism. *Acta Ophthalmologica, 97*(6), 608–615.

Kassem, I. S., Rubin, S. E., & Kodsi, S. R. (2012). Exotropia in children with high hyperopia. *Journal of AAPOS, 16*(5), 437–440.

Kavitha, V., Heralgi, M. M., Harishkumar, P. D., Harogoppa, S., Shivaswamy, H. M., & Geetha, H. (2019). Analysis of macular, foveal, and retinal nerve fiber layer thickness in children with unilateral anisometropic amblyopia and their changes following occlusion therapy. *Indian Journal of Ophthalmology, 67*(7), 1016–1022.

Kedzia, B., Pieczyrak, D., Tondel, G., & Maples, W. C. (1999). Factors affecting the clinical testing of accommodative facility. *Ophthalmic and Physiological Optics, 19,* 12–21.

Keech, R. V., & Kutschke, P. J. (1995). Upper age limit for the development of amblyopia. *Journal of Pediatric Ophthalmology and Strabismus, 32,* 89–93.

Kelly, S. L., & Buckingham, T. J. (1998). Movement hyperacuity in childhood amblyopia. *The British Journal of Ophthalmology, 82,* 991–995.

Khan, A. O. (2008). Persistent diplopia following secondary intraocular lens placement in patients with sensory strabismus from uncorrected monocular aphakia. *British Journal of Ophthalmology, 92*(1), 51–53.

Kim, H., Kim, D. H., Ahn, H., & Lim, H. T. (2017). Proposing a new scoring system in intermittent exotropia: towards a better assessment of control. *Canadian Journal of Ophthalmology, 52*(3), 235–239.

Kim, J. H., & Hwang, J. M. (2005). Presence of the abducens nerve according to the type of Duane's retraction syndrome. *Ophthalmology, 112*, 109–113.

King, A. J., Stacey, E., Stephenson, G., & Trimble, R. G. (1995). Spontaneous recovery rates for unilateral sixth nerve palsies. *Eye, 9*, 476–478.

Kiorpes, L., Carlson, M. R., & Alfi, D. (1989). Development of visual acuity in experimentally strabismic monkeys. *Clinical Vision Sciences, 4*, 950.

Kirsch, I. (1996). Hypnosis in psychotherapy: efficacy and mechanisms. *Contemporary Hypnosis, 13*, 109–114.

Kirschen, D. G. (1983). Auditory feedback in the control of congenital nystagmus. *American Journal of Optometry and Physiological Optics, 60*(5), 364–368.

Kirschen, D. G. (1999). Understanding sensory evaluation. In A. L. Rosenbaum, & A. P. Santiago (Eds.), *Clinical strabismus management* (pp. 22–36). Philadelphia: W.B. Saunders Company.

Kirwan, C., O'Keefe, M., O'Mullane, G. M., & Sheehan, C. (2010). Refractive surgery in patients with accommodative and non-accommodative strabismus: 1-year prospective follow-up. *The British Journal of Ophthalmology, 94*(7), 898–902.

Kitaguchi, Y., Bessho, K., Yamaguchi, T., Nakazawa, N., Mihashi, T., & Fujikado, T. (2007). In vivo measurements of cone photoreceptor spacing in myopic eyes from images obtained by an adaptive optics fundus camera. *Japanese Journal of Ophthalmology, 51*(6), 456–461.

Koc, F., Ozal, H., & Firat, E. (2003). Is it possible to differentiate early-onset accommodative esotropia from early-onset essential esotropia? *Eye, 17*, 1–4.

Koc, F., Ozal, H., Yasar, H., & Firat, E. (2005). Resolution in partially accommodative esotropia during occlusion treatment for amblyopia. *Eye, 20*(3), 325–328.

Koklanis, K., Abel, L. A., & Aroni, R. (2006). Psychosocial impact of amblyopia and its treatment: a multidisciplinary study. *Clinical & Experimental Ophthalmology, 34*(8), 743–750.

Kommerell, G., Horn, R., & Bach, M. (1986). Motion perception in congenital nystagmus. In E. L. Keller, & D. S. Zee (Eds.), *Adaptive processes in visual and oculomotor systems* (pp. 485–491). Oxford: Pergamon Press.

Kommerell, G., Kromeier, M., Scharff, F., & Bach, M. (2015). Asthenopia, associated phoria, and self-selected prism. *Strabismus, 23*(2), 51–65.

Konig, H. H., & Barry, J. C. (2004). Cost effectiveness of treatment for amblyopia: an analysis based on a probabilistic Markov model. *The British Journal of Ophthalmology, 88*, 606–612.

Kono, R., Poukens, V., & Demer, J. L. (2002). Quantitative analysis of the structure of the human extraocular muscle pulley system. *Investigative Ophthalmology & Visual Science, 43*(9), 2923–2932.

Kora, T., Awaya, S., & Sato, M. (1997). Evaluation of motor and sensory function in patients with esotropia followed for more than 13 years after surgery. *Folia Ophthalmologica Japonica, 48*, 495–501.

Korah, S., Philip, S., Jasper, S., Antonio-Santos, A., & Braganza, A. (2014). Strabismus surgery before versus after completion of amblyopia therapy in children. *Cochrane Database of Systematic Reviews, 10*, CD009272.

Kosmorsky, G. S., & Diskin, D. (1991). Examination of the pupil. In B. K. Farris (Ed.), *The basics of neuro-ophthalmology* (pp. 9–45). St. Louis: Mosby.

Kothari, M. (2007). Clinical characteristics of spontaneous late-onset comitant acute nonaccommodative esotropia in children. *Indian Journal of Ophthalmology, 55*(2), 117–120.

Kothari, M., Mody, K., Walinjkar, J., Madia, J., & Kaul, S. (2009). Paralysis of the near-vision triad in a child. *Journal of AAPOS, 13*(2), 202–203.

Kowal, L., Battu, R., & Kushner, B. (2005). Refractive surgery and strabismus. *Clinical & Experimental Ophthalmology, 33*, 90–96.

Kraft, S. P., O'Reilly, C., Quigley, P. L., Allan, K., & Eustis, H. S. (1993). Cyclotorsion in unilateral and bilateral superior oblique paresis. *Journal of Pediatric Ophthalmology and Strabismus, 30*, 361–367.

Kramer, P., Shippman, S., Bennett, G., Meininger, D., & Lubkin, V. (1999). A study of aniseikonia and Knapp's law using a projection space eikonometer. *Binocular Vision & Strabismus Quarterly, 14*(3), 197–201.

Krimsky, E. (1943). The binocular examination of the young child. *American Journal of Ophthalmology*, *26*, 624.

Kromeier, M., Schmitt, C., Bach, M., & Kommerell, G. (2001). Heterophoria measured with white, dark-grey and dark-red Maddox rods. *Graefes Archive for Clinical and Experimental Ophthalmology*, *239*, 937–940.

Kulp, M. T., Ciner, E., Maguire, M., Moore, B., Pentimonti, J., Pistilli, M., ... Ying, G.-S. (2016). Uncorrected hyperopia and preschool early literacy. *Ophthalmology*, *123*(4), 681–689.

Kulp, M. T., Ciner, E., Maguire, M., Pistilli, M., Candy, T. R., Ying, G.-S., ... Group f.t.V.i.P.-H.i.P.S.. (2017). Attention and visual motor integration in young children with uncorrected hyperopia. *Optometry and Vision Science*, *94*(10), 965–970.

Kulp, M. T., Foster, N. C., Holmes, J. M., Kraker, R. T., Melia, B. M., Repka, M. X., & Tien, D. R. (2012). Effect of ocular alignment on emmetropization in children <10 years with amblyopia. *American Journal of Ophthalmology*, *154*(2), 297–302.e1.

Kushner, B. J., & Kowal, L. (2003). Diplopia after refractive surgery: occurrence and prevention. *Archives of Ophthalmology*, *121*, 315–321.

Kushner, B. J. (1995). Fixation switch diplopia. *Archives of Ophthalmology*, *113*, 896–899.

Kushner, B. J. (2002). Intractable diplopia after strabismus surgery in adults. *Archives of Ophthalmology*, *120*, 1498–1504.

Kushner, B. J. (2005). The treatment of convergence insufficiency. *Archives of Ophthalmology*, *123*, 100–101.

Kushner, B. J. (2007). The inferior oblique muscle adherence syndrome. *Archives of Ophthalmology*, *125*(11), 1510–1514.

Kushner, B. J. (2013). Vertical strabismus. In C. S. Hoyt, & D. Taylor (Eds.), *Pediatric ophthalmology and strabismus*. Elsevier Saunders.

Kushner, B. J., & Hariharan, L. (2009). Observations about objective and subjective ocular torsion. *Ophthalmology*, *116*(10), 2001–2010.

Kutschke, P. J., & Scott, W. E. (2004). Prism adaptation in visually mature patients with esotropia of childhood onset. *Ophthalmology*, *111*, 177–179.

Kutschke, P. J., Scott, W. E., & Keech, R. V. (1991). Anisometropic amblyopia. *Ophthalmology*, *98*, 258–263.

Kvarnstrom, G., Jakobsson, P., & Lennerstrand, G. (2001). Visual screening of Swedish children: an ophthalmological evaluation. *Acta Ophthalmologica Scandinavica*, *79*, 240–244.

Laidlaw, D. A., Abbott, A., & Rosser, D. A. (2003). Development of a clinically feasible logMAR alternative to the Snellen chart: performance of the "compact reduced logMAR" visual acuity chart in amblyopic children. *British Journal of Ophthalmology*, *87*, 1232–1234.

Lal, V., Sahota, P., Singh, P., Gupta, A., & Prabhakar, S. (2009). Ophthalmoplegia with migraine in adults: is it ophthalmoplegic migraine? *Headache*, *49*(6), 838–850.

Lambooij, M., Fortuin, M., Ijsselsteijn, W., Evans, B., & Heynderickx, I. (2010). Measuring visual fatigue and visual discomfort associated with 3-D displays. *Journal of the Society for Information Display*, *18*(11), 931–943.

Lanca, C. C., & Rowe, F. J. (2019). Measurement of fusional vergence: a systematic review. *Strabismus*, *27*(2), 88–113.

Lang, J. (1966). Evaluation in small angle strabismus or microtropia. In A. Arruga (Ed.), *International strabismus symposium* (p. 219). Basel: University of Giessen.

Lang, J. (1994). The weak points of prismatic correction with the Polatest. *Klinische Monatsblatter fur Augenheilkunde*, *204*, 378–380.

Lang, J. I., & Lang, T. J. (1988). Eye screening with the Lang Stereotest. *American Orthoptic Journal*, *38*, 38–50.

Laria, C., Alio, J. L., & Pinero, D. N. (2010). Intrastromal corneal tattooing as treatment in a case of intractable strabismic diplopia (double binocular vision). *Binocular Vision & Strabismus Quarterly*, *25*(4), 238–242.

Larson, S. A., Keech, R. V., & Verdick, R. E. (2003). The threshold for the detection of strabismus. *Journal of AAPOS*, *7*, 418–422.

Larson, W. L., & Faubert, J. (1992). Stereolatency: a stereopsis test for everyday depth perception. *Optometry and Vision Science*, *69*(12), 926–930.

Leat, S. J. (2011). To prescribe or not to prescribe? Guidelines for spectacle prescribing in infants and children. *Clinical and Experimental Optometry, 94*(6), 514−527.

Lederer, P., Poltavski, D., & Biberdorf, D. (2015). Confusion inside Panum's area and symptomatic convergence insufficiency. *Vision Development Rehabilitation, 1*(1), 46−60.

Lee, J. (1999). Management of selected forms of neurogenic strabismus. In A. L. Rosenbaum, & A. P. Santiago (Eds.), *Clinical strabismus management* (pp. 380−392). Philadelphia: Saunders.

Lee, J., & Flynn, J. T. (1985). Bilateral superior oblique palsies. *The British Journal of Ophthalmology, 69*, 508−513.

Lee, J. J., Chun, K. I., Baek, S. H., & Kim, U. S. (2013). Relationship of hypertropia and excyclotorsion in superior oblique palsy. *Korean Journal of Ophthalmology, 27*(1), 39−43.

Lee, P. P., Spritzer, K., & Hays, R. (1997). The impact of blurred vision on functioning and well-being. *Ophthalmology, 104*, 390−396.

Lee, S. Y., & Isenberg, S. J. (2003). The relationship between stereopsis and visual acuity after occlusion therapy for amblyopia. *Ophthalmology, 110*, 2088−2092.

Leguire, L. E., Rogers, G. L., & Bremer, D. L. (1990). Amblyopia: the normal eye is not normal. *Journal of Pediatric Ophthalmology and Strabismus, 27*(1), 32−38.

Leguire, L. E., Rogers, G. L., & Bremer, D. L. (1991). Visual-evoked response binocular summation in normal and strabismic infants: defining the critical period. *Investigative Ophthalmology & Visual Science, 32*, 126−133.

Leigh, R. J., Rushton, D. N., Thurston, S. E., Hertle, R. W., & Yaniglos, S. S. (1988). Effects of retinal image stabilization in acquired nystagmus due to neurologic disease. *Neurology, 38*, 122−127.

Lempert, P. (2000). Optic nerve hypoplasia and small eyes in presumed amblyopia. *Journal of American Association for Pediatric Ophthalmology and Strabismus, 4*, 258−266.

Lempert, P. (2004). The axial length/disc area ratio in anisometropic hyperopic amblyopia*1: A hypothesis for decreased unilateral vision associated with hyperopic anisometropia. *Ophthalmology, 111*, 304−308.

Lennerstrand, G., & Samuelson, B. (1983). Amblyopia in 4-year-old children treated with grating stimulation and full-time occlusion; a comparative study. *British Journal of Ophthalmology, 67*, 181−190.

Leske, D. A., & Holmes, J. M. (2004). Maximum angle of horizontal strabismus consistent with true stereopsis. *Journal of AAPOS, 8*(1), 28−34.

Lesueur, L. C., & Arne, J. L. (2002). Phakic intraocular lens to correct high myopic amblyopia in children. *Journal of Refractive Surgery, 18*, 519−523.

Leung, V., Wick, B., & Bedell, H. E. (1996). Multifaceted treatment of congenital nystagmus: a report of 6 cases. *Optometry and Vision Science, 73*, 114−124.

Levartovsky, S., Oliver, M., Gottesman, N., & Shimshoni, M. (1995). Factors affecting long term results of successfully treated amblyopia: initial visual acuity and type of amblyopia. *The British Journal of Ophthalmology, 79*, 225−228.

Levi, D., & Saarinen, J. (2004). Perception of mirror symmetry in amblyopic vision. *Vision Research, 44*(21), 2475−2482.

Levi, D. M. (1994). Pathophysiology of binocular vision and amblyopia. *Current Opinion in Ophthalmology, 5*(5), 3−10.

Levi, D. M. (2008). Crowding--an essential bottleneck for object recognition: a mini-review. *Vision Research, 48*(5), 635−654.

Lew, H., Kim, C. H., Yun, Y. S., & Han, S. H. (2007). Binocular photophobia after surgical treatment in intermittent exotropia. *Optometry and Vision Science, 84*(12), 1101−1103.

Lewis, A. R., Kline, L. B., & Sharpe, J. A. (1996). Acquired esotropia due to Arnold-Chiari I malformation. *Journal of Neuro-Ophthalmology, 16*, 49−54.

Li, J., Hess, R. F., Chan, L. Y., Deng, D., Yang, X., Chen, X., ... Thompson, B. (2013). Quantitative measurement of interocular suppression in anisometropic amblyopia: a case-control study. *Ophthalmology, 120*(8), 1672−1680.

Li, J., Thompson, B., Deng, D., Chan, L. Y. L., Yu, M., & Hess, R. F. (2013). Dichoptic training enables the adult amblyopic brain to learn. *Current Biology, 23*(8), R308−R309.

Li, J., Thompson, B., Ding, Z., Chan, L. Y., Chen, X., Yu, M., ... Hess, R. F. (2012). Does partial occlusion promote normal binocular function? *Investigative Ophthalmology & Visual Science, 53*(11), 6818−6827.

Li, T., Qureshi, R., & Taylor, K. (2019). Conventional occlusion versus pharmacologic penalization for amblyopia. *Cochrane Database of Systematic Reviews (Online)*, *8*, CD006460.

Li, X., Dumoulin, S. O., Mansouri, B., & Hess, R. F. (2007). Cortical deficits in human amblyopia: their regional distribution and their relationship to the contrast detection deficit. *Investigative Ophthalmology Visual Science*, *48*(4), 1575–1591.

Lie, I., & Opheim, A. (1985). Long-term acceptance of prisms by heterophorics. *Journal of the American Optometric Association*, *56*, 272–278.

Lie, I., & Opheim, A. (1990). Long-term stability of prism correction of heterophorics and heterotropics; a 5 year follow-up. *Journal of the American Optometric Association*, *61*, 491–498.

Lie, I., Watten, R., & Fostervold, K. I. (2000). Accommodation/vergence/fixation disparity and synergism of head, neck and shoulders. In O. Fransen, H. Richter, & L. Stark (Eds.), *Accommodation and vergence mechanisms in the visual system*. Basel, Switzerland: Birkhauser.

Lim, L. (1999). Divergence paralysis. In A. L. Rosenbaum, & A. P. Santiago (Eds.), *Clinical strabismus management* (pp. 159–162). Philadelphia: W.B. Saunders Company.

Lim, S. A., Siatkowski, R. M., & Farris, B. K. (2005). Functional visual loss in adults and children: patient characteristics, management, and outcomes. *Ophthalmology*, *112*, 1821–1828.

Lindblom, B., Westheimer, G., & Hoyt, W. F. (1997). Torsional diplopia and its perceptual consequences: a 'user-friendly' test for oblique eye muscle palsies. *Neuro-Ophthalmology*, *18*, 105–110.

Lindqvist, S., Vik, T., Indredavik, M. S., & Brubakk, A. M. (2007). Visual acuity, contrast sensitivity, peripheral vision and refraction in low birthweight teenagers. *Acta Ophthalmologica Scandinavica*, *85*(2), 157–164.

Lindsay, R. (1941). *Neuro-ophthalmology* (p. 49) London: Heinemann.

Lithander, J., & Sjostrand, J. (1991). Anisometropic and strabismic amblyopia in the age group 2 years and above: a prospective study of the results of treatment. *The British Journal of Ophthalmology*, *75*, 111–116.

Little, J.-A. (2018). Vision in children with autism spectrum disorder: a critical review. *Clinical and Experimental Optometry*, *101*(4), 504–513.

Locke, L. C., & Somers, W. (1989). A comparison study of dynamic retinoscopy techniques. *Optometry and Vision Science*, *66*(8), 540–544.

Logan, N., Gilmartin, B., Marr, J. E., Stevenson, M. R., & Ainsworth, J. R. (2004). Community-based study of the association of high myopia in children with ocular and systemic disease. *Optometry and Vision Science*, *81*, 11–13.

Logan, N. S., Davies, L. N., Mallen, E. A., & Gilmartin, B. (2005). Ametropia and ocular biometry in a U. K. university student population. *Optometry and Vision Science*, *82*(4), 261–266.

London, R. (1987). Monovision correction for diplopia. *Journal of the American Optometric Association*, *58*, 568–570.

London, R., & Crelier, R. S. (2006). Fixation disparity analysis: sensory and motor approaches. *Optometry (St. Louis, Mo.)*, *77*(12), 590–608.

London, R. F., & Wick, B. (1987). Vertical fixation disparity correction: effect on the horizontal forced-vergence fixation disparity curve. *American Journal of Optometry and Physiological Optics*, *64*(9), 653–656.

London, R. F., & Wick, B. (1987). Vertical fixation disparity correction: effect on the horizontal forced-vergence fixation disparity curve. *American Journal of Optometry*, *64*(9), 653–655.

Long, J., Cheung, R., Duong, S., Paynter, R., & Asper, L. (2017). Viewing distance and eyestrain symptoms with prolonged viewing of smartphones. *Clinical and Experimental Optometry*, *100*(2), 133–137.

Lord, S. R., & Dayhew, J. (2001). Visual risk factors for falls in older people. *Journal of the American Geriatrics Society*, *49*, 508–515.

Lord, S. R., Dayhew, J., & Howland, A. (2002). Multifocal glasses impair edge-contrast sensitivity and depth perception and increase the risk of falls in older people. *Journal of the American Geriatrics Society*, *50*, 1760–1766.

Louwagie, C. R., Diehl, N. N., Greenberg, A. E., & Mohney, B. G. (2009). Is the incidence of infantile esotropia declining? A population-based study from Olmsted County, Minnesota, 1965 to 1994. *Archives of Ophthalmology*, *127*(2), 200–203.

Ludlow, A. K., Wilkins, A. J., & Heaton, P. (2008). Colored overlays enhance visual perceptual performance in children with autism spectrum disorders. *Research in Autism Spectrum Disorders*, *2*(3), 498–515.

Lueder, G. T., & Norman, A. A. (2006). Strabismus surgery for elimination of bifocals in accommodative esotropia. *American Journal of Ophthalmology, 142*(4), 632–635.

Lukman, H., Kiat, J. E., Ganesan, A., Chua, W. L., Khor, K. L., & Choong, Y. F. (2010). Strabismus-related prejudice in 5-6-year-old children. *The British Journal of Ophthalmology, 94*(10), 1348–1351.

Luu, C. D., Green, J. F., & Abel, L. (2000). Vertical fixation disparity curve and the effects of vergence training in a normal young adult population. *Optometry and Vision Science, 77*, 663–669.

Lyle, T. K., & Wybar, K. C. (1967). *Lyle and Jackson's practical orthoptics in the treatment of squint (and other anomalies of binocular vision)*. London: Lewis.

Lyons, J. G. (1966). Fixation disparity researches: Part 1-8. *The Optician, 151*, 152, 665-672; 4-8, 86-89, 110-113, 163-167, 189-193, 216-219, 243-246.

Ma, M. M., Kang, Y., Scheiman, M., & Chen, X. (2019). Office-based vergence and accommodative therapy for the treatment of intermittent exotropia: a pilot study. *Optometry and Vision Science, 96*(12), 925–933.

MacEwen, C. J., & Chakrabarti, H. S. (2004). Why is squint surgery in children in decline? *British Journal of Ophthalmology, 88*, 509–511.

MacEwen, C. J., Lymburn, E. G., & Ho, W. O. (2008). Is the maximum hypermetropic correction necessary in children with fully accommodative esotropia? *British Journal of Ophthalmology, 92*(10), 1329–1332.

Maconachie, G. D., Farooq, S., Bush, G., Kempton, J., Proudlock, F. A., & Gottlob, I. (2016). Association between adherence to glasses wearing during amblyopia treatment and improvement in visual acuity. *JAMA Ophthalmol, 134*(12), 1347–1353.

Magli, A., Forte, R., Gallo, F., & Carelli, R. (2014). Refractive surgery for accommodative esotropia: 5-year follow-up. *Journal of Refractive Surgery, 30*(2), 116–120.

Major, A., Maples, W. C., Toomey, S., DeRosier, W., & Gahn, D. (2007). Variables associated with the incidence of infantile esotropia. *Optometry (St. Louis, Mo.), 78*(10), 534–541.

Mallett, R. F. J. (1979a). Effect of fixation disparity (letter to Editor). *The Ophthalmic Optician, 19*, 818–819.

Mallett, R. (1988a). Techniques of investigation of binocular vision anomalies. In K. Edwards, & R. Llewellyn (Eds.), *Optometry* (pp. 238–269). London: Butterworths.

Mallett, R. (1988b). The management of binocular vision anomalies. In K. Edwards, & R. Llewellyn (Eds.), *Optometry* (pp. 270–284). London: Butterworths.

Mallett, R. F. (1979b). The use of prisms in the treatment of concomitant strabismus. *The Ophthalmic Optician, t9*, 793–798.

Mallett, R. F. J. (1964). The investigation of heterophoria at near and a new fixation disparity technique. *The Optician, l48*, 547–551.

Mallett, R. F. J. (1966). A fixation disparity test for distance use. *The Optician, 152*, 1–4.

Mallett, R. F. J. (1969). The sequelae of ocular muscle palsy. *Ophthalmic Optician, 6 September*, 920–923.

Mallett, R. F. J. (1969). The sequelae of ocular muscle palsy. *Ophthalmic Optician, 6 September*, 920–923.

Mallett, R. F. J. (1970). Anomalous retinal correspondence: the new outlook. *The Ophthalmic Optician, 13 June*, 606–624.

Mallett, R. F. J. (1975). Using after-images in the investigation and treatment of strabismus. *The Ophthalmic Optician, 15*, 727–729.

Mallett, R. F. J. (1977). Aspects of the investigation and treatment of strabismus. *The Ophthalmic Optician, May 28*, 432–433.

Mallett, R. F. J. (1983). The treatment of congenital idiopathic nystagmus by intermittent photic stimulation. *Ophthalmic and Physiological Optics, 3*, 341–356.

Mallett, R. F. J. (1985). A unit for treating amblyopia and congenital nystagmus by intermittent photic stimulation. *Optometry Today, 25*(8), 260–264.

Mallett, R.F.J., Radnam, R. (1992). Congenital nystagmus: improvement in sensory aspects of vision with a new method of treatment. *Unpublished manuscript presented at American Academy Europe meeting, Stratford*, UK.

Mallett, R. F. J., & Radnan-Skibin, R. (1994). The new dual fixation disparity test. *Optometry Today, Mar 14*, 32–34.

Manchandia, A. M., & Demer, J. L. (2014). Sensitivity of the three-step test in diagnosis of superior oblique palsy. *Journal of AAPOS, 18*(6), 567–571.

Manny, R. E., Hussein, M., Gwiazda, J., Marsh-Tootle, W., & COMET study group. (2003). Repeatability of ETDRS visual acuity in children. *Investigative Ophthalmology and Visual Science, 44*, 3294–3300.

Marran, L. F., De Land, P. N., & Nguyen, A. L. (2006). Accommodative insufficiency is the primary source of symptoms in children diagnosed with convergence insufficiency. *Optometry and Vision Science*, *83*, 281−289.

Marshman, W. E., Dawson, E., Neveu, M. M., Morgan, M. J., & Sloper, J. J. (2001). Increased binocular enhancement of contrast sensitivity and reduced stereoacuity in Duane syndrome. *Investigative Ophthalmology & Visual Science*, *42*, 2821−2825.

Marton, H. B. (1954). Some clinical aspects of heterophoria. *British Journal of Physiological Optics*, *11*(3), 170−175.

Matheron, E., & Kapoula, Z. (2011). Vertical heterophoria and postural control in nonspecific chronic low back pain. *PLoS One*, *6*(3), e18110.

Matilla, M. T., Pickwell, D., & Gilchrist, J. (1995). Research note: The effect of red and neutral density filters on the degree of eccentric fixation. *Ophthalmic and Physiological Optics*, *15*(3), 223−226.

Maybodi, M. (2003). Infantile-onset nystagmus. *Current Opinion in Ophthalmology*, *14*, 276−285.

McCulloch, D. L. (1998). The infant patient. *Ophthalmic and Physiological Optics*, *18*, 140−146.

McCullough, S. J., O'Donoghue, L., & Saunders, K. J. (2016). Six-year refractive change among white children and young adults: evidence for significant increase in myopia among white UK children. *PLoS One*, *11*(1), e0146332.

McIntyre, A., & Fells, P. (1996). Use of Bangerter foils in the treatment of intractable diplopia. *British Orthoptic of Journal*, *53*, 43−47.

McKenzie, K. M., Kerr, S. R., Rouse, M. W., & DeLand, P. N. (1987). Study of accommodative facility testing reliability. *American Journal of Optometry and Physiological Optics*, *64*(3), 186−194.

McKeon, C., Wick, B., Aday, L. U., & Begley, C. (1997). A case comparison of intermittent exotropia and quality of life measurement. *Optometry and Vision Science*, *74*, 105−110.

Medland, C., Walter, H., & Margaret Woodhouse, J. (2010). Eye movements and poor reading: does the Developmental Eye Movement test measure cause or effect? *Ophthalmic and Physiological Optics*, *30*(6), 740−747.

Mehta, A. (1999). Chief complaint, history, and physical examination. In A. L. Rosenbaum, & A. P. Santiago (Eds.), *Clinical Strabismus Management* (pp. 3−21). Philadelphia: W.B. Saunders Company.

Mehta, A. M., & Demer, J. L. (1994). Magnetic resonance imaging of the superior oblique muscle in superior oblique myokymia. *Journal of Pediatric Ophthalmology And Strabismus*, *31*, 378−383.

Membreno, J. H., Brown, M. M., Brown, G. C., Sharma, S., & Beauchamp, G. R. (2002). A cost-utility analysis of therapy for amblyopia. *Ophthalmology*, *109*, 2265−2271.

Menon, V., Saha, J., Tandon, R., Mehta, M., & Khokhar, S. (2002). Study of the psychosocial aspects of strabismus. *Journal of Pediatric Ophthalmology and Strabismus*, *39*, 197.

Mestre, C., Otero, C., Díaz-Doutón, F., Gautier, J., & Pujol, J. (2018). An automated and objective cover test to measure heterophoria. *PLoS One*, *13*(11), e0206674.

Methling, D., & Jaschinski, W. (1996). Contrast sensitivity after wearing prisms to correct heterophoria. *Ophthalmic and Physiological Optics*, *16*, 211−215.

Metz, H. S. (1986). Think superior oblique palsy. *Journal of Pediatric Ophthalmology and Strabismus*, *23*, 166−169.

Metzler, U., Ham, O., Flores, V., Claramunt, M., Sepulveda, C., & Casanova, D. (1998). Blue filter amblyopia treatment protocol for strabismic amblyopia: a prospective comparative study of 50 cases. *Binocular Vision & Strabismus Quarterly*, *13*, 241−248.

Mezer, E., Meyer, E., Wygnansi-Jaffe, T., Haase, W., Shauly, Y., & Biglan, A. W. (2015). The long-term outcome of the refractive error in children with hypermetropia. *Graefe's Archive for Clinical and Experimental Ophthalmology*, *253*(7), 1013−1019.

Mezer, E., & Wygnanski-Jaffe, T. (2012). Do children and adolescents with attention deficit hyperactivity disorder have ocular abnormalities? *European Journal of Ophthalmology*, *22*(6), 931−935.

Middleton, E. M., Sinason, M. D. A., & Davids, Z. (2007). Blurred vision due to psychosocial difficulties: a case series. *Eye*, *22*(2), 316−317.

Migneco, M. K. (2008). Alleviating vertical diplopia through contact lenses without the use of prism. *Eye & Contact Lens*, *34*(5), 297−298.

Miki, T., Ito, H., Kawai, H., & Nakanishi, T. (1999). Chiari malformation (type I) associated with bilateral abducens nerve palsy: case report. *No Shinkei Geka. Neurological Surgery*, *27*, 1037−1042.

Miles, C., Krall, J., Thompson, V., & Colvard, D. M. (2015). A new treatment for refractory chronic migraine headaches. Costa Mesa, CA: eyeBrain Medical, Inc.

Miller, N. R. (2011). Functional neuro-ophthalmology. *Handbook of Clinical Neurology, 102*, 493–513.

Millodot, M. (1993). *Dictionary of optometry* (3rd ed.). Oxford: Butterworth-Heinemann.

Millodot, M. (2009). *Dictionary of optometry* (7th ed.). Oxford: Butterworth-Heinemann.

Mills, M. D., Coats, D. K., Donahue, S. P., & Wheeler, D. T. (2004). Strabismus surgery for adults: a report by the American Academy of Ophthalmology. *Ophthalmology, 111*, 1255–1262.

Minnal, V. R., & Rosenberg, J. B. (2011). Refractive surgery: a treatment for and a cause of strabismus. *Current Opinion in Ophthalmology, 22*(4), 222–225.

Mirabella, G., Hay, S., & Wong, A. M. (2011). Deficits in perception of images of real-world scenes in patients with a history of amblyopia. *Archives of Ophthalmology, 129*(2), 176–183.

Mittelman, D. (2006). Age-related distance esotropia. *Journal of AAPOS, 10*(3), 212–213.

Mohan, K., Saroha, V., & Sharma, A. (2004). Successful occlusion therapy for amblyopia in 11- to 15-year-old children. *Journal of Pediatric Ophthalmology and Strabismus, 41*, 89–95.

Mohindra, I., & Molinari, J. F. (1979). Near retinoscopy and cycloplegic retinoscopy in early primary grade schoolchildren. *American Journal of Optometry and Physiological Optics, 56*, 34–38.

Mohney, B. G., & Huffaker, R. K. (2003). Common forms of childhood exotropia. *Ophthalmology, 110*, 2093–2096.

Mohney, B. G., Cotter, S. A., Chandler, D. L., Holmes, J. M., Wallace, D. K., Yamada, T., ... Wu, R. (2019). Three-year observation of children 3 to 10 years of age with untreated intermittent exotropia. *Ophthalmology, 126*(9), 1249–1260.

Momeni-Moghaddam, H., Eperjesi, F., Kundart, J., & Sabbaghi, H. (2014a). Induced vertical disparity effects on local and global stereopsis. *Current Eye Research, 39*(4), 411–415.

Momeni-Moghaddam, H., Goss, D. A., & Sobhani, M. (2014b). Accommodative response under monocular and binocular conditions as a function of phoria in symptomatic and asymptomatic subjects. *Clinical and Experimental Optometry, 97*(1), 36–42.

Monger, L., Wilkins, A., & Allen, P. (2015). Identifying visual stress during a routine eye examination. *Journal of Optometry, 8*(2), 140–145.

Montes-Mico, R. (2001). Prevalence of general dysfunctions in binocular vision. *Annals of Ophthalmology, 33*, 205–208.

Mon-Williams, M., Plooy, A., Burgess-Limerick, R., & Wann, J. (1998). Gaze angle: a possible mechanism of visual stress in virtual reality headsets. *Ergonomics, 41*(3), 280–285.

Mon-Williams, M., Wann, J. P., & Rushton, S. (1993). Research note: binocular vision in a virtual world: visual deficits following the wearing of a head-mounted display. *Ophthalmic and Physiological Optics, 3*, 387–391.

Moore, C., & Drack, A. V. (2000). Prism adaptation in decompensated monofixation syndrome. *American Orthoptic Journal, 50*, 80–84.

Moore, S., & Cohen, R. L. (1985). Congenital exotropia. *American Orthoptic Journal, 35*, 68–70.

Morgan, M. W. (1944). Analysis of clinical data. *American journal of optometry and archives of American Academy of Optometry, 21*(12), 477–491.

Morris, R. J. (1991). Double vision as a presenting symptom in an ophthalmic casualty department. *Eye, 5*, 124–129.

Morrison, L. C. (1993). Adapting to aniseikonia: Part 1. *Optometry Today, July 23*, 24–27.

Morse, S. E., & Jiang, B. (1999). Oculomotor function after virtual reality use differentiates symptomatic from asymptomatic individuals. *Optometry and Vision Science, 76*, 637–642.

Morton, V., & Torgerson, D. J. (2003). Effect of regression to the mean on decision making in health care. *BMJ, 326*(7398), 1083–1084.

Mulvihill, A., MacCann, A., Flitcroft, I., & O'Keefe, M. (2000). Outcome in refractive accommodative esotropia. *The British Journal of Ophthalmology, 84*(7), 746–749.

Mutti, D. O. (2007). To emmetropize or not to emmetropize? The question for hyperopic development. *Optometry and Vision Science, 84*(2), 97–102.

Mutti, D. O., Mitchell, G. L., Jones-Jordan, L. A., Cotter, S. A., Kleinstein, R. N., Manny, R. E., ... Group, C. S. (2017). The response AC/A ratio before and after the onset of myopia. *Investigative Ophthalmology & Visual Science, 58*(3), 1594–1602.

Myklebust, A., & Riddell, P. (2016). Fusional stamina: an alternative to Sheard's criterion. *Scandinavian Journal of Optometry and Visual Science, 9*(2), 7.

Nabovati, P., Kamali, M., Mirzajani, A., Jafarzadehpur, E., & Khabazkhoob, M. (2020). The effect of base-in prism on vision-related symptoms and clinical characteristics of young adults with convergence insufficiency; a placebo-controlled randomised clinical trial. *Ophthalmic & Physiological Optics, 40*(1), 8–16.

Nahar, N. K., Gowrisankaran, S., Hayes, J. R., & Sheedy, J. E. (2011). Interactions of visual and cognitive stress. *Optometry, 82*(11), 689–696.

Naylor, R. J. (2005). The ocular effects of Parkinsonism and its treatment. *Optometry in Practice, 6*, 19–31.

Neetens, A., & Janssens, M. (1979). The superior oblique: a challenging extraocular muscle. *Documenta Ophthalmologica, 46*(2), 295–303.

Neikter, B. (1994a). Effects of diagnostic occlusion on ocular alignment in normal subjects. *Strabismus, 2*, 67–77.

Neikter, B. (1994b). Horizontal and vertical deviations after prism neutralization and diagnostic occlusion in intermittent exotropia. *Strabismus, 2*, 13–22.

Nelson, J. (1988a). Amblyopia: the cortical basis of binocularity and vision loss in strabismus. In K. Edwards, & R. Llewellyn (Eds.), *Optometry* (pp. 189–216). London: Butterworths.

Nelson, J. (1988b). Binocular vision: disparity detection and anomalous correspondence. In K. Edwards, & R. Llewellyn (Eds.), *Optometry* (pp. 217–237). London: Butterworths.

Neuenschwander, E., Rohrbach, L., Schroth, V. (2018). Improvement of the NPC in subjects with convergence insufficiency after IFS exercises, ed. Institute of Optometry, Switzerland. Alten, Switzerland.

Newsham, D. (2002). A randomised controlled trial of written information: the effect on parental non-concordance with occlusion therapy. *British Journal of Ophthalmology, 86*, 787–791.

Newsham, D., O'Connor, A. R., & Harrad, R. A. (2018). Incidence, risk factors and management of intractable diplopia. *The British Journal of Ophthalmology, 102*(3), 393–397.

Ng, Y. S., & Lyons, C. J. (2005). Oculomotor nerve palsy in childhood. *Canadian Journal of Ophthalmology, 40*, 645–653.

Ngan, J., Goss, D. A., & Despirito, J. (2005). Comparison of fixation disparity curve parameters obtained with the Wesson and Saladin fixation disparity cards. *Optometry and Vision Science, 82*, 69–74.

Noorden, G. K. V., & Campos, E. (2002). *Binocular vision and ocular motility: theory and management of strabismus.* St Louis: Mosby.

Noorden, G. Kvon, & Campos, E. (2004). Patching regimens (letter). *Ophthalmology, 111*, 1063.

Noorden, G. Kvon, Murray, E., & Wong, S. Y. (1986). Superior oblique paresis. A review of 270 cases. *Archives of Ophthalmology, 104*, 1771.

Noorden, G. Kvon (1976). The nystagmus compensation (blocking) syndrome. *American Journal of Ophthalmology, 82*, 283–290.

Noorden, G. Kvon (1996). *Binocular vision and ocular motility* (5th ed.). St. Louis: Mosby.

Norbis, A. L., & Malbran, E. (1956). Concomitant esotropia of late onset; pathological report of four cases in siblings. *The British Journal of Ophthalmology, 40*(6), 373–380.

Norn, N. S. (1964). Congenital idiopathic nystagmus. Incidence and occupational prognosis. *Acta Ophthalmologica, 42*, 889–896.

North, R. (1986). Atropine penalisation for treatment of amblyopia. *The Optician, February 28*, 32–33.

North, R., & Henson, D. B. (1985). Adaptation to lens-induced heterophorias. *American Journal of Optometry and Physiological Optics, 62*(11), 774–780.

North, R. V., & Henson, D. B. (1981). Adaptation to prism induced heterophoria in subjects with abnormal binocular vision or asthenopia. *American Journal of Optometry, 58*(9), 746–752.

North, R. V., & Henson, D. B. (1982). Effect of orthoptics upon the ability of patients to adapt to prism induced heterophoria. *American Journal of Optometry, 59*, 983–990.

North, R. V., & Henson, D. B. (1992). The effect of orthoptic treatment upon the vergence adaptation mechanism. *Optometry and Vision Sciences, 69*, 294–299.

North, R. V., Henson, D. B., & Smith, T. J. (1993). Influence of proximal, accommodative and disparity stimuli upon the vergence system. *Ophthalmic and Physiological Optics, 13*, 239–243.

Nucci, P., Kushner, B. J., Serafino, M., & Orzalesi, N. (2005). A multi-disciplinary study of the ocular, orthopedic, and neurologic causes of abnormal head postures in children. *American Journal of Ophthalmology, 140*, 65–68.

Numa, W. A., Desai, U., Gold, D. R., Heher, K. L., & Annino, D. J. (2005). Silent sinus syndrome: a case presentation and comprehensive review of all 84 reported cases. *The Annals of Otology, Rhinology, and Laryngology*, *114*(9), 688−694.

Nusz, K. J., Mohney, B. G., & Diehl, N. N. (2006). The course of intermittent exotropia in a population-based cohort. *Ophthalmology*, *113*(7), 1154−1158.

Nuzzi, G., & Cantu, C. (2003). Spatial perception in normal and strabismic subjects: role of stereopsis and monocular clues. *European Journal of Ophthalmology*, *13*(6), 507−514.

Nyman, K. G., Singh, G., Rydberg, A., & Fornander, M. (1983). Controlled study comparing CAM treatment with occlusion therapy. *British Journal of Ophthalmology*, *67*, 178−180.

O'Donoghue, L., Rudnicka, A. R., McClelland, J. F., Logan, N. S., & Saunders, K. J. (2012). Visual acuity measures do not reliably detect childhood refractive error--an epidemiological study. *PLoS One*, *7*(3), e34441.

O'Leary, C. I., & Evans, B. J. W. (2003). Criteria for prescribing optometric interventions: literature review and practitioner survey. *Ophthalmic and Physiological Optics*, *23*, 429−439.

O'Connor, A. R., Birch, E. E., Anderson, S., & Draper, H. (2010). The functional significance of stereopsis. *Investigative Ophthalmology & Visual Science*, *51*(4), 2019−2023.

Odell, N. V., Hatt, S. R., Leske, D. A., Adams, W. E., & Holmes, J. M. (2009). The effect of induced monocular blur on measures of stereoacuity. *Journal of AAPOS*, *13*(2), 136−141.

Ogle, K. N. (1950). *Researches in binocular vision* (pp. 68−93). Philadelphia and London: W. B. Saunders.

Ogle, K. N., Mussey, F., & Prangen, A. H. (1949). Fixation disparity and the fusional processes in binocular single vision. *American Journal of Ophthalmology*, *32*, 1069-1027.

Ohlsson, J., Baumann, M., Sjostrand, J., & Abrahamsson, M. (2002). Long-term visual outcome in amblyopia treatment. *British Journal of Ophthalmology*, *86*, 1148−1151.

Ohlsson, J., Villarreal, G., Abrahamsson, M., Cavazos, H., Sjostrom, A., & Sjostrand, J. (2001). Screening merits of the Lang II, Frisby, Randot, Titmus, and TNO stereo tests. *Journal of AAPOS*, *5*, 316−322.

Ohlsson, J., Villarreal, G., Sjostrom, A., Abrahamsson, M., & Sjostrand, J. (2002). Screening for amblyopia and strabismus with the Lang II stereo card. *Acta Ophthalmologica*, *80*, 163−166.

Ohtsuka, K., Maeda, S., & Oguri, N. (2002). Accommodation and convergence palsy caused by lesions in the bilateral rostral superior colliculus. *American Journal of Ophthalmology*, *133*, 425−427.

Okuda, F. C., Apt, A., & Wanter, B. S. (1977). Evaluation of the random dot stereogram tests. *American Orthoptic Journal*, *28*, 124−130.

O'Leary, C. I., & Evans, B. J. W. (2003). Criteria for prescribing optometric interventions: literature review and practitioner survey. *Ophthalmic and Physiological Optics*, *23*, 429−439.

O'Leary, C. I., & Evans, B. J. W. (2006). Double-masked randomised placebo-controlled trial of the effect of prismatic corrections on rate of reading and the relationship with symptoms. *Ophthalmic and Physiological Optics*, *26*(6), 555−565.

O'Leary, C. I., & Evans, B. J. W. (2006). Double-masked randomised placebo-controlled trial of the effect of prismatic corrections on rate of reading and the relationship with symptoms. *Ophthalmic and Physiological Optics*, *26*(6), 555−565.

Oliver, M., Neumann, R., Chaimovitch, Y., Gotesman, N., & Shimshoni, M. (1986). Compliance and results of treatment for amblyopia in children more than 8 years old. *American Journal of Ophthalmology*, *102*, 340−345.

Olsson, M., Fahnehjelm, K. T., Rydberg, A., & Ygge, J. (2015). Ocular motor score (OMS): a clinical tool to evaluating ocular motor functions in children. Intrarater and inter-rater agreement. *Acta Ophthalmologica*, *93*, 444−449.

Ong, E., Ciuffreda, K. J., & Tannen, B. (1993). Static accommodation in congenital nystagmus. *Investigative Ophthalmology and Visual Science*, *34*, 194−204.

Osborne, D. C., Greenhalgh, K. M., Evans, M. J. E., & Self, J. E. (2018). Atropine penalization versus occlusion therapies for unilateral amblyopia after the critical period of visual development: a systematic review. *Ophthalmology and Therapy*, *7*(2), 323−332.

Otto, J. M., Bach, M., & Kommerell, G. (2008). The prism that aligns fixation disparity does not predict the self-selected prism. *Ophthalmic & Physiological Optics*, *28*(6), 550−557.

Otto, J. M., Bach, M., & Kommerell, G. (2010). Advantage of binocularity in the presence of external visual noise. *Graefe's Archive for Clinical and Experimental Ophthalmology*, *248*(4), 535−541.

Otto, J. M., Kromeier, M., Bach, M., & Kommerell, G. (2008). Do dissociated or associated phoria predict the comfortable prism? *Graefe's Archive for Clinical and Experimental Ophthalmology, 246*(5), 631–639.

Pacheco, M., & Peris, E. (1994). Validity of the Lang, Frisby and Random Dot E stereotests for screening of pre-school children. *Optometry and Vision Science* (Supplement), 657.

Packwood, E. A., Cruz, O. A., Rychwalski, P. J., & Keech, R. V. (1999). The psychosocial effects of amblyopia study. *Journal of American Association for Pediatric Ophthalmology and Strabismus, 3*, 15–17.

Palomo, A. C., Puell, M. C., Sanchez-Ramos, C., & Villena, C. (2006). Normal values of distance hetero-phoria and fusional vergence ranges and effects of age. *Graefe's Archive for Clinical and Experimental Ophthalmology, V244*(7), 821–824.

Palomo-Alvarez, C., & Puell, M. C. (2010). Binocular function in school children with reading difficulties. *Graefe's Archive for Clinical and Experimental Ophthalmology, 248*(6), 885–892.

Papadopoulos, M., Brookes, J. L., & Khaw, P. T. (2005). Childhood glaucoma. In C. S. Hoyt, & D. Taylor (Eds.), *Pediatric ophthalmology and strabismus* (4th ed., pp. 353–367). Elsevier Saunders.

Papageorgiou, E., Asproudis, I., Maconachie, G., Tsironi, E. E., & Gottlob, I. (2019). The treatment of amblyopia: current practice and emerging trends. *Graefe's Archive for Clinical and Experimental Ophthalmology, 257*(6), 1061–1078.

Park, K. A., Kim, S. M., & Oh, S. Y. (2011). The maximal tolerable reduction in hyperopic correction in patients with refractive accommodative esotropia: a 6-month follow-up study. *American Journal of Ophthalmology, 151*(3), 535–541.

Parkes, L. C. (2001). An investigation of the impact of occlusion therapy on children with amblyopia, its effect on their families, and compliance with treatment. *British Orthoptic Journal, 58*, 30–37.

Parks, M. M. (1969). The monofixational syndrome. *Transactions of the American Ophthalmological Society, 67*, 609.

Parks, M. M., & Eustis, A. J. (1961). Monofixational phoria. *American Orthoptic Journal, 11*, 38–42.

Parmar, K. R., Dickinson, C., & Evans, B. J. W. (2019). Does an iPad fixation disparity test give equivalent results to the Mallett near fixation disparity test? *Journal of Optometry, 12*(4), 222–231.

Patsopoulos, N. A. (2011). A pragmatic view on pragmatic trials. *Dialogues in Clinical Neuroscience, 13*(2), 217–224.

Paula, J. S., Ibrahim, F. M., Martins, M. C., Bicas, H. E., & Velasco e Cruz, A. A. (2009). Refractive error changes in children with intermittent exotropia under overminus lens therapy. *Arquivos Brasileiros de Oftalmologia, 72*(6), 751–754.

Payne, C. R., Grisham, J. D., & Thomas, K. L. (1974). A clinical examination of fixation disparity. *American Journal of Ophthalmic and Physiological Optics, 51*, 88–90.

Paysse, E. A., Coats, D. K., Hussein, M. A. W., Hamill, M. B., & Koch, D. D. (2006). Long-term out-comes of photorefractive keratectomy for anisometropic amblyopia in children. *Ophthalmology, 113*, 169–176.

Paysse, E. A., Hamill, M. B., Hussein, M. A., & Koch, D. D. (2004). Photorefractive keratectomy for pediatric anisometropia: safety and impact on refractive error, visual acuity, and stereopsis. *American Journal of Ophthalmology, 138*, 70–78.

Pearson, R. M. (1994). Letter. *Optometry Today, December 19*, 6.

Pediatric Eye Disease Investigator Group (PEDIG). (2002a). The clinical spectrum of early-onset esotropia: experience of the Congenital Esotropia Observational Study. *American Journal of Ophthalmology, 133*, 102–108.

Pediatric Eye Disease Investigator Group (PEDIG). (2002b). Spontaneous resolution of early-onset esotro-pia: experience of the congenital esotropia: observational study. *American Journal of Ophthalmology, 133*, 109–118.

Pediatric Eye Disease Investigator Group (PEDIG). (2003). The course of moderate amblyopia treated with patching in children: experience of the amblyopia treatment study. *American Journal of Ophthalmology, 136*(4), 620–629.

PEDIG., Cotter, S. A., Mohney, B. G., Chandler, D. L., Holmes, J. M., Repka, M. X., ... Birch, E. E., et al. (2014). A randomized trial comparing part-time patching with observation for children 3 to 10 years of age with intermittent exotropia. *Ophthalmology, 121*(12), 2299–2310.

Peli, E., & McCormack, G. (1983). Dynamics of cover test eye movements. *American Journal of Optometry and Physiological Optics, 60*(8), 712–724.

Pellizzer, S., & Siderov, J. (1998). Assessment of vergence facility in a sample of older adults with presbyopia. *Optometry and Vision Science, 75,* 817–821.

Percival, A. S. (1928). *Faulty tendencies and deviations of the ocular muscles. The prescribing of spectacles* (pp. 81–139). Bristol: Wright, Chapter III.

Phillips, P. H. (2007). Treatment of diplopia. *Seminars in Neurology, 27*(3), 288–298.

Phillips, P. H., Fray, K. J., & Brodsky, M. C. (2005). Intermittent exotropia increasing with near fixation: a "soft" sign of neurological disease. *The British Journal of Ophthalmology, 89,* 1120–1122.

Phillips, P. H., & Hunter, D. G. (1999). *Evaluation of ocular torsion and principles of management. Clinical strabismus management* (pp. 52–72). Philadelphia: Saunders.

Pickwell, D. (1984a). *Binocular vision anomalies.* Oxford: Butterworth.

Pickwell, D. (1984b). *Binocular vision anomalies* (1st ed.). Oxford: Butterworth.

Pickwell, D., Jenkins, T. C. A., & Yekta, A. A. (1987). The effect on fixation disparity and associated heterophoria of reading at an abnormally close distance. *Ophthalmic and Physiological Optics, 7*(4), 345–347.

Pickwell, L. D. (1971). Simple methods in everyday orthoptics. *The Optician, 161*(4177), 10–12.

Pickwell, L. D. (1976). The management of amblyopia without occlusion. *British Journal of Physiological Optics, 31*(2), 115–118.

Pickwell, L. D. (1977a). Binocular vision: the Berlin outlook. *The Optician, 174*(8), 11, 35.

Pickwell, L. D. (1977b). The management of amblyopia: a review. *The Ophthalmic Optician, 17,* 743–745.

Pickwell, L. D. (1979a). The effect of fixation disparity. *The Ophthalmic Optician, 19,* 709, 716.

Pickwell, L. D. (1979b). Prevalence and management of divergence excess. *American Journal of Optometry, 56*(2), 78–81.

Pickwell, L. D. (1981). A suggestion for the origin of eccentric fixation. *Ophthalmic and Physiological Optics, 1,* 55–57.

Pickwell, L. D. (1984). Significance of the central binocular lock in fixation disparity and associated heterophoria. *Transactions of First International Congress of British College of Opthalmic Opticians (Optometrists), 1,* 108–113.

Pickwell, L. D. (1985). The increase in convergence inadequacy with age. *Ophthalmic and Physiological Optics, 5*(3), 347–348.

Pickwell, L. D. (1989). *Binocular vision anomalies* (2nd ed.). Oxford: Butterworth-Heinemann.

Pickwell, L. D., Gilchrist, J. M., & Hesler, J. (1988). Comparison of associated heterophoria measurements using the Mallett test for near vision and the Sheedy Disparometer. *Ophthalmic & Physiological Optics, 8*(1), 19–25.

Pickwell, L. D., & Hampshire, R. (1981a). The significance of inadequate convergence. *Ophthalmic and Physiological Optics, 1,* 13–18.

Pickwell, L. D., & Hampshire, R. (1981b). Jump convergence test in strabismus. *Ophthalmic and Physiological Optics, 1,* 123–124.

Pickwell, L. D., & Hampshire, R. (1984). Convergence insufficiency in patients taking medicines. *Ophthalmic and Physiological Optics, 4*(2), 151–154.

Pickwell, L. D., & Jenkins, T. C. (1982). Orthoptic treatment in teenage patients. *Ophthalmic & Physiological Optics, 2*(3), 221–225.

Pickwell, L. D., & Jenkins, T. C. A. (1978). Using the Titmus stereotest. *The Optician, 175,* 17, 19.

Pickwell, L. D., & Jenkins, T. C. A. (1982). Orthoptic treatment in teenage patients. *Ophthalmic and Physiological Optics, 2*(3), 221–225.

Pickwell, L. D., & Jenkins, T. C. A. (1983). Response to amblyopia treatment. *Australian Journal of Optometry, 66*(1), 29–33.

Pickwell, L. D., Kaye, N. A., & Jenkins, T. C. A. (1991). Distance and near readings of associated heterophoria taken on 500 patients. *Ophthalmic and Physiological Optics, 11,* 291–296.

Pickwell, L. D., & Kurtz, B. H. (1986). Lateral short-term prism adaptation in clinical evaluation. *Ophthalmic and Physiological Optics, 6*(1), 67–73.

Pickwell, L. D., & Sheridan, M. (1973). The management of ARC. *The Ophthalmic Optician, 13*(11), 588–592.

Pickwell, L. D., & Stephens, L. C. (1975). Inadequate convergence. *British Journal of Physiological Optics, 30,* 34–37.

Pickwell, L. D., & Stockley, L. A. F. (1960). The position of the retinal image at the limits of fusion. *British Journal of Physiological Optics, 17*(2), 89–94.

Pickwell, L. D., Viggars, M. A., & Jenkins, T. C. A. (1986). Convergence insufficiency in a rural population. *Ophthalmic and Physiological Optics, 6*(3), 339–340.

Pickwell, L. D., Yekta, A. A., & Jenkins, T. C. A. (1987). The effect of reading in low illumination on fixation disparity. *American Journal of Optometry, 64*(7), 513–518.

Pineles, S. L., Aakalu, V. K., Hutchinson, A. K., Galvin, J. A., Heidary, G., Binenbaum, G., … Lambert, S. R. (2020). Binocular treatment of amblyopia: a report by the American Academy of Ophthalmology. *Ophthalmology, 127*(2), 261–272.

Pirouzian, A., & Ip, K. C. (2010). Anterior chamber phakic intraocular lens implantation in children to treat severe anisometropic myopia and amblyopia: 3-year clinical results. *Journal of Cataract and Refractive Surgery, 36*(9), 1486–1493.

Pitts, J. F. (1996). Orbital blow-out fractures. *Eye News, 3*, 12–14.

Plager, D. A. (1999). Superior oblique palsy and superior oblique myokymia. In A. L. Rosenbaum, & A. P. Santiago (Eds.), *Clinical strabismus management* (pp. 219–229). Philadelphia: Saunders.

Pointer, J. S. (2001). Sighting dominance, handedness, and visual acuity preference: three mutually exclusive modalities? *Ophthalmic and Physiological Optics, 21*, 117–126.

Pointer, J. S. (2005). An enhancement to the Maddox Wing test for the reliable measurement of horizontal heterophoria. *Ophthalmic and Physiological Optics, 25*, 446–451.

Polat, U., Mizobe, K., Pettet, M. W., Kasamatsu, T., & Norcia, A. M. (1998). Collinear stimuli regulate visual responses depending on cell's contrast threshold. *Nature, 391*(6667), 580–584.

Polensek, S. H., & Tusa, R. J. (2009). Nystagmus during attacks of vestibular migraine: an aid in diagnosis. *Audiology & Neuro-otology, 15*(4), 241–246.

Pollard, Z. F., Greenberg, M. F., Bordenca, M., Elliott, J., & Hsu, V. (2011). Strabismus precipitated by monovision. *American Journal of Ophthalmology, 152*(3), 479–482.

Porcar, E., & Martinez-Palomera, A. (1997). Prevalence of general binocular dysfunctions in a population of university students. *Optometry and Vision Science, 74*, 111–113.

Portela-Camino, J. A., Martin-Gonzalez, S., Ruiz-Alcocer, J., Illarramendi-Mendicute, I., & Garrido-Mercado, R. (2018). A random dot computer video game improves stereopsis. *Optometry and Vision Science, 95*(6), 523–535.

Preslan, M. W., & Novak, A. (1998). Baltimore vision screening project. Phase 2. *Ophthalmology, 105*(1), 150–153.

Press, L. J. (2000). Letter responding to: a randomized trial of the effect of single vision vs. bifocal lenses on myopia progression in children with esophoria. *Optometry and Vision Science, 77*, 630–632.

Press, L. J., Overton, M., & Leslie, S. (2016). A discussion and analysis, in the context of current research to May 2016, of "A critical evaluation of the evidence supporting the practice of behavioural vision therapy" by Brendan T Barrett (2009). *Australasian College of Behavioural Optometrists*.

Przekoracka-Krawczyk, A., Michalak, K. P., & Pyzalska, P. (2019). Deficient vergence prism adaptation in subjects with decompensated heterophoria. *PLoS One, 14*(1), e0211039.

Quaid, P., & Simpson, T. (2013). Association between reading speed, cycloplegic refractive error, and oculomotor function in reading disabled children versus controls. *Graefe's Archive for Clinical and Experimental Ophthalmology, 251*(1), 169–187.

Raab, E. L. (2001). Follow-up monitoring of accommodative esotropia. *Journal of AAPOS, 5*, 246–249.

Rabbetts, R. B. (1972). A comparison of astigmatism and cyclophoria in distance and near vision. *The British Journal of Physiological Optics, 27*, 161–190.

Rabbetts, R. B. (2007). *Bennett & Rabbetts' clinical visual optics*. Edinburgh: Butterworth Heinemann Elsevier.

Rae, S. (2015). Evidence-based management of convergence insufficiency. *Optometry in Practice, 16*(1), 1–10.

Rahi, J. S., Logan, S., Borja, M., Timms, C., Russell-Eggitt, I., & Taylor, D. (2002). Prediction of improved vision in the amblyopic eye after visual loss in the non-amblyopic eye (Research letter). *The Lancet, 360*, 621–622.

Rahi, J. S., Logan, S., Timms, C., Russell-Eggitt, I., & Taylor, D. (2002). Risk, causes, and outcomes of visual impairment after loss of vision in the non-amblyopic eye: a population-based study. *The Lancet, 360*, 597–602.

Rainey, B. B. (2000). The effect of prism adaptation on the response AC/A ratio. *Ophthalmic and Physiological Optics, 20*, 199–206.

Rainey, B. B., Schroeder, T. L., Goss, D. A., & Grosvenor, T. P. (1998). Clinical research note: Reliability of and comparisons among three variations of the alternating cover test. *Ophthalmic and Physiological Optics*, *18*, 430–437.

Ramadan, N. M. (1996). Headache caused by raised intracranial pressure and intracranial hypotension. *Current Opinion in Neurology*, *9*, 214–218.

Ranka, M. P., & Steele, M. A. (2015). Esotropia associated with high myopia. *Current Opinion in Ophthalmology*, *26*(5), 362–365.

Reading, R. W. (1988). Near point testing. In K. Edwards, & R. Llewellyn (Eds.), *Optometry* (pp. 150–160). London: Butterworths.

Reading, R. W. (1992). Vergence errors: some hitherto unreported aspects of fixation disparity. *Optometry and Vision Science*, *69*(7), 538–543.

Reddy, A. K., Freeman, C. H., Paysse, E. A., & Coats, D. K. (2009). A data-driven approach to the management of accommodative esotropia. *American Journal of Ophthalmology*, *148*(3), 466–470.

Repka, M., Simons, K., & Kraker, R. (2010). Laterality of amblyopia. *American Journal of Ophthalmology*, *150*(2), 270–274.

Repka, M. X. (1999). Nystagmus: clinical evaluation and surgical management. In A. L. Rosenbaum, & A. P. Santiago (Eds.), *Clinical strabismus management* (pp. 404–420). Philadelphia: Saunders.

Repka, M. X., Wallace, D. K., Beck, R. W., Kraker, R. T., Birch, E. E., Cotter, S. A., ... Holmes, J. M., et al. (2005). Two-year follow-up of a 6-month randomized trial of atropine vs patching for treatment of moderate amblyopia in children. *Archives of Ophthalmology*, *123*, 149–157.

Revell, M. J. (1971). *Strabismus: the history of orthoptic techniques*. London: Barrie & Jenkins Ltd.

Richman, J., Garzia, R., & Cron, M. (1992). Annual review of the literature: 1991. *Journal of Optometric Vision Development*, *23*, 3–37.

Riddell, P. M., Horwood, A. M., Houston, S. M., & Turner, J. E. (1999). The response to prism deviations in human infants. *Current Biology*, *9*, 1050–1052.

Robaei, D., Huynh, S. C., Kifley, A., & Mitchell, P. (2006). Correctable and non-correctable visual impairment in a population-based sample of 12-year-old Australian children. *American Journal of Ophthalmology*, *142*, 112.

Robaei, D., Rose, K. A., Kifley, A., Cosstick, M., Ip, J. M., & Mitchell, P. (2006). factors associated with childhood strabismus: findings from a population-based study. *Ophthalmology*, *113*(7), 1146–1153.

Roch-Levecq, A. C., Brody, B. L., Thomas, R. G., & Brown, S. I. (2008). Ametropia, preschoolers' cognitive abilities, and effects of spectacle correction. *Archives of Ophthalmology*, *126*(2), 252–258.

Romano, P. E. (1999). Aniseikonia. *Binocular Vision & Strabismus Quarterly*, *14*, 173–176.

Romano, P. E., & von Noorden, G. K. (1969). Atypical responses to the four diopter prism test. *American Journal of Ophthalmology*, *67*, 935–941.

Romano, P. E., Romano, J. A., & Puklin, J. E. (1975). Stereoacuity development in children with normal binocular single vision. *American Journal of Ophthalmology*, *79*, 966–971.

Romero-Apis, D., & Herrera-Gonsalez, B. (1995). Guest editorial: some considerations with regard to Huber's classification of Duane's retraction syndrome. *Binocular Vision quarter Binocular Vision Quarterly Eye Muscle surgery*, *10*, 13.

Rose, K., Younan, C., Morgan, I., & Mitchell, P. (2003). Prevalence of undetected ocular conditions in a pilot sample of school children. *Clinical & Experimental Ophthalmology*, *31*, 237.

Rosenfield, M. (1997). Tonic vergence and vergence adaptation. *Optometry and Vision Science*, *74*, 303–328.

Rosenfield, M. (2016). Computer vision syndrome (aka digital eye strain). *Optometry in Practice*, *17*(1), 1–10.

Rosenfield, M., Chun, T. W., & Fischer, S. E. (1997). Effect of prolonged dissociation on the subjective measurement of near heterophoria. *Ophthalmic and Physiological Optics*, *17*, 478–482.

Rosenfield, M., & Ciuffreda, K. J. (1991). Does the gradient AC/A ratio vary with target distance? *Optometry and Vision Science (supplement)*, *68*(12s), 151.

Rosenfield, M., Ciuffreda, K. J., Ong, E., & Super, S. (1995). Vergence adaptation and the order of clinical vergence range testing. *Optometry and Vision Science*, *72*(4), 219–223.

Rosenfield, M., Rappon, J. M., & Carrel, M. F. (2000). Vergence adaptation and the clinical AC/A ratio. *Ophthalmic and Physiological Optics*, *20*, 207–211.

Roszkowska, A. M., Biondi, S., Chisari, G., Messina, A., Ferreri, F. M., & Meduri, A. (2006). Visual outcome after excimer laser refractive surgery in adult patients with amblyopia. *Journal of Ophthalmology*, *16*, 214–218.

Rouse, M., Borsting, E., Mitchell, G. L., Kulp, M. T., Scheiman, M., Amster, D., ... Gallaway, M. (2009). Academic behaviors in children with convergence insufficiency with and without parent-reported ADHD. *Optometry and Vision Science, 86*(10), 1169–1177.

Rouse, M. W. (1987). Management of binocular anomalies: efficacy of vision therapy in the treatment of accommodative deficiencies. *American Journal of Optometry and Physiological Optics, 64,* 415–420.

Rouse, M. W., Borsting, E., Hyman, L., Hussein, M., Cotter, S., Flynn, M., ... De Land, P. (1999). Frequency of convergence insufficiency among fifth and sixth graders. *Optometry and Vision Science, 76,* 643–649.

Rouse, M. W., Borsting, E. J., Mitchell, G. L., Scheiman, M., Cotter, S. A., Cooper, J., ... Wensveen, J. (2004). Validity and reliability of the revised convergence insufficiency symptom survey in adults. *Ophthalmic & Physiological Optics, 24,* 384–390.

Rouse, M. W., Nestor, E. M., Parot, C. J., & DeLand, P. N. (2004). A reevaluation of the Developmental Eye Movement (DEM) test's repeatability. *Optometry and Vision Science, 81,* 934–938.

Rouse, M. W., Tittle, J. S., & Braunstein, M. L. (1989). Stereoscopic depth perception by static stereo-deficient observers in dynamic displays with constant and changing disparity. *Optometry and Vision Science, 66,* 355–362.

Rowe, E., & Evans, B. J. W. (2018). Are commonplace optometric activities evidence-based? *Optometry in Practice, 18*(4), 207–218.

Rowe, F. (2004). *Clinical Orthoptics* (2nd ed.). Oxford: Blackwell.

Rowe, F. J., Hanna, K., Evans, J. R., Noonan, C. P., Garcia-Finana, M., Dodridge, C. S., ... Maan, T., et al. (2018). Interventions for eye movement disorders due to acquired brain injury. *Cochrane Database of Systematic Reviews* (3).

Rowe, F. J., & Noonan, C. P. (2017). Botulinum toxin for the treatment of strabismus. *Cochrane Database of Systematic Reviews, 3,* CD006499.

Rowe, F. J., Noonan, C. P., Freeman, G., & DeBell, J. (2009). Intervention for intermittent distance exotropia with overcorrecting minus lenses. *Eye, 32*(2), 320–325.

Rueff, E. M., King-Smith, P. E., & Bailey, M. D. (2015). Can binocular vision disorders contribute to contact lens discomfort? *Optometry & Vision Science, 92*(9), e214–e221.

Rundstrom, M., & Eperjesi, F. (1995). Is there a need for binocular vision evaluation in low vision? *Ophthalmic and Physiological Optics, 15,* 525–528.

Russell, G. E., Wick, B., & Tang, R. A. (1992). Arnold-Chiari malformation. *Optometry and Vision Science, 69,* 242–247.

Rutstein, R. P. (2000). Spasm of the near reflex mimicking deteriorating accommodative esotropia. *Optometry and Vision Science, 77,* 344–346.

Rutstein, R. P., & Corliss, D. (1999). Relationship between anisometropia, amblyopia, and binocularity. *Optometry and Vision Science, 76,* 229–233.

Rutstein, R. P., & Corliss, D. A. (2003). The clinical course of intermittent exotropia. *Optometry and Vision Science, 80,* 644–649.

Rutstein, R. P., Corliss, D. A., & Fullard, R. J. (2006). Comparison of aniseikonia as measured by the aniseikonia inspector and the space eikonometer. *Optometry and Vision Science, 83*(11), 836–842.

Rutstein, R. P., & Eskridge, J. B. (1984). Stereopsis in small-angle strabismus. *American Journal of Optometry Vision Science, 61,* 491–498.

Rutstein, R. P., & Eskridge, J. B. (1990). Effect of cyclodeviations on the axis of astigmatism (for patients with superior oblique paresis). *Optometry and Vision Science, 67*(2), 80–83.

Rutstein, R. P., Fuhr, P., & Schaafsma, D. (1994). Distance stereopsis in orthophores, heterophores, and intermittent strabismics. *Optometry and Vision Science, 71*(7), 415–421.

Rutstein, R. P., & Marsh-Tootle, W. (1998). Clinical course of accommodative esotropia. *Optometry and Vision Science, 75,* 97–102.

Rutstein, R. P., Marsh-Tootle, W., & London, R. (1989). Changes in refractive error for exotropes treated with overminus lenses. *Optometry and Vision Science, 66,* 487–491.

Rutstein, R. P., Marsh-Tootle, W., Scheiman, M. M., & Eskridge, J. B. (1991). Changes in retinal correspondence after changes in ocular alignment. *Optometry and Vision Science, 68,* 325–330.

Rutstein, R. P., Quinn, G. E., Lazar, E. L., Beck, R. W., Bonsall, D. J., Cotter, S. A., ... Leske, D. A., et al. (2010). A randomized trial comparing Bangerter filters and patching for the treatment of moderate amblyopia in children. *Ophthalmology, 117*(5), 998–1004.

Ruttum, M. S., Bence, S. M., & Alcorn, D. (1986). Stereopsis testing in a preschool vision screening program. *Journal of Pediatric Ophthalmology and Strabismus, 23,* 298–302.

Rydberg, A., & Ericson, B. (1998). Assessing visual function in children younger than 1.5 years with normal and subnormal vision: evaluation of methods. *Journal of Pediatric Ophthalmology and Strabismus, 35,* 312–319.

Sabri, K., Knapp, C. M., Thompson, J. R., & Gottlob, I. (2006). The VF-14 and psychological impact of amblyopia and strabismus. *Investigative Ophthalmology Visual Science, 47*(10), 4386–4392.

Saladin, J. J. (2005). Stereopsis from a performance perspective. *Optometry and Vision Science, 82,* 186–205.

Salam, A., Meligonis, G., & Malhotra, R. (2008). Superior oblique myositis as an early feature of orbital Wegener's granulomatosis. *Orbit, 27*(3), 203–206.

Salt, A. T., Sonksen, P. M., Wade, A., & Jayatunga, R. (1995). The maturation of linear acuity and compliance with the Sonksen-Silver acuity system in young children. *Developmental Medicine and Child Neurology, 37,* 505–514.

Sampath, V., & Bedell, H. E. (2002). Distribution of refractive errors in albinos and persons with idiopathic congenital nystagmus. *Optometry and Vision Science, 79,* 292–299.

Santi, K. L., Francis, D. J., Currie, D., & Wang, Q. (2014). Visual-motor integration skills: accuracy of predicting reading. *Optometry and Vision Science, 92*(2), 217–226.

Santiago, A. P., Ing, M. R., Kushner, B. J., & Rosenbaum, A. L. (1999). Intermittent exotropia. In A. L. Rosenbaum, & A. P. Santiago (Eds.), *Clinical strabismus management* (pp. 163–175). Philadelphia: W. B. Saunders Company.

Santiago, A. P., & Rosenbaum, A. L. (1999). Sixth cranial nerve palsy. In A. L. Rosenbaum, & A. P. Santiago (Eds.), *Clinical strabismus management* (pp. 259–271). Philadelphia: W.B. Saunders Company.

Savino, G., Di Nicola, D., Bolzani, R., & Dickmann, A. (1998). Four diopters prism test recording in small angle esotropia: a quantitative study using a magnetic search coil. *Strabismus, 6*(2), 59–69.

Scheiman, M., Cotter, S., Kulp, M. T., Mitchell, G. L., Cooper, J., Gallaway, M., ... Chung, I. (2011). Treatment of accommodative dysfunction in children: results from a randomized clinical trial. *Optometry and Vision Science, 88*(11), 1343–1352.

Scheiman, M., Cotter, S., Rouse, M., Mitchell, G. L., Kulp, M., Cooper, J., & Borsting, E. (2005). Randomised clinical trial of the effectiveness of base-in prism reading glasses versus placebo reading glasses for symptomatic convergence insufficiency in children. *The British Journal of Ophthalmology, 89* (10), 1318–1323.

Scheiman, M., Denton, C., Borsting, E., Kulp, M., Cotter, S., Mitchell, G., ... Hertle, R., et al. (2019). Effect of vergence/accommodative therapy on reading in children with convergence insufficiency: a randomized clinical trial CITT-ART Investigator Group. *Optometry and Vision Science, 96*(11), 836–849.

Scheiman, M., Gallaway, M., Coulter, R., Reinstein, F., Ciner, E., Herzberg, C., & Parisi, M. (1996). Prevalence of vision and ocular disease conditions in a clinical pediatric population. *Journal of the American Optometric Association, 67*(4), 193–202.

Scheiman, M., Gallaway, M., Frantz, K. A., Peters, R. J., Hatch, S., Cuff, M., & Mitchell, G. L. (2003). Nearpoint of convergence: test procedure, target selection, and normative data. *Optometry and Vision Science, 80*(3), 214–225.

Scheiman, M., Kulp, M. T., Cotter, S., Mitchell, G. L., Gallaway, M., Boas, M., ... Tamkins, S. (2010). Vision therapy/orthoptics for symptomatic convergence insufficiency in children: treatment kinetics. *Optometry and Vision Science, 87*(8), 593–603.

Scheiman, M., Mitchell, G. L., Cotter, S., Cooper, J., Kulp, M., Rouse, M., ... Wensveen, J. (2005). A randomized clinical trial of treatments for convergence insufficiency in children. *Archives of Ophthalmology, 123*(1), 14–24.

Scheiman, M., Mitchell, G. L., Cotter, S., Kulp, M. T., Cooper, J., Rouse, M., ... Wensveen, J. (2005). A randomized clinical trial of vision therapy/orthoptics versus pencil pushups for the treatment of convergence insufficiency in young adults. *Optometry and Vision Science, 82*(7), 583–595.

Scheiman, M., & Wick, B. (1994). *Clinical management of binocular vision.* Philadelphia: Lippincott.

Scheiman, M. M., Hertle, R. W., Beck, R. W., Edwards, A. R., Birch, E., Cotter, S. A., ... Donahue, S., et al. (2005). Randomized trial of treatment of amblyopia in children aged 7 to 17 years. *Archives of Ophthalmology, 123,* 437–447.

Schimitzek, T., & Haase, W. (2002). Efficiency of a video-autorefractometer used as a screening device for amblyogenic factors. *Graefes Archive for Clinical and Experimental Ophthalmology, 240*, 710–716.

Schmid, K. L., Beavis, S. D., Wallace, S. I., Chen, J., Chien, Y. T., Nguyen, T., ... Atchison, D. A. (2019). The effect of vertically yoked prisms on binocular vision and accommodation. *Optometry and Vision Science, 96*(6), 414–423.

Schmidt, D., & Stapp, M. (1977). [The effect of euthyscope- and occlusion therapy in cases of convergent strabismus. Comparative, prospective examinations (author's transl)]. *Klinische Monatsblatter fur Augenheilkunde, 171*, 105–117.

Schmidt, P. P. (1994). Vision screening with the RDE Stereotest in pediatric populations. *Optometry and Vision Science, 71*(4), 273–281.

Schneck, M. E., Haegerstrom-Portnoy, G., Lott, L. A., & Brabyn, J. A. (2000). Ocular contributions to age-related loss in coarse stereopsis. *Optometry and Vision Science, 77*, 531–536.

Schor, C. (1978). A motor theory for monocular eccentric fixation of amblyopic eyes. *American Journal of Optometry, 55*, 183–186.

Schor, C., & Horner, D. (1989). Adaptive disorders of accommodation and vergence in binocular dysfunction. *Ophthalmic and Physiological Optics, 9*, 264–268.

Schor, C. M. (1979). The relation between fusional eye movements and fixation disparity. *Vision Research, 19*(12), 1359–1367.

Schor, C. M. (1993). Oculomotor function: introduction. In K. Simons (Ed.), Early visual development: normal and abnormal (pp. 39–45). New York: Oxford University Press.

Schoser, B. G. H., & Pongratz, D. (2006). Extraocular mitochondrial myopathies and their differential diagnoses. *Strabismus, 14*(2), 107–113.

Schroeder, T. L., Rainey, B. B., Goss, D. A., & Grosvenor, T. P. (1996). Review: Reliability of and comparisons among methods of measuring dissociated phoria. *Optometry and Vision Science, 73*, 389–397.

Schroth, V., Joos, R., & Jaschinski, W. (2015). Effects of prism eyeglasses on objective and subjective fixation disparity. *PLoS One, 10*(10), e0138871.

Schuler, E., Silverberg, M., Beade, P., & Moadel, K. (1999). Decompensated strabismus after laser in situ keratomileusis. *Journal of Cataract and Refractive Surgery, 25*, 1552–1553.

Schweers, M. A., & Baker, J. D. (1992). Comparison of Titmus and two Randot tests in monofixation. *American Orthoptic Journal, 42*, 135–141.

Scobee, R. G. (1952). *The oculorotary muscles* (pp. 188–190). London: Henry Kimpton.

Scott, J. A., & Egan, R. A. (2003). Prevalence of organic neuro-ophthalmologic disease in patients with functional visual loss. *American Journal of Ophthalmology, 135*(5), 670–675.

Searle, A., Norman, P., Harrad, P., & Vedhara, K. (2002). Psychosocial and clinical determinants of compliance with occlusion therapy for amblyopic children. *Eye, 16*, 150–155.

Self, J. E., Dunn, M. J., Erichsen, J. T., Gottlob, I., Griffiths, H. J., Harris, C., ... Shawkat, F., et al. (2020). Management of nystagmus in children: a review of the literature and current practice in UK specialist services. *Eye, 34*, 1515–1534.

Serrano-Pedraza, I., Clarke, M. P., & Read, J. C. (2011). Single vision during ocular deviation in intermittent exotropia. *Ophthalmic & Physiological Optics, 31*(1), 45–55.

Sethi, B., & North, R. V. (1987). Vergence adaptive changes with varying magnitudes of prism-induced disparities and fusional amplitudes. *American Journal of Optometry and Physiological Optics, 64*, 263–268.

Shah, R., Edgar, D. F., & Evans, B. J. W. (2007). A survey of the availability of state funded primary eyecare in the UK. *Ophthalmic & Physiological Optics, 27*(5), 473–481.

Shan, Y., Moster, M. L., Roemer, R. A., & Siegfried, J. B. (2000). Abnormal function of the parvocellular visual system in anisometropic amblyopia. *Journal of Pediatric Ophthalmology and Strabismus, 37*, 73–78.

Shapiro, I. J. (1995). Parallel-testing infinity balance. Instrument and technique for the parallel testing of binocular vision. *Optometry and Vision Science, 72*, 916–923.

Shapiro, J. (1998). A new instrument and technique of refraction and binocular balancing. *The Optician, 215*, 34–40.

Sheard, C. (1934). The prescription of prisms. *American Journal of Optometry, 11*(10), 364–378.

Sheard, C. (1923). A dozen worthwhile points in ocular refraction. *American Journal of Physiology Optics, 4*, 443.

Sheard, C. (1930). Zones of ocular comfort. *American Journal of Optometry, 7*, 9–25.

Sheard, C. (1930). Zones of ocular comfort. *American Journal of Optometry*, 7, 9–25.

Sheard, C. (1931). Ocular discomfort and its relief. *Eye, Ear, Nose, and Throat Monthly*, July.

Sheedy, J., Hayes, J., & Engle, J. (2003). Is all asthenopia the same? *Optometry and Vision Science*, 81, 732–739.

Sheedy, J., Truong, S. D., & Hayes, J. R. (2003). What are the visual benefits of eyelid squinting? *Optometry and Vision Science*, 80, 740–744.

Sheedy, J. E., Bailey, I. L., Buri, M., & Bass, E. (1986). Binocular vs monocular task performance. *American Journal of Optometry and Physiological Optics*, 63, 839–846.

Sheedy, J. E., & Saladin, J. J. (1978). Association of symptoms with measurements of oculomotor deficiencies. *American Journal of Optometry*, 55, 670–676.

Sheppard, A. L., & Wolffsohn, J. S. (2018). Digital eye strain: prevalence, measurement and amelioration. *BMJ Open Ophthalmol*, 3(1), e000146.

Shery, T., Proudlock, F. A., Sarvananthan, N., McLean, R. J., & Gottlob, I. (2006). The effects of gabapentin and memantine in acquired and congenital nystagmus - a retrospective study. *British Journal of Ophthalmology*, 90(7), 839–843.

Sheth, N. V., Dell'Osso, L. F., Leigh, R. J., Van Doren, C. L., & Peckham, H. P. (1995). The effects of afferent stimulation on congenital nystagmus foveation periods. *Vision Research*, 35(16), 2371–2382.

Shin, H. S., Park, S. C., & Park, C. M. (2009). Relationship between accommodative and vergence dysfunctions and academic achievement for primary school children. *Ophthalmic & Physiological Optics*, 29(6), 615–624.

Shiono, T., Mutoh, T., Chida, Y., & Tamai, M. (1994). Ocular albinism with unilateral sectorial pigmentation in the fundus. *British Journal of Ophthalmology*, 78, 412–413.

Shneor, E., Evans, B. J., Fine, Y., Shapira, Y., Gantz, L., & Gordon-Shaag, A. (2016). A survey of the criteria for prescribing in cases of borderline refractive errors. *Journal of Optometry*, 9(1), 22–31.

Shute, R., Candy, R., Westall, C., & Woodhouse, J. M. (1990). Success rates in testing monocular acuity and stereopsis in infants and young children. *Ophthalmic and Physiological Optics*, 10, 133–136.

Siatkowski, R. M. (2011). The decompensated monofixation syndrome (an American ophthalmological society thesis). *Transactions of the American Ophthalmological Society*, 109, 232–250.

Siderov, J. (2001). Suppression: clinical characteristics, assessment and treatment. In B. Evans, & S. Doshi (Eds.), Binocular vision and orthoptics ((pp. 58–64). Oxford: Butterworth-Heinemann.

Silverberg, M., Schuler, E., Veronneau-Troutman, S., Wald, K., Schlossman, A., & Medow, N. (1999). Nonsurgical management of binocular diplopia induced by macular pathology. *Archives of Ophthalmology*, 117, 900–903.

Simmers, A. J., & Dulley, P. (2014). Amblyopia and the relevance of uncorrected refractive error in childhood. *Optometry in Practice*, 15(4), 169–176.

Simmons, K. (2017). Oculomotor dysfunction: where's the evidence? *Optometry Visual Performance*, 5(5), 198–202.

Simons, K., & Preslan, M. (1999). Natural history of amblyopia untreated owing to lack of compliance. *The British Journal of Ophthalmology*, 83, 582–587.

Simons, K. (1981). Stereoacuity norms in young children. *Archives of Ophthalmology*, 99, 439–445.

Simons, K., Arnoldi, K., & Brown, M. H. (1994). Color dissociation artifacts in double Maddox rod cyolodeviation testing. *Ophthalmology*, 101, 1897–1901.

Simons, K., Stein, L., Sener, E. C., Vitale, S., & Guyton, D. L. (1997). Full-time atropine, intermittent atropine, and optical penalization and binocular outcome in treatment of strabismic amblyopia. *Ophthalmology*, 104, 2143–2155.

Singh, N. K., Mani, R., & Hussaindeen, J. R. (2017). Changes in stimulus and response AC/A ratio with vision therapy in convergence insufficiency. *Journal of Optometry*, 10(3), 169–175.

Sireteanu, R., Baumer, C. C., & Iftime, A. (2008). Temporal instability in amblyopic vision: relationship to a displacement map of visual space. *Investigative Ophthalmology & Visual Science*, 49(9), 3940–3954.

Slavin, M. L. (1989). Hyperdeviation associated with isolated unilateral abducens palsy. *Ophthalmology*, 96, 512–516.

Sloper, J. J., Garnham, C., Gous, P., Dyason, R., & Plunkett, D. (2001). Reduced binocular beat visual evoked responses and stereoacuity in patients with Duane syndrome. *Investigative Ophthalmology and Visual Science*, 42, 2826–2830.

Smith, D. R. (1979). Restricted Lees screen fields in patients with asthenopia, with and without psychogenic disorders. *Ophthalmology, 86*, 2126–2133.

Smith, E. L., Fern, K., Manny, R., & Harwerth, R. S. (1994). Interocular suppression produced by rivalry stimuli: a comparison of normal and abnormal binocular vision. *Optometry and Vision Science, 71*(8), 479–491.

Smith, E. L., Hung, L. F., Arumugam, B., Wensveen, J. M., Chino, Y. M., & Harwerth, R. S. (2017). Observations on the relationship between anisometropia, amblyopia and strabismus. *Vision Research, 134*, 26–42.

Smith, G. (2006). Refraction and visual acuity measurements: what are their measurement uncertainties? *Clinical and Experimental Optometry, 89*(2), 66–72.

Smith, L. K., Thompson, J. R., Woodruff, G., & Hiscox, F. (1994). Social deprivation and age at presentation in amblyopia. *Journal of Public Health Medicine, 16*, 348–351.

Snowdon, S., & Stewart-Brown, S. (1997). Preschool vision screening: results of a systematic review. *NHS Centre for Reviews and Dissemination: CRD Report 9.*

Solebo, A. L. (2019). Identification of visual impairments. In A. Edmond (Ed.), *Health For All Children* (5th ed.). Oxford: Oxford University Press.

Solebo, A. L., Rahi, J. S. (2013). Vision screening in children aged 4-5 years: external review against programme appraisal criteria for the UK National Screening Committee (UK NSC), May 2013 ed. National Screening Committee, UK.

Solomons, H. (1978). *Binocular vision: a programmed text.* London: Heinemann.

Somer, D., Budak, K., Demirci, S., & Duman, S. (2002). Against-the-rule (ATR) astigmatism as a predicting factor for the outcome of amblyopia treatment. *American Journal of Ophthalmology, 133*, 741–745.

Somer, D., Cinar, F. G., & Duman, S. (2006). The accommodative element in accommodative esotropia. *American Journal of Ophthalmology, 141*, 819–826.

Sondhi, N., Archer, S. M., & Helveston, E. (1990). Development of normal ocular alignment. *Journal of Pediatric Ophthalmology and Strabismus, 25*, 210–211.

Spalton, D. J., Hitchings, R. A., & Hunter, P. A. (1984). *Atlas of clinical ophthalmology.* Edinburgh: Churchill Livingstone.

Spector, R. H. (1993). Vertical diplopia. *Survey of Ophthalmology, 38*(1), 31–62.

Spielmann, A. (1994). Nystagmus. *Current Opinion in Ophthalmology, 5*, 20–24.

Spierer, A. (1991). Etiology of reduced visual acuity in congenital nystagmus. *Annals of Ophthalmology, 23* (10), 393–397.

Spierer, A. (2003). Acute concomitant esotropia of adulthood. *Ophthalmology, 110*, 1053–1056.

Spierer, A., Priel, A., & Sachs, D. (2005). Strabismus in senile cataract patients. *Journal of AAPOS, 9*(5), 422–425.

Spiritus, M. (1994). Comitant strabismus. *Current Opinion in Ophthalmology, 5*(5), 11–16.

Stafford, M., & Morris, J. (1993). Retinoscopy in the eye examination. *Optometry Today, February 8*, 17–25.

Stankovic, B., & Milenkovic, S. (2007). Continuous full-time occlusion of the sound eye vs full-time occlusion of the sound eye periodically alternating with occlusion of the amblyopic eye in treatment of amblyopia: a prospective randomized study. *European Journal of Ophthalmology, 17*(1), 11–19.

Stark, L. R., & Atchison, D. A. (1994). Subject instructions and methods of target presentation in accommodation research. *Investigative Ophthalmology & Visual Science, 35*, 528–537.

Stayte, M., Johnson, A., & Wortham, C. (1990). Ocular and visual defects in a geographically defined population of 2-year-old children. *British Journal of Ophthalmology, 74*, 465–468.

Steffen, H., Krugel, U., Holz, F. G., & Kolling, G. H. (1996). Acquired vertical diplopia in macular dystrophy as a model for obligate fixation disparity. *Der Ophthalmologe, 93*, 383–386.

Stegall, F. W. (1973). Orthoptic aspects of nystagmus. *American Orthoptic Journal, 23*, 30–34.

Stein, J. F., Riddell, P. M., & Fowler, S. (1988). Disordered vergence control in dyslexic children. *British Journal of Ophthalmology, 72*, 162–166.

Sterner, B., Abrahamsson, M., & Sjostrom, A. (2001). The effects of accommodative facility training on a group of children with impaired relative accommodation - a comparison between dioptric treatment and sham treatment. *Ophthalmic and Physiological Optics, 21*, 470–476.

Sterner, B., Gellerstedt, M., & Sjostrom, A. (2006). Accommodation and the relationship to subjective symptoms with near work for young school children. *Ophthalmic and Physiological Optics, 26*(2), 148–155.

Stevenson, S. B., Lott, L. A., & Yang, J. (1997). The influence of subject instruction on horizontal and vertical vergence tracking. *Vision Research, 37*, 2891–2898.

Stewart, C. E., Fielder, A. R., Stephens, D. A., & Moseley, M. J. (2005). Treatment of unilateral amblyopia: factors influencing visual outcome. *Investigative Ophthalmology & Visual Science, 46*, 3152–3160.

Stewart, C. E., Moseley, M. J., & Fielder, A. R. (2003). Defining and measuring treatment outcome in unilateral amblyopia. *British Journal of Ophthalmology, 87*, 1229–1231.

Stewart, C. E., Moseley, M. J., Stephens, D. A., & Fielder, A. R. (2004). Treatment dose-response in amblyopia therapy: the monitored occlusion treatment of amblyopia study (MOTAS). *Investigative Ophthalmology Visual Science, 45*, 3048–3054.

Stewart, C. E., Shah, S., Wren, S., & Roberts, C. J. (2016). Paediatric eye services: how much of the workload is amblyopia-related? *Strabismus, 24*(3), 109–112.

Stewart-Brown, S., Haslum, M. N., & Butler, N. (1985). Educational attainment of 10-year-old children with treated and untreated visual defects. *Developmental Medicine and Child Neurology, 27*(4), 504–513.

Stidwill, D. (1997). Clinical survey: epidemiology of strabismus. *Ophthalmic and Physiological Optics, 17*, 536–539.

Stidwill, D. (1998). *Orthoptic Assessment and Management.* Oxford: Blackwell Science.

Stifter, E., Burggasser, G., Hirmann, E., Thaler, A., & Radner, W. (2005). Monocular and binocular reading performance in children with microstrabismic amblyopia. *The British Journal of Ophthalmology, 89*, 1324–1329.

Stohler, T. (1973). Afterimage treatment in nystagmus. *American Orthoptic Journal, 23*, 65–67.

Stone, N. M., Somner, J. E. A., & Jay, J. L. (2008). Intractable diplopia: a new indication for corneal tattooing. *British Journal of Ophthalmology, 92*(11), 1445.

Strupp, M., Dieterich, M., Brandt, T., & Feil, K. (2016). Therapy of vestibular paroxysmia, superior oblique myokymia, and ocular neuromyotonia. *Current Treatment Options in Neurology, 18*(7), 34.

Sturm, V., Berger, R. W., & Zangemeister, W. H. (2007). Alcohol as an alternative therapy in accommodative and convergence insufficiency. *Canadian Journal of Ophthalmology, 42*(6), 880.

Sturm, V., Landau, K., Grossglauser, B., & Sturmer, J. (2008). Bilateral Brown syndrome related to sinusitis. *Canadian Journal of Ophthalmology, 43*(6), 721–722.

Sucher, D. F. (1991). Variability of monocular visual acuity during binocular viewing. *Optometry and Vision Science, 68*(12), 966–971.

Sucher, D. F. (1994). The association of headache and monocular blur effect in a clinical population. *Optometry and Vision Science, 71*(11), 707–712.

Sulley, A., Hawke, R., Lorenz, K. O., Toubouti, Y., & Olivares, G. (2015). Resultant vertical prism in toric soft contact lenses. *Contact Lens & Anterior Eye, 38*(4), 253–257.

Sun, P. Y., Leske, D. A., Holmes, J. M., & Khanna, C. L. (2016). Diplopia in medically and surgically treated patients with glaucoma. *Ophthalmology, 124*(2), 257–262.

Sundaram, P. M., Jayakumar, N., & Noronha, V. (2004). Extraocular muscle cysticercosis – a clinical challenge to the ophthalmologists. *Orbit, 23*(4), 255–262.

Surdacki, M., & Wick, B. (1991). Diagnostic occlusion and clinical management of latent hyperphoria. *Optometry and Vision Science, 68*(4), 261–269.

Suter, P. S., Bass, B. L., & Suter, S. (1993). Early and late VEPs for reading stimuli are altered by common binocular misalignments. *Psychophysiology, 30*(5), 475–485.

Suttle, C., Alexander, J., Liu, M., Ng, S., Poon, J., & Tran, T. (2009). Sensory ocular dominance based on resolution acuity, contrast sensitivity and alignment sensitivity. *Clinical & Experimental Optometry, 92*(1), 2–8.

Swann, P. G. (2001). Some aspects of paralytic strabismus. *Optometry Today, March 23*, 38–40.

Tacagni, D. J., Stewart, C. E., Moseley, M. J., & Fielder, A. R. (2007). Factors affecting the stability of visual function following cessation of occlusion therapy for amblyopia. *Graefe's Archive for Clinical and Experimental Ophthalmology, 245*(6), 811–816.

Tailor, V., Bossi, M., Bunce, C., Greenwood, J. A., & Dahlmann-Noor, A. (2015). Binocular versus standard occlusion or blurring treatment for unilateral amblyopia in children aged three to eight years. *Cochrane Database of Systematic Reviews* (8).

Tait, E. F. (1951). Accommodative convergence. *American Journal of Ophthalmology, 34*, 1093–1107.

Tamhankar, M. A., Kim, J. H., Ying, G. S., & Volpe, N. J. (2011). Adult hypertropia: a guide to diagnostic evaluation based on review of 300 patients. *Eye (Lond), 25*(1), 91–96.

Tang, S. T. W., & Evans, B. J. W. (2007). The Near Mallett Unit Foveal Suppression Test: a cross-sectional study to establish test norms and relationship with other optometric tests. *Ophthalmic and Physiological Optics, 27*(1), 31–43.

Tarczy-Hornoch, K., & Repka, M. X. (2004). Superior oblique palsy or paresis in pediatric patients. *Journal of AAPOS, 8,* 133–140.

Tassinari, J. T. (2002). Monocular estimate retinoscopy: central tendency measures and relationship to refractive status and heterophoria. *Optometry and Vision Science, 79,* 708–714.

Taylor, D. (1997). Peculiar visual images. In D. Taylor (Ed.), *Paediatric ophthalmology* (pp. 1071–1075). Oxford: Blackwell Science.

Taylor, K., & Elliott, S. (2014). Interventions for strabismic amblyopia. *Cochrane Database of Systematic Reviews* (7).

Taylor-Kulp, M., & Schmidt, P. P. (1997). The relation of clinical saccadic eye movement testing to reading in kindergartners and first graders. *Optometry and Vision Science, 74,* 37–42.

Teitelbaum, B., Pang, Y., & Krall, J. (2009). Effectiveness of base in prism for presbyopes with convergence insufficiency. *Optometry and Vision Science, 86*(2), 153–156.

Teller, D. Y. (1990). The development of visual function in infants. In B. Cohen, & I. Bodis-Wollner (Eds.), *Vision and the brain* (pp. 109–118). New York: Raven Press.

Terao, Y., Fukuda, H., & Hikosaka, O. (2017). What do eye movements tell us about patients with neurological disorders? — An introduction to saccade recording in the clinical setting. *Proceedings of the Japan Academy, Series B Physical Biology Science, 93*(10), 772–801.

Theodorou, M., Quartilho, A., Xing, W., Bunce, C., Rubin, G., Adams, G., & Dahlmann-Noor, A. (2018). Soft contact lenses to optimize vision in adults with idiopathic infantile nystagmus: a pilot parallel randomized controlled trial. *Strabismus, 26*(1), 11–21.

Thiagarajan, P., Ciuffreda, K. J., & Ludlam, D. P. (2011). Vergence dysfunction in mild traumatic brain injury (mTBI): a review. *Ophthalmic & Physiological Optics, 31*(5), 456–468.

Thimbleby, H., & Neesham, C. (1993). How to play tricks with dots. *New Scientist, 9 October,* 26–29.

Thomas, S., Farooq, S. J., Proudlock, F. A., & Gottlob, I. (2005). Vertical deviation exacerbated by convergence and accommodation. *The British Journal of Ophthalmology, 89,* 1371–1372.

Thompson, C. (1993). Assessment of child vision and refractive error. In T. Buckingham (Ed.), *Visual problems in childhood* (pp. 159–210). Oxford: Butterworth-Heinemann.

Thomson, D. (2000). Test Chart 2000. *The Optician, 220,* 28–31.

Thomson, D. (2002). Child vision screening survey. *The Optician, 224*(5863), 16–20.

Thomson, D. (2002). Child vision screening survey. *The Optician, 224,* 16–20.

Thomson, D. EMedInfo. https://www.thomson-software-solutions.com/emedinfo/. Accessed 26-10-2020.

Thomson, W. D., Desai, N., & Russell-Eggitt, I. (1990). A new system for the measurement of ocular motility using a personal computer. *Ophthalmic and Physiological Optics, 10,* 137–143.

Thomson, W. D., & Evans, B. (1999). A new approach to vision screening in schools. *Ophthalmic and Physiological Optics, 19,* 196–209.

Thomson, W. D., & Evans, B. J. W. (1999). A new approach to vision screening in schools. *Ophthalmic and Physiological Optics, 19*(3), 196–209.

Tkalcevic, L. A., & Abel, L. A. (2005). The effects of increased visual task demand on foveation in congenital nystagmus. *Vision Research, 45,* 1139–1146.

Tollefson, M. M., Mohney, B. G., Diehl, N. N., & Burke, J. P. (2006). Incidence and types of childhood hypertropia: a population-based study. *Ophthalmology, 113*(7), 1142–1145.

Tomac, S., & Birdal, E. (2001). Effects of anisometropia on binocularity. *Journal of Pediatric Ophthalmology and Strabismus, 38*(1), 27–33.

Tomac, S., Mutlu, F. M., & Altinsoy, H. I. (2007). Duane's retraction syndrome: its sensory features. *Ophthalmic & Physiological Optics, 27*(6), 579–583.

Tomac, S., Sener, E. C., & Sanac, A. S. (2002). Clinical and sensorial characteristics of microtropia. *Japanese Journal of Ophthalmology, 46*(1), 52–58.

Tomlinson, A. (1969). Alignment errors. *The Ophthalmic Optician, 5th April,* 330–341.

Tomsak, R. L., Kosmorsky, G. S., & Leigh, R. J. (2002). Gabapentin attenuates superior oblique myokymia. *American Journal of Ophthalmology, 133,* 721–723.

Toor, S., Horwood, A., & Riddell, P. (2019). The effect of asymmetrical accommodation on anisometropic amblyopia treatment outcomes. *Journal of American Association for Pediatric Ophthalmology and Strabismus, 23*(4), 203.e201–203.e205.

Toor, S., Horwood, A. M., & Riddell, P. (2018). Asymmetrical accommodation in hyperopic anisometropic amblyopia. *British Journal of Ophthalmology, 102*(6), 772–778.

Townshend, A. M., Holmes, J. M., & Evans, L. S. (1993). Depth of anisometropic amblyopia and difference in refraction. *American Journal of Ophthalmology, 116*, 431–436.

Tran, T. M., McClelland, C. M., & Lee, M. S. (2019). Diagnosis and management of trochleodynia, trochleitis, and trochlear headache. *Frontiers in Neurology, 10*, 361.

Trbovich, A. M., Sherry, N. K., Henley, J., Emami, K., & Kontos, A. P. (2019). The utility of the Convergence Insufficiency Symptom Survey (CISS) post-concussion. *Brain Injury, 33*(12), 1545–1551.

Troyer, M. E., Sreenivasan, V., Peper, T. J., & Candy, T. R. (2017). The heterophoria of 3–5 year old children as a function of viewing distance and target type. *Ophthalmic and Physiological Optics, 37*(1), 7–15.

Tsukuda, S., Murai, Y. (1988). A case report of manifest esotropia after viewing anagryph stereoscopic movie. *Unknown [Japanese]*.

Turnbull, P. R., Vingrys, A. J., & Kalloniatis, M. (2007). Short- and long-term vertical diplopia secondary to blunt trauma. *Clinical and Experimental Optometry, 90*(6), 457–462.

Twelker, J. D., & Mutti, D. O. (2001). Retinoscopy in infants using a near noncycloplegic technique, cycloplegia with tropicamide 1%, and cycloplegia with cyclopentolate 1%. *Optometry and Vision Science, 78*, 215–222.

Tytla, M. E., & Labow-Daily, L. S. (1981). Evaluation of the CAM treatment for amblyopia: a controlled study. *Investigative Ophthalmology and Visual Science, 20*(3), 400–406.

Ukwade, M. T. (2000). Effects of nonius line and fusion lock parameters on fixation disparity. *Optometry and Vision Science, 77*, 309–320.

Ukwade, M. T., & Bedell, H. E. (1992). Variation of congenital nystagmus with viewing distance. *Optometry and Vision Science, 69*, 976–985.

Ukwade, M. T., & Bedell, H. E. (1993). Stability of oculomotor fixation as a function of target contrast and blur. *Optometry and Vision Science, 70*(2), 123–126.

Ukwade, M. T., Bedell, H. E., & Harwerth, R. S. (2003). Stereopsis is perturbed by vergence error. *Vision Research, 43*, 181–193.

Uretmen, O., Civan, B. B., Kose, S., Yuce, B., & Egrilmez, S. (2007). Accommodative esotropia following surgical treatment of infantile esotropia: frequency and risk factors. *Acta Ophthalmologica Scandinavica, 86*(3), 279–283.

Utine, C. A., Cakir, H., Egemenoglu, A., & Perente, I. (2008). LASIK in children with hyperopic anisometropic amblyopia. *Journal of Refractive Surgery, 24*(5), 464–472.

Vaegan., & Taylor, D. (1979). Critical period for deprivation amblyopia in children. *Trans. Ophthalmol Soc. UK, 99*, 432–439.

Vaegan. (1979). Convergence and divergence show large and sustained improvement after short isometric exercises. *American Journal of Optometry and Physiological Optics, 56*, 23–33.

Valente, P., Buzzonetti, L., Dickmann, A., Rebecchi, M. T., Petrocelli, G., & Balestrazzi, E. (2006). Refractive surgery in patients with high myopic anisometropia. *Journal of Refractive Surgery, 22*(5), 461–466.

van Doorn, L. L. A., Evans, B. J. W., Edgar, D. F., & Fortuin, M. F. (2014). Manufacturer changes lead to clinically important differences between two editions of the TNO stereotest. *Ophthalmic and Physiological Optics, 34*(2), 243–249.

Van Haeringen, R., McClurg, P., & Cameron, K. D. (1986). Comparison of Wesson and Modified Sheedy fixation disparity tests. Do fixation disparity measures relate to normal binocular status? *Ophthalmic and Physiological Optics, 6*, 397–400.

van Leeuwen, R., Eijkemans, M. J. C., Vingerling, J. R., Hofman, A., de Jong, P. T. V. M., & Simonsz, H. J. (2007). Risk of bilateral visual impairment in individuals with amblyopia: the Rotterdam study. *British Journal of Ophthalmology, 91*(11), 1450–1451.

van Rijn, L. J., Krijnen, J. S., Nefkens-Molster, A. E., Wensing, K., Gutker, E., & Knol, D. L. (2014). Spectacles may improve reading speed in children with hyperopia. *Optometry and Vision Science, 91*(4), 397–403.

Vancleef, K., Read, J. C. A., Herbert, W., Goodship, N., Woodhouse, M., & Serrano-Pedraza, I. (2017). Overestimation of stereo thresholds by the TNO stereotest is not due to global stereopsis. *Ophthalmic and Physiological Optics, 37*(4), 507−520.

Vazquez, R. L. (1984). A graphical three-step-test. *Archives of Ophthalmology, 102,* 98−99.

Vera, J., Jiménez, R., García, J. A., & Cárdenas, D. (2017). Simultaneous physical and mental effort alters visual function. *Optometry and Vision Science, 94*(8), 797−806.

Veverka, K. K., Hatt, S. R., Leske, D. A., Brown, W. L., Iezzi, R., Jr., & Holmes, J. M. (2017). Causes of diplopia in patients with epiretinal membranes. *American Journal of Ophthalmology, 179,* 39−45.

Vivian, A. J., Lyons, C. J., & Burke, J. (2002). Controversy in the management of convergence excess esotropia. *British Journal of Ophthalmology, 86,* 923−929.

Vogt, U. (2003). Kersley lecture: eye believe in contact lenses: contact lenses and/or refractive surgery. *Eye & Contact Lens, 29,* 201−206.

Waddingham, P. E., Butler, T. K., Cobb, S. V., Moody, A. D., Comaish, I. F., Haworth, S. M., … Griffiths, G. D. (2006). Preliminary results from the use of the novel Interactive Binocular Treatment (I-BiTtrade mark) system, in the treatment of strabismic and anisometropic amblyopia. *Eye, 20,* 375−378.

Wahlberg, M., Abdi, S., & Brautaset, R. (2010). Treatment of accommodative insufficiency with plus lens reading addition: is +1.00 D better than +2.00 D? *Strabismus, 18*(2), 67−71.

Wakayama, A., Nakada, K., Abe, K., Matsumoto, C., & Shimomura, Y. (2013). Effect of suppression during tropia and phoria on phoria maintenance in intermittent exotropia. *Graefe's Archive for Clinical and Experimental Ophthalmology, 251*(10), 2463−2469.

Walker, M., Duvall, A., Daniels, M., Doan, M., Edmondson, L. E., Cheeseman, E. W., … Peterseim, M. M. W. (2020). Effectiveness of the iPhone GoCheck Kids smartphone vision screener in detecting amblyopia risk factors. *Journal of AAPOS, 24*(1), 16 e11−16 e15.

Wallace, D. K., Chandler, D. L., Beck, R. W., Arnold, R. W., Bacal, D. A., Birch, E. E., … Hoover, D., et al. (2007). Treatment of bilateral refractive amblyopia in children three to less than 10 years of age. *American Journal of Ophthalmology, 144*(4), 487−496.

Walline, J. J., Mutti, D. O., Zadnik, K., & Jones, L. A. (1998). Development of phoria in children. *Optometry and Vision Science, 75,* 605−610.

Walraven, J., & Janzen, P. (1993). TNO stereopsis test as an aid to the prevention of amblyopia. *Ophthalmic and Physiological Optics, 13,* 350−356.

Wang, F. M., & Chryssanthou, G. (1988). Monocular eye closure in intermittent exotropia. *Archives of Ophthalmology, 106/7,* 941−942.

Wang, J., Wyatt, L. M., Felius, J., Stager, D. R., Jr., Stager, D. R., Sr., Birch, E. E., & Bedell, H. E. (2010). Onset and progression of with-the-rule astigmatism in children with infantile nystagmus syndrome. *Investigative Ophthalmology & Visual Science, 51*(1), 594−601.

Wann, J. P., Rushton, S., & Mon-Williams, M. (1995). Natural problems for stereoscopic depth perception in virtual environments. *Vision Research, 35,* 2731−2736.

Warwick, R. (1976). *Eugene Wolff's anatomy of the eye and orbit* (7th ed.). London: H.K. Lewis and Co. Ltd..

Watson, P. G., Sanac, A. S., & Pickering, M. S. (1985). A comparison of various methods of treatment of amblyopia. A block study. *Transactions of the Ophthalmological Societies of the United Kingdom, 104*(Pt 3), 319−328.

Watten, R. G., & Lie, I. (1996). Visual functions and acute ingestion of alcohol. *Ophthalmic and Physiological Optics, 16,* 460−466.

Waugh, S. J., & Bedell, H. E. (1992). Sensitivity to temporal luminance modulation in congenital nystagmus. *Investigative Ophthalmology and Visual Science, 33,* 2316−2324.

Weakley, D. R. (2001). The association between nonstrabismic anisometropia, amblyopia, and subnormal binocularity. *Ophthalmology, 108,* 163−171.

Weakley, D. R., Stager, D. R., & Stager, D. R. (1999). Brown syndrome. In A. L. Rosenbaum, & A. P. Santiago (Eds.), *Clinical strabismus management* (pp. 347−357). Philadelphia: Saunders.

Webber, A., Wood, J., Gole, G., & Brown, B. (2011). DEM Test, visagraph eye movement recordings, and reading ability in children. *Optometry and Vision Science, 88*(2), 295−302.

Webber, A. L., Wood, J. M., Gole, G. A., & Brown, B. (2008). The effect of amblyopia on fine motor skills in children. *Investigative Ophthalmology & Visual Science, 49*(2), 594−603.

Webber, A. L., Wood, J. M., Thompson, B., & Birch, E. E. (2019). From suppression to stereoacuity: a composite binocular function score for clinical research. *Ophthalmic and Physiological Optics, 39*(1), 53–62.

Weiler, D. L. (2017). Thyroid eye disease: a review. *Clinical & Experimental Optometry, 100*(1), 20–25.

Wesson, M. D., & Amos, J. F. (1985). Norms for hand-held rotary prism vergences. *American Journal of Optometry and Physiological Optics, 62*, 88–94.

West, S., & Williams, C. (2016). Amblyopia in children (aged 7 years or less). *BMJ Clinical Evidence, 2016*.

Westall, C. (1993). Measurement of binocular function in infants. Presented at: *Infant Vision: 4th Meeting of the Child Vision Research Society*, Lyon.

Whitman, M. C., MacNeill, K., & Hunter, D. G. (2016). Bifocals fail to improve stereopsis outcomes in high AC/A accommodative esotropia. *Ophthalmology, 123*(4), 690–696.

Whyte, M. B., & Kelly, P. (2018). The normal range: it is not normal and it is not a range. *Postgraduate Medical Journal, 94*(1117), 613–616.

Wick, B. (1977). Vision training for presbyopic nonstrabismic patients. *American Journal of Optometry and Physiological Optics, 54*, 244–247.

Wick, B. (1990). Vision therapy for preschool children. In A. A. Rosenbloom, & M. W. Morgan (Eds.), *Pediatric optometry* (pp. 274–292). Philadelphia: Lippincott.

Wick, B., Wingard, M., Cotter, S., & Scheiman, M. (1992). Anisometropic amblyopia: is the patient ever too old to treat? *Optometry and Vision Science, 69*(11), 866–878.

Wiessberg, E., Suckow, M., & Thorn, F. (2004). Minimal angle horizontal strabismus detectable by lay observers. *Optometry and Vision Science, 81*, 505–509.

Wiggins, D., Woodhouse, J. M., Margrain, T. H., Harris, C. M., & Erichsen, J. T. (2007). Infantile nystagmus adapts to visual demand. *Investigative Ophthalmology Visual Science, 48*(5), 2089–2094.

Wiggins, R. E., & von Noorden, G. K. (1990). Monocular eye closure in sunlight. *Journal of Pediatric Ophthalmology and Strabismus, 27*, 16–20.

Wildsoet, C., Wood, J., Maag, H., & Sabdia, S. (1998). The effect of different forms of monocular occlusion on measures of central visual function. *Ophthalmic and Physiological Optics, 18*, 263–268.

Wildsoet, C. F., & Cameron, K. D. (1985). The effect of illumination and foveal fusion lock on clinical fixation disparity measurements with the Sheedy Disparometer. *Ophthalmic and Physiological Optics, 5*, 171–178.

Wildsoet, C. F., Chia, A., Cho, P., Guggenheim, J. A., Polling, J. R., Read, S., ... Walline, J. J., et al. (2019). IMI - Interventions Myopia Institute: interventions for controlling myopia onset and progression report. *Investigative Ophthalmology & Visual Science, 60*(3), M106–M131.

Wilker, S. C., Rucker, J. C., Newman, N. J., Biousse, V., & Tomsak, R. L. (2009). Pain in ischemic ocular motor cranial nerve palsies. *The British Journal of Ophthalmology, 93*(12), 1657–1659.

Wilkins, A. J. (2018). A theory of visual stress and its application to the use of coloured filters for reading. In L. W. MacDonald, C. P. Biggam, & G. V. Paramei (Eds.), *Progress in colour studies: cognition, language and beyond* (pp. 319–338). Philadelphia: John Benjamins Publishing Company.

Wilkins, A. J. (1995). *Visual stress*. Oxford: Oxford University Press.

Wilkins, A. J., Baker, A., Smith, S., Bradford, J., Zaiwalla, Z., Besag, F. M., ... Fish, D. (1999). Treatment of photosensitive epilepsy using coloured glasses. *Seizure, 8*(8), 444–449.

Wilkins, A. J., Evans, B. J. W., Brown, J., Busby, A., Wingfield, A. E., Jeanes, R., & Bald, J. (1994). Double-masked placebo-controlled trial of precision spectral filters in children who use coloured overlays. *Ophthalmic and Physiological Optics, 14*, 365–370.

Wilkins, A. J., Patel, R., Adjamian, P., & Evans, B. J. W. (2002). Tinted spectacles and visually sensitive migraine. *Cephalalgia, 22*, 711–719.

Williams, C., Harrad, R. A., Harvey, I., Sparrow, J. M., & ALSPAC Study Team. (2001). Screening for amblyopia in preschool children: results of a population-based, randomized controlled trial. *Ophthalmic Epidemiology, 8*, 279–295.

Williams, C., Northstone, K., Harrad, R. A., Parr, J. M., Harvey, I., & ALSPAC Study Team. (2003). Amblyopia treatment outcomes after preschool screening v school entry screening: observational data from a prospective cohort study. *British Journal of Ophthalmology, 87*, 988–993.

Williams, C., Northstone, K., Harrad, R. A., Sparrow, J. M., Harvey, I., & ALSPAC Study Team. (2002). Amblyopia treatment outcomes after screening before or at age 3 years: follow up from randomised trial. *British Medical Journal, 324*.

Williams, C., Northstone, K., Howard, M., Harvey, I., Harrad, R. A., & Sparrow, J. M. (2008). Prevalence and risk factors for common vision problems in children: data from the ALSPAC study. *British Journal of Ophthalmology*, *92*(7), 959–964.

Williams, W. R., Latif, A. H., Hannington, L., & Watkins, D. R. (2005). Hyperopia and educational attainment in a primary school cohort. *Archives of Disease in Childhood*, *90*(2), 150–153.

Wilmer, J. B., & Buchanan, G. M. (2009). Nearpoint phorias after nearwork predict ADHD symptoms in college students. *Optometry and Vision Science*, *86*(8), 971–978.

Wingate, P. (1976). *The penguin medical encyclopedia* (2nd ed.). Harmondsworth: Penguin.

Winn, B., Ackerley, R. G., Brown, C. A., Murray, F. K., Prais, J., St., & John, M. F. (1988). Reduced aniseikonia in axial anisometropia with contact lens correction. *Ophthalmic and Physiological Optics*, *8*, 341–344.

Winn, B., Gilmartin, B., Sculfor, D. L., & Bamford, J. C. (1994). Vergence adaptation and senescence. *Optometry and Vision Science*, *71*, 797–800.

Wong, A. M. (2008). Timing of surgery for infantile esotropia: sensory and motor outcomes. *Canadian Journal of Ophthalmology*, *43*(6), 643–651.

Wong, A. M., Lueder, G. T., Burkhalter, A., & Tychsen, L. (2000). Anomalous retinal correspondence: neuroanatomic mechanism in strabismic monkeys and clinical findings in strabismic children. *Journal of American Association for Pediatric Ophthalmology and Strabismus*, *4*, 168–174.

Wong, A. M., Tweed, D., & Sharpe, J. A. (2002). Vertical misalignment in unilateral sixth nerve palsy. *Ophthalmology*, *109*, 1315–1325.

Wong, E. P., Fricke, T. R., & Dinardo, C. (2002). Interexaminer repeatability of a new, modified prentice card compared with established phoria tests. *Optometry and Vision Science*, *79*(6), 370–375.

Wood, I. C. J. (1983). Stereopsis with spatially-degraded images. *Ophthalmic and Physiological Optics*, *3*, 337–340.

Wood, J. M., & Abernethy, B. (1997). An assessment of the efficacy of sports vision training programs. *Optometry and Vision Science*, *74*, 646–659.

Wood, J. M., Black, A. A., Hopkins, S., & White, S. L. J. (2018). Vision and academic performance in primary school children. *Ophthalmic and Physiological Optics*, *38*(5), 516–524.

Woodruff, G., Hiscox, F., Thompson, J. R., & Smith, L. K. (1994a). Factors affecting the outcome of children treated for amblyopia. *Eye*, *8*(Pt 6), 627–631.

Woodruff, G., Hiscox, F., Thompson, J. R., & Smith, L. K. (1994b). The presentation of children with amblyopia. *Eye*, *8*(Pt 6), 623–626.

Worfolk, R. (1993). Control of eye movements. *Optometry Today*, *March 8*, 30–32.

Worrell, B. E., Hirsch, M. J., & Morgan, M. W. (1971). An evaluation of prism prescribed by Sheard's criterion. *American Journal of Optometry and Archives of the American Academy of Optometry*, *48*, 373–376.

Worth, C. (1905). *Squint: Its causes, pathology, and treatment*. London: Bale.

Worth, C. (1903). *Squint*. London: Baillière, Tindall & Cox.

Wright, K. W. (1994). Strabismus management. *Current Opinion in Ophthalmology*, *5*(5), 25–29.

Wright, L. (1998). Common drugs for treatment of the dry eye. *Optometry Today*, *February 13*, 23–26.

Wright, M. C., Colville, D. J., & Oberklaid, F. (1995). Is community screening for amblyopia possible, or appropriate? *Archives of Disease in Childhood*, *73*, 192–195.

Wu, H., Sun, J., Xia, X., Xu, L., & Xu, X. (2006). Binocular status after surgery for constant and intermittent exotropia. *American Journal of Ophthalmology*, *142*(5), 822-822.

Wu, Y. T., Cafiero-Chin, M., & Marques, C. (2015). Wall-eyed bilateral internuclear ophthalmoplegia: review of pathogenesis, diagnosis, prognosis and management. *Clinical & Experimental Optometry*, *98*(1), 25–30.

Wutthiphan, S. (2005). Guidelines for prescribing optical correction in children. *Journal of the Medical Association of Thailand*, *88*(Suppl 9), S163–169.

Yammouni, R., & Evans, B. J. (2020). An investigation of low power convex lenses (adds) for eyestrain in the digital age (CLEDA). *J Optom*, *13*(3), 198–209.

Yang, H. K., Choi, J. Y., Kim, D. H., & Hwang, J. M. (2014). Changes in refractive errors related to spectacle correction of hyperopia. *PLoS One*, *9*(11), e110663.

Yang, H. K., & Hwang, J. M. (2011). The effect of target size and accommodation on the distant angle of deviation in intermittent exotropia. *American Journal of Ophthalmology*, *151*(5), 907–913.e1.

Yaniglos, S. S., & Leigh, R. J. (1992). Refinement of an optical device that stabilizes vision in patients with nystagmus. *Optometry and Vision Science, 69,* 447–450.

Yanoff, M., & Duker, J. S. (1999). *Ophthalmology* (p. 115) London: Mosby.

Yekta, A. A., & Pickwell, L. D. (1986). The relationship between heterophoria and fixation disparity. *Clinical & Experimental Optometry, 69,* 228–231.

Yekta, A. A., Jenkins, T., & Pickwell, D. (1987). The clinical assessment of binocular vision before and after a working day. *Ophthalmic and Physiological Optics, 7,* 349–352.

Yekta, A. A., Pickwell, L. D., & Jenkins, T. C. A. (1989). Binocular vision without visual stress. *Optometry and Vision Science, 66,* 815–817.

Yekta, A. A., Pickwell, L. D., & Jenkins, T. C. A. (1989). Binocular vision, age and symptoms. *Ophthalmic and Physiological Optics, 9,* 115–120.

Ygge, J. (2000). Vertical vergence - normal function and plasticity. In O. Fransen, H. Richter, & L. Stark (Eds.), *Accommodation and vergence mechanisms in the visual system.* Basel, Switzerland: Birkhauser.

Young, R. W. (1994). Review: the family of sunlight-related eye diseases. *Optometry and Vision Science, 71* (2), 125–144.

Yu, R., & Chen, L. (2014). The need to control for regression to the mean in social psychology studies. *Frontiers in Psychology, 5,* 1574.

Yudkin, P. L., & Stratton, I. M. (1996). How to deal with regression to the mean in intervention studies. *Lancet, 347*(8996), 241–243.

Zaroff, C. M., Knutelska, M., & Frumkes, T. E. (2003). Variation in stereoacuity: normative description, fixation disparity, and the roles of aging and gender. *Investigative Ophthalmology & Visual Science, 44*(2), 891–900.

Zellers, J. A., Alpert, T. L., & Rouse, M. W. (1984). A review of the literature and a normative study of accommodative facility. *Journal of the American Optometric Association, 55,* 31–74.

Ziakas, N. G., Woodruff, G., Smith, L. K., & Thompson, J. R. (2002). A study of hereditary as a risk factor in strabismus. *Eye, 16,* 519–521.

Zinkernagel, S. M., & Mojon, D. S. (2009). Distance doubling visual acuity test: a reliable test for nonorganic visual loss. *Graefe's Archive for Clinical and Experimental Ophthalmology, 247*(6), 855–858.

Ziylan, S., Yabas, O., Zorlutuna, N., & Serin, D. (2007). Isometropic amblyopia in highly hyperopic children. *Acta Ophthalmologica Scandinavica, 85*(1), 111–113.

Zurcher, B., & Lang, J. (1980). Reading capacity in cases of 'cured' strabismic amblyopia. *Transactions of the Ophthalmological Societies of the United Kingdom, 100,* 501–503.

Related words or phrases that are cross-referenced and described elsewhere in the glossary are given in bold. The abbreviation 'c.f.' is used to highlight related terms. Commonly used abbreviations for words or phrases are included in parentheses and italics. Most terms in the glossary are described in detail elsewhere in the book and the relevant page numbers can be found in the Index.

A-pattern. A binocular anomaly characterised by, relatively speaking, excessive divergence on downward gaze and/or excessive convergence on upward gaze. Synonyms: A-phenomenon, A-syndrome.

Abduction. When an eye moves in a temporalward direction.

Abnormal correspondence. See **retinal correspondence**.

Abnormal retinal correspondence. See **retinal correspondence**.

Absolute hypermetropia. Hypermetropia for which accommodation cannot compensate.

AC/A ratio. The accommodative-convergence to accommodation ratio. See **accommodation**.

Accidental alternator. A rarely used to term to describe most cases of alternating strabismus where one eye usually fixates. c.f., **Essential alternator**.

Accommodation. Alteration in the dioptric power of the eye to enable it to focus at different distances. Accommodation is linked to convergence and the amount of convergence that occurs reflexly in response to a change in accommodation is called the accommodative convergence. The amplitude of accommodation (*Amp. Acc.*) is a measure of the closest point at which a person can focus and is measured in dioptres (D), with any significant spectacle correction in place.

Accommodative esotropia. A strabismus in which accommodation has a major influence on the deviation, through accommodative convergence. Accommodative esotropia is characterised by a significant degree of hypermetropia and/or a high AC/A ratio.

Accommodative facility (*Acc. Fac.*). The ability of the eyes to rapidly change their accommodation.

Active position. The position of the eyes characterised by foveal fixation of an object by both eyes.

Adduction. When an eye moves in a nasalward direction.

Agonist. A muscle receiving primary innervation to contract, to move the eye into a new direction of gaze.

Aligning prism (*A.P.*). The prismatic correction required to eliminate a fixation disparity. This term has been recommended as a replacement for associated heterophoria. If no prism is required, the appropriate symbol is an X with a vertical and/or horizontal line through it (Rabbetts, 2007).

Alternating deorsumduction. A type of **Dissociated vertical deviation** where either eye deviates downward under cover. Synonym: alternating hypophoria (see also **kataphoria**).

Alternating strabismus. A strabismus where, at a given distance, either eye is sometimes used for fixation.

Alternating sursumduction. A type of **Dissociated vertical deviation** where either eye deviates upwards under cover. Synonym: alternating hyperphoria (see also **anaphoria**).

Amblyopia (*amb.*). A visual loss resulting from an impediment or disturbance to the normal development of vision. Clinically, visual acuity worse than 6/9 and/or two lines worse than the better eye, which is not due to immediately correctable refraction errors, ophthalmoscopically detectable anomalies of the fundus, or pathology of the visual pathway.

Amblyoscope. See **synoptophore**.

Amp. Acc. Amplitude of accommodation.

Anaglyph. The creation of binocularly fusible, usually stereoscopic, images using stimuli of complementary colours that are viewed through coloured filters (usually, red and green). Sometimes, the term **tranaglyph** is used synonymously with anaglyph.

Anaphoria. Sometimes anaphoria is used as a synonym of **alternating sursumduction** (Millodot, 1993). Alternatively, the term anaphoria is defined differently as a type of **gaze palsy** in which the eyes have limited ability for depression, so that both eyes turn upwards in the absence of a fixation stimulus (Rabbetts, 2007).

Angle alpha. The angle between the visual axis (which passes through the object of regard and fovea) and the optical axis (which passes through the optical centres of the refracting surfaces of the eye). The visual axis usually lies nasal to the optical axis on the plane of the cornea (a positive angle alpha).

Angle gamma. The angle between the optical axis and the fixation axis (which passes through the object of regard and the centre of rotation of the eye).

Angle kappa. The angle between the optical axis and the line of sight (which passes through the object of regard and centre of the entrance pupil).

Angle lambda. The angle between the pupillary axis (which passes through the centre of the entrance pupil and is normal to the corneal surface) and the line of sight.

Angle of anomaly. The difference between the **subjective angle of deviation** and the **objective angle of deviation**. The angle of anomaly is usually zero: when it is other than zero this implies that unharmonious anomalous retinal correspondence (UARC) is present, which is usually an artefact resulting from unnatural viewing conditions during clinical testing.

Angle of deviation. The angle between the two visual axes when the eyes are deviated in strabismus or dissociation (e.g., when measuring heterophoria). See **subjective angle of deviation** and **objective angle of deviation**.

Angular visual acuity (*Ang. V/A*). The visual acuity when viewing single letters (c.f. **morphoscopic or linear visual acuity**). The letters lack any significant **crowding effect**.

Aniseikonia. When the retinal image size of an object in one eye is significantly different to that in the other eye.

Anisometropia. A **refractive error** differing in the two eyes. Usually, anisometropia is considered to be relevant when it is greater than 0.75D in any meridian.

Anisophoria. An unequal heterophoria in the two eyes. Optical anisophoria results from anisometropia, when there can be different accommodative demands in each eye and differing prismatic effects induced by spectacle lenses. Essential anisophoria occurs in incomitancy.

Anisotropia. An unequal strabismus in the two eyes. For classification, see **anisophoria**.

Anomalous (abnormal) retinal correspondence. (*ARC*). See **retinal correspondence**.

Antagonist. The muscle which receives primary innervation to relax when the **agonist** contracts.

APD. Afferent pupillary defect. In the swinging flashlight test (carried out in a darkened room), when the light is swung to the normal eye both pupils constrict and when the light is swung to the affected eye there is a small bilateral dilation.

Associated heterophoria. See **aligning prism** (preferred term).

Asthenopia. A term used to describe any symptoms associated with the use of the eyes, typically eyestrain and headache. Literally, the term means weakness, or debility, of the eyes or vision.

Astigmatism (*astig.*). A refractive error in which the image of a point object is not a single point but two orthogonal lines at different distances from the optical system.

Bangerter foils. Opaque (frosted) films, which can be pressed onto spectacle lenses. They are available in a series of differing degrees of opacification and are used to treat amblyopia and intractable diplopia.

Behavioural optometry. A controversial (Barrett, 2009) philosophy of optometric management emphasising aspects related to visual information processing, visualisation, visual awareness, visual attention, visual cognitive, visual motor, and visual spatial functions (Birnbaum, 1993). Behavioural optometry aims to enhance visual information processing in individuals who may not appear to have a specific ocular or vision defect. The philosophy of behavioural optometry has been criticised because of the high proportion of patients who are treated and for the paucity of controlled trials (Barrett, 2009).

Bielschowsky's phenomenon. A phenomenon which occurs in **dissociated vertical deviation** (DVD). If one eye is occluded and a **neutral density filter** bar is placed before the fixating eye, as the filter density is increased there comes a point when the eye behind the cover moves down. This phenomenon can be used to test for DVD.

Bielschowsky's head tilt test. A test to determine which of the inferior or superior extraocular muscles is paretic.

Binocular. Pertaining to both eyes.

Binocular instability. A heterophoric condition in which the alignment of the visual axes, at a given fixation distance, is unstable. The condition is characterised by an unstable heterophoria and low fusional reserves. Synonym: fusional vergence dysfunction.

Binocular lock. The visual input which is common to both eyes, and thus helps to maintain fusion.

Binocular vision (BV). The ability to use the two eyes together simultaneously. In normal binocular single vision, sensory and motor fusion result in a single percept and stereopsis.

Biocular. Pertaining to the use of the two eyes but without fusion or stereopsis.

Blind spot syndrome. See **Swann's syndrome**.

Brown's superior oblique tendon sheath syndrome. A condition believed to be caused by a short tendon sheath of the superior oblique muscle and an apparent anomaly of the inferior oblique muscle. There is a limitation of elevation of the eye in adduction, but normal or near normal elevation when the eye is abducted.

Chiastopic fusion. A patient over-converges, for example when using the three-cats card to train convergent fusional reserves, so that the visual axes cross in front of the card. The term is derived from the Greek letter chi, which resembles the letter X. c.f., **orthopic fusion**.

Comitant (com.). In optometry, this term is used to describe the normal situation when, for a given fixation distance, the angle between the visual axes remains constant, no matter to which part of the visual field the eyes are directed. Synonym: concomitant.

Concomitant. See **comitant**.

Confusion. The visual disturbance created in strabismus by dissimilar images falling on each fovea and being projected to the same position in space.

Congenital (congen.). A condition that is present at or shortly after birth.

Conjugate eye movements. See **version**.

Contracture. Inability of an extraocular muscle to relax may result in permanent structural changes with irreversible inelasticity.

Contour interaction. See **crowding effect**.

Contrast sensitivity function (CSF). Measurement of the detection of objects of varying spatial frequencies by varying contrast. This is a more complete assessment of vision than standard visual acuity measurement.

Convergence (con.). A turning in of the visual axes, usually to maintain fixation upon an object as it approaches. An example of a **vergence** eye movement.

Convergence excess. An eso-deviation greater for near vision than for distance fixation.

Convergence insufficiency (CI). A subnormal power of convergence; often associated with **exophoria** at near. Two different conditions are variously described as CI, **convergence insufficiency exophoria syndrome (CIES)** and **near point of convergence insufficiency (NPCI)**.

Convergence insufficiency exophoria syndrome (CIES). A syndrome characterised as a greater exophoria at near than distance, remote near point of convergence, and inadequate convergent near fusional reserve all producing symptoms.

Covariation. The ability of a person to maintain harmonious anomalous **retinal correspondence** despite changes in the objective angle of strabismus.

Cover test. A dissociation test in which each eye is covered in turn whilst the patient fixates a target at a given fixation distance. The practitioner observes the eye movements, from which the type of binocular vision anomaly can be diagnosed.

Crètes prism. See **rotary prism**.

Crowding effect. The phenomenon whereby visual acuity when looking at a letter surrounded by other contours (e.g., in a line of letters) is worse than when looking at individual letters (because of 'contour interaction'). The crowding effect is exaggerated in strabismic amblyopia. Synonym: crowding phenomenon.

Cycloparesis. A weakness of the ciliary muscle.

Cyclophoria. A type of **heterophoria** in which there is a tendency, which becomes manifest when the eyes are dissociated, for the eyes to rotate about their anterior-posterior axis. In excyclophoria, the top of the eye tends to rotate outwards (temporalwards); in incyclophoria, inwards. This tendency is controlled (i.e., there is no **strabismus**).

Cycloplegic. A drug which causes temporary paralysis of the ciliary muscle, and therefore of accommodation. *Cyclo* is often used to describe a cycloplegic refraction.

Cyclospasm. A spasm of the ciliary muscle.

Cyclotropia. A type of **strabismus** in which one eye is rotated about its anterior-posterior axis relative to the other.

Cyclovergence. A type of **vergence** eye movement in which the eyes rotate about their anterior/posterior axis. In excyclovergence the top of the eye is rotated outwards (temporalwards) and in incyclovergence it is rotated inwards (nasalwards).

D, DV. Distance vision.

Decompensation. A failure of the vergence eye movement system to overcome adequately a deviation that has been hitherto compensated. Most commonly, decompensation describes a heterophoria that has not previously caused problems becoming a decompensated heterophoria. Decompensation can also describe, for example, an incomitant deviation that has been stable for some time and then worsens.

Deviation. A generic term for any type of deviation of the visual axes, whether in strabismus or, during dissociation, in heterophoria.

Diplopia (*dip*.). Double vision owing to the stimulation of noncorresponding retinal points by the same object. This results in the simultaneous appreciation of two images of one object. Diplopia of a nonfixated target is physiological (see **physiological diplopia**), and of a fixated target is pathological.

Disjunctive eye movements. See **vergence**. Synonym: disjugate eye movements.

Dissociated heterophoria (*diss. phoria*). The size, in prism dioptres, of the heterophoria measured using a **dissociation test**.

Dissociated vertical deviation (divergence) (*DVD*). A condition in which each eye, when covered, turns upwards (sursumduction) or downwards (deorsurmduction).

Dissociation test (*dissoc. test*). A test in which fusion is prevented by presenting the two eyes with dissimilar or nonfusible objects.

Divergence (*div*.). A turning outwards of the eyes, typically to maintain fixation upon an object as it moves away from the observer. An example of a **vergence** eye movement.

Divergence excess. An exodeviation greater for distance vision than for near fixation.

Divergence weakness. An esodeviation greater for distance vision than for near fixation.

Donders squint. An **accommodative esotropia**.

Duane's retraction syndrome. An ocular disorder consisting of retraction of the globe with narrowing of the palpebral aperture in attempted **adduction**, frequent **abduction** deficiency, with variable limitation to adduction and upshoot and/or downshoot of the affected eye on adduction.

Duction. A consideration of the movement of one eye alone, e.g., **abduction, adduction**, depression, elevation. Sometimes, confusingly, the term duction is used as a synonym of vergence.

Eccentric fixation (*EF*). A monocular condition when the image of the point of fixation is not formed on the foveola. This often occurs in strabismic eyes and the angle of eccentric fixation is correlated with visual acuity loss. The eccentrically fixating area is usually nasal to the foveola in esotropia, but can be temporalward (paradoxical eccentric fixation); and vice versa in exotropia.

Egocentric localisation. See **localisation**.

Emmetropisation. A process whereby the components of the optical system of the eye develop in such a way as to reduce ametropia.

Enophthalmos. Posterior displacement of the globe within the orbit due to changes in the volume of the orbit relative to its contents, or loss of function of the orbitalis muscle.

Entoptic image. An image arising from within the eye.

Esophoria (*SOP*). A type of **heterophoria** in which there is a tendency which becomes manifest when the eyes are dissociated for the eyes to turn inwards. This tendency is controlled (i.e., there is no **strabismus**).

Esotropia (*SOT*). A type of **strabismus** in which one eye is deviated inwards relative to the other. Sometimes called convergent strabismus (e.g., right convergent strabismus, right convergent squint, *RCS*).

Essential alternators. (1) Conventionally used to refer to alternating strabismus in which all efforts to obtain fusion prove unavailing. (2) Common usage is to describe unusual cases of alternating strabismus when, at a specified distance, either eye is equally likely to be used for fixation.

Excyclophoria. See **cyclophoria**.

Excyclovergence. See **cyclovergence**.

Exophoria (*XOP*). A type of **heterophoria** in which there is a tendency, which becomes manifest when the eyes are dissociated, for the eyes to turn outwards. This tendency is controlled (i.e., there is no **strabismus**).

Exotropia (*XOT*). A type of **strabismus** in which one eye deviates outwards. An exotropia is sometimes called a divergent strabismus (e.g., left divergent strabismus, left divergent squint, *LDS*).

Extraocular muscles. The six striated muscles that control the movement of each eye: medial rectus, lateral rectus, superior rectus, inferior rectus, superior oblique, and inferior oblique muscles. Synonym: oculorotatory muscles.

Extrinsic muscles. The **extraocular muscles** and the **lid muscles**.

Extrinsic suppression. Suppression of one eye which has been acquired because of long periods of monocular vision. The suppression results from extrinsic, or environmental factors, such as using a monocular eyepiece for prolonged periods.

Facultative suppression. See **suppression**.

Field of fixation. The area in space over which an eye can fixate when the head remains stationary. It extends to approximately 47 degrees temporally, 45 degrees nasally, 43 degrees upwards, and 50 degrees downwards.

Fixation axis. The line joining the object of regard to the centre of rotation of the eye. A synonym is line of fixation.

Fixation disparity (*FD*). When both eyes are fixating a point which is seen in binocular single vision, the eyes can be minutely misaligned without causing diplopia. This misalignment is called a fixation disparity and usually occurs in the direction of the heterophoria, within Panum's fusional areas.

Free-space. Objects are viewed in free-space when they are observed under natural viewing conditions (c.f., in a **synoptophore** or **stereogram**). Synonym: true-space.

Fresnel prism. A type of prismatic lens consisting of many small prismatic elements parallel to one another. This allows for a high prismatic correction in a thin lens, although there is some loss of optical clarity.

Fusion. In vision, the act of combining the monocular images into a single percept. Sensory fusion is the neural process of synthesising or integrating the monocular percepts into a single binocular percept. Motor fusion refers to the act of moving the eyes so the object of regard falls on corresponding retinal areas.

Fusional reserves. The maximum amount by which the eyes can converge (positive or base-out fusional reserves) or diverge (negative or base-in fusional reserves) whilst still maintaining binocular single vision at a given fixation distance. Normally when the vergence changes, the accommodation changes by a linked amount. Relative fusional reserves are the amount by which the vergence can change without changing the accommodation. Vertical fusional reserves can also be measured but are small. Synonyms: vergence reserves, prism vergences.

Fusional vergence dysfunction. See **binocular instability**.

Gaze palsy. The inability to move the eyes conjugately, either laterally or vertically, due to involvement of cortical or subcortical ocular motor centres.

Global stereopsis. The perception of depth in features that can only be detected binocularly: they have no monocularly recognisable form. Global stereopsis is tested with random dot stereograms; e.g., TNO test. c.f., **local stereopsis**.

Habitual angle of strabismus. In a strabismic patient, the angle between the two visual axes which is usually present during natural, everyday, viewing conditions.

Haidinger's brushes. An entoptic phenomenon which tags the projected location of the centre of the macula and can be used in detecting and treating eccentric fixation.

Haploscope. The generic term for an instrument which presents separate fields of view to the two eyes. There are many specially designed haploscopes for clinical and experimental use, which allow considerable manipulation of the fixation targets, accommodation, and vergence. Synoptophores and stereoscopes are examples of haploscopic instruments.

Harmonious anomalous retinal correspondence (*HARC*). Synonym: harmonious anomalous retinal correspondence. See **retinal correspondence**.

Hering's law of equal innervation. Nerve impulses stimulating an **agonist** are equal to those stimulating its contralateral **synergist**.

Herschel prism. See **rotary prism**.

Hess screen. An instrument used to quantify an incomitancy of the **extraocular muscles**.

Heterophoria (*phoria*). A tendency for the eyes to move out of alignment when one is covered or when they view dissimilar objects. Types of heterophoria are **exophoria, esophoria, hyperphoria,** and **cyclophoria**. Previously called 'latent strabismus' or 'latent squint'. If there is no heterophoria, the appropriate symbol is a circle with a horizontal and/or vertical line through it.

Heterotropia (*tropia*). See **strabismus**.

Horopter. The surface in physical space upon which objects lie which stimulate corresponding retinal points in each eye for a given fixation distance.

Horror fusionis. An irrepressible motor movement to prevent bi-foveal fixation of an object, even when bi-foveal stimulation is attempted taking account of the angle of deviation (c.f., **sensory fusion disruption syndrome**).

Hypermetropia. Refractive error where distant objects are focused behind the retina when the accommodation is relaxed. Synonyms of hypermetropia are far- or long-sightedness or hyperopia.

Hyperopia. See **hypermetropia**.

Hyperphoria (*HYPERP*). A type of **heterophoria** in which there is a tendency, which becomes manifest when the eyes are dissociated, for one eye to turn upwards relative to the other.

Hypertropia (*HYPERT*). A type of **strabismus** in which the visual axis of one eye is raised relative to the other.

Hypoglobus. Inferior displacement of the globe in the orbit. It may or may not be associated with enophthalmos.

Hypotropia (*HYPOT*). A type of **strabismus** in which the visual axis of one eye is lowered relative to the other.

Iatrogenic. A condition which arises from the treatment of another illness.

Incomitant (*incom.*). In optometry, this term describes the abnormal situation when the two eyes do not move in a parallel, yoked, fashion when looking at equidistant objects in various positions of gaze; the angle between the visual axis changes. Additionally, the angle of deviation differs according to which eye is fixating. Synonym: Inconcomitant.

Inconcomitant. See **incomitant**.

Incyclophoria. See **cyclophoria**.

Incyclovergence. See **cyclovergence**.

Internuclear ophthalmoplegia. A condition resulting from a lesion in the medial longitudinal fasciculus and characterised by poor adduction of the eye on the affected side and abducting nystagmus in the contralateral eye. Convergence is often, but not always, intact.

Irlen syndrome. See **sensory visual stress**.

Kataphoria. Sometimes, kataphoria is used as a synonym of **alternating deorsumduction** (Millodot, 1993). Alternatively, the term kataphoria is defined differently as a type of **gaze palsy** in which the eyes have limited ability for elevation, so that both eyes turn downwards in the absence of a fixation stimulus (Rabbetts, 2007).

Krimsky's test. A coarse objective method of estimating the deviation of an eye in which prisms are used to move the corneal reflex.

Latent strabismus (latent squint). See **heterophoria**.

Lees screen. An instrument used to quantify an incomitancy.

Line of sight. Line joining the point of fixation to the centre of the entrance pupil of the eye.

Linear visual acuity. See **morphoscopic visual acuity**.

Local stereopsis. The perception of depth in features that can be seen both monocularly and binocularly. Local stereopsis is tested with contoured stereograms (e.g., Titmus circles test). c.f., **global stereopsis**.

Localisation. Perception of the direction of an object in space with respect to either the eye (oculocentric localisation) or the self (egocentric localisation).

Magnocellular visual system. The sensory visual system can be subclassified into pathways, two of which are the parvocellular and magnocellular pathways, named after ganglion cell types. The magnocellular pathway detects movement and gross structures, which may then be examined in more detail by the **parvocellular system**. Synonym: transient visual system.

Major amblyoscope. See **synoptophore**.

MARCS test. Mallett ARC and suppression in strabismus test. On the Mallett near vision unit, the fixation disparity (small OXO) test should not be used for detecting and assessing ARC and suppression. The Mallett unit has a large OXO test (approximately, twice the size of the fixation disparity test) that is designed to assess ARC and suppression, called the Mallett ARC and suppression in strabismus (MARCS) test.

Maxwell's spot. An entoptic phenomenon which can be used in the assessment of eccentric fixation.

Meares-Irlen Syndrome. See **sensory visual stress**.

Mental effort. A method of orthoptic treatment based on the wilful production of voluntary vergence.

Microtropia. A small (less than 6Δ or 10Δ) strabismus, which may be difficult or impossible to detect by cover testing. A microtropia with identity occurs when the angles of the deviation, anomaly, and of eccentric fixation are equal.

Middle third technique. A method of exploring the functions of accommodation and convergence. It is used to determine whether a heterophoria is likely to be compensated and can be used as an aid when prescribing prisms. The original middle third technique, proposed by Percival, was later modified by Sheard. See **Sheard's criterion**, **Percival's criterion**.

Monofixational heterophoria. See **Parks' monofixational syndrome**.

Morphoscopic visual acuity (*Morph. VA*). The visual acuity when viewing a line of letters (c.f., **angular visual acuity** when viewing isolated single letters). The morphoscopic visual acuity is normally slightly worse (much worse in strabismus) than the angular visual acuity due to the **crowding effect**.

Motor field. See **field of fixation**.

Motor fusion. See **fusion**.

Myectomy. Removal of all or part (strictly, a partial myectomy) of a muscle.

Myopia. A refractive error in which distant objects are focused in front of the retina. Distant objects are blurred. Synonyms: short- or near-sightedness.

Myotomy. Surgical procedure to weaken the action of a muscle, commonly the inferior oblique muscle.

N, NV. Near vision.

Near point of accommodation. The nearest point at which an object can be seen clearly.

Near point of convergence. The nearest point at which an object can be seen singly (not in diplopia).

Near point of convergence insufficiency (*NPCI*). An unusually remote near point of convergence. NPCI is used in this book to differentiate an isolated finding of a remote near point of convergence from **convergence insufficiency exophoria syndrome (CIES)**, which is diagnosed as a syndrome of symptoms and clinical signs (including a significant near exophoria and, sometimes, NPCI).

Neutral density filter (*ND filter*). A grey filter that reduces all wavelengths of light equally, so of neutral (grey) colour. They are available in various depths or transmittance. There are several schemata for grading ND filters, sometimes described as ND1number (lightest ND 101 to darkest ND 113), ND.number (lightest ND 0.3 to darker ND 5.0; used most in optics), and NDnumber (ND2 to ND100000; used most in photography). The ND.number is a logarithmic scale: ND 0.0 is clear, ND 0.3 reduces transmittance to 50%, ND 0.6 to 25%, ND 0.9 to 12.5%, ND 1.0 to 10%, ND 2.0 to 1%, ND 3.0 to 0.1%, etc. Alternatively, two linear polarising filters can be placed in a trial frame, one in front of the other, initially with coincident axes of polarisation. If one is rotated in a trial frame, the transmittance will vary with the cosine squared of the angle.

Normal retinal correspondence (NRC). See **retinal correspondence**.

Nystagmus (*nystag*.). An eye movement disorder characterised by abnormal, involuntary rhythmic oscillations of one or both eyes, initiated by a slow phase.

Objective angle of deviation. The angle of deviation between the visual axes in strabismus, as measured objectively, e.g., with a cover test.

Obligatory suppression. See **suppression**.

Ocular flutter. A burst of horizontal back to back saccades with no resting interval between them.

Ocular motor. The term motor refers to that which imparts motion, so ocular motor describes the neurological, muscular, and associated structures and functions involved in movements of part or all of one or both eyes. See also **oculomotor**.

Ocular myopathy. See **ophthalmoplegia**.

Ocular torticollis. The adoption of an abnormal head posture (usually from early infancy) to compensate for an ocular condition (e.g., **extraocular muscle palsy, nystagmus**).

Oculocentric localisation. See **localisation**.

Oculomotor. Strictly speaking, this term refers only to the functioning of the third cranial nerve. Some authors use oculomotor as a synonym of **ocular motor**. This can cause confusion and the literal definitions are used in this book.

Oculorotatory muscles. See **extraocular muscles**.

Ophthalmoplegia. Paralysis of the extraocular muscles. Ophthalmoplegia can be external, referring to one or more of the extraocular muscles (if the levator palpebrae are involved, this is usually called ocular myopathy); internal, referring to the muscles of the iris and ciliary muscle; or total (all the muscles, including the levator palpebrae).

Opsoclonus. A type of **ocular flutter** in which the saccades are multidirectional.

Optic nerve hypoplasia. Underdevelopment of the optic nerve. In severe cases, there will be a small optic disc and poor acuity. In subtle cases, the optic nerve may appear normal and the vision may be minimally affected.

Optical axis of the eye. The line joining the optical centres of the refractive surfaces of the eye.

Optometry. A healthcare profession that is autonomous, educated, and regulated (licensed/registered). Optometrists are the primary healthcare practitioners of the eye and visual system who provide comprehensive eye and vision care, which includes refraction and dispensing, detection/diagnosis and management of disease in the eye, and the rehabilitation of conditions of the visual system. Definition of the World Council of Optometry.

Orthopic fusion. A patient under-converges, for example when a patient with an eso-deviation uses the three-cats card to train divergent fusional reserves, so the visual axes cross behind the card (c.f., **chiastopic fusion**).

Orthophoria. A perfect alignment of the visual axes, both when fused and dissociated; i.e., no **heterophoria** or **strabismus** is present.

Orthophorisation. A natural process that acts to reduce or eliminate any **heterophoria**. Orthophorisation is believed to account for the greater prevalence of orthophoria than would be predicted by chance.

Orthoptics. The study, diagnosis, and nonsurgical treatment of binocular vision anomalies. It is practised mostly by optometrists and orthoptists.

Palsy. Generic term to describe a **paralysis** or a **paresis**.

Panum's area. An area (notionally) in the retina of one eye, any point of which, when stimulated simultaneously with a single point in the retina of the other eye, will give rise to a single percept. It is the range of disparities allowing fusion and stereopsis. Synonym: Panum's fusional space.

Paradoxical diplopia. Diplopia in which the images occupy a relative position opposite to that normally expected, e.g., uncrossed (homonymous) in divergent strabismus. Paradoxical diplopia results from unharmonious **anomalous retinal correspondence**, usually temporarily after surgery.

Paralysis. Complete loss of action of a muscle (c.f., **paresis**).

Paresis. Partial loss of action of a muscle (c.f., **paralysis**).

Parinaud's syndrome. A condition characterised by: gaze palsy for elevation or depression or both for saccades and later pursuit, convergence retraction nystagmus, upper eyelid retraction, pupil abnormalities, and papilloedema.

Parks' monofixational syndrome. The appearance, during cover testing, of an esophoria superimposed upon a microtropia.

Park's three-step test. A method for determining which of the vertical extraocular muscles is paretic.

Parvocellular visual system. The sensory visual system can be subclassified into pathways, two of which are the parvocellular and magnocellular pathways, named after the type of ganglion cell. The parvocellular system is responsible for the detailed analysis of an object. Synonym: sustained visual system.

Passive position. The position the eyes adopt when they fixate at a given distance without any stimulus to achieve fusion; e.g., during a **dissociation test**.

Past pointing. The inability to accurately point to a fixated object; commonly seen in **eccentric fixation** and recent onset **strabismus**, especially when **incomitant**.

Penalisation. A method of treating **amblyopia** and **eccentric fixation** in which the vision of the nonamblyopic eye is reduced (e.g., by topical drugs, optical overcorrection) to compel the amblyopic eye to fixate.

Percival's criterion. For a heterophoria to be asymptomatic, the point of fixation should lie within the middle third of the vergence range (measured between break, diplopia, points).

Phi movement. The illusion of movement created when one object disappears, and an identical object appears in a neighbouring region of the same plane. A similar phenomenon can result in the subjective impression of movement during the alternating cover test. Rabbetts (2007) argued that the term should not be used for binocular vision, because the physiological mechanism is different to the simple movement illusion to which the term usually refers.

Phoria. See **heterophoria**.

Physiological diplopia. Diplopia which exists during normal binocular single vision. It is the appreciation that a near object appears double when a distant object is fixated and vice versa. The diplopia is crossed (heteronymous) when the more distant of the two objects is fixated and uncrossed (homonymous) when the nearer is fixated.

Pleoptics. A method of treating (usually severe) amblyopia using bright lights to dazzle the eccentrically fixating area.

Polyopia. Appreciation of a number of images of a single object.

Position of anatomical rest. The position the eyes take up when they are completely devoid of tonus, as in death.

Primary angle of deviation. The **angle of deviation** when the nonparetic eye is fixating.

Primary position. The direction of gaze when both eyes fixate an object at infinity, on the midline, at eye level.

Prism. A type of lens which deviates light in one direction without bringing it to a focus. A prism is wedge-shaped (or made up of wedge-shaped components, a **Fresnel prism**) with a base and an apex. Prisms always deviate light towards their base, resulting in an apparent shift of the image towards the apex. Thus, base-in prisms can be used to relieve an exo-deviation, or can be used to force the eyes to diverge when measuring the divergent **fusional reserves**.

Prism dioptre (Δ). A prism of power one prism dioptre will deviate parallel rays of light by a distance of 1 cm on a flat surface at a distance of 1 m from the prism. $1\Delta = 0.57294°$ or 34.4 minutes of arc.

Prism reflection test. See **Krimsky's test**.

Prism vergences. See **fusional reserves**.

Ptosis. A drooping of the upper eyelid resulting in a narrowing of the palpebral fissure.

Pursuit. A type of eye movement where the eyes follow smoothly a relatively slowly moving target. If the target moves too quickly, the eyes start making saccadic movements to 'catch up' with the target (saccadation of pursuit).

Random dot stereograms. A **stereogram** in which the eyes see an array of small characters or dots containing no recognisable shape or contours. Some characters are displaced and, although this is monocularly imperceptible, it facilitates **global stereopsis**.

Randomised controlled trial (*RCT*). A study in which participants are allocated at random to receive one of two (or more) clinical interventions. One of these interventions is the intervention(s) under investigation and another a control (which may be a placebo). Typically, the experimenters measuring the outcome(s) and participants and experimenters are masked (blinded) to the identity of the interventions.

Range of fusion. See **fusional reserves**.

Recession. A surgical procedure to weaken the action of a muscle by moving its insertion nearer to the origin of the muscle.

Recidivism. A relapse (usually relapsing into crime). In amblyopia treatment, recidivism describes a relapse of acuity following apparently successful treatment.

Refraction. The process of measuring the **refractive error** of the eyes.

Refractive error (Rx). The power of lenses required to correct any anomalies of the refractive state of the eye.

Relative fusional convergence/divergence. See **fusional reserves**.

Relative vergences. See **fusional reserves**.

Resection. A surgical procedure to increase the action of a muscle by excising a portion of the muscle to shorten it.

Retinal correspondence. Describes the concept that retinal points (or areas) in similar positions in the two eyes give rise to a common visual direction. When the visual axes are perfectly aligned, an object falling on a certain point on the retina of one eye will fall on the same corresponding point in the other eye. In fact, a point on the retina of one eye innately corresponds with an area (**Panum's area**) on the retina of the other eye. This is **normal retinal correspondence** (*NRC*). If the visual axes become significantly misaligned (strabismus), an object will no longer be imaged on corresponding retinal points. These innately noncorresponding retinal points may become associated with one another through a cortical adaptation resulting in **anomalous (abnormal) retinal correspondence** (*ARC*). Nearly always, this is **harmonious anomalous retinal correspondence** (*HARC*): the angle between the abnormally corresponding points and innately corresponding points is equal to the habitual angle of the strabismus so diplopia and suppression are prevented. **Unharmonious anomalous retinal correspondence** (*UARC*) describes the rare condition where the angle between abnormally corresponding points and innately corresponding points is not equal to the habitual angle of strabismus. Usually, UARC is an artefact from using tests that interfere with normal viewing conditions. UARC can also result from a second strabismus developing 'on top of' an initial strabismus, sometimes after surgery.

Retinal rivalry. A condition that occurs when dissimilar images fall on corresponding retinal areas and the subject perceives an unstable perception comprising alternation and occasional mixing of the monocular images.

Retinoscopy. An objective method of measuring the refractive error of the eye by neutralising (with lenses) light reflected from the retina.

Risley prism. See **rotary prism**.

Rotary prism. A type of prismatic lens whose power can be smoothly altered. Synonyms: Risley prism, Crétès prism, Herschel prism.

Saccade. A rapid conjugate movement of the eyes to fixate a point of interest.

SAFE. Acronym to describe ocular motility test results: smooth, accurate, full, extensive.

Scobee's three-step test. A method for determining which of the vertical extraocular muscles is palsied.

Scotoma. An area of partial or complete blindness surrounded by normal or relatively normal visual field.

Secondary angle of deviation. In **incomitant** deviations, the **angle of deviation** when the paretic eye is fixating.

Sensory fusion. See **fusion**.

Sensory fusion disruption syndrome. A condition in which a patient, in a haploscopic device or with prisms, can achieve superimposition of each eye's image (c.f., **horror fusionis**), but cannot achieve sensory fusion.

Sensory visual stress (Meares-Irlen Syndrome). A controversial condition characterised by symptoms on viewing certain stimuli, typically text, that are alleviated by using coloured filters of a specific tint. Synonyms: visual stress, Meares-Irlen syndrome, Irlen syndrome, scotopic sensitivity syndrome.

Separation difficulties. See **crowding phenomenon**.

Sheard's criterion. States that, for a **heterophoria** to be compensated, the opposing **fusional reserve** (to blur point) should be at least twice the heterophoria.

Sherrington's law of reciprocal innervation. The contraction of a muscle is accompanied by simultaneous and proportional relaxation of its **antagonist**. Sherrington's law applies to the muscles of one eye.

SILO. Acronym for Small In, Large Out (c.f., **SOLI**). It refers to the perception that some people experience when horizontal prisms are introduced whilst they maintain fusion. When the eyes move inwards (converge) with base-out prisms, typically the object appears to become smaller and closer. Conversely, when the eyes move outwards (diverge) with base-in prisms, the object appears larger and further away. Note: the acronym refers to the movement of the eyes, not the prism base direction.

Single mirror haploscope. An adjustable **stereoscope** used for the measurement and treatment of binocular vision anomalies.

Skew deviation. A usually transient hypertropia in which the eyes move in opposite directions equally: one eye is elevated and the other depressed; an acquired hypertropia, often fairly comitant; often due to a brain stem or cerebellar lesion.

SOLI. Acronym for Small Out, Large In (c.f., **SILO**). It refers to the perception that a few people experience when horizontal prisms are introduced whilst they maintain fusion. When the eyes move outwards (diverge) with base-in prisms, sometimes the object appears to become smaller. Conversely, when the eyes move inwards (converge) with base-out prisms, the object may appear larger. Note: the acronym refers to the movement of the eyes, not the prism base direction.

Square wave jerks. A relatively common phenomenon in which a small horizontal saccade takes the eye off the fixation point and is quickly corrected by a second saccade.

Squint. Synonym of **strabismus**. The term 'squint' is deprecated because it is often used by patients to describe signs other than strabismus.

Stanworth synoptiscope. A modification of a **synoptophore** which allows objects to be viewed in free-space. It represents an attempt, only partially successful, to give the synoptophore a less artificial viewing environment.

Stereoacuity (*stereo.*). A measure of **stereopsis**. The method of measurement influences the result obtained.

Stereogram. Two separate images of an object (e.g., letters, photographs, drawings, or pseudo-random dots) with parallax differences between them which, when fused, give a stereoscopic percept. The targets can be fused in a **stereoscope** or, using over- or under-convergence, in **free-space**.

Stereopsis. Depth perception due to retinal disparity; i.e., arising from binocular vision.

Stereoscope. An instrument (type of **haploscope**) that allows targets to be presented independently to the two eyes.

Strabismus (*strab.*). A condition where the visual axes are misaligned by a deviation that is too great for sensory fusion within Panum's fusional areas. Types of strabismus are **exotropia, esotropia, hypertropia, hypotropia,** and **cyclotropia**. Synonyms of strabismus include heterotropia, turning eye, squint, and cast. The last two terms have other meanings and are deprecated.

Strabismus fixus. A congenital condition in which the affected eye is 'anchored' in a position because of fibrous tightening of an extraocular muscle.

Subjective angle of deviation. In **strabismus**, the angle between the two visually perceived directions (angle of diplopia), when measured subjectively. Conventionally, it has been measured using artificial instruments, such as the **synoptophore**, but if a strabismic patient does not have complete **suppression** of one eye's binocular field and does not experience **diplopia** and **confusion**, the subjective angle of deviation in everyday life must be zero.

Superior oblique myokymia. An episodic small amplitude nystagmoid intorsion and depression of one eye, accompanied by visual shimmer and oscillopsia. The condition was originally called 'unilateral rotary nystagmus'.

Superior oblique tendon sheath syndrome. A congenital condition caused by a fibrous unyielding superior oblique muscle, resulting in the appearance of a paralysis of the inferior oblique muscle. Synonym: **Brown syndrome**.

Suppression (*supp.*). A binocular condition in which the image of an object formed upon the retina is not perceived but is mentally ignored or neglected, either partially or completely, due to an incongruous image in the other eye. Suppression is one mechanism of avoiding **diplopia** in **strabismus**. Suppression can be further classified into facultative, which ceases when the fixating eye is occluded, and obligatory, which is operative under all conditions.

Suspension. An archaic term used to describe minor degrees of central suppression, occurring mainly during binocular vision. Now referred to as **foveal suppression**.

Sustained visual system. See **parvocellular visual system**.

Swann's syndrome. An esotropia where the angle of deviation is such that the retinal image of the object of regard in the deviated eye falls on the optic disc (blind spot). Synonyms: blind spot syndrome, blind spot mechanism.

Synergist. Muscles are synergists if they normally act together. When a muscle contracts then its synergists contract at the same time. c.f., **antagonist**.

Synoptophore. An instrument used to investigate binocular vision. A large range of different targets can be used in each eye individually, or similar targets to investigate **sensory fusion**. The target for each eye can be moved independently to investigate **motor fusion**. The main disadvantage of the instrument is that it creates an artificial visual environment, causing the eyes to behave atypically. Synonym: major amblyoscope.

Tangent scale. A simple scale calibrated in **prism dioptres**. It is sometimes used at 6 or 3 metres in the Maddox rod test. A spotlight is at the centre of a horizontal and vertical scale and the patient reports the number on the appropriate scale through which the streak from the rod passes.

Tenotomy. The operation of cutting a muscle tendon.

Tenoplication. The surgical procedure of tucking a muscle tendon to shorten it.

Three-step test. A method of diagnosing incomitant deviations of cyclovertical muscles. The best known is Park's three-step test; another is Scobee's three-step test.

Torsion. A rotatory movement of an eye about its anterior-posterior axis.

Torticollis. Head tilting usually accompanied by a rotation of the neck. Ordinarily, torticollis is caused by congenital unilateral contracture of the sternomastoid muscle in the neck. However, 'ocular torticollis' can also occur as a result of an ocular condition (e.g., incomitancy, nystagmus).

Total angle of strabismus. The angle of **strabismus** measured after the patient's habitual viewing conditions are degraded, for example by prolonged or repeated occlusion. This is larger than the **habitual angle of strabismus**.

Tranaglyph. See **anaglyph**.

Transient visual system. See **magnocellular visual system**.

Triplopia. Appreciation of three images of a single object.

Trochleitis. See **trochleodynia**.

Trochleodynia. A spectrum of disorders characterised by pain arising from the trochlear region.

True-space. See **free-space**.

Typoscope. A reading shield made of black material in which there is a rectangular aperture allowing one or more lines of print to be seen.

Unharmonious abnormal retinal correspondence. See **retinal correspondence**.

V-pattern. A binocular vision anomaly characterised by, relatively speaking, excessive convergence on downgaze and/or excessive divergence on upgaze. Synonym: V-syndrome.

Vectogram. A polarised **stereogram** consisting of two cross-polarised images.

Vergence eye movements. Eye movements in which the eyes move in opposite directions to maintain fixation on an object that is moving in depth. The movements are sometimes described as disjunctive.

Vergence facility (Verg. Fac.). The ability of the eyes to rapidly change their vergence.

Vergence reserves. See **fusional reserves**.

Version eye movements. Conjugate movement of both eyes in the same direction.

Vision Screeners. Instruments designed to screen for visual defects. Usually these are used by personnel who are not professionally trained in vision care.

Vision and Visual acuity. Classically, **vision** (V) refers to unaided (without glasses) Snellen (letter chart) acuity, and visual acuity (VA) refers to acuity with optimum correction. These parameters are usually represented as a fraction; the decimal equivalent of this relates to the normal of 1.0., e.g., 6/6 = 20/20 = 1.0 (decimal), 6/12 = 0.5 (person only able to resolve at 50% of normal), 6/3 = 2.0 (person able to resolve detail half the size of that resolved by a hypothetical 'average' person). The numerator of the fraction refers to the distance at which the test is carried out (usually 6 m in the UK or 20 ft in the USA).

Vision training. Training methods aimed at improving visual function. Vision training is sometimes used as an extension of orthoptic techniques in an attempt to enhance visual perception and ocular motor performance in those who would, by conventional criteria, be considered to already have normal or supra-normal visual function. Synonym: vision therapy.

Visual axis. The line joining the object of regard to the foveola.

Visual stress. See **sensory visual stress.**

Visual conversion reaction. Reduced visual function where the origin is psychogenic (subconscious).

Visuscope. An ophthalmoscope specially modified for the measurement of eccentric fixation.

Yoked prisms. Identical prisms placed before each eye in the same base direction (e.g., base-up both eyes, base-down both eyes, base-out one eye and base-in for the other eye).

Appendices 2–9 are clinical worksheets and diagnostic algorithms to assist in clinical practice. Some of the worksheets include several tests for assessing an aspect of orthoptic function. Students may find it useful to work through these, and experienced practitioners, although most likely to use their preferred approach, may find other methods useful as confirmatory tests. Students may find it helps to work through the worksheets as preparation for examinations, especially Appendix 1 which explains some confusing aspects of binocular vision testing. Appendix 11 is a headache diary which can be issued to patients to help them identify visual triggers to their headaches. Appendix 12 is a non-exhaustive list of suppliers of many items of equipment mentioned in this book. For explanations of abbreviations used in the appendices, please see the relevant section of the book.

Appendix 1: Confusing Aspects of Binocular Vision Tests

There are several potentially confusing aspects of binocular vision tests. This appendix aims to remove some of this confusion and to provide useful mnemonics and 'memory hooks'.

BINOCULAR VISION TESTS: PRACTITIONER'S PERSPECTIVE

Rule	Mnemonic
Light is deviated towards the base of a prism	Imagine a prism standing on its base with light parallel to the ground: it will be deviated down by gravity
If eye is OUT, need base IN prism	OUT – IN IN – OUT
i.e., EXO needs base in to correct	IN'XS' (in excess)
If eye is UP, need base DOWN	UP – DOWN DOWN – UP
i.e., R hyper needs base down RE	
GENERAL RULE: (1) prism base to relieve a deviation is in opposite direction to the deviation or (2) 'the base of the prism must be on the side of the inefficient muscle' (Percival, 1928).	

BINOCULAR VISION TESTS: PATIENT'S PERSPECTIVE

Rule	Mnemonic
EXO deviations give crossed disparity	eXo X = cross(ed)
exo: RE image is seen on left of LE image	
eso: RE image is seen on right of LE image	
R hyper: RE image is seen below LE image	
FD: if RE image goes to the left, then exo: introduce base in	
FD: if RE image goes up, then R hypo: introduce base up RE	
Maddox rod: if RE rod image is to left of LE spot, then exo: introduce base in	LOSEX: L of spot if exo ROSES: R of spot if eso
Maddox rod: if RE rod image is up, then R hypo: need base up RE	
In NPC or fusional reserve tests, if suppression is present:	Target appears to jump towards the side of the suppressing eye
Subjective cover (Phi) test: image moves with cover = exo image moves against cover = eso	Phite against it: it = inward turn
Subjective cover test: if image appears to be down when RE uncovered, then R hyper	
CYCLO deviations: a line is perceived to be tilted in the direction in which the underacting muscle would rotate the eye In double Maddox rod test, if top of Maddox rod has to be rotated outwards, then excyclotorsion	If patient perceives intorsion, the eye is extorted. The lens has to be rotated in the direction in which the eye has moved.
GENERAL RULE: image is seen in opposite direction to the deviation of the eye; prism base required is in the opposite direction to the deviation of the eye	

FD, Fixation disparity; L, left; LE, left eye; NPC, near point of convergence; R, right; RE, right eye.

MOTILITY TESTING

- In motility, the image furthest out is seen by the under-acting eye (i.e., the image is seen in the opposite direction to the deviation of the eye).
- **Secondary & tertiary actions**: the vertical Recti muscles both ADduct and the Superior recti and superior oblique muscles both INtort (Mnemonic: RADSIN).

CONFUSING FEATURES

- When measuring fusional reserves, use base in prism to make the eyes diverge. This is because you are forcing the eye to move, so use the opposite prism to that which would be used to relieve a deviation.

Appendix 2: Worksheet for Investigation of Infant/Toddler

See Chapter 3.

Each test has space to record the quality of response obtained from the infant, reflecting the practitioner's confidence in the test result.

SYMPTOMS & HISTORY

PARENTAL REPORTS: ....

BIRTH: ....FH: ....

VISUAL ACUITY

METHOD 1: ....RE ....LE ....BE ....   good/moderate/poor

METHOD 2: ....RE ....LE ....BE ....   good/moderate/poor

Reaction to occlusion:

tolerant/equally intolerant to R or L occlusion/intolerant of occlusion of RE/LE

REFRACTION (RETINOSCOPY)

STATIC METHOD: ....| DYNAMIC METHOD: ....

RE ....| RE ....

LE ....| LE ....

response: good/moderate/poor | response: good/moderate/poor

OCULAR ALIGNMENT (METHODS: COVER TEST; HIRSCHBERG, KRIMSKY, BRUCKNER)

D: method 1: ....result: .... good/moderate/poor

D: method 2: ....result: .... good/moderate/poor

N: method 1: ....result: .... good/moderate/poor

N: method 2: ....result: .... good/moderate/poor

NPC: ....cm   Response: good/moderate/poor

MOTILITY: .... good/moderate/poor

FUSIONAL RESERVE (NEAR)

METHOD: ....Δ base out   eye movements: brisk/moderate/slow/none

METHOD: ....Δ base in   eye movements: brisk/moderate/slow/none

Estimated validity of result: good/moderate/poor

STEREOACUITY

METHOD: ....RESULT: ....seconds good/moderate/poor

OCULAR HEALTH

PUPILS: ....HVID: R: ....mm L: ....mm
MEDIA: ....
FUNDUS: red reflex/some fundus seen & normal/most fundus seen & normal/all fundus
seen & normal
DISCS: R: seen/not seen: ....L: seen/not seen: ....
MACS: R: seen/not seen: ....L: seen/not seen: ....
OTHER OBSERVATIONS: ....

NORMS
Visual acuity

Method (based on Table 3.1)	Minimum normal acuity for age (months)						
	1	3	6	12	24	36	48
Vertical prism test	With 10 Δ up one eye, should alternate freely						
Grating preferential looking (Telle1990)	6/180	6/90	6/30	6/24	6/12	6/6	6/6
Cardiff cards				6/48	6/15	6/12	6/9
Snellen chart letter matching						6/12	6/9

Refractive error
Based on Leat (2011); see p. 41

Refractive error	Age (y) Criterion		Adjustment
Hypermetropia	1+	≥3.50D in any meridian	Give partial Rx
	4+	≥2.50D in any meridian	Reduce by 1 to 1.50D
	School	≥1.50D	Nearly fully correct
Astigmatism	1.25+	≥2.50DC	Give partial Rx
	2+	≥2.00DC	Give partial Rx
Oblique astigmatism	1+	≥1.00DC	Correct ~¾
	4+	≥1.50DC	Give full cylinder
	School	≥0.75	Fully correct
Anisometropia	If amblyopia, correct the full level of anisometropia		
	1+	≥3.00	Reduce by 1.00D aniso
	3.5	≥1.00 if hypermetropia ≥2.00 if myopia ≥1.50 if astigmatism	Fully correct the anisometropic element of Rx
Myopia	0–1	<−5.00	Undercorrect by 2.00D
	1–walking	<−2.00	Undercorrect by 0.50 to 1.00
	4–school	<−1.00	Full correction
	School any myopia		Full correction[a]

[a]Consider myopia control (p. 101)

Fusional reserve to 20Δ base out

AGE (MONTHS)	TEST	RESPONSE
0–3	20 Δ out	Unlikely to make any response
by 6	20 Δ out	Should be overcome; if can only overcome 10Δ, monitor

Stereoacuity

AGE	TEST	RESPONSE
0–3 mo.	Any	Unlikely to make any response
6–18 mo.	Lang 1	Observe patient's eyes: may see fixations indicating sees pictures
18–24 mo.	Lang 1 or 2	Should fixate and may point at pictures
>24 mo.	Lang 1 or 2	Should be able to point and name pictures
≥ 24 mo.	Randot (shapes)	If sees shapes on random dot background indicates no strabismus
≥ 24 mo.	Randot (animals)	Should be able to see all animals
3–5 yrs.	Randot (circles)	70″
>5 yrs.	Randot (circles)	40″ or better
3.5 yrs.	Titmus	3000″ (Romano et al., 1975)
5 yrs.	Titmus	140″ (Romano et al., 1975)
6 yrs.	Titmus	80″ (Romano et al., 1975)
7 yrs.	Titmus	60″ (Romano et al., 1975)
9 yrs.	Titmus	40″ (Romano et al., 1975)
3–5 yrs.	Frisby	250″
3–5 yrs.	TNO	120″

Visual behavioural signs

Infants should be attending to faces by about 1 month and fixating and following targets of interest by the age of 2 months.

Iris diameter (HVID) (Papadopoulos et al., 2005)

Refer if neonate: >11 mm or age 6–12 months: >12 mm or any age: >13 mm or asymmetric

Appendix 3: Worksheet for Diagnosis of Decompensated Heterophoria and Binocular Instability

Follow the table, ticking as appropriate and entering 'scores' in the right-hand column. The table is for horizontal phorias. If a vertical aligning prism of 0.5Δ or more is detected then, after checking trial frame alignment, measure the vertical dissociated phoria. If this is $\geq$ aligning prism and there are symptoms, likely diagnosis: decompensated hyperphoria. See Chapters 4 and 5.

DISTANCE/NEAR (DELETE)	SCORE
1. Does the patient have one or more of the symptoms of decompensated heterophoria (headache, aching eyes, diplopia, blurred vision, distortions, reduced stereopsis, monocular comfort, sore eyes, general irritation; associated with visual tasks at the relevant distance)? *If so, score +3 (+2 or +1 if borderline)* Are the symptoms at D □ or N □ *(if both ticked, complete 2 worksheets)*	
2. Is the patient orthophoric on cover testing? Yes □ or No □ *If no, score +1*	
3. Is the cover test recovery rapid and smooth? Yes □ or No □ *If no, score +2 (+1 if borderline)*	
4. Is the Mallett Hz aligning prism: $<1\Delta$ for patients under 40, or $<2\Delta$ for patients 40 + ? Yes □ or No □ *If no, score +2*	
5. Is the Mallett aligning prism stable (Nonius strips stationary with any required prism)? Yes □ or No □ *If no, score +1*	
6. Using the polarised letters binocular status test, is any foveal suppression < 1 line? Yes □ or No □ *If no, score +2*	
Add up score so far and enter in right hand column *If score: ≤ 3 probably normal; ≥ 6 treat; 4–5 continue down table adding to score so far*	
7. Sheard's criterion: (a) Measure the dissociated phoria; record size & stability. (b) Measure the fusional reserve opposing the heterophoria (i.e., convergent, or base out, in exophoria). Record as blur/break/recovery in Δ. Is the blur point, or if no blur point the break point, in (b) at least twice the phoria in (a)? Yes □ or No □ *If no, score +2*	
8. Percival's criterion (near vision only): measure the other fusional reserve and compare the two break points. Is the larger break point less than twice the smaller break point? Yes □ or No □ *If no, score +1*	
9. When you measured the dissociated heterophoria, was the result stable, or unstable (varying over a range of $\pm 2\Delta$ or more)? Stable □ or Unstable □ *If unstable, score +1*	
10. Using the fusional reserve measurements, add the divergent break point to the convergent break point. Is the total (=fusional amplitude) at least 20Δ? Yes □ or No □ *If no, score +1*	
Add up total score (from both sections of table) and enter in right hand column. If total score: ≤ 5 then probably OK, monitor; if >5 likely to benefit from treatment.	

Appendix 4: Specific Learning Difficulties (Dyslexia)

The flow chart summarises the role of the optometrist in detecting and treating visual factors that may co-occur with specific learning difficulties (see p. 64). The Delphi criteria are described in Evans et al. (2017) and examples given in Evans (2018a,b).

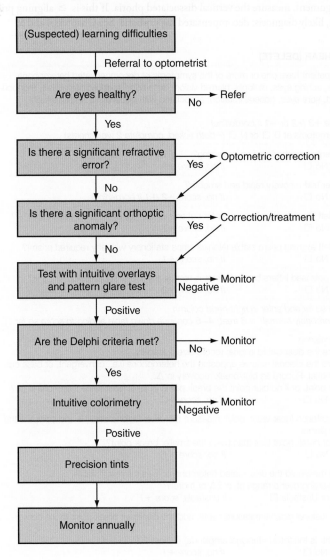

Appendix 5: Worksheet for the Investigation of Strabismus

See Chapters 12 and 14.

N.B., Pathology must be carefully excluded: check pupil reactions, fundus, fields, motility, etc.

1. (a) *MOTOR*: COVER TEST
(to diagnose and quantify, by estimation, motor deviation)

Distance: ....

Near: ....

N.B., The above should include: direction; estimate of size; is angle stable/variable, constant/intermittent, unilateral/alternating

If strabismus is intermittent, see also heterophoria worksheet

(b) *MOTOR*: DISSOCIATION TEST
(to quantify motor deviation, e.g., Maddox rod, Maddox wing)

Distance: test: .... result .... was covering required? ....

Near: test: .... result .... was covering required? ....

2. (a) *SENSORY*: MARCS test (large OXO) (to investigate sensory status)

Test distance: 1 m/near
Result: HARC/suppression/diplopia
During test, check motor status with cover test.

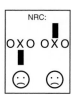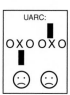

If diplopia, is the angle between the two OXOs similar to/same as that in 1(b)?

- If so → HARC
- If not → UARC (very unlikely: is the patient usually diplopic? If not, UARC is test artefact)

If HARC, use ND filter bar in front of strabismic eye: depth of filter to disrupt HARC: ....ND units

If suppression, use ND filter bar in front of good eye: depth of filter to disrupt suppression: ....ND units

(b) *SENSORY*: BAGOLINI LENS (to investigate sensory status)
If unilateral strabismus, use Bagolini lens before strabismic eye
If alternating strabismus, use two Bagolini lenses at 45°/135°

During test, check motor response with cover test.
Test distance: 6 m/near
Result: HARC/suppression/diplopia

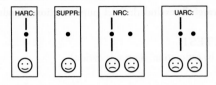

If diplopia, is the angle between the two spots similar to the angle in 1(b)?

- If so → HARC
- If not → UARC (very unlikely: is the patient usually diplopic? If not, UARC is test artefact)

If HARC, use ND filter bar in front of strabismic eye: depth of filter to disrupt HARC: ....ND units

If suppression, use ND filter bar in front of good eye: depth of filter to disrupt suppression: ....ND units

Diagnosis: HARC/suppression/diplopia/UARC
(UARC is very unlikely, possibly secondary to surgery)

Appendix 6: Worksheet for the Investigation of Amblyopia

See Chapter 13. Pathology must be carefully excluded: check pupil reactions, fundus, fields, motility, etc.

VISUAL ACUITIES

Line of letters: R ....   L ....   Single letters: R ....   L ....
Is the linear acuity of worse eye 2 lines + worse than other? yes/no
Yes ⇒ amblyopia

Is the poorer eye worse than 6/9? yes/no
Yes ⇒ amblyopia

Is linear acuity >1 line worse than single letter acuity? yes/no
Yes ⇒ strabismic amblyopia

Line with 2.0 ND: R ....   L ....   B ....   chart: ....
Is mesopic acuity worse (∼1 line) than normal acuity? yes/no No ⇒ strabismic amblyopia

REFRACTIVE ERROR (DELETE: RET/SUB CYCLO/DRY)

R: ....   L: ....
Is there >1.00D anisometropia yes/no
Yes ⇒ anisometropic amblyopia

COVER TEST

Distance: ....   Near: ....
Is the patient strabismic at distance & near yes/no
Yes ⇒ strabismic amblyopia

ECCENTRIC FIXATION

Ophthalmoscope method
1. Check 'good eye' fixates centrally (to train patient and check response)
2. Draw what you see in strabismic eye, marking position of fixation mark with X
   - macula reflex represented by ○
   - estimate the distance between reflex and fixation mark ....mins/disc diameters

Amsler chart method

Look for evidence of a one-sided scotoma

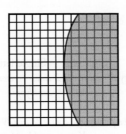

Other method (e.g., after-image)

Method: ....   Result: ....

Is eccentric fixation present? yes/no
Yes ⇒ strabismic amblyopia

N.B., if eccentric fixation is present but there is no apparent strabismus, consider **microtropia**

Appendix 7: Treatment of Amblyopia

The flow chart that follows is a general guide to the treatment of amblyopia (see Chapter 13). The values (e.g., refractive errors and ages) are approximate, and other factors (e.g., motivation) should influence decisions. Orthotropic refractive amblyopia is likely to respond to treatment at any age (Chapter 13). If the visual acuity in anisometropia does not improve with spectacles, it might with contact lenses, otherwise patching will be required. Asymptomatic adults with anisometropic amblyopia may prefer not to receive treatment, unless symptoms or vocational requirements suggest otherwise. For strabismic patients over the age of about 8 years, patching is usually contraindicated and any marked change in their refractive correction should be accompanied by instructions to cease wear and return if diplopia occurs. Indeed, any patient receiving amblyopia treatment should receive these instructions.

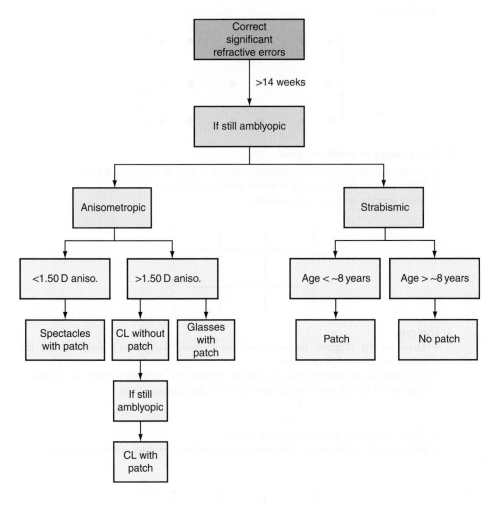

Appendix 8: Worksheet for the Investigation of Incomitancy

See Chapter 17.

MOTILITY

1. **Observation of pupil reflexes:**
   - Each pair of stars represent the patient's pair of pupil reflexes in different positions of gaze.
   - Where the pupil reflexes suggest that the visual axes are non-parallel, mark the deviation of the eye with an arrow.

   N.B., Recorded as the patient sees it (like visual field), with their left field on the left side of the diagram

   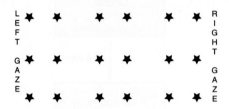

2. **Cover testing in peripheral gaze:**
   - Write cover test results in peripheral positions of gaze in the relevant box.
   - Make sure the fixation target is always visible to both eyes.
   - Make sure the occluder fully occludes.

   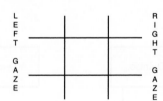

3. **Diplopia:**
   - Draw on the diagram, for each position of gaze, the patient's perspective of the separation of the diplopic image.
   - For example, if in right gaze the patient reports that their right image is up and to their left of the left eye's image, then record in the relevant box as:

     R
       L
   - Mark * where greatest separation of images
   - In this position, the paretic eye's image is furthest out. ⇒ paretic muscle(s): ....

   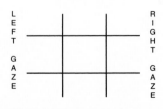

HESS SCREEN: (attach plot)

1. Which eye is deviated (which is strabismic during the cover test)? R/L/B
2. Which is the smaller plot (=paretic eye): R/L
3. In the paretic eye's plot, which muscle appears to be under-acting the most [=paretic muscle(s)]? ....

Is there overaction of the contralateral synergist? yes/no (if no, rethink; there may be two palsies) ....

CONCLUSION: PARETIC MUSCLE(S): ....

4. (a) If the paretic eye is the usually deviated eye, is there contracture (enlarged plot in field of action) of ipsilateral antagonist? yes/no
   (b) If the paretic eye is not the usually deviated eye, is there a restriction of the plot in the field of action of the contralateral antagonist? yes/no
5. Are the right and left eye plots a similar size? yes/no

IF THE ANSWER TO 4 (A) OR (B) IS YES AND THE ANSWER TO 5 IS YES, THE PARESIS IS LIKELY TO BE OLD

CONCLUSION: OLD/NEW/UNCERTAIN

....

If vertically acting muscle may be affected, proceed below:

MADDOX	DISTANCE						NEAR	
ROD	(a)	(b)	(c)	(d)	(e)	(f)	(g)	(h)
	Horizontal	Vertical	Vertical	Vertical	Vertical	Vertical	Horizontal	Vertical
Gaze/ head tilt	Primary	Primary	R gaze	L gaze	R tilt	L tilt	Primary	Primary
RE fixing (rod LE)								
LE fixing (rod RE)								

PARKS THREE-STEPS METHOD: (consider R hypodeviation to be L hyperdeviation)

1. Is it R/L or L/R [from column (b) and (h)]? ....
   R/L: RSO, RIR, LIO, LSR   L/R: RIO, RSR, LSO, LIR
2. Is the vertical deviation greater in R or L gaze [columns (c) and (d)]? ....
   R gaze: RSR, RIR, LIO, LSO   L gaze: RIO, RSO, LSR, LIR,
3. Is the vertical deviation greater with head tilt to R or L [columns (e) and (f)]? ....
   R tilt: RSO, RSR, LIO, LIR   L tilt: RIO, RIR, LSO, LSR

CONCLUSION: PARETIC MUSCLE(S): ....

SCOBEE'S METHOD:

1. Is it R/L or L/R [from column (b) and (h)]? ....
   R/L: RSO, RIR, LIO, LSR L/R: RIO, RSR, LSO, LIR
2. Is the vertical deviation greater at D (primary pos'n [column (b)]) or N (adducted [column (h)])? ....
   D: RSR, RIR, LSR, LIR N: RSO, RIO, LSO, LIO

3. Which eye is fixating when there is the greatest vertical deviation [column (b) and (h)]?

....

R: RSR, RIR, RSO, RIO   L: LSR, LIR, LSO, LIO

CONCLUSION: PARETIC MUSCLE(S): ....

LINDBLOM'S METHOD: patient views a 70 cm horizontal rod at 1 m. If no vertical diplopia, use 2 Maddox rods with vertical prism (with double Maddox rods, perceived tilt is in direction that affected muscle would rotate eye, <10 degrees suggests one superior oblique muscle likely to be involved, ≥ 10 degrees suggests bilateral)

1. Where is the vertical diplopia greatest? ....
upgaze: RSR, RIO, LSR, LIO   downgaze: RIR, RSO, LIR, LSO

2. Where there is maximum diplopia, are the two images parallel or torsional? ....
parallel: RSR, RIR, LSR, LIR   torsional: RSO, RIO, LSO, LIO

3. If parallel, does the separation increase on R or L gaze? ....
R: RSR, RIR   L: LSR, LIR

4. If tilted, does the illusion of tilt increase in upgaze or downgaze?
upgaze: RIO, LIO   downgaze: RSO, LSO

5. If tilted, the position of intersection of the 2 rods (resembling an arrow) points to the side of the paretic eye. Does the intersection of the rods point to the patient's R or L, or is it crossed like an X?
R: RSO, RIO   L: LSO, LIO

6. If crossed, does the tilt angle increase in upward gaze or downward?
upgaze: bilateral IO paresis (very unlikely)   downgaze: bilateral SO paresis

CONCLUSION: PARETIC MUSCLE(S): ....

ANOMALOUS HEAD POSITION: N.B. rarely, this can be paradoxical (opposite to below)
HEAD TILT (tipped on one side) ....degrees [estimate], top tipped to
    patient's: right/left [delete as appropriate]
Right: LSO (likely) or (unlikely) LSR/RIO/RIR   Left: RSO (likely) or (unlikely) RSR/
    LIO/LIR
HEAD ELEVATION (chin up or down) ....degrees [estimate], chin: up/down
    [delete as appropriate]
Up: RSR/RIO/LSR/LIO   Down: RSO/LSO (likely) or RIR/LIR (unlikely)
HEAD TURN (turn to one side) ....degrees [estimate], nose turned to
    patient's: right/left [delete as appropriate]
Right: RLR (likely) or LMR/RSR/RIR/LSO/LIO (unlikely)   Left: LLR (likely) or
    RMR/LSR/LIR/RSO/RIO (unlikely) OR Duane's syndrome

Appendix 9: Investigation of Reduced Visual Acuity From a Suspected Visual Conversion Reaction (p. 18)

INTRODUCTION

- Health checks → refer if abnormal
- If monocular:
  - occlude with refractor head
  - polarisation
  - anaglyph
  - fogging
- If binocular:
  - refractive checks
    - pinhole
    - plano placebo lens
    - placebo grey lens
    - cf. subjective and objective: is patient consistent?
    - comparison with opposite of preferred lens
  - other tests
    - reduce testing distance
    - 4Δ vertical prism test (Table 2.2)
    - paired cylinders test (Table 2.3)
    - forced choice preferential looking
    - kinetic perimetry: is there a spiral field?
    - kinetic perimetry: 'look at the other stick'
    - refer for visual evoked potentials (VEP) (? only if VAs < 6/24)

Appendix 10: Norms and Formulae

NORMS

The table below gives norms for orthoptic tests. Typically, norms vary little from age 6–12 years (Jimenez et al., 2004b); for younger children, see Appendix 2. Values for fusional reserves are quoted in prism diopters and the near test distance is 40 cm. Assuming a normal distribution, 68% of the population lie within 1 standard deviation (SD) of the mean and 98% within 2 standard deviations. It should be noted that lying outside the normal range does not necessarily mean a person requires treatment (Whyte & Kelly, 2018).

Variable	Mean	SD	Source
Heterophoria (Δ)			
Distance	1 XOP	2	Goss (1995)
Near	3 XOP	5	
Distance aligning prism (Δ with Mallett test)			
Rare for readings to be larger than 1			Pickwell et al. (1991)
Near aligning prism (Δ on Mallett unit)			
Pre-presbyopes: 1 or more is abnormal			Jenkins et al. (1989)
Presbyopes: 2 or more is abnormal			
Distance divergent fusional reserves (Δ)			
Blur	–	–	Morgan (1944)
Break	7	3	
Recovery	4	2	
Distance convergent fusional reserves (Δ)			
Blur	9	4	
Break	19	8	
Recovery	10	4	
Near divergent fusional reserves (Δ)			
Blur	13	4	
Break	21	4	
Recovery	13	5	
Near convergent fusional reserves (Δ)			
Blur	17	5	
Break	21	6	
Recovery	11	7	
Vertical (distance & near; Δ)			
Important that they are balanced (base up limits similar to base down).	2–4		Pickwell (1989)
NPC: normal range 6–10 cm			Hayes et al. (1998)
Accommodation (D)			
Average amplitude = 18.5 – (0.3 × age)			
Minimum amplitude = 15.0 – (0.25 × age)			
Plus to blur at 40 cm (negative relative accomm.)	+ 2.00	0.50	Hofstetter, cited by
Minus to blur at 40 cm (positive relative accomm.)	– 2.37	1.12	Reading (1988)
Monocular facility (± 2.00)	11	5	Goss (1995)
Binocular facility (± 2.00)	7.7	5	Zellers et al. (1984)
Lag (MEM)	+ 0.35	0.34	Tassinari (2002)
AC/A (gradient, +1.00 & –1.00, Δ/D)	2.2	0.8	Jimenez et al. (2004b)[a]

[a]Morgan's (1944) norms are often cited for the AC/A ratio, but he does not state the power of trial lenses. The data used here are from Jimenez et al. (2004b); the mean of results from 7 groups aged 6–12 years, which showed minimal developmental trend.

FORMULAE

The formula for calculating the AC/A ratio by the heterophoria method is:

$$AC/A = PD - \frac{(\text{Dist phoria} - \text{Nr phoria})}{F} \quad (\text{Jennings, 2001a})$$

where PD is interpupillary distance in cm and F is dioptric distance from distance to near. Exo-deviations are entered as negative values and eso-deviations as positive values.

The formula for converting the NPC in cm to a value for the convergent amplitude at this point in Δ is:

$$\Delta = \frac{10 \times PD}{NPC} + 2.7 \ (\text{Goss, 1995})$$

where PD is interpupillary distance in mm, NPC is near point of convergence in cm

....

Prismatic effect for free-space stereograms = 2.5 $\times$ separation of identical points (cm)

Appendix 11: Headache Diary

INSTRUCTIONS TO PATIENT

This sheet has been designed as a diary for you to record factors associated with your headaches. This can help to discover causes and in turn assist in preventing headaches in the future.

Enter every headache you experience in the table below. Intensity ratings can be graded as: mild, moderate, severe, very severe. In the next column, state if you need to rest or stop work because of the headache. Tick any of the 'triggers' that describe your activities before the headache. 'Hormonal' refers to certain times in women's monthly cycle; 'flickering' refers to flickering fluorescent lights, night clubs, or lights flickering through, for example, trees; 'patterns' refers to striped patterns. When you have completed the table, if any frequent triggers become apparent, try avoiding these. If visual stimuli (flickering, patterns, or reading) are triggers, consult your optometrist.

Date	Time	Intensity: mild, moderate, severe, very severe	Had to rest? yes/no	Name of medicine taken	Dosage	Time to relief	Triggers																Comments
							Reading	Patterns	Flickering	Other drinks	Caffeine	Red wine	Other food	Cheese	Chocolate	Smells	Tiredness	Noise	Stress	Hormonal	

Appendix 12: Equipment Suppliers

The following list is indicative, not exhaustive. Other suppliers may be available and it is recommended the reader carries out an internet search.

Equipment	Available from:
Aperture rule trainer	Bernell VTP www.bernell.com https://louisstone.co.uk/pdfs/Bernell_2020_Catalog_LS.pdf
Bagolini lenses	Sussex Vision www.sussex-vision.co.uk Haag-Streit UK eshop.haagstreituk.com
Bangerter foils	Hilco Vision www.hilcovision.com Haag-Streit UK eshop.haagstreituk.com
Bar readers	Bernell VTP www.bernell.com https://louisstone.co.uk/pdfs/Bernell_2020_Catalog_LS.pdf
Bar reading anaglyph (red green) charts	Bernell VTP www.bernell.com https://louisstone.co.uk/pdfs/Bernell_2020_Catalog_LS.pdf
Bernell-O-scope Bernell mirror stereoscope	Bernell VTP www.bernell.com https://louisstone.co.uk/pdfs/Bernell_2020_Catalog_LS.pdf
Cardiff acuity test (Keeler Cardiff test)	Sussex Vision www.sussex-vision.co.uk
Flippers	Sussex Vision www.sussex-vision.co.uk
Fresnel prisms	Norville Optical www.norville.co.uk Hilco Vision www.hilcovision.com Haag-Streit UK www.haagstreituk.com
Frisby stereoacuity test	Frisby stereotests www.frisbystereotest.co.uk Hilco Vision www.hilcovision.com
LogMAR crowded test	Keeler Instruments www.keeler.co.uk
IFS exercises (see declaration below)	I.O.O. Sales www.ioosales.co.uk
Keeler acuity cards	Keeler Instruments www.keeler.co.uk
Lang stereopsis test	Hilco Vision www.hilcovision.com Sussex Vision www.sussex-vision.co.uk
Lea gratings paddles	Sussex Vision www.sussex-vision.co.uk
Maddox wing	iOO Sales Ltd www.ioosales.co.uk Hilco Vision www.hilcovision.com Sussex Vision www.sussex-vision.co.uk
Mallett unit (fixation disparity, foveal suppression, stereopsis, modified OXO test)	*Keeler Instruments www.keeler.co.uk
Neutral density filter bar	iOO Sales Ltd www.ioosales.co.uk Hilco Vision www.hilcovision.com
Orthoweb	www.academy.org.uk/orthoweb
Pattern glare test	iOO Sales Ltd www.ioosales.co.uk
PC Hess screen	Thomson Software Solutions www.thomson-software-solutions.com

(Continued)

Equipment	Available from:
Prism bar	Hilco Vision www.hilcovision.com Sussex Vision www.sussex-vision.co.uk
RAF rule	Keeler Instruments www.keeler.co.uk Sussex Vision www.sussex-vision.co.uk
Randot stereopsis test	Hilco Vision www.hilcovision.com Sussex Vision www.sussex-vision.co.uk
Test chart 2000	Thomson Software Solutions www.thomson-software-solutions.com
Three cats exercise	Hilco Vision www.hilcovision.com
Titmus stereoacuity test	Keeler Instruments www.keeler.co.uk Hilco Vision www.hilcovision.com
TNO stereoacuity test	Haag-Streit UK www.haagstreituk.com
Translucent occluder (Spielmann)	I.O.O. Sales www.ioosales.co.uk Hilco Vision www.hilcovision.com
Vectograms	Bernell VTP www.bernell.com https://louisstone.co.uk/pdfs/Bernell_2020_Catalog_LS.pdf
Vergence facility prism	Bernell VTP www.bernell.com https://louisstone.co.uk/pdfs/Bernell_2020_Catalog_LS.pdf Hilco Vision www.hilcovision.com
Wilkins intuitive overlays	I.O.O. Sales www.ioosales.co.uk
Wilkins intuitive colorimeter & precision tints	Cerium Visual Technologies www.ceriumvistech.co.uk

*genuine Mallett units are not currently available, but a close copy is made by Evans Instruments Ltd (not related to the author) and is available from Keeler and other suppliers.

Declaration of interest: The author developed the IFS exercises at the Institute of Optometry, which is a charity. The exercises are marketed by I.O.O. Sales Ltd., which raises funds for the Institute of Optometry. I.O.O. Sales Ltd pays a small 'award to inventor' to the author based on sales of the IFS exercises.

Appendix 13: Guide to the Digital Resource

The **Digital Resource** accompanying this book is intended as a supplement to Chapter 17 on incomitant deviations. The primary method of detecting and diagnosing incomitant deviations is the motility test, and observations during this test can be difficult to interpret. Photographs of the eyes in peripheral positions of gaze often give stylised images of incomitancies, and it is hoped that the inclusion of video clips will assist readers in interpreting motility results as they are actually observed in clinical practice. Some of the cases show subtle incomitancies, others are more obvious.

The **Digital Resource** should run automatically, starting with the Introduction page. Blue text indicates links, allowing the user to choose which elements of the resource to access and their preferred order. At any time, the user can select the appropriate link to return to the first slide and select other incomitant deviations to study.

The video clips are taken from patients encountered in routine primary eyecare practice, so they reflect the types of incomitant deviations most likely to be encountered in clinical practice.

Note: Page numbers followed by *b* indicate boxes; *f*, figures; *t*, tables.